Critical Care Neurology and Neurosurgery

D1556594

CURRENT CLINICAL NEUROLOGY

Daniel Tarsy, MD, SERIES EDITOR

Critical Care Neurology and Neurosurgery

Edited by

Jose I. Suarez, MD

Neurosciences Critical Care, University Hospitals of Cleveland,
Case Western Reserve University, Cleveland, OH

Foreword by

Daniel Tarsy, MD

Department of Neurology, Beth Israel Deaconess Medical Center,
Harvard Medical School, Boston, MA

SPRINGER SCIENCE+BUSINESS MEDIA, LLC

© 2004 Springer Science+Business Media New York
Originally published by Humana Press Inc. in 2004
Softcover reprint of the hardcover 1st edition 2004

humanapress.com

All rights reserved. No part of this book may be reproduced, stored in a retrieval system, or transmitted in any form or by any means, electronic, mechanical, photocopying, microfilming, recording, or otherwise without written permission from the Publisher.

All papers, comments, opinions, conclusions, or recommendations are those of the author(s), and do not necessarily reflect the views of the publisher.

Due diligence has been taken by the publishers, editors, and authors of this book to assure the accuracy of the information published and to describe generally accepted practices. The contributors herein have carefully checked to ensure that the drug selections and dosages set forth in this text are accurate and in accord with the standards accepted at the time of publication. Notwithstanding, as new research, changes in government regulations, and knowledge from clinical experience relating to drug therapy and drug reactions constantly occurs, the reader is advised to check the product information provided by the manufacturer of each drug for any change in dosages or for additional warnings and contraindications. This is of utmost importance when the recommended drug herein is a new or infrequently used drug. It is the responsibility of the treating physician to determine dosages and treatment strategies for individual patients. Further it is the responsibility of the health care provider to ascertain the Food and Drug Administration status of each drug or device used in their clinical practice. The publisher, editors, and authors are not responsible for errors or omissions or for any consequences from the application of the information presented in this book and make no warranty, express or implied, with respect to the contents in this publication.

This publication is printed on acid-free paper. ∞
ANSI Z39.48-1984 (American Standards Institute) Permanence of Paper for Printed Library Materials.

Cover illustration: Figure 2 from Chapter 4, "Cerebral Metabolism: Implications for Neurocritically Ill Patients," by M. Briones-Galang and C. Robertson and Figure 1A from Chapter 22, "Traumatic Head Injury," by S. Kuniyoshi and J. I. Suarez.

Cover design by Patricia F. Cleary.

Production Editor: Jessica Jannicelli.

Additional material to this book can be downloaded from http://extras.springer.com

Photocopy Authorization Policy:
Authorization to photocopy items for internal or personal use, or the internal or personal use of specific clients, is granted by Springer Science+Business Media, LLC provided that the base fee of US $25.00 per copy is paid directly to the Copyright Clearance Center at 222 Rosewood Drive, Danvers, MA 01923. For those organizations that have been granted a photocopy license from the CCC, a separate system of payment has been arranged and is acceptable to Springer Science+Business Media, LLC.
The fee code for users of the Transactional Reporting Service is: [1-58829-089-1/04 $25.00].

ISBN 978-1-61737-350-3

Library of Congress Cataloging in Publication Data

Critical care neurology and neurosurgery / edited by Jose I. Suarez.
      p. cm. -- (Current clinical neurology)
Includes bibliographical references and index.
   ISBN 978-1-61737-350-3   ISBN 978-1-59259-660-7 (eBook)
   DOI 10.1007/978-1-59259-660-7
   1. Neurological intensive care. 2. Nervous system--Surgery. I.
Suarez, Jose I., 1951- II. Series.
   RC350.N49C753 2003
   616.8'0428--dc22
                                        2003024501

Dedication

To Ana Maria, my wife, companion, and best friend, for being my major pillar of support. To my family and friends who have been a constant source of encouragement.

"Era tanto o que havia para contar, tantas as novidades, tantos os altos e baixos de esperança e de ânimo vividos nestes dias...
O primeiro acto da função terminou, os adereços de cena foram retirados, os actores descansam do esforço da apoteose..."

José Saramago, *A caverna*, 2000

"There were so many things to tell, so much news, so many highs and lows in hopes and spirits...
The first act of the play is over, the scenery has been removed, the actors are retiring from their exertions in the final climatic scene..."

José Saramago, *The Cavern*

Jose I. Suarez, MD

Foreword

Historically, neurology has not been particularly well known as a treatment-oriented specialty. Diagnosis and patient management have been its main areas of interest, whereas therapeutics traditionally have not been considered a strong suit. This has changed considerably in the past two decades as a result of new medical and surgical developments in many of the neurological subspecialties. Perhaps the most dramatic example of rapidly evolving neurologic therapeutics has been in the area of critical care neurology. The classic monograph on *Stupor and Coma* by Plum and Posner emphasized diagnosis. Since then, knowledge regarding the management of critically ill patients in general, and neurological and neurosurgical patients in particular, has rapidly evolved. This has inevitably led to the establishment of increasing numbers of neurology critical care training programs and units which have, in turn, spawned CME courses and books on the subject that emphasize therapeutics. In addition to basic neurology and neurosurgery, care of the critically ill neurologic or neurosurgical patient requires sophisticated knowledge and understanding of neurophysiology, cerebrovascular and cardiovascular physiology, general physiology, anesthesia, respiratory medicine, peripheral and brain metabolism, neuroropharmacology, neuromonitoring, and even bioethics.

For *Critical Care Neurology and Neurosurgery*, Dr. Jose Suarez has brought together an impressive and experienced group of experts in the field of critical care medicine, neurology, and neurosurgery who deliver this complex knowledge in dazzling detail. The basic neuroscientific underpinnings of neurocritical care are emphasized in great detail, thereby justifying the use of the term *neurosciences critical care unit*. The chapters abound with useful tables and are accompanied by the very latest references. Authors from several highly respected institutions participated in this ouvre, but a particular strength of the book is the fact that many practice together with Dr. Suarez at University Hospitals of Cleveland, thereby lending a reassuring consistency to their approach. Dr. Suarez's participation in one-third of the chapters also lends useful uniformity to the subject. Although this is a multiauthored volume, the chapters are organized very consistently with useful attention to background and pathophysiology in addition to therapeutics. In the end, the entire range of topics one needs to know about in order to work in or even direct a successful neurosciences critical care unit are provided in impressive detail. This book admirably describes the current state of the art in neurocritical care and should be a benchmark in the field for some time to come.

Daniel Tarsy, MD

Preface

Modern neurocritical care probably started with the polio epidemics of 1916, and the introduction of the iron lung in the late 1920s, to provide ventilatory support to patients with weak respiratory muscles. At that time, neurologists were the primary treating physicians of these patients. However, the advent of polio vaccines and subsequent eradication of this disease from the Western Hemisphere led to a decline of interest in critical care within the neurological community. At the same time, a lack of important developments in neurosurgical techniques helped foster a nihilistic approach to critically ill neurologic and neurosurgical patients. For the last 20 years, we have seen significant enhancement of neurocritical care as a result of improved monitoring techniques, microsurgical approaches, and therapies for various complex neurologic and neurosurgical conditions.

Critical Care Neurology and Neurosurgery begins with recommendations for the organization of a modern and efficient neurosciences critical care unit, which is followed by discussions of intracranial physiology, and current neuromonitoring techniques. The concepts reviewed are paramount to understanding the management of critically ill neurologic and neurosurgical patients. Subsequently, we discuss the latest developments in monitoring of different body systems, emphasizing the management of cardiorespiratory complications and other medical conditions that may threaten the patient's life. This part serves as a useful guide for physicians caring for these patients who are faced with difficult dilemmas, agitated or nutritionally at-risk patients.

The last chapters of the book deal with commonly encountered conditions in the neurosciences critical care unit for which we have several therapeutic alternatives and the importance of good nursing care in our units. *Critical Care Neurology and Neurosurgery* concludes with a discussion on outcomes research in this field and an Appendix of different useful equations for neurointensivists and house officers caring for these patients.

I would like to acknowledge all the contributors who were chosen because of their recognized achievements in furthering our understanding of neurocritical care.

Jose I. Suarez, MD

Contents

Contributors

DINESH ARAB, MD • Division of Cardiology, Department of Medicine, School of Medicine and Biomedical Sciences, University at Buffalo, State University of New York, Buffalo, NY

NEERAJ BADJATIA, MD • Neurointensive Care Neurology, Massachusetts General Hospital, Boston, MA

NICHOLAS C. BAMBAKIDIS, MD • Department of Neurosurgery, University Hospitals of Cleveland, Case Western Reserve University, Cleveland, OH

ANISH BHARDWAJ, MD • Neurosciences Critical Care Division, Johns Hopkins University School of Medicine, Baltimore, MD

THOMAS P. BLECK, MD, FCCM • Neurosciences Intensive Care Unit, University of Virginia Health Sciences Center, Charlottesville, VA

CECIL O. BOREL, MD • Neurosciences Critical Care Unit, Duke University Medical Center, Durham, NC

MARIA BRIONES-GALANG, MD • Department of Neurosurgery, Baylor College of Medicine, Houston, TX

MAREK BUCZEK, MD, PhD • Fellow Autonomic Disorders, Department of Neurology, University Hospitals of Cleveland, Case Western Reserve University, Cleveland, OH

J. RICARDO CARHUAPOMA, MD • Neurosciences Critical Care Program, Wayne State University, Detroit, MI

JULIO A. CHALELA, MD • National Institute of Neurological Disorders and Stroke, National Institutes of Health, Bethesda, MD

CHERE MONIQUE CHASE, MD • Fellow Neurosciences Critical Care, Johns Hopkins Hospital, Baltimore, MD

THOMAS C. CHELIMSKY, MD • Autonomic Disorders Laboratory, Department of Neurology, University Hospitals of Cleveland, Case Western Reserve University, Cleveland, OH

JOY DERWENSKUS, DO • Department of Neurology, University Hospitals of Cleveland, Case Western Reserve University, Cleveland, OH

JOSE L. DIAZ, MD • Clinica Universitaria Bolivariana, Clinica Medellin, Medellin, Colombia

MATTHEW ECCHER, MD • Department of Neurology, University Hospitals of Cleveland, Case Western Reserve University, Cleveland, OH

ELIAHU S. FEEN, MD • Department of Neurology, University Hospitals of Cleveland, Louis Stokes Veterans Affairs Medical Center, Case Western Reserve University, Cleveland, OH

ROMERGRYKO GEOCADIN, MD • Neuroscience Critical Care Division, Johns Hopkins University School of Medicine, Baltimore, MD

ALEXANDROS L. GEORGIADIS, MD • Department of Neurology, University Hospitals of Cleveland, Case Western Reserve University, Cleveland, OH

MARCELA GRANADOS, MD, FCCM • Fundacion Clinica Valle del Lili, Universidad del Valle, Cali, Colombia

DAKSHIN GULLAPALLI, MD • Veterans Affairs Medical Center, University of Virginia School of Medicine, Salem, VA

LOTFI HACEIN-BEY, MD • Interventional Neuroradiology, Medical College of Wisconsin, Milwaukee, WI

RICARDO A. HANEL, MD • Department of Neurosurgery and Toshiba Stroke Research Center, School of Medicine and Biomedical Sciences, University at Buffalo, State University of New York, Buffalo, NY

MITZI K. HEMSTREET, MD, PhD • Division of Neuroanesthesiology and Neurosciences Critical Care, Department of Anesthesiology and Critical Care Medicine, Johns Hopkins University, Baltimore, MD

JANICE L. HICKMAN, RN, MSN, CS • Neurosciences Critical Care Unit, University Hospitals of Cleveland, Cleveland, OH

NAZLI JANJUA, MD • Department of Neurology, Columbia-Presbyterian Medical Center, New York, NY

ABEL D. JARELL, MD • Neurosurgery, Walter Reed Army Medical Center, Washington, DC

JAWAD F. KIRMANI, MD • Department of Neurosurgery and Toshiba Stroke Research Center, School of Medicine and Biomedical Sciences, University at Buffalo, State University of New York, Buffalo, NY

WALTER J. KOROSHETZ, MD • Neurointensive Care Neurology, Massachusetts General Hospital, Harvard University School of Medicine, Boston, MA

SANDRA KUNIYOSHI, MD • Department of Neurology, University Hospitals of Cleveland, Case Western Reserve University, Cleveland, OH

ALEKSANDYR W. LAVERY, MD • Department of Neurosurgery, University Hospitals of Cleveland, Louis Stokes Veterans Affairs Medical Center, Case Western Reserve University, Cleveland, OH

R. JOHN LEIGH, MD • Department of Veterans Affairs Medical Center, University Hospitals of Cleveland, Case Western Reserve University, Cleveland, OH

GEOFFREY S. F. LING, MD, PhD • Neurocritical Care, Walter Reed Army Medical Center, Uniformed Services University of the Health Sciences, Bethesda, MD

ZEYAD MARCOS, MD • Department of Neurology, University Hospitals of Cleveland, Case Western Reserve University, Cleveland, OH

STEPHAN A. MAYER, MD • Clinical Neurology and Neurosurgery, Columbia-Presbyterian Medical Center, New York, NY

MAREK A. MIRSKI, MD, PhD • Neurosciences Critical Care Unit/Neuroanesthesiology, Johns Hopkins University, Baltimore, MD

DAVID L. McDONAGH, MD • Fellow Neuroanesthesia/Neurocritical Care, Department of Anesthesiology, Duke University Medical Center, Durham, NC

DANIEL W. MILLER, MD • Department of Neurology, University Hospitals of Cleveland, Case Western Reserve University, Cleveland, OH

NANCY A. NEWMAN, RD, LD • Department of Nutrition Services, University Hospitals of Cleveland, Cleveland, OH

THANH N. NGUYEN, MD • Neurointensive Care Neurology, Massachusetts General Hospital, Boston, MA

ADNAN I. QURESHI, MD • Department of Neurosurgery and Toshiba Stroke Research Center, School of Medicine and Biomedical Sciences, University at Buffalo, State University of New York, Buffalo, NY

RONALD G. RIECHERS, II, MD • Neurology, Walter Reed Army Medical Center, Washington, DC

CLAUDIA ROBERTSON, MD • Department of Neurosurgery, Baylor College of Medicine, Houston, TX

TINA RODRIGUE, MD • Department of Neurosurgery, University Hospitals of Cleveland, Case Western Reserve University, Cleveland, OH

WARREN R. SELMAN, MD • Department of Neurosurgery, University Hospitals of Cleveland, Case Western Reserve University, Cleveland, OH

JOSE I. SUAREZ, MD • Neurosciences Critical Care, University Hospitals of Cleveland, Louis Stokes Veterans Affairs Medical Center, Case Western Reserve University, Cleveland, OH

SOPHIA SUNDARARAJAN, MD, PhD • Department of Neurology, University Hospitals of Cleveland, Case Western Reserve University, Cleveland, OH

GENE SUNG, MD, MPH • Neurocritical Care and Stroke Program, University of Southern California, Los Angeles, CA

JEFFREY L. SUNSHINE, MD, PhD • Departments of Radiology, Neurology, and Neurosurgery, University Hospitals of Cleveland, Case Western Reserve University, Cleveland, OH

ROBERT W. TARR, MD • Departments of Radiology, Neurology, and Neurosurgery, University Hospitals of Cleveland, Case Western Reserve University, Cleveland, OH

MICHEL T. TORBEY, MD, MPH • Neurosciences Critical Care Division, Johns Hopkins University School of Medicine, Baltimore, MD

EROBOGHENE E. UBOGU, MD • Department of Neurology, Department of Veterans Affairs Medical Center, University Hospitals of Cleveland, Case Western Reserve University, Cleveland, OH

JOHN A. ULATOWSKI, MD, PhD, MBA • Neuroscience Critical Care Unit, Johns Hopkins Hospital, Baltimore, MD

PANAYIOTIS N. VARELAS, MD, PhD • Neurosciences Critical Care Unit, Medical College of Wisconsin, Milwaukee, WI

ANDREW R. XAVIER, MD • Department of Neurosurgery and Toshiba Stroke Research Center, School of Medicine and Biomedical Sciences, University at Buffalo, State University of New York, Buffalo, NY

ABUTAHER M. YAHIA, MD • Department of Neurosurgery and Toshiba Stroke Research Center, School of Medicine and Biomedical Sciences, University at Buffalo, State University of New York, Buffalo, NY

STUART YOUNGNER, MD • Center for Biomedical Ethics, Case Western Reserve University, Cleveland, OH

OSAMA O. ZAIDAT, MD, MSc • Clinical Associate, Duke University Medical Center, Durham, NC

WENDY C. ZIAI, MD • Division of Neurosciences Critical Care, Department of Anesthesia and Critical Care Medicine, and Neurology, Johns Hopkins University School of Medicine, Baltimore, MD

Introduction

Jose I. Suarez

DEFINITIONS OF NEUROSCIENCES CRITICAL CARE

Neurosciences critical care units (NSU) were designed for the care of critically ill adolescent, adult, and geriatric neurology and neurosurgery patients requiring specialized intensive nursing and medical care. The creation of NSU arose from the awareness of special and different needs that these patients have, which require treatment by a team acutely versed in the interactions between systemic and central nervous system (CNS) alterations. A discussion on the organization of NSU is presented in Chapter 2.

The birth of NSU brought along the need for a critical care subspecialty made up of intensivists from different medical and surgical backgrounds but with a keen interest in impacting on short- and long-term neurological outcome of patients. This subspecialty has been called Neurosciences Critical Care or Critical Care Neurology and Neurosurgery, which is dealt with in more detail in Chapter 34. The role of the neurointensivists would primarily involve caring for the critically ill neurological and neurosurgical patient, as well as discussing with families their loved one's clinical condition and prognosis. However, they should also actively participate in the teaching and training of residents, fellows, nursing staff, and medical students to make them more competent in this area. Other important functions are the consultation in other critical care areas to prognosticate neurological outcome and determine brain death, active participation in institutional critical care councils to develop and enforce policies, and attendance of national and international meetings to expand awareness and recognition of this subspecialty.

This introductory chapter to this book concentrates on the delineation of brain injury and outlines proposed admission and discharge criteria for NSU.

BRAIN INJURY

CNS insults have been categorized as primary and secondary (Table 1; *1–19*). Primary insults refer to direct pathological changes resulting from the impact and severity of the injury itself. Examples of this primary injury include cell necrosis in the core of a brain infarct or diffuse vascular damage after severe traumatic brain injury (TBI). In many cases, this primary injury has already occurred when patients are admitted to the NSU and is therefore not amenable to treatment. The establishment of preventive measures is the best method to reduce the incidence of primary CNS insults. However, it is important to note that primary brain insults are not simply one-time events, but rather an ongoing phenomenon that starts with the initial impact and evolves over hours or maybe days, and this process may be stopped or improved *(1)*. For instance, early treatment of acute ischemic stroke can reverse the cytotoxic and inflammatory cascade triggered by the lack of cerebral blood flow to the brain, which translates into improved clinical outcome *(20)*.

From: *Current Clinical Neurology*
Critical Care Neurology and Neurosurgery
Edited by: J. I. Suarez © Humana Press Inc., Totowa, NJ

Table 1
Primary and Secondary Brain Insults

Type of injury	Most common conditions
Primary brain insult Best remedy: prevention of risk factors and early treatment	Acute ischemic stroke, intracranial hemorrhage, subarachnoid hemorrhage, traumatic brain injury, spinal cord injury or compression, neoplasm, meningitis or encephalitis
Secondary brain insult Best remedy: early detection and treatment; protocol-driven management may help; team approach useful (nurse-physician cooperation)	Hypoxemia, elevated intracranial pressure, hydrocephalus, hypotension, seizures and status epilepticus (overt or subtle), hyperthermia (usually > 37.5°C), hyperglycemia (usually blood glucose > 150 mg/dL), infections, acidosis, vasospasm

Secondary CNS insults, on the other hand, present after the primary insult and unless corrected promptly and aggressively can worsen neurological damage and clinical outcome (Table 1). Such secondary insults can be prevented *(4,5,8,10,12)*. This can be best accomplished when patients are closely monitored and managed in NSU where the appropriate equipment and expert personnel are available. The main goals of NSU patient management is the treatment of primary insults whenever possible and prevention of secondary insults to guarantee the best possible outcome. Throughout this book, these concepts are emphasized and useful guidelines are provided to help treating physicians deal with them effectively.

TRIAGE OF PATIENTS WITH BRAIN INSULTS

Initial Evaluation

The first steps in the assessment of the critically ill neurological and neurosurgical patient should be, like in any other medical conditions, the ABC. These include the determination and maintenance of a patent airway, adequate breathing and ventilation, and sufficient circulation to ensure CNS perfusion and oxygenation *(5,10)*. Patients with a Glasgow Coma Scale (GCS) score less than 8 or with signs of respiratory distress should be intubated emergently. A detailed description of airway management and mechanical ventilation is presented in Chapter 9.

Once the ABCs are dealt with, physicians should perform a general physical and neurologic examination to obtain clues regarding the patient's current status *(21;* Table 2). Important information can be obtained just by observing the patient's breathing pattern, spontaneous movements, and skin discoloration. Always look for signs of trauma on the physical examination. Performing quick neurological scales at the bedside such as the GCS or the National Institutes of Health Stroke Scale (NIHSS) can be very useful when it comes to urgent triaging and treatment-decision making *(10,20)*. Examination of the eyes is of the utmost importance because of the enormous amount of information that can be obtained. Because of this, a separate chapter is dedicated to this topic (*see* Chapter 30). It cannot be emphasized enough the fact that information obtained from witnesses or relatives should also provide medical personnel with useful data to better treat the patient.

Establishing venous access should also be part of the initial assessment and may include placement of central venous lines. At the time of venous catheter insertion, blood samples should be

Table 2
General and Neurological Examination Findings That May Help With Treatment Decision Making at the Bedside in Critically Ill Neurologic and Neurosurgical Patients

Frequent findings on examination	Disease association
General appearance:	
Disheveled or unkempt	Dementia, assault or neglect syndromes
Agitation	Delirium (pain, psychosis, hyperthryroidism, postictal)
Vomitus	Elevated intracranial pressure
Urinary and fecal incontinence	Seizures or spinal cord lesions
Breathing pattern:	
Cheyne-Stokes	Bilateral cerebral dysfunction
Hyperventilation	Low midbrain or upper pons dysfunction
Apneusis	Middle and caudal pons dysfunction (Tegmentum)
Cluster	Lower pons dysfunction (Tegmentum)
Ataxia	Dorsomedial medullary dysfunction
Skin and teguments:	
Skin discoloration:	
Pale	Anemia
Bluish tinge	Methemoglobin
Pink	CO poisoning
Yellow	Jaundice, high beta carotenes
Sallow with brownish tinge	Uremia
Retro-auricular echymosis or "raccoon eyes"	Trauma, skull base fractures
Antecubital needle marks	Drug use
Tegument changes:	
Splinter hemorrhages under nails	Vasculitis, subacute bacterial endocarditis
Finger clubbing	Chronic obstructive pulmonary disease neoplasms

(Continued on next page)

Table 2 *(Continued)*

Frequent findings on examination	Disease association
Eye movements and pupils:	
Fixed unreactive puils	Pharmacologic bilateral tectal dysfunction, brain death
Anisocoria	Transtentorial herniation, pharmacological, Horner's syndrome
Absent eye movements	Muscle paralysis, pontine dysfunction
Gaze preference	Hemispheric infarct, seizures, pontine dysfunction
Spontaneous movements:	
Clonic or tonic focal or generalized activity	Seizures
Hemiparesis	Hemispheric or brainstem dysfunction
Paraparesis	Spinal cord or bifrontal dysfunction
Bedside neurologic scales:	
GCS < 8	Coma of any cause
NIHSS	Triaging of acute stroke patients
Response to noxious stimuli in unconscious patients:	
Bilateral extensior posturing	Bilateral midbrain or pontine dysfunction
Flexion of upper limbs and extension of lower limbs	Many locations above midbrain

CO, carbon monoxide; GCS, Glasgow Coma Scale; NIHSS, National Institutes of Health Stroke Scale.

obtained to be analyzed in the laboratory. The most common and useful laboratory tests include complete blood cell count (CBC), coagulation screening, blood type and screen, electrolytes, blood glucose, hepatic and renal panels, blood and urine toxicology screen, arterial blood gases, and determination of anticonvulsant drugs serum concentration.

If neurologic compromise is established in the triaging area, then neuroimaging evaluation is indicated. As indicated in Chapter 7, head computed tomography (CT) scanning or magnetic resonance imaging are the most commonly used techniques and the ones with the highest yield acutely. For instance, these should determine whether a patient is suffering from a hemorrhagic or an ischemic cerebral infarct. They may also help determine, in conjunction with the physical examination, whether

Table 3
NSU Admission Criteria at the University Hospitals of Cleveland

1. Acute respiratory failure:
   Patients with COPD, aspiration pneumonia or PE: persistent tachypnea (respiratory rate > 35/min), respiratory muscle fatigue (abdominal paradox), acute respiratory acidosis, persistent or poorly responsive hypoxemia, requiring $FiO_2 > 50\%$
   Patients with pulmonary edema: cardiogenic (not responsive to treatment, requiring $FiO_2 > 50\%$, persistent tachypnea), noncardiogenic, and acute myocardial infarction
   Imminent intubation or acutely intubated patients
2. Hemodynamic instability:
   Inability to maintain blood pressure without vasoactive drugs, large volume infusions, and other invasive cardiovascular monitoring
   Requirement of pulmonary artery monitoring and cardiac output recordings
   Unstable cardiac rhythms requiring frequent drug or mechanical interventions
   Requirement of arterial line for blood pressure monitoring
   Shock: mean arterial blood pressure < 60 mmHg; evidence of clinically significant hypoperfusion as manifested by peripheral vasoconstriction, oliguria, altered mentation or unexplained hypothermia
3. Hypertensive crisis:
   Clinically unresponsive to oral agents
   Requirement of intravenous agents
4. Massive gastrointestinal bleeding
5. Drug overdose:
   Compromised mentation (GCS < 8)
   Hemodynamic instability
   Requiring mechanical ventilation
   Cardiac arrythmias
6. Metabolic emergencies:
   Severe hyperkalemia (> 6 mEq/L or > 5.5 mEq/L with ECG changes)
   Hypercalcemia
   Acute hyponatremia
   Addisonian crisis
   Diabetic ketoacidosis or hyperosmolar states
7. Coma of any etiology in need of intensive medical and/or nursing care
8. Status epilepticus
9. Craniospinal postoperative patient, including endovascular procedures
10. Untreated craniospinal mass effect
11. Patient with acute ischemic stroke undergoing thrombolysis
12. Patients with intracranial hemorrhage
13. Patients with acute, treatable, or diagnostically uncertain unstable neuromuscular disease
14. Patients with critical, reversible cerebral ischemia
15. Patients with severe head and spinal cord injury
16. Patients requiring external ventricular drainage or neuromonitoring that can only be provided in the NSU
17. Patients who have "Do Not Resuscitate" orders who are admitted to the NSU must be candidates for, and committed to, aggressive care short of resuscitation

COPD, chronic obstructive pulmonary disease; PE, pulmonary embolism; GCS, Glasgow Coma Scale; ECG, electrocardiography; FiO_2, inspired fraction of oxygen.

a patient needs emergent neurosurgical evaluation and transport to the operating room. It is essential that the cervical spine be immobilized until fractures or dislocations are excluded (*see* Chapter 23). Other imaging studies, such as chest radiology or chest and abdomen CT scanning, are also useful because they can detect systemic abnormalities that may require immediate attention such as pneumonias, pneumothorax, or pulmonary edema, or intra-abdominal catastrophes.

Table 4
NSU Discharge Criteria at the University Hospitals of Cleveland

1. Respiratory stability
   Patient does not require mechanical ventilation or endotracheal intubation
   Patient has independent and adequate respiratory function
   Patient does not require respiratory therapy intervention more often than every 4 h
   Patient is capable of maintaining adequate oxygenation: $SaO_2 > 92\%$
2. Hemodynamic stability
   Patient does not require vasoactive drugs
   Patient does not require drug or mechanical agents for life threatening cardiac dysrhythmia
   No need for pulmonary artery catheter
   No need for arterial line for blood pressure monitoring
   Patient has stable vital signs for at least 12 h
3. Neurological system and signs are without unexpected change
4. Patient has nursing needs requiring interventions no greater than every 3 h and requires vital sign monitoring on a "routine" basis no more frequently than every 4 h
5. It has been determined that because of the terminal irreversible nature of the patients' condition, it is no longer appropriate to care for them in the NSU

SaO_2, arterial oxygen saturation.

Admission to the NSU

NSU resources are expensive and scarce. Therefore, appropriate patient selection is important *(22–25)*. In general, patients admitted to the NSU should include those that are likely to benefit from this level of care as compared to those who are not because they are not sick enough to warrant critical care or they have catastrophic conditions that results in impending death. Although no clear data exist to validate the usefulness of establishing admission criteria, the Society of Critical Care Medicine has provided guidelines to this effect *(22)*. NSU should create policies and mission statements specific to each hospital and level of expertise available.

In the NSU at the University Hospitals of Cleveland, we have determined that regardless of the underlying pathology, patients should fall into one or more of the following categories to be admitted: (1) patients should be at risk of serious event as a result of the disease process; (2) patients require highly specialized and concentrated nursing and medical care; and (3) patients require specific interventions or techniques not appropriate or not available for use on the other in-patient divisions (i.e., continuous cardiac monitoring, mechanical ventilation, intracranial pressure monitoring, and so forth). We have developed NSU admission criteria that combine specific diagnoses and objective parameters (Table 3). It is important to remember that these criteria are presented as guidelines. It is also equally important to maintain adequate track records of compliance with these criteria for performance evaluation.

Discharge from the NSU

From the moment patients arrive in the NSU, they are aggressively managed and monitored for medical and neurologic stability. Once they are deemed stable enough to not require intensive care or monitoring, they are usually discharged from the NSU *(22–25)*. In the setting of an open or semi-open NSU, this should be discussed with the primary neurology or neurosurgical teams and a careful treatment plan should be outlined before discharge to minimize the number of readmissions. We present in Table 4 the discharge criteria for NSU patients at the University Hospitals of Cleveland. These patients may be discharged to intermediate or regular floor levels of care. Similar to admission criteria, records should be kept because it has been shown that the identification of patients at risk of dying after discharge is important to reduce mortality *(26)*. Such patients should be monitored for longer periods in the critical care areas.

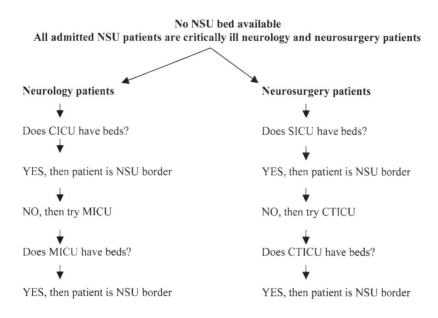

Fig. 1. Algorithm for triaging NSU patients at the University Hospitals of Cleveland. CICU, cardiac intensive care unit; MICU, medical intensive care unit; SICU, surgical intensive care unit; CVICU, cardiothoracic intensive care unit; border refers to a patient who is cared for by the NSU team but is housed in another unit other than the NSU.

Dealing With "The Last Bed" or "No Beds"

Many times we are faced with situations when admission of new patients to the NSU becomes problematic because of high occupancy or high acuity. In such cases triaging is the only choice *(22,27)*. Ideally, the least sick patients should be discharged from the NSU to accommodate more acutely ill ones. However, often times disease severity is significant in all patients and discharge may not be appropriate. We have developed a triaging algorithm to tackle these issues (Fig. 1). This basically entails making all vacant critical care beds in the hospital available to NSU patients. We prefer to prioritize neurology patients to medical units and neurosurgical patients to surgical units. All these decisions should be made in conjunction with the nursing staff to guarantee smooth transition of patient care. The NSU medical staff continues caring for these patients to avoid disruptions of continuity of treatment.

CONCLUSION

NSU have become an integral part of critical care in major academic centers. One of the main goals of treatment in NSU is the prevention of secondary CNS insults to prevent further damage. Like other critical care areas, admission and discharge criteria need to be developed. These should be unique to each medical center, but keeping the general guidelines given by the Society of Critical Care Medicine. Performance evaluations of NSU should consider these criteria as an integral part of the process.

REFERENCES

1. Reilly PL. Brain injury: the pathophysiology of the first hours. "Talk and Die revisited." *J. Clin. Neurosci.* 2001;8:398–403.
2. Hatton J. Pharmacological treatment of traumatic brain injury: a review of agents in development. *CNS Drugs* 2001;15:553–581.
3. Varelas PN, Mirski MA. Seizures in the adult intensive care unit. *J. Neurosurg. Anesthesiol.* 2001;163–175.

4. Coplin WM. Intracranial pressure and surgical decompression for traumatic brain injury: biological rationale and protocol for a randomized clinical trial. *Neurol. Res.* 2001;23:277–290.
5. The Brain Trauma Foundation. The American Association of Neurological Surgeons. The Joint Section on Neurotrauma and Critical Care. Hypotension. *J. Neurotrauma* 2000;17:591–595.
6. Menon DK. Cerebral protection in severe brain injury: physiological determinants of outcome and their optimisation. *Br. Med. Bull.* 1999;55:226–258.
7. Glass TF, Fabian MJ, Schweitzer JB, Weinberg JA, Proctor KG. Secondary neurologic injury from nonhypotensive hemorrhage combined with mild traumatic injury. *J. Neurotrauma* 1999;16:771–782.
8. Chamberlain DJ. The critical care nurse's role in preventing secondary brain injury in severe head trauma: achieving the balance. *Aust. Crit. Care* 1998;11:123–129.
9. Dearden NM. Mechanisms and prevention of secondary brain damage during intensive care. *Clin. Neuropathol.* 1998;17:221–228.
10. Abrams KJ. Airway management and mechanical ventilation. *New Horiz.* 1995;3:479–487.
11. Hovda DA, Becker DP, Katayama Y. Secondary injury and acidosis. *J. Neurotrauma* 1992;9 Suppl 1:S47–S60.
12. Robertson CS, Valadka AB, Hannay HJ, et al. Prevention of secondary ischemic insults after severe head injury. *Crit. Care Med.* 1999;27:2086–2095.
13. Struchen MA, Hannay HJ, Contant CF, Robertson CS. The relation between acute physiological variables and outcome on the Glasgow Outcome Scale and Disability Rating Scale following severe traumatic brain injury. *J. Neurotrauma* 2001;18:115–125.
14. Rovlias A, Kotsou S. The influence of hyperglycemia on neurological outcome in patients with severe head injury. *Neurosurgery* 2000;46:335–342.
15. Markgraf CG, Clifton GL, Moody MR. Treatment window for hypothermia in brain injury. *J. Neurosurg.* 2001;95:979–983.
16. The Hypothermia after Cardia Arrest Study Group. Mild therapeutic hypothermia to improve neurologic outcome after cardiac arrest. *N. Engl. J. Med.* 2002;346:549–556.
17. Bernard SA, Gray TW, Buist MD, et al. Treatment of comatose survivors of out-of-hospital cardiac arrest with induced hypothermia. *N. Engl. J. Med.* 2002;346:557–563.
18. Wolach B, Sazbon L, Gavrieli R, Broda A, Schlesinger M. Early immunological defects in comatose patients after acute brain injury. *J. Neurosurg.* 2001;94:706–711.
19. Suarez JI, Qureshi AI, Yahia AB, et al. Symptomatic vasospasm diagnosis after subarachnoid hemorrhage: evaluation of transcranial Doppler ultrasound and cerebral angiography as related to compromised vascular distribution. *Crit. Care Med.* 2002;30:1348–1355.
20. The National Institute of Neurological Disorders and Stroke rt-PA study group. Tissue plasminogen activator for acute ischemic stroke. *N. Engl. J. Med.* 1995;333:1581–1587.
21. Macleod J, Munro J, eds. Clinical Examination, 7th ed. Edinburgh: Churchill Livingstone, 1986.
22. Guidelines for intensive care unit admission, discharge, and triage. Task Force of the American College of Critical Care Medicine, Society of Critical Care Medicine. *Crit. Care Med.* 1999;27:633–638.
23. Nasraway SA, Cohen IL, Dennis RC, et al. Guidelines on admission and discharge for adult intermediate care units. American College of Critical Care Medicine of the Society of Critical Care Medicine. *Crit. Care Med.* 1998;26:607–610.
24. Dawson JA. Admission, discharge, and triage in critical care. *Crit. Care Clin.* 1993;9:555–574.
25. Bone RC, McElwee NE, Eubanks DH, Gluck EH. Analysis of indications for intensive care unit admission. Clinical efficacy assessment project: American College of Physicians. *Chest* 1993;104:1806–1811.
26. Daly K, Beale R, Chang RW. Reduction in mortality after inappropriate early discharge from intensive care unit: logistic regression triage model. *BMJ* 2001;322:1274–1276.
27. Teres D. Civilian triage in the intensive care unit: the ritual of the last bed. *Crit. Care Med.* 1993;21:598–606.

2

Organization of a Neuroscience Critical Care Unit

Historical Perspectives and Vision for the Future

Chere Monique Chase and John A. Ulatowski

Of greater human interest than the details of design and equipment [is] ... the need to appreciate the emotional strain to which members of the ... [critical care] staff are exposed when, hour by hour, their whole attention is focused on patients who are immediately and constantly dependent on their vigilance. *(1)*

INTRODUCTION

Medical historians date the beginning of neurocritical care back to the 16th century. In delineating the history of critical care, some quote biblical passages, philosophers, and historians, and ethicists indicate historically early end-of-life discussions, and attempts at resuscitation and artificial ventilation *(2)*. Pictorial illustrations of early artificial respiration devices and descriptions of resuscitation practices appear primitive and comical *(3)*. However, these devices and methods set the foundation for significant advances in the 19th century. In the first half of the 20th century, when neurologists were challenged by the poliomyelitis epidemics, they had the groundwork for the first large-scale use of mechanical ventilation *(4)*. Modern neurological intensive care began with the use of respiratory care principles established during European poliomyelitis epidemics and expanded into a broad field that encompasses all acute and serious aspects of neurological and neurosurgical disease *(5)*.

As the development of neurocritical care was defined by historical events, so too were the roles of neurosurgeons, neurologists, and neuroanesthesiologists in the field. When the American Academy of Neurology (AAN) was founded, most poliomyelitis victims primarily received their care from neurologists. Dr. A. B. Baker, a founding AAN member and vocal proponent of neurosciences, strongly advocated for the role of neurologists in the care of polio victims and other critically ill neurological patients *(4)*. During that time, the issue of infectious disease as the precipitating factor or secondarily related to the neurologic critical illness was debated. Baker contended that neurologists of his era provided more comprehensive care than infectious disease specialists. Because of patient acuity, early 20th century neurology practices required critical care medicine. Neurologists performed tracheotomies, rigid bronchoscopes, and other minor surgical procedures *(4)*.

Early neurologists played an active role in the instruction of critical care skills. Neurologists not only played an active role in neurocritical care training and development of neurocritical care as a specialty, but they also played key roles in growth of general critical care. In the 1970s, Dr. David Jackson, a neurologist at Case Western Reserve University, directed one of the first general critical

From: *Current Clinical Neurology*
Critical Care Neurology and Neurosurgery
Edited by: J. I. Suarez © Humana Press Inc., Totowa, NJ

care training programs. While furthering general critical care, he also instituted the American Academy of Neurology's annual course in critical care.

History demonstrates a fluctuation in the level of interest and degree to which neurologists have participated in the care of the critically ill. Once the vaccine for poliomyelitis was discovered and incidence of poliomyelitis rapidly declined, neurologists returned to general neurology consultation *(4)*. However, a resurgence of neurology interest in critically ill patients became apparent when Dr. Allan Ropper, internist and neurologist, founded the neurological–neurosurgical critical care service at Massachusetts General Hospital in the late 1970s. In 1983, Ropper was one of the authors of the first American textbook of neurocritical care. Other early neurocritical care training programs were founded by internist–neurologists, such as Dr. Daniel Hanley at Johns Hopkins, Dr. Matthew Fink at Columbia, and Dr. Thomas Bleck at the University of Virginia.

Interest in the potential benefits of neurosciences critical care units (NSUs) has also increased. Challenges that face the new generation of neurologists and critical care physicians are the rapidly aging population, increase in neurosurgical volumes, and rapid advancement of acute therapies for neurological and neurosurgical patients. Neurointensivists must be trained to enhance medical care by combining the knowledge of neurologic disease and intraoperative care with techniques of intensive care.

Arguments regarding the necessity of neurospecialty trained intensivists have been ongoing throughout American and European literature *(6–8)*. Those arguments in favor of NSUs tend to highlight trends toward more accurate and efficient practice patterns designed for neurological and neurosurgical patients *(7)*. The assertion is that the care of neuroscience patients requires training in clinical physiology of intracranial pressure (ICP), cerebral blood flow (CBF), brain electrical activity; systemic abnormalities and medical complications of nervous system diseases; postoperative care; and management of neuromuscular respiratory failure. Acute stroke, intracerebral hemorrhage (ICH), brain death, ethical dilemmas of severe neurologic illnesses, and neurologic features of critically ill medical patients now fall well under the auspices of neurosciences intensive care.

Critical care has an important and permanent place in neurological and neurosurgical research, education, and practice. In the past, neurocritical care was only useful for cardiopulmonary support while nervous tissue recovered. Now, therapies for brain resuscitation and brain-sparing methods impact outcomes in neurological and neurosurgical emergencies. Specific advances in monitoring of electrophysiological and intracranial physiological indices brought laboratory physiology to the bedside and allowed standardization of diagnosis and prognosis. Modern NSUs are not only a place for sick neuroscience patients but also a place to incorporate advanced medical technology with understanding of the organ dysfunction that follows brain and nerve failure.

HISTORICAL PERSPECTIVES

Development of Medical and Surgical Intensive Care Medicine

Close observation of critically ill patients dates back to ancient time; however, with the advent of modern technology, monitoring functions and evidence-based clinical care are recent phenomena *(9)*. Along with improved technology, clinicians better understand the needs of patients with acute, life-threatening illnesses or injury. Health providers' personal papers and autobiographies can be used to trace the emergence of the "grouped patient" approach to care. Nurses were some of the first to appreciate that very sick patients receive more attention if they are grouped together. In the 1860s, Florence Nightingale wrote about advantages of establishing separate areas of the hospital in which patients recovered from surgery.

Intensive care units had their origin in the postoperative recovery room. The first surgical intensive care unit (SICU) was also the first NSU. In 1923, Dr. W.E. Dandy created a three-bed unit for the postoperative neurosurgical patients at the Johns Hopkins Hospital in Baltimore, Maryland. The concept of intensive care units further developed during World War II. Areas designated as "shock wards" were established to resuscitate and care for soldiers injured in battle or undergoing surgery. Historically, the fluctuation in demand for nursing care and the supply of nurses greatly facilitated the development of such units. Directly after World War II, there was a nursing shortage that sparked a nationwide initiative to recruit and train nurses *(10)*. In the meantime, grouping of postoperative and seriously ill patients in recovery rooms to ensure attentive care was necessary.

When the polio epidemic struck Europe and the United States, healthcare providers were confronted with staggering fatality rates. Interest in improving treatment of patients dying from respiratory paralysis fueled scientific and medical endeavors. Initially, many patients with bulbar poliomyelitis were treated with iron lungs. At the peak of the epidemic, the supply of iron lungs could not meet the demand. In response, the European market answered the challenge with the invention of positive pressure ventilation administered through an endotracheal tube, popularized in Denmark *(11)*. The Denmark experience stimulated research in automated machines capable of intermittent positive pressure ventilation and during the 1950s, development of mechanical ventilation led to organization of respiratory intensive care units in many European and American hospitals. Not surprisingly, care and monitoring of ventilated patients proved to be more efficient when patients were grouped in a single location *(12)*.

There was a flurry of medical advances during the two decades that followed the polio epidemic. Higher expectations and standards for rate of survival lead to formation of designated areas in hospitals for continuous physiologic monitoring and life-saving interventions. In 1956, the first external defibrillator and synchronized direct-current cardioversion to treat refractory tachyarrhythmia was introduced. Peter Safar and W.B. Kouwenhoven advanced care of the critically ill patient to a new realm when they introduced the combined technique of rhythmic lower sternal pressure and mouth-to-mouth breathing, which we now refer to as cardiopulmonary resuscitation (CPR; *13*).

Technological inventions and special triage areas were only the first steps toward improved outcomes. In 1942, the fire at Boston's Coconut Grove nightclub, one of the worst civilian disasters in American history, marked a unique time in the history of intensive care. Advances in the areas of burn care, resuscitation of shock, use of antibiotics, and understanding metabolic response to injury resulted from the Boston experience *(14)*. During the mid-1960s, resuscitative techniques with intravenous fluids and blood products for shock were improved allowing for increased patient stability and evacuation to facilities that were suitably equipped to address their needs. By the late 1960s, health care witnessed a rapid spread of resuscitation and surgical techniques and the creation of recovery rooms in nearly every hospital. Coincidentally, in 1958, only 25% of community hospitals with more than 300 beds reported having an ICU but by the late 1960s, close to 95% of all acute care hospitals in the United States had some sort of critical care unit *(15)*.

In the 1960s, the government began to pay for the health services of poor and elderly patients through Medicaid and Medicare. These programs enabled access to health care for a larger segment of the population and allowed hospitals to purchase the cutting-edge technology. More specialized units came into favor and cardiologists emerged as the directors of coronary care units. As a result, by the end of the 1960s, the mortality rate of cardiac patients was reduced 20%. Early successes of specialty-trained intensivists have evolved into evidence-based, outcome studies that show that units managed by specialty-trained intensivists with protocol based care result in better outcomes *(15,16)*.

Development of Neuroanesthesiology and Medical Monitoring

In the 1960s, neuroanesthesiology developed as a definitive subspecialty. During this development, advances and standardization of methods to measure CBF, cerebral oxygen saturation, ICP, electrophysiology, and neurochemical indices were introduced *(17)*. With these contributions from general anesthesiologists and neuroanethesiologists, ICUs became a gathering place for expensive technology to supplement and improve the cardiopulmonary support patients received. Professor

Andrew Hunter, the author of the first book on neuroanesthesia, is considered one of the pioneers in his field. Unfortunately, the earliest minutes of the historic discussions and accounts of the developments are lost. However, much of the progress in anesthesia from the "rag-and-bottle inhalation era" to the use of intravenous anesthetics, neuromuscular blocking agents, ventilators and monitoring can be credited to anesthesiologists like Maurice Albin and Thomas Langfitt. Concurrently through cooperative efforts with surgeons, such as Cushing and Halsted, thoracic and neurosurgical anesthesia were revolutionized, cardiac surgery became possible, and resuscitation with intravenous (IV) fluids, blood, and plasma was further developed *(18)*.

Development of Intravenous Techniques and Nutrition

Early efforts in cardiac resuscitation and critical care included assessment and management of volume status and were markedly advanced by development of IV techniques. Neurologic patients present with a combination of derangements. Patients with hypertensive crisis have high blood pressure but may be volume-depleted. Alternatively patients with spinal shock and dysautonomia may have normal blood volume but are hypotensive due to vasoparalysis. The pulmonary artery catheter and echocardiography has assisted intensivists with determination of vascular volume and cardiovascular function. Vascular resuscitation essential for maintenance of cerebral and spinal perfusion pressure involves use of vasopressors and inotropic agents guided by these monitoring techniques (*see also* Chapters 8, 10, and 13).

Nutrition was an often-overlooked aspect of critical care illness. Through the years, nutritional status, including energy and protein requirements, has been carefully correlated with outcomes in neurologic patients. Intensivists now recognize syndromes associated with the phenomena of underfeeding and overfeeding. Experience with IV nutritional therapies led to a better understanding of the increased caloric demands of neuroscience patients, particularly after head trauma *(19–22)*. By virtue of their condition, many neuroscience patients are at greater risk for aspiration (*see also* Chapter 11). Because enteral feeding is still favorable, nasogastric and percutaneous gastric tubes came into use. Occasionally, total parenteral nutrition is necessary for patients in coma with poor gut motility. Nutritional consultation and services are an integral part of the NSU design and staffing providing specialized formulations for the catabolic brain injured patient (*see* Chapter 14).

Development of Hygiene Guidelines and Infection Control

Despite fastidious attention to sterile technique, infections occur. In distinction to other ICU patients, an NSU patient rarely has open wounds, fractures and markedly altered skin barriers. The risk of wound infection after craniotomy is low *(23)*. Infections usually occur in lung, bladder, blood, and brain or meninges after trauma, surgery, or placement of extraventricular devices. Infections within the CNS are particularly difficult to treat given the generally poor antibiotic penetration of the blood-brain barrier (*see* Chapter 29).

Critical care nursing has played an important role in the development of infection control standards. Florence Nightingale observed that hand washing reduced the spread of infection. The European Prevalence of Infection in Intensive Care (EPIC) study conducted by the European Society of Critical Care Medicine suggested that minimizing the nurse-patient ratio reduced spread of ICU-acquired infections *(11)*. Institution of infection control standards for monitoring strict hand washing, use of sterile technique during bedside procedures, and patient isolation have become as important as pharmacotherapy. Adequate amount of appropriate supplies must be on hand in each room to reduce the traffic between patients and supply areas. However, careful calculations for supply requirements are necessary to avoid waste from contamination.

Care of the critically ill and immune compromised has incorporated the use of broad-spectrum antibiotics. Unfortunately, the repeated use and misuse of antibiotics has resulted in antimicrobial resistance *(24)*. Future ICU design and construction must facilitate safety and infection control requirements. Staff education should target infection control as management of infection can lead to shortened length of stay, improved outcomes *(25)*, and increase ICU throughput.

Development of NSU as a Subspecialty

Over the past two to three decades, ICUs caring for neonatal, trauma, burn, cancer, neurologic, and postoperative cardiac patients have evolved. The argument is made that care in specialized units is of a higher quality because of focus on the special needs of the patients. Recent reports suggest that outcome is improved in stroke patients cared for in stroke units *(26,27)* and ICH patients cared for by specialty-trained physicians and nurses in NSUs *(7,28)*. As technology supporting more advanced and invasive care of brain injured patients has improved, a specific and in-depth knowledge base has become a sought after commodity. As a result, the number of specialty ICUs for care of neurological and/or neurosurgical patients has been growing rapidly. Training programs have grown in number to meet the need for specialty-trained physicians and nurses *(7)*. An important development has been the foundation of the Neurocritical Care Society in February 2003. This society is an international organization composed of healthcare workers from various disciplines interested in caring for critically ill neurological and neurosurgical patients. We anticipate a promising future for further NSU growth and research.

ORGANIZATION

Admission, Triage, and Discharge for an NSU

The success of intensive care is not measured only by statistics of survival, as though each death were a medical failure. It is measured by the quality of lives preserved or restored, the quality of the dying of those whose interest it is to die and by the quality of relationships involved in each death. *(29)*

Patients admitted to an NSU usually have one or a combination of the following abnormalities: altered level of consciousness, mechanical ventilatory insufficiency, loss of airway protective reflexes, risk of rapid deterioration in neurologic function, or cardiovascular instability associated with neurological injury.

In 1977, Marsh et al. listed stroke, head injury, brain tumor, post-hypoxic encephalopathy, and admission for immediate postoperative observation as the most common admitting diagnoses. Less commonly admitted patients were those with spinal cord injury, status epilepticus, myasthenia gravis and various infectious, and metabolic and hypertensive encephalopathies. Although admitting diagnoses have not changed, emergence of new means of diagnosing and treating acute neurological diseases increases the number of patients that are candidates for NSU care.

Acute management of stroke, until recently, was characterized by supportive therapy alone. Although advances in cardiorespiratory care have allowed improved outcomes, it has taken new therapies directed at the brain to improve function. For example, patients with vertebrobasilar territory infarcts uniformly died before techniques to support ventilation and treat cardiovascular collapse. Now with these techniques, patients live to be candidates for intra-arterial thrombolysis and neuroprotective drug trials (*see* Chapters 17 and 18). On the other hand, aggressive therapies, such as intravenous, intra-arterial or combined tissue plasminogen administration have led to increased risk of hemorrhage. Judicious blood pressure control *(29)* and close observation can modify this risk by specially trained staff. Sequelae of ICH and subarachnoid hemorrhage (SAH) are more likely to be identified and result in early and directed medical and surgical interventions in an ICU staffed by individuals specifically trained in the area of neuroscience. Head trauma patients are also more like to have better outcomes in a specialty ICU *(30)*.

In the past, neurologic and neurosurgical intensive care developed in parallel. However, common pathways of brain and whole body response to a variety of inciting neurological injuries have brought these two disciplines closer. Neurologists' interests in acute medical care and neurosurgical concentration on new operative techniques have resulted in new expansive knowledge, making collaboration necessary for the future. A multidisciplinary team comprised of a combination of neurologists, neurointensivists, neurosurgeons, and neuroradiologists is frequently seen in the NSUs of the academic medical center of today.

The intensivist is unit/hospital based and can serve many roles including medical direction, consultant, triage, and manager of ICU resources. The administrative role of the intensivist includes teaching, institution of protocols for health outcome improvement, reduction of length of stay and readmission, and maintenance of staff milieu. Protocols are being established as guidelines for unit functions and bed control. This allows for the appropriate nurse staffing and bed availability. Several studies have looked at various aspects of admission, discharge, and triage. Hyman et al. designed criteria that have been adapted and further expanded *(31)*. These criteria are summarized in Tables 1–3. Sample detailed admission, discharge, and triage criteria for an actual NSU are presented in Chapter 1.

Design of an NSU

Design of modern ICUs present unique challenges to both physicians and administrators in the current health care environment. Cost-effective and cost-beneficial design is essential for all ICUs. There are specific needs of the neuroscience patient that necessitate both financial and human resource investments.

The NSU can be a geographically separate area of the hospital or housed within a multispecialty unit. Number of beds should be based on referral and admission patterns as well as available staffing. Adequate floor space for traffic patterns, and easy movement through the unit and around patients are required. Ideally designed NSUs provide for the best visualization of monitors and direct patient observation. Unique floor plan design including windowed walls and remote camera monitoring provide high-frequency visibility.

Present-day design mandates private rooms or adequate space between patients to provide privacy and confidentiality. Experts have reported the necessity of a minimum of 200 to 330 ft^2 per bed area *(32,33)* to accommodate ancillary equipment. Floor space should allow for positioning of bed and equipment to facilitate traffic, workflow patterns and access to the patient from all angles (Fig. 1). Specific to NSUs, the room layout must allow 270–360 degrees access to the head because of frequent minor surgical interventions and cerebral monitoring (Fig. 2). Adequate supplies of oxygen, air, suction, electricity, and lighting are clustered, along with back-facilities in the event of supply failure. In addition to routine monitoring and call/signal systems, NSUs should include systems that do not depend on patient-generated activation. Systems activated by ventilator disconnect, motion detectors, and video observation should be considered.

Design can facilitate fluctuations in patient acuity. As the acuity of patients increases, a higher nurse to patient ratio (1:1, 1:2) is required and more personnel may need to be at the bedside. Concomitantly, the nurse-to-patient ratio may need to transiently decrease (1:3) for lower acuity patients. Therefore, the floor plan becomes important to ensure multiple forms of visibility of patients and changing staffing patterns. There are several architectural models to consider (Fig. 3). Staffing, projected occupancy and constraints of the building floor plan determine the ideal layout. Most ICUs were built into an existing building footprint and configuration was limited. Rectangular design with a central nursing station limits visibility at the ends. The need for storage and conference space limits patient directed care resources. Family waiting and grieving areas were never planned and are located in other areas of the hospital. Perhaps the best designs take advantage of circular array of beds around a central nursing core. However, circular designs do not necessarily fit well in hospital floor plans.

Staffing of an NSU

Several models of care (e.g., open vs closed ICUs, resident/fellows vs physician extenders, nurses only) are used throughout the country, with varying degrees of success. Although all care models

Table 1
NSU Admission Criteria

1. Postoperative patients who need neurological and cardiopulmonary assessment at least every 2 h; patients may be admitted directly from the operating room or recovery room
2. Patients needing brain and/or spinal cord assessment more frequently than every 2 h
3. Patients with uncontrolled seizures requiring assessment at least every hour
4. Patients who need frequent monitoring or treatments unavailable in general care areas (electrocardiogram, invasive pressure monitoring, drug infusions, respiratory monitoring, mechanical ventilation, and so on)
5. Overflow from other intensive care areas; these patients may not always have neurological diseases

Table 2
NSU Discharge Criteria

Discharged to	Patients
General care floor	There is no neurological change for 24 h, seizures are controlled with medications, metabolic homeostasis is present, intravascular volume is adequate; there is no life-threatening arrhythmia or hemodynamic instability, respiratory status is stable, assessments and therapies (e.g., suctioning) are required every 4 h or less, care withdrawn for comfort measures
Intermediate care unit	There is no life-threatening arrhythmia or hemodynamic instability, but may still require intermittent IV bolus of antiarrhythmic or antihypertensive agent. Respiratory status is stable but requires ventilatory support or frequent respiratory treatment; intracranial monitoring is stopped

Table 3
NSU Triage Criteria

1. When the NSU census is full, the unit director generates a triage list of patients who could be adequately managed on an alternate level unit.
2. If the NSU is full, and all possible patients have been transferred to a general or intermediate unit, any patient needing NSU should be referred to an alternate ICU with close NSU follow-up.
3. It may be preferable to triage more stable patients to other ICUs to make space for a more acute NSU patient.

may work, the ideal model for a given ICU can be found only through ongoing performance improvement *(34)*. There are several standard staffing issues in the design of any NSU.

All intensivists have knowledge of acute circulatory, respiratory, and metabolic disturbances and general skills required for advanced cardiac life support, cardioversion, intubation and ventilator management, and insertion of invasive hemodynamic monitoring. There is debate regarding the role of general critical care physicians versus specially trained neurointensivists in NSUs. Both models can work but optimally the general intensivist should have special training in neuroscience and neuroscientists have taken the time to train in general ICU issues through a formal fellowship. Neurocritical care physicians are especially adept in discussion of cerebrovascular pathophysiology and complex end-of-life issues. With experience in defining brain death and prognosis in severe brain injury, currently neurocritical care specialists are leading the way as an interface for organ procurement and donation.

Observational studies of ICU directors identified five characteristics that were thought to result in effective leadership: clinical credibility; an active clinical presence in the unit; a supportive approach

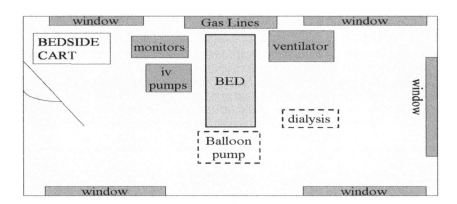

Fig. 1. General ICU bed orientation.

that encouraged input and suggestions; an ability to accept responsibility and be accountable; and a dedication to continuous teaching, improvement and excellence in patient care *(34)*.

Staffing should facilitate training of junior staff members in different aspects of intensive care. Both physicians and nurses depend on a hierarchical model of transferring knowledge and experience. Given the high turnover of personnel in ICUs this approach serves to insure a ready supply of developing practitioners. Even those who agree that neuroscience specialty training is essential are unclear as to what standardized criteria should be introduced into training programs. National standards and a curriculum are under development.

Efficiency and core proficiency of any NSU depends on a central core of nurses with neurocritical care training. This may be one of the most difficult staffing issues faced in the NSU. Care of neurological and neurosurgical patients requires perseverance as they often do not improve and the gratification of successful outcome is rare. The nursing profession is exhibiting a severe shortage in qualified caregivers and the average age of critical care nurses is over 40 yr. Aging of the experienced nursing cohort will worsen the staffing shortages in the coming years. Despite the rise of professional and academic standard of nurses, the profession continues to lose its appeal for a variety of reasons including shift work, lack of employment benefits, and increased interest in administrative positions and out-of-hospital job opportunities. Recruitment and retention of nursing staff must play an integral role in staffing and budget planning (*see also* Chapter 33). An expansion of the role of advanced clinical nurses could potentially increase job interest as well as improve care in the setting of limited staffing. Thus, when there is a limited in-house medical staff, no full-time medical director, or only nominal medical leadership, expansion of nursing roles is essential *(11)*.

Staffing of an ICU demands special relationships within the ICU team and with other teams in the hospital. There is ongoing debate about whether ICUs require a dedicated, full time team. Some referring physicians will wish to be involved in decisions of any magnitude and others to leave management entirely to the ICU team. This dynamic is typically characterized as "open" and "closed" unit management designs, respectively. Lustbadder and Fein *(35)* describe advantages and disadvantages of each design as follows:

Open Unit
    Advantages
- May have ICU Director
- Private physicians manage cases
- May be appropriate for smaller nonteaching hospitals
- Intensivist may be involved in case (as a consultant)
- Greater private physician satisfaction

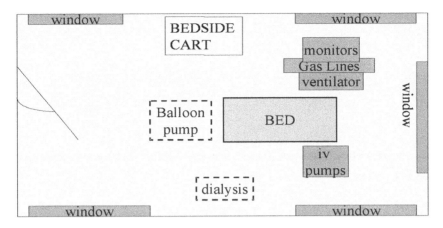

Fig. 2. Ideal NSU bed orientation.

Disadvantages
- Frequently lacks team leader
- Variable coverage nights and weekends
- Intensivist may not be involved in the case
- Physicians manage cases
- Less efficient and prolonged ICU length of stay

Closed Unit
Advantages
- ICU Director
- Single intensivist manages all cases and is team leader
- House staff usually present
- Improved efficiency and reduced length of stay
- Reduced resource utilization
- Facilitates protocols (weaning, medication)
- Formal ICU rounds
- Greater nursing satisfaction

Disadvantages
- May cause physician conflict
- No pre-existing relationship with patients and their families
- May not have details and nuances of patient's medical history
- May alienate referring physicians
- Primary physician may not want patient back on transfer from ICU to floor

Favoring an open system is increased continuity of care as patients are moved to and from ICU and general wards. However, several studies have shown that closed units result in a decrease in morbidity and mortality rates *(36,37)*, average ventilation time, length of stay *(38,39)*, and cost *(40)*. In addition, most of the stated disadvantages to a closed system can be easily resolved with a concerted effort to communicate with referring physicians, patients and families.

FUTURE DESIGN: EVERYTHING FROM TELECOMMUNICATION SYSTEMS TO ROBOTICS

With the advent of affordable and more portable technology, changes will occur in the structure and function of ICUs. Units were created as quarantined areas of the hospital in times of epidemics and were kept separate to cluster patients in areas where high-cost monitoring and specially trained personnel could be concentrated. With the advancement of the information age, some of these physi-

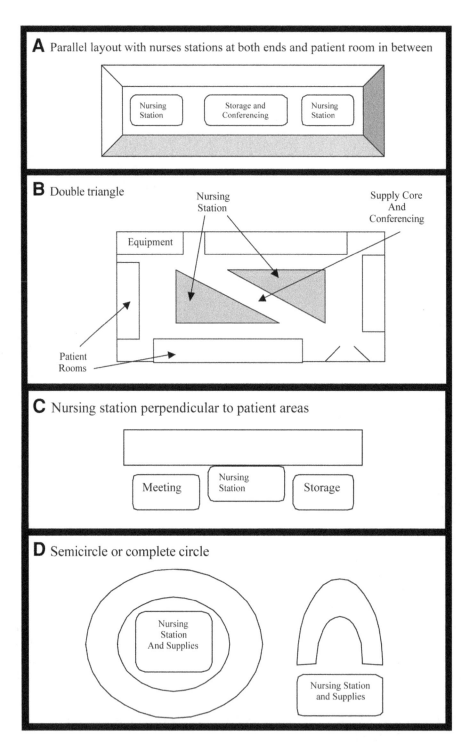

Fig. 3. Different ICU designs.

cal barriers may disappear. Education is online and available for all medical professionals making all healthcare workers more informed. There may be a time when every patient in a hospital is "wired" and information transmitted wirelessly to remote stations for monitoring of a variety of health parameters by nurses and hospitalist physicians trained to recognize signs of worsening. Critical care may be delivered on site in wardrooms capable of being converted to a high-monitored setting with the flip of a switch.

Rapid advances in telemedicine have paralleled the growth in general medicine. In 1897, the telephone was used to help diagnose croup in a child. Einthoven used an ordinary analog phone in 1910 to transmit electroencephalograms and electrocardiograms. In 1959, the US government helped fund the first functional telemedicine program, providing outpatient psychiatric patient care and medical education in Nebraska *(41)*. Several other projects were initiated throughout the 1960s and 1970s. These earlier efforts were hindered by the high cost of technology, poor image quality, and increased time required to train medical personnel. During the past two decades, considerable improvements in telecommunication devices (including powerful computers with high-speed connections, satellite systems, and digital technology) have again resurrected interest in use of this exciting and valuable adjunct to practice and delivery health care, particularly in rural areas *(42)*. In addition, there has been broader usage in neuroscience *(43)*.

Preliminary studies provide data that demonstrate favorable outcomes. Telemedicine reduces mortality, length of stay, ICU complications, and costs when remote interventionist provides care in comparison to care not directed by an interventionist. There are no studies regarding use of telemedicine in neurocritical care specifically. However, the Telemedical Emergency Neurosurgical Network (TENN) was developed in the early 1990s. Collected data suggest a potentially exciting role for neurocritical specialists. The clinical efficacy and cost effectiveness noted in the TENN study suggest an immeasurable promise for new relationships between intensivists, community providers and "at-risk" underserved populations *(44)*.

Several large medical centers have adopted computer-based monitoring systems. The first of which was seen at Case Western Reserve University Hospital in the 1970s. Now, these systems are frequently used to assist in record keeping and collection of medical data for research. Such systems also function as flowsheets for charting purposes and minimize use of paper records and daily notes. These offer a more accessible, legible, permanent, and legal record of medical data. As these systems are placed at the bedside, nurses will spend more time and attention on patients *(45)*.

Neuroscience has been at the forefront of technology since the creation of the CT scanner. The need to transport critically ill patients has decreased by having portable CT scanners housed in the ICU. Magnetic resonance imaging and positron emission tomography scanners are being built in proximity to ICUs. Robotic surgical devices are appearing in hospitals across the country. It will not be long before detailed neuroanatomic knowledge will be programmed into robots at the bedside to guide invasive techniques formerly done in the operating rooms and interventional suites. Robots will play important roles in hospital and ICU daily operations to perform routine fetch and carry tasks, handle difficult and hazardous materials, assist healthcare professionals to provide improved standards of treatment and care, and perhaps solve the shortage in healthcare workers associated with the advancing age of the population *(46)*.

The high cost of health care will continue to change the face of care delivery and reimbursement. Consolidation of hospitals has occurred throughout the country. Regional provision of critical care services is likely to become the norm. As provider organizations come to control a large number of beds in a geographic area, centralization of critically ill patients in well-managed, technologically sophisticated, and specialized ICUs will become more attractive than less efficient alternatives. Institutions will need to opt for practice patterns that demonstrably lower costs and improve outcomes *(36)*.

REFERENCES

1. [No authors listed]. Intensive therapy and care. *Br. J. Anaesth.* 1965;37:465.
2. Cowley LT. Care of the dying: an ethical and historical perspective. *Crit. Care Med.* 1992;20:1473–1482.
3. Meyer JA. A practical mechanical respirator, 1929: "The iron lung." *Ann. Thorac. Surg.* 1990;50:490–493.
4. Bleck T. Critical care and emergency neurology. In: Cohen MM, ed. *The American Academy of Neurology: The First 50 Years 1948-1998.* St Paul, MN, The American Academy of Neurology, 1998;225–227.
5. Ropper AH. Neurologic intensive care. *Ann. Neurol.* 1992;32:564–569.
6. Kochanek PM, Snyder JV, Sirio CA, Saxena S, Bircher NG. Specialty neurointensive care: Is it just a name or a way of life? *Crit. Care Med.* 2001;29:692–693.
7. Diringer MN, Edwards DF. Admission to a neurologic/neurosurgical intensive care unit is associated with reduced mortality rate after intracerebral hemorrhage. *Crit. Care Med.* 2001;29:635–640.
8. Zulch KJ. Does a neurology department need its own intensive care unit? *Z. Neurol.* 1972;201:1–5.
9. Calvin JE, Habet K, Parrillo JE. Critical care in the United States: Who are we and how did we get here? *Crit. Care Med.* 1997;13:363–376.
10. Abedellah FG. The nursing shortage: dynamics and solutions. Reflections on recurring theme. *Nurs. Clin. North Am.* 1990;25:5009–5016.
11. Byran-Brown CW, Dracup K. Millenial solutions. *Am. J. Crit. Care* 2000;9:3–5.
12. Society of Critical Care Medicine: The Society of Critical Care Professionals. Available at: www.sccm.org.
13. Safar PJ. *Careers in Anesthesiology: An Autobiographical Memoir.* Wood Library—Museum of Anesthesiology. Park Ridge, IL: 2000.
14. Saffle JR. The 1942 fire at Boston's Coconut Grove nightclub. *Am. J. Surg.* 1993;166:581–591.
15. Shackford SR, Hollingworth-Fridlund P, Cooper GF, et al. The effect of regionalization upon the quality of trauma care as assessed by concurrent audit before and after institution of a trauma center: a preliminary report. *J. Trauma* 1986;26:812–820.
16. Guidelines Committee of American College of Critical Care Medicine. Society of Critical Care Medicine and American Association of Critical Care Nurses Transfer Guidelines Task Force: Guidelines for the transfer of critically ill patients. *Crit. Care Med.* 1993;21:931–937.
17. Albin MS. Celebrating silver: the genesis of neuroanesthesiology society. *J. Neurosurg. Anesth.* 1997;9:296–307.
18. Norman J. An informal history of the first 25 years. *Br. J. Anaesth.* 2002;88:445–450.
19. Donaldson J, Borzetta MA, Matossian D. Nutrition strategies in neurotrauma. *Crit. Care Nurs. Clin. North Am.* 2000;12:465–475.
20. Yanagawa T, Bunn F, Roberts I, Wentz R, Pierro A. Nutrition support for head-injured patients. *Cochrane Database Syst. Rev.* 2002;CD001530.
21. Roberts PR. Nutrition in head-injured patients. *New Horiz.* 1995;3:506–517.
22. Rapp RP, Young B, Twyman D, et al. The favorable effect of early parenteral feeding on survival in head-injured patients. *J. Neurosurg.* 1983;58:906–912.
23. Blomstedt GC. Craniotomy infections. *Neurosurg. Clin. North Am.* 1992;3:375–385.
24. Wester CW, Durairaj L, Evans AT, et al. Antibiotic resistance: a survey of physician perceptions. *Arch. Intern. Med.* 2002;162:2210–2216.
25. Berenholtz SM, Dorman T, Ngo K, et al. Qualitative review of intensive care unit quality indicators. *J. Crit. Care* 2002;17:12–15.
26. Webb DJ, Faya PB, Wilbur C, et al. Effects of specialized team on stroke care: the first two years of the Yale Stroke Program decreases hospitalization costs and length of stay. *Stroke* 1998;26:1353–1357.
27. Wentworth DA, Atkinson RP. Implementation of an acute stroke program decreases hospitalization costs and length of stay. *Stroke* 1998;27:1040–1043.
28. Mirski M, Chang CW, Cowan R. Impact of a neurosciences intensive care unit on neurosurgical patient outcomes and cost of care. *J. Neurosurg. Anesth.* 2001;13:83–92.
29. Dustan GR. Hard questions in intensive care. *Anaesthesia* 1985;40:479–482.
30. Patel HC, Menon DK, Tebbs S, et al. Specialist neurocritical care and outcome from head injury. *Intensive Care Med.* 2002;28:547–553.
31. Hyman S, William V, Maciunas RJ. Neurosurgical intensive care unit organization and function: an American experience. *J. Neurosurg. Anesth.* 1993;5:71–80.
32. Bell JA, Bradley RD, Jenkins BS, Spencer GT. Six years of multidisciplinary intensive care. *BMJ* 1974;2:483–488.
33. Hospital Building Note Number 27. Intensive therapy unit. Department of Health and Social Security. London: H.M.S.O., 1970.
34. Barie PS, Bacchetta MD, Eachempati SR. The contemporary surgical intensive care unit. Structure, staffing, and issues. *Surg. Clin. North Am.* 2000;80:791–804.
35. Lustbader D, Fein A. ICU bedside technology: emerging trends in ICU management and staffing. *Crit. Care Clin.* 2000;16:735–748.

36. Ghorra S, Reinert SE, Cioffi W, et al. What's new in general surgery: Analysis of the effect of conversion from open to closed surgical intensive care unit. *Ann. Surg.* 1999;229:163–171.

37. Carlson RW, Weiland DE, Srivathsan K. Does a full-time 24-hour intensivist improve care and efficiency? *Crit. Care Clin.* 1996;12:525–551.

38. Bach PB, Carson SS, Jeff A. Outcomes and resource utilization for patients with prolonged critical illness managed by university based or community based subspecialties. *Am. J. Respir. Crit. Care Med.* 1989;158:1410–1415.

39. Multz A, Chalfin DB, Samson IM, et al. A 'closed' medical intensive care unit (MICU) improves resource utilization when compared with an 'open' MICU. *Am. J. Respir. Crit. Care Med.* 1978;157:1468–1473.

40. Hanson CW III, Deutschman CS, Anderson HL III, et al. Effects of an organized critical care service on outcomes and resource utilization: a cohort study. *Crit. Care Med.* 1999;27:270–274.

41. Shafazand S, Shigemitsu H, Weinacker AB. A brave new world: remote intensive care unit for the 21st century. *Crit. Care Med.* 2000;28:3945–3946.

42. Kesler C, Balch D. Development of telemedicine and distance learning network in rural North Carolina. *J. Telemed. Telecare* 1995;1:178–182.

43. Chua R, Craig J, Esmonde T, et al. Telemedicine for new neurological outpatients: Putting a randomized controlled trial in the context of everyday practice. *J. Telemed. Telecare* 2002;8:270–273.

44. Chodroff PH. A three-year review of telemedicine at the community level- Clinical and fiscal results. *J. Telemed. Telecare* 1999;5:28S–30S.

45. Franklin DF, Bargsley L. Comprehensive patient monitoring in a neurosurgical intensive care unit. *J. Neurosurg. Nurs.* 1983;15:205–212.

46. Finlay PA. Medical robots in intensive care. *Intensive Care World* 1990;7:30–31.

3

Cerebral Blood Flow Physiology and Monitoring

Michel T. Torbey and Anish Bhardwaj

INTRODUCTION

For optimal therapy of patients with brain injury, a thorough knowledge of the underlying cerebral blood flow (CBF) physiology is essential. This chapter reviews the relationship between CBF and brain metabolism and summarizes the therapeutic implications of this interaction in patients with brain injury.

PHYSIOLOGY OF CEREBRAL CIRCULATION

The adult brain (1200–1400 g) comprises 2–3% of total body weight and receives 15–20% of cardiac output. The central nervous system has a high metabolic rate for oxygen ($CMRO_2$) and uses glucose predominantly as the substrate for its energy needs. Although glial cells make up almost 50% of the brain, they consume less than 10% of total cerebral energy due to their low metabolic rate [1]. Neurons expend most of the available energy [1]. Fifty percent of the total energy generated is used for maintenance and restoration of ion gradients across the cell membrane, and the remaining 25% is used for molecular transport, synaptic transmission and other processes [1]. Normal CBF in humans averages 50 mL/100 g brain tissue per minute [2]. It is usually higher in children and adolescents and drops further with age [3,4]. Irreversible neuronal damage occurs when CBF drops below 10–15 cc/100 g/min, whereas reversible neuronal injury occurs with CBF between 15 and 20 cc/100 g/min [5,6].

Because the brain has no significant storage capacity, cerebral metabolism, CBF, and oxygen extraction are tightly coupled. This relationship is expressed by the Fick's equation: $CMRO_2 = CBF \times AVDO_2$, in which $CMRO_2$ represents cerebral metabolic rate for oxygen and $AVDO_2$, arterio-venous difference of oxygen [2]. Under normal conditions, the brain maintains a constant $AVDO_2$ by responding to changes in metabolism, cerebral perfusion pressure (CPP), and blood viscosity with changes in vessel caliber, a phenomenon referred to as *autoregulation* [7,8].

Mechanisms of Autoregulation

The precise mechanism(s) of autoregulation have not been fully elucidated. Two theories have been postulated [9]; myogenic and metabolic [10,11]. The evidence supporting the *myogenic theory* consists of experiments in which alterations in transmural pressures have been shown to trigger immediate changes in the autoregulatory response [9,12]. The *metabolic theory* is based on the hypothesis that changes in the microenvironment alter vasomotor responses. Variations in the partial pressure of arterial carbon dioxide ($PaCO_2$) exert a profound influence on CBF. At $PaCO_2$ levels within the normal range, CBF changes by approx 3–4% for every 1% change in pCO_2 [10,11], and there is an increment of approx 4% in CBF for every increase of 1 mmHg between $PaCO_2$ values of 25 and 100

From: *Current Clinical Neurology*
Critical Care Neurology and Neurosurgery
Edited by: J. I. Suarez © Humana Press Inc., Totowa, NJ

mmHg. The arteriolar responses that follow changes in $PaCO_2$ are believed to be mediated by a local effect of H^+ or, in turn, pH variations of the extracellular fluid surrounding resistance vessels in the brain *(13)*. However, $PaCO_2$-induced effects on CBF are transient and diminish because of adaptive changes in bicarbonate concentration of the cerebrospinal fluid (CSF).

Other physiologic factors that alter CBF include the partial pressure of arterial oxygen (PaO_2) and temperature. Within the normal physiologic range, changes in PaO_2 do not affect CBF. However, CBF increases dramatically when PaO_2 falls below 50 mmHg. Temperature has a profound effect on $CMRO_2$ by 6–7% for every 1°C increase in temperature. Conversely, $CMRO_2$ is reduced by the same percentage with hypothermia.

Limits of CBF Autoregulation

Autoregulation of CBF is effective over a wide range of perfusion pressures with lower and upper limits estimated to be at a mean arterial pressure (MAP) of 60–150 mmHg, respectively *(14,15*; Fig. 1). Outside this range of autoregulation, CBF varies directly with perfusion pressure. Below the lower limit, CBF decreases as vasodilation becomes insufficient, consequently resulting in ischemia *(16)*. Above the upper limit, increased intraluminal pressure results in a forceful dilation of arterioles ("luxury" perfusion), leading to disruption of blood brain barrier and brain edema *(17,18)*.

Neurogenic Effect on CBF

In addition to myogenic control and the chemical influences, this mechanism is believed to play a small role in controlling CBF. Although the specific mechanism(s) remains unclear, anatomic studies have shown the existence of an extensive nerve supply to the extracranial and intracranial vessels *(11)*. Activation of the α-adrenergic sympathetic nerves shifts the limits of autoregulation toward higher pressures and acute denervation shifts the limits of autoregulation toward lower pressures *(19–21)*. Experimental evidence supports that sympathetic innervation plays an important modulating role during acute hypertensive episodes, resulting in vasoconstriction of the cerebral vasculature *(22)*.

CBF in Chronic Hypertension

Chronic arterial hypertension causes both structural *(23,24)* and functional hemodynamic changes in cerebral resistance vessels *(14)*. These adaptive changes are partly reversible after chronic treatment with antihypertensive treatment *(25)*. In the muscular arteries, the media is thickened and undergo fibrosis, with patchy degeneration of smooth muscle cells and fibrous thickening of the intimal layer. The thickening is usually caused by medial cell hypertrophy and possibly hyperplasia, and later by degeneration of the muscle cells and deposition of hyaline material and fibrin *(23,24,26)*. Autoregulation of CBF is preserved in uncomplicated arterial hypertension, but the lower and upper limits are shifted toward higher values of arterial pressure in proportion to the severity of hypertension *(27)*. This shift of the lower limit is also reflected by the fact that the lowest tolerated arterial pressure is higher in hypertensive than in normotensive patients *(27)*. The hypertensive vascular changes that impair the tolerance to acute hypotension concomitantly improve the tolerance of the brain to hypertension *(28)*. Consequently, acute pharmacologic reduction of systemic arterial pressures should be gradual and mild enough to avoid drops in arterial pressure below the lower limit of autoregulation. The choice of antihypertensive agent is important because some agents, in addition to their antihypertensive effect, may affect or abolish CBF autoregulation, making the acute lowering of arterial pressure even hazardous and further exacerbate ischemic brain injury *(29)*.

Effects of Blood Rheology on CBF

Under normal conditions in healthy subjects, the pressure gradient and radius of the cerebral blood vessels are the major determinants of CBF *(30)*. However, in areas of focal cerebral ischemia that have lost the capacity to pressure autoregulate and in which vessel radius is maximal, viscosity of blood assumes greater importance in the determination of CBF *(30,31)*.

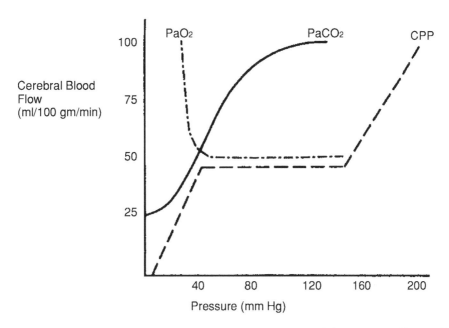

Fig. 1. In normal brain, CBF is kept constant through autoregulation of CPP between 40 and 140 mmHg. Other factors that independently affect CBF include $PaCO_2$ and PaO_2. Adapted from ref. *15* with permission.

Blood viscosity is determined by several factors, including hematocrit, erythrocyte aggregation, erythrocyte flexibility, platelet aggregation, and plasma viscosity *(32)*. Hematocrit is the major factor influencing blood viscosity *(33)*. Under normotension, a decrease in hematocrit from 35% to 25% is associated with a 30% increase in CBF *(34)*. This relationship is not maintained at low perfusion pressure, suggesting that the increase in CBF following hemodilution is caused by compensatory vasodilatation and not by reduction of blood viscosity *(35)*. This may imply that hemodilution may not improve CBF in areas of impaired autoregulation *(34)*. Compensatory vasodilatory mechanisms are exhausted at hematocrit of 19% as indicated by a reduction of CBF and cerebral oxygen delivery *(36)*. Although hemodilution plays some role in therapy for cerebral vasospasm following subarachnoid hemorrhage, its therapeutic role in ischemic stroke is still not well established. Several studies have demonstrated that hemoglobin level greater than 15 g/L is a risk factor for stroke or other occlusive disease *(37–39)*; however, no trials to date have demonstrated a therapeutic effect *(40,41)*.

Relationship Between Intracranial Pressure and CBF

The contents of the skull can be conceptualized as a three-compartment model composed of brain and interstitial fluid (80%), CSF (10%), and blood (10%), all of which are largely incompressible. Cerebral perfusion pressure (CPP), defined as MAP-ICP, is well maintained in healthy subjects. However, in pathological states, such as in space occupying lesions, initially small increases in intracranial volume can be accommodated by translocation of CSF into distensible spinal subarachnoid space with little effect on ICP. However, with exhaustion of this compensatory mechanism, can result in large increases in ICP, leading to decreased CPP or CBF. Thus, factors that influence ICP can have profound effects on CBF by altering CBF.

RATIONALE FOR CBF MEASUREMENT

Unlike intracranial pressure monitoring, bedside evaluation and monitoring of CBF in ICU patients is difficult. Yet, bedside measurement of CBF remains a longstanding goal of neurointensivists. Frequent or continuous monitoring of CBF allows the intensive care team to identify progression of pathophyisological mechanisms involved, intervene to halt or reverse this progression, and identify the response to treatment to modify the intervention if necessary.

Techniques for Measuring CBF

The ideal CBF measurement technique in the ICU should be portable, have the capacity for continuous monitoring or at least be easily repeatable, noninvasive, and inexpensive. No currently available method comes close to having these ideal characteristics. However, several methods can provide quantitative measurement of absolute or relative global or regional CBF. Currently available techniques are summarized in Table 1 with their advantages and disadvantages. The majority of these techniques are not available in the ICU and may be associated with the risk of transporting critically ill patients out of the ICU and back *(42)*.

Serial Neurologic Examinations

It is the most common and easily available qualitative indirect guide to CBF at the bedside. A change in the level of consciousness or onset of a focal neurological deficit suggests that CBF has fallen almost to a threshold level for development of permanent neuronal damage from cerebral ischemia. Unfortunately it is not sensitive enough to provide early warning of CBF impairment and hence not very specific as an indicator of CBF impairment.

Neurophysiologic Monitoring

Electroencephalography (EEG) and evoked potentials (EP) testing can be used as a supplement to serial neurological examinations and other diagnostic studies in critically ill patients with cerebrovascular disease for early identification of ischemia. EEG and EP change predictably with cerebral ischemia, and recognition of these changes may allow intervention before tissue infarction *(43,44)*. Slowing of EEG occurs with CBF of 16–22 mL/100 g/min *(45)*; EEG amplitude is diminished with CBF of 11–19 mL/100 g/min *(5)*; and EEG activity is profoundly diminished or absent with CBF ≤ 10 mL/100 g/min *(46)*. Similarly, somatosensory EP (SSEP) undergo predictable changes in amplitude, latency, and central conduction time at reduced levels of CBF. Cortical amplitude of SSEP is decreased by 50% when CBF is reduced to 16 mL/100 g/min, and is abolished when CBF is 12 mL/100 g/min *(44)*. In summary, EEG and EP monitoring can be powerful tools for identifying neurophysiologic changes in patients with cerebrovascular disease. Neurophysiologic techniques in the ICU are likely to gain an expanded role with the development of better computing equipment and growing expertise in following neurophysiologic data over time.

Cerebral Perfusion Pressure

CBF is equal to CPP divided by the cerebral vascular resistance (CVR) [CBF=CPP/CVR]. Because measurement of CBF is technically difficult, CPP has been monitored in an attempt to assess the adequacy of CBF. Normal values for CPP are between 70 and 100 mmHg. However, a normal CPP represents a normal CBF only if CVR is normal. If CVR is high, because of stenosis or spasm, a normal CPP may be accompanied by ischemia. Alternatively, if CVR is low, a normal CPP may be associated with hyperemia and increased ICP. Thus it is imperative to maintain CPP in any situation especially if in situations where autoregulation is impaired.

Kety and Schmidt Technique

This is the first technique described to quantify CBF and is based on the Fick's principle, which uses nitrous oxide as a tracer of CBF. This gas is an ideal tracer because it is metabolically inert and diffuses rapidly into the brain *(47)*. In this method nitrous oxide is introduced into inspired air while serial samples of arterial and jugular venous blood are taken and analyzed for its concentration. By defining the time course of the change in nitrous oxide concentration in arterial and venous blood samples, and by using previous measurements of the blood/brain partition coefficient, global CBF can be calculated. This technique is based on two assumptions: continuous blood flow, and absence

Table 1
Advantages and Disadvantages of Different Techniques for CBF Measurements

Method	Advantages	Disadvantages
Neurologic examination	• Can be performed repeatedly	• Not sensitive for early CBF changes
Neurophysiologic monitoring	• Allows continuous monitoring	• Subject to artifact • Require expensive computing equipment for data analysis and storage
Fick's method	• Direct measure of CBF • Gold standard	• Measures only global CBF • Invasive • Requires manual, sequential sampling
Xenon-133	• Reproducible • Limited radioactive exposure	• Not suitable for deeper brain structures • Limited resolution
Xenon CT	• Can monitor specific regions over several studies	• Expensive • Technically difficult • Anesthetic effects from Xenon
PET scan	• Measures CBV • Calculates $CMRO_2$	• Limited availability • Expensive • Requires highly trained personnel
MRI and CT perfusion	• Can measure CBV and CBF	• It is qualitative comparing hemispheres
TCD	• Inexpensive • Portable • Allows continuous monitoring	• Requires stable arterial diameter and perfusion territories • Poor temporal windows in some patients • Insonation of large vessels in the Circle of Willis only

CT, computed tomography; MRI, magnetic resonance imaging; PET, positron emission tomography; TCD, transcranial Doppler.

27

of extracerebral contamination of jugular venous blood. A special apparatus is required for mixing the tracer with inspired air and best results are obtained in intubated patients.

Xenon-133

Intravenous or inhalation ^{133}Xe *(48,49)* has been used to measure CBF. Calculation of CBF using this technique requires measurement of the arterial concentration of the tracer, estimated by measuring radioactivity in end-tidal expired air, and determination of the dynamic change in the concentration of tracer in the brain, measured by extracranial detectors. A small, cart-mounted portable unit is currently available for bedside CBF measurement in the ICU. The quantitative accuracy of this technique may be compromised in pathological conditions by the fact that the blood-brain partition coefficient for ^{133}Xe can be abnormal.

Xenon Computed Tomography

Xenon computed tomography (CT) is another technique that can be used for critically ill patients in the ICU. Stable xenon is inhaled and acts as a contrast agent during CT imaging of the brain. Xenon CT provides a high degree of spatial resolution and differential regional CBF measurements of cortical and subcortical structures in a "CT CBF map" *(50)*.

Other Radiographic Techniques

Several in vivo methods, such as positron emission tomography (PET) *(51)*, single-photon emission computed tomography (SPECT) *(52)*, magnetic resonance (MR) imaging *(53,54)*, and CT perfusion *(55–58)* are presently available to measure CBF and cerebral blood volume (CBV). However, high costs coupled with limited accessibility and difficulty in obtaining quantitative values by using SPECT and MR and CT imaging have restricted the widespread clinical use of these imaging modalities.

Transcranial Doppler Ultrasound

Transcranial Doppler Ultrasound (TCD) represents a noninvasive method to estimate cerebral volume flow in larger conducting vessels at the base of the brain. Estimations of global CBF can be made using TCD if the amount of flow through all cerebral vessels is measured simultaneously. When rCBF is being estimated, the amount of blood flow through one cerebral vessel can be used as an estimate of blood flow only if the perfusion territory of that artery is known. By properly obtaining and analyzing the cerebral blood flow velocity (CBFV), resistance index, or pulsatility index of intracranial and extracranial arteries, and by performing arterial compression tests when appropriate, one can monitor the development of vasospasm following subarachnoid hemorrhage *(59)*, pattern of collateral circulation through the circle of Willis *(60)*, state of cerebral arterial patency during or following thrombolytic therapy *(61)*, or development of and progression to brain death *(62)*.

While the fundamental concept of maintaining adequate CBF or CPP is the cornerstone of management of patients with brain injury from diverse etiologies, many of the pathologic states pose additional concerns that must be considered to render optimal care.

CBF IN VARIOUS PATHOLOGICAL CONDITIONS

Traumatic Brain Surgery

Secondary ischemia, cerebral edema, and elevated ICP have been shown to contribute to neurologic injury after head trauma. Hence, a thorough understanding of immediate and delayed changes in CBF is paramount in the treatment of patients with traumatic brain injury (TBI). A drop in CBF has been reported in 50–60% of patients in the first few hours following TBI *(63–66)*. AVDO$_2$ measurements demonstrate that CBF exceeds metabolic requirements in majority of patients and hence a diminution in CBF does not represent ischemia in these patients *(2,67,68)*. In only 27% of patients, with CBF as low as 18 mL/100 g per min, AVDO$_2$ measurement revealed that CBF did not meet metabolic demands of the injured brain *(65)*. Hyperemia or "luxury perfusion" *(2,69,70)*, usually a delayed process, occurs in the first few days following severe TBI and is believed to be an important factor in the development of high ICP. From the uncoupling of CBF and cerebral metabolism, hyperemia cannot be defined by CBF criteria alone. AVDO$_2$ and CMRO$_2$ must be taken into account as well *(2)*. During the acute phase of the illness, sustained ICP elevation greater than 20 mmHg developed in 47% of patients, 77% of whom had hyperemic flow, and only 23% had reduced flow. This prompted the following suggested classification: (1) reduced flow (CBF below 33 mL/100 g/min) (2) relative hyperemia (CBF between 33 and 55 mL/100 g/min), and (3) absolute hyperemia (CBF 55 mL/100 g/min).

Ischemia after severe TBI has been clearly associated with poor prognosis *(66)*. Optimization and maintenance of CBF is therefore a cornerstone of contemporary management in patients with TBI. Maintenance of adequate CPP is critical in patients with defective as well as those with intact auto-regulation. In the defective autoregulation group, CBF will decrease linearly with CPP and may reach ischemic levels *(71)*, whereas decreased CPP in patients with intact autoregulation results in vasodilation (and CBV), which consequently leads to increases in ICP due to decreased intracranial compliance *(71)*.

There is still debate concerning the target CPP in patients with TBI. Several clinical studies recommend CPP of 70–80 mmHg as the clinical threshold below which there may be a significant risk of cerebral ischemia, particularly if CPP falls any further *(72,73)*. A recent study demonstrated that CPP < 60 mmHg appears to be hazardous in adults with TBI, but failed to demonstrate that CPP above 70–80 mmHg is beneficial *(74)*. Based on its safety and efficacy profile, CPP-directed therapy is being incorporated in standard treatment protocols for TBI patients currently *(72,75)*. Several studies have demonstrated a better outcome using this strategy *(71–74)*.

CBF and Seizures

Penfield's observations in the 1930s provided the first systematic evidence of changes in regional CBF associated with focal seizures *(76)*. Further studies in humans and animals have confirmed increases in CBF and metabolism during generalized seizures followed by a postictal depression *(77,78)*. The interictal, ictal, and postictal changes in focal epilepsy have begun to be elucidated in the last decade with the advent of in vivo imaging techniques, such as PET and SPECT. In focal seizures, the characteristic finding has been interictal reduction in CBF or metabolism in the affected temporal lobe, or more extensively in the ipsilateral hemisphere *(79)*. Few studies to date have investigated ictal or postictal changes in rCBF using SPECT that demonstrate hyperperfusion of the entire temporal lobe and the hippocampus during the ictus, combined with hypoperfusion of lateral structures in the immediate postictal period *(80,81)*. Later in the postictal period, hypoperfusion alone is seen *(82)*. Limited studies of coupling between CBF and metabolism in humans have suggested that CBF during seizures is adequate for metabolic demands *(83,84)*, although some animal studies have suggested localized areas of uncoupling *(85)*.

CBF and Subarachnoid Hemorrhage

Symptomatic vasospasm (VSP) remains a major complication associated with aneurysmal SAH, resulting in delayed ischemic deficits (DID) in 2–52% of all cases *(86–89)*. Hence, an understanding of CBF changes following SAH is crucial for optimal therapy of VSP. Decline in CBF is usually seen as early as 2 d after SAH, which continues to fall progressively during the first 2 wk, and remaining abnormally low throughout the 3 wk following SAH. In general, CBF falls no further after the 14th day, although it remains well below normal levels for at least 3 wk after SAH *(3,90)*. This decline in CBF appears to be global and not affected by age, clinical grade, arterial blood pressure, end-tidal partial pressure of carbon dioxide, aneurysm location, and drug therapy. In addition, the drop in CBF occurs with or without a demonstrable aneurysm angiographically *(3)*. The progressive decline in CBF is least in those patients who subsequently made the best clinical recovery.

It is clear that patient age is extremely important in determining the precise level of CBF after recent SAH. The normal inverse relationship between CBF and a subject's age is preserved after

SAH, although CBF is reduced. After SAH, therefore the lowest values of resting CBF tend to occur in older patients. The fall in blood after SAH means that the resting CBF is displaced toward the ischemic threshold of the brain *(91,92)*. For older SAH patients (whose resting CBF tends to be the lowest), the margin between CBF and the ischemic threshold may become especially narrow. Accordingly, ischemic neurologic deficit would be likely in these patients if the CBF were to fall still further, for example, with vasopsasm or arterial hypotension when cerebral autoregulation is impaired as a result of SAH *(91)*.

Volby et al. similarly noted a decrease in $CMRO_2$ but reported an early uncoupling of flow to cerebral metabolism following SAH. This uncoupling appears to follow two patterns. In patients with larger amount of blood deposited in the subarachnoid space, CBF is initially depressed that increases with time. Lower-grade SAH patients have a higher initial CBF that decreases with time *(93)*. Flow metabolism coupling begins to normalize over the course of a week *(94)*.

Patients with cerebral VSP are often treated with hypervolemia and induced hypertension with good results leading to improved neurological status in 60% of patients *(89,95,96)*. The therapeutic rationale of these medical therapies is to increase CBF. It has been demonstrated that during hypervolemic hemodilution therapy, CBF returns to baseline in both hemispheres *(86)*. The goal of hypertensive therapy is to titrate MAP to a threshold that reverses neurological deficit(s) or raise MAP 20% above baseline. Cerebral edema and hemorrhage are uncommon complications of hypertensive therapy, because the cerebral microcirculation is "insulated" from high systemic arterial pressures by the blunting effect of vasospasm *(97)*.

CBF and Ischemic Stroke

In normal brain, CBF and $CMRO_2$ have a linear relationship and oxygen extraction fraction (OEF) is similar over the entire brain. Four types of changes on PET scan occurring during focal brain ischemia have been described: (1) increase in CBV to maintain CBF (normal autoregulation), (2) increase in OEF in a response to a CBF decline to maintain $CMRO_2$ (oligemia), (3) increased OEF in regions with reduced CBF and $CMRO_2$ (ischemia), and (4) very low CBF and $CMRO_2$ levels with poor OEF (irreversible ischemic injury) *(98)*. Several studies provide a strong evidence for the existence of an ischemic penumbra surrounding infarcted tissue and this region persists for much longer than originally thought *(99–101)*. Further studies have demonstrated that autoregulation is impaired within this ischemic penumbra and there is a linear relationship between systemic MAP and rCBF *(102)*. Consequently, raising systemic blood pressure can restore perfusion to this vulnerable region *(103)*. Small patient studies *(104–106)* have provided preliminary data indicating that blood pressure (BP) augmentation with intravenous vasopressors may be relatively safe and effective in improving neurological function in acute stroke.

Initially, elevated BP in a stroke patient may be beneficial *(104)* because it enhances CBF to the ischemic penumbra. But if sustained, hypertension may increase the likelihood of cerebral edema and hemorrhagic transformation *(107)*. For patients with perfusion deficit who are not candidates for recombinant tissue plasminogen activator therapy or angioplasty or with documented critical extracranial or intracranial vascular stenosis, BP augmentation may be beneficial. MAP is judiciously titrated with vasopressors to 120–140 mmHg with frequent neurologic assessment. If no clinical improvement is seen over 48 h of therapy, pressors are tapered. In patients who have improvement with BP augmentation, an oral agent, such as midodrine may be beneficial for long-term management.

CBF and Intracerebral Hemorrhage

In several animal models of acute intracerebral hemorrhage (ICH), reduced CBF has been demonstrated both globally and in the area immediately surrounding the hematoma *(108,109)*. However, not all experimental data support these findings *(110)*. A similar zone of hypoperfusion surrounding the hematoma has been demonstrated in patients with acute ICH *(111,112)*. In these studies, both perihematomal CBF and $CMRO_2$ were significantly reduced compared to contralateral anatomical regions. $CMRO_2$ was reduced to a greater extent than CBF in the perihematomal region in acute ICH, resulting in reduced OEF rather than the increased OEF that occurs in ischemia *(113)*.

Arterial hypertension is common in the first 24 h after acute ICH *(114,115)*. Arguments against treatment of hypertension in patients with acute ICH are based primarily on the concern that reducing arterial BP will lead to reduced CBF *(116,117)*. Under normal conditions, changes in MAP have no effect on CBF due to intact autoregulation. In patients with small-to-medium sized acute ICH, autoregulation of CBF is preserved with reduction in MAP by 15% of baseline *(118)*. Reductions of MAP in excess of 20% *(119)* or below 84 mmHg *(120)* may reduce CBF. Thus, judicious treatment of HTN in patients with ICH is very important with the objective of preventing secondary brain injury.

SUMMARY

Knowledge of normal CBF physiology and alterations caused by specific diseases is paramount in the treatment of critically ill patients with acute brain injury. Although subtle changes in serial neurologic examinations may suggest alterations in CBF, its sensitivity is enhanced by careful attention to other bedside indicators, such as CPP. Although conventional methods for measuring and monitoring CBF are tedious and not readily available, TCD ultrasonography is a reliable bedside technique that can provide indirect measure of CBF on intermittent or continuous basis.

ACKNOWLEDGMENT

Dr. Bhardwaj is supported in part by the *Established Investigator Award* from the American Heart Association.

REFERENCES

1. Siesjo BK. Cerebral circulation and metabolism. *J. Neurosurg.* 1984;60(5):883–908.
2. Obrist WD, Langfitt TW, Jaggi JL, Cruz J, Gennarelli TA. Cerebral blood flow and metabolism in comatose patients with acute head injury. Relationship to intracranial hypertension. *J. Neurosurg.* 1984;61(2):241–253.
3. Meyer CH, Lowe D, Meyer M, Richardson PL, Neil-Dwyer G. Progressive change in cerebral blood flow during the first three weeks after subarachnoid hemorrhage. *Neurosurgery* 1983;12(1):58–76.
4. Melamed E, Lavy S, Bentin S, Cooper G, Rinot Y. Reduction in regional cerebral blood flow during normal aging in man. *Stroke* 1980;11(1):31–35.
5. Astrup J, Siesjo BK, Symon L. Thresholds in cerebral ischemia - the ischemic penumbra. *Stroke* 1981;12(6):723–735.
6. Hossmann KA. Viability thresholds and the penumbra of focal ischemia. *Ann. Neurol.* 1994;36(4):557–565.
7. Lassen N. Cerebral blood flow and oxygen consumption in man. *Physiol. Rev.* 1959;39:183–238.
8. Fog M. Cerebral circulation. The reaction of the pial arteries to a fall in blood pressure. *Arch. Neurol. Psych.* 1937;37:351–364.
9. Symon L, Held K, Dorsch NW. A study of regional autoregulation in the cerebral circulation to increased perfusion pressure in normocapnia and hypercapnia. *Stroke* 1973;4(2):139–147.
10. Davis SM, Ackerman RH, Correia JA, et al. Cerebral blood flow and cerebrovascular CO2 reactivity in stroke-age normal controls. *Neurology* 1983;33(4):391–399.
11. Obrist WD, Thompson HK Jr, Wang HS, Wilkinson WE. Regional cerebral blood flow estimated by 133-xenon inhalation. *Stroke* 1975;6(3):245–256.
12. Osol G, Halpern W. Myogenic properties of cerebral blood vessels from normotensive and hypertensive rats. *Am. J. Physiol.* 1985;249(5 Pt 2):H914–H921.
13. Pannier JL, Weyne J, Leusen I. Effects of changes in acid-base composition in the cerebral ventricles on local and general cerebral blood flow. *Eur. Neurol.* 1971;6(1):123–126.
14. Strandgaard S, Olesen J, Skinhoj E, Lassen NA. Autoregulation of brain circulation in severe arterial hypertension. *BMJ* 1973;1(852):507–510.
15. Miller R. Anesthesia for neurosurgery. In: Firestone L, Lebowitz P, Cook C, editors. *Clinical Anesthesia Procedures of the Massachusetts General Hospital.* 3rd ed. Boston: Little Brown; 1988.
16. Paulson OB, Waldemar G, Schmidt JF, Strandgaard S. Cerebral circulation under normal and pathologic conditions. *Am. J. Cardiol.* 1989;63(6):2C–5C.

17. Westergaard E, van Deurs B, Brondsted HE. Increased vesicular transfer of horseradish peroxidase across cerebral endothelium, evoked by acute hypertension. *Acta. Neuropathol. (Berl.)* 1977;37(2):141–152.
18. Sokrab TE, Johansson BB, Kalimo H, Olsson Y. A transient hypertensive opening of the blood-brain barrier can lead to brain damage. Extravasation of serum proteins and cellular changes in rats subjected to aortic compression. *Acta. Neuropathol.* 1988;75(6):557–565.
19. Gross PM, Heistad DD, Strait MR, Marcus ML, Brody MJ. Cerebral vascular responses to physiological stimulation of sympathetic pathways in cats. *Circ. Res.* 1979;44(2):288–294.
20. Edvinsson L, Owman C, Siesjo B. Physiological role of cerebrovascular sympathetic nerves in the autoregulation of cerebral blood flow. *Brain Res.* 1976;117(3):519–523.
21. Bill A, Linder J. Sympathetic control of cerebral blood flow in acute arterial hypertension. *Acta. Physiol. Scand.* 1976;96(1):114–121.
22. Heistad DD. Protection of cerebral vessels by sympathetic nerves. *Physiologist* 1980;23(5):44–49.
23. Nordborg C, Johansson BB. Morphometric study on cerebral vessels in spontaneously hypertensive rats. *Stroke* 1980;11(3):266–270.
24. Hart MN, Heistad DD, Brody MJ. Effect of chronic hypertension and sympathetic denervation on wall/lumen ratio of cerebral vessels. *Hypertension* 1980;2(4):419–423.
25. Hoffman WE, Miletich DJ, Albrecht RF. The influence of antihypertensive therapy on cerebral autoregulation in aged hypertensive rats. *Stroke* 1982;13(5):701–704.
26. Mayhan WG, Werber AH, Heistad DD. Protection of cerebral vessels by sympathetic nerves and vascular hypertrophy. *Circulation* 1987;75(1 Pt 2):I107–I112.
27. Strandgaard S. Autoregulation of cerebral blood flow in hypertensive patients. The modifying influence of prolonged antihypertensive treatment on the tolerance to acute, drug-induced hypotension. *Circulation* 1976;53(4):720–727.
28. Strandgaard S, Jones JV, MacKenzie ET, Harper AM. Upper limit of cerebral blood flow autoregulation in experimental renovascular hypertension in the baboon. *Circ. Res.* 1975;37(2):164–167.
29. Barry DI. Cerebrovascular aspects of antihypertensive treatment. *Am. J. Cardiol.* 1989;63(6):14C–18C.
30. Kee DB Jr, Wood JH. Rheology of the cerebral circulation. *Neurosurgery* 1984;15(1):125–131.
31. Symon L, Branston NM, Strong AJ. Autoregulation in acute focal ischemia. An experimental study. *Stroke* 1976;7(6):547–554.
32. Sakuta S. Blood filtrability in cerebrovascular disorders, with special reference to erythrocyte deformability and ATP content. *Stroke* 1981;12(6):824–828.
33. Grotta J, Ackerman R, Correia J, Fallick G, Chang J. Whole blood viscosity parameters and cerebral blood flow. *Stroke* 1982;13(3):296–301.
34. von Kummer R, Scharf J, Back T, Reich H, Machens HG, Wildemann B. Autoregulatory capacity and the effect of isovolemic hemodilution on local cerebral blood flow. *Stroke* 1988;19(5):594–597.
35. Brown MM, Marshall J. Regulation of cerebral blood flow in response to changes in blood viscosity. *Lancet* 1985;1:604–609.
36. Rebel A, Lenz C, Krieter H, Waschke KF, Van Ackern K, Kuschinsky W. Oxygen delivery at high blood viscosity and decreased arterial oxygen content to brains of conscious rats. *Am. J. Physiol. Heart Circ. Physiol.* 2001;280(6):H2591–H25917.
37. Harrison MJ, Pollock S, Thomas D, Marshall J. Haematocrit, hypertension and smoking in patients with transient ischaemic attacks and in age and sex matched controls. *J. Neurol. Neurosurg. Psychiatry* 1982;45(6):550–551.
38. Wade JP, Taylor DW, Barnett HJ, Hachinski VC. Hemoglobin concentration and prognosis in symptomatic obstructive cerebrovascular disease. *Stroke* 1987;18(1):68–71.
39. Toghi M, Uchiyama S, Ogawa M, Tabuchi M, Nagura H, Yamanouchi H. The role of blood constitutents in the pathogenesis of cerebral infarction. *Acta. Neurol. Scand.* 1979;72:616–617.
40. Multicenter trial of hemodilution in acute ischemic stroke. I. Results in the total patient population. Scandinavian Stroke Study Group. *Stroke* 1987;18(4):691–699.
41. Haemodilution in acute stroke: Results of the Italian haemodilution trial. Italian Acute Stroke Study Group. *Lancet* 1988;1:318–321.
42. Andrews PJ, Piper IR, Dearden NM, Miller JD. Secondary insults during intrahospital transport of head-injured patients. *Lancet* 1990;335:327–330.
43. Macdonell RA, Donnan GA, Bladin PF, Berkovic SF, Wriedt CH. The electroencephalogram and acute ischemic stroke. Distinguishing cortical from lacunar infarction. *Arch. Neurol.* 1988;45(5):520–524.
44. Symon L. The relationship between CBF, evoked potentials and the clinical features in cerebral ischaemia. *Acta. Neurol. Scand. Suppl.* 1980;78:175–190.
45. Sundt TM Jr, Sharbrough FW, Anderson RE, Michenfelder JD. Cerebral blood flow measurements and electroencephalograms during carotid endarterectomy. *J. Neurosurg.* 1974;41(3):310–320.
46. Sundt TM Jr, Sharbrough FW, Piepgras DG, Kearns TP, Messick JM Jr, O'Fallon WM. Correlation of cerebral blood flow and electroencephalographic changes during carotid endarterectomy: with results of surgery and hemodynamics of cerebral ischemia. *Mayo Clin. Proc.* 1981;56(9):533–543.

47. Kety S, Schmidt C. The determination of cerebral blood flow in man by the use of nitrous oxide in low concentrations. *Am. J. Physiol.* 1945;143:53–66.

48. Obrist WD, Thompson HK Jr, King CH, Wang HS. Determination of regional cerebral blood flow by inhalation of 133-Xenon. *Circ. Res.* 1967;20(1):124–135.

49. Obrist WD, Wilkinson WE. Regional cerebral blood flow measurement in humans by xenon-133 clearance. *Cerebrovasc. Brain Metab. Rev.* 1990;2(4):283–327.

50. Gur D, Yonas H, Good WF. Local cerebral blood flow by xenon-enhanced CT: Current status, potential improvements, and future directions. *Cerebrovasc. Brain Metab. Rev.* 1989;1(1):68–86.

51. Leenders KL, Perani D, Lammertsma AA, et al. Cerebral blood flow, blood volume and oxygen utilization. Normal values and effect of age. *Brain* 1990;113(Pt 1):27–47.

52. Sakai F, Nakazawa K, Tazaki Y, et al. Regional cerebral blood volume and hematocrit measured in normal human volunteers by single-photon emission computed tomography. *J. Cereb. Blood Flow Metab.* 1985;5(2):207–213.

53. Rempp KA, Brix G, Wenz F, Becker CR, Guckel F, Lorenz WJ. Quantification of regional cerebral blood flow and volume with dynamic susceptibility contrast-enhanced MR imaging. *Radiology* 1994;193(3):637–641.

54. Baird AE, Warach S. Magnetic resonance imaging of acute stroke. *J. Cereb. Blood Flow Metab.* 1998;18(6):583–609.

55. Nabavi DG, Cenic A, Craen RA, et al. CT assessment of cerebral perfusion: experimental validation and initial clinical experience. *Radiology* 1999;213(1):141–149.

56. Cenic A, Nabavi DG, Craen RA, Gelb AW, Lee TY. Dynamic CT measurement of cerebral blood flow: A validation study. *AJNR* 1999;20(1):63–73.

57. Muizelaar JP, Fatouros PP, Schroder ML. A new method for quantitative regional cerebral blood volume measurements using computed tomography. *Stroke* 1997;28(10):1998–2005.

58. Wintermark M, Thiran JP, Maeder P, Schnyder P, Meuli R. Simultaneous measurement of regional cerebral blood flow by perfusion CT and stable xenon CT: A validation study. *AJNR* 2001;22(5):905–914.

59. Lindegaard KF, Nornes H, Bakke SJ, Sorteberg W, Nakstad P. Cerebral vasospasm diagnosis by means of angiography and blood velocity measurements. *Acta. Neurochir.* 1989;100(1–2):12–24.

60. Lindegaard KF, Bakke SJ, Grolimund P, Aaslid R, Huber P, Nornes H. Assessment of intracranial hemodynamics in carotid artery disease by transcranial Doppler ultrasound. *J. Neurosurg.* 1985;63(6):890–898.

61. Karnik R, Stelzer P, Slany J. Transcranial Doppler sonography monitoring of local intra-arterial thrombolysis in acute occlusion of the middle cerebral artery. *Stroke* 1992;23(2):284–287.

62. Hassler W, Steinmetz H, Pirschel J. Transcranial Doppler study of intracranial circulatory arrest. *J. Neurosurg.* 1989;71(2):195–201.

63. Mendelow AD, Teasdale GM, Russell T, Flood J, Patterson J, Murray GD. Effect of mannitol on cerebral blood flow and cerebral perfusion pressure in human head injury. *J. Neurosurg.* 1985;63(1):43–48.

64. Yoshino E, Yamaki T, Higuchi T, Horikawa Y, Hirakawa K. Acute brain edema in fatal head injury: Analysis by dynamic CT scanning. *J. Neurosurg.* 1985;63(6):830–839.

65. Bouma GJ, Muizelaar JP, Stringer WA, Choi SC, Fatouros P, Young HF. Ultra-early evaluation of regional cerebral blood flow in severely head-injured patients using xenon-enhanced computerized tomography. *J. Neurosurg.* 1992;77(3):360–368.

66. Bouma GJ, Muizelaar JP, Choi SC, Newlon PG, Young HF. Cerebral circulation and metabolism after severe traumatic brain injury: the elusive role of ischemia. *J. Neurosurg.* 1991;75(5):685–693.

67. DeSalles AA, Kontos HA, Becker DP, et al. Prognostic significance of ventricular CSF lactic acidosis in severe head injury. *J. Neurosurg.* 1986;65(5):615–624.

68. Robertson CS, Grossman RG, Goodman JC, Narayan RK. The predictive value of cerebral anaerobic metabolism with cerebral infarction after head injury. *J. Neurosurg.* 1987;67(3):361–368.

69. Langfitt TW, Marshall WJ, Kassell NF, Schutta HS. The pathophysiology of brain swelling produced by mechanical trauma and hypertension. *Scand. J. Clin. Lab. Invest. Suppl.* 1968;102.

70. Muizelaar JP, Ward JD, Marmarou A, Newlon PG, Wachi A. Cerebral blood flow and metabolism in severely head-injured children. Part 2: Autoregulation. *J. Neurosurg.* 1989;71(1):72–76.

71. Bouma GJ, Muizelaar JP, Bandoh K, Marmarou A. Blood pressure and intracranial pressure-volume dynamics in severe head injury: relationship with cerebral blood flow. *J. Neurosurg.* 1992;77(1):15–19.

72. Rosner MJ, Rosner SD, Johnson AH. Cerebral perfusion pressure: management protocol and clinical results [see comments]. *J. Neurosurg.* 1995;83(6):949–962.

73. Andrews P, Souter M, Mascia L. Cerebral blood flow in acute brain injury. In Vincent J, editor. *Year Book of Intensive Care and Emergency Medicine.* Heidelberg: Springer; 1997, pp. 739–748.

74. Juul N, Morris GF, Marshall SB, Marshall LF. Intracranial hypertension and cerebral perfusion pressure: influence on neurological deterioration and outcome in severe head injury. The Executive Committee of the International Selfotel Trial. *J. Neurosurg.* 2000;92(1):1–6.

75. Bullock R, Chesnut R, Clifton G, et al. *Guidlines for the Management of Severe Head Injury.* Brain Trauma Foundation, New York; 1995.

76. Penfield W, Von Santha K, Cipriani A. Cerebral blood flow during induced epileptiform seizures in animals and man. *J. Neurophysiol.* 1939;2:257–267.

77. Posner JB, Plum F, Van Poznak A. Cerebral metabolism during electrically induced seizures in man. *Arch. Neurol.* 1969;20(4):388–395.

78. Meldrum BS, Nilsson B. Cerebral blood flow and metabolic rate early and late in prolonged epileptic seizures induced in rats by bicuculline. *Brain* 1976;99(3):523–542.

79. Bernardi S, Trimble MR, Frackowiak RS, Wise RJ, Jones T. An interictal study of partial epilepsy using positron emission tomography and the oxygen—15 inhalation technique. *J. Neurol. Neurosurg. Psychiatry* 1983;46(6):473–477.

80. Engel J Jr, Kuhl DE, Phelps ME. Patterns of human local cerebral glucose metabolism during epileptic seizures. *Science* 1982;218:64–66.

81. Engel J, Jr., Kuhl DE, Phelps ME, Rausch R, Nuwer M. Local cerebral metabolism during partial seizures. *Neurology* 1983;33(4):400–413.

82. Duncan R. Epilepsy, cerebral blood flow, and cerebral metabolic rate. *Cerebrovasc. Brain Metab. Rev.* 1992;4(2):105–121.

83. Kuhl DE, Engel J Jr, Phelps ME, Selin C. Epileptic patterns of local cerebral metabolism and perfusion in humans determined by emission computed tomography of 18FDG and 13NH3. *Ann. Neurol.* 1980;8(4):348–360.

84. Plum F, Posner JB, Troy B. Cerebral metabolic and circulatory responses to induced convulsions in animals. *Arch. Neurol.* 1968;18(1):1–13.

85. Ingvar M, Siesjo BK. Local blood flow and glucose consumption in the rat brain during sustained bicuculline-induced seizures. *Acta. Neurol. Scand.* 1983;68(3):129–144.

86. Mori K, Arai H, Nakajima K, Tajima A, Maeda M. Hemorheological and hemodynamic analysis of hypervolemic hemodilution therapy for cerebral vasospasm after aneurysmal subarachnoid hemorrhage. *Stroke* 1995;26(9):1620–1626.

87. Torbey MT, Hauser TK, Bhardwaj A, et al. Effect of age on cerebral blood flow velocity and incidence of vasospasm after aneurysmal subarachnoid hemorrhage. *Stroke* 2001;32(9):2005–2011.

88. Allen GS, Ahn HS, Preziosi TJ, et al. Cerebral arterial spasm—a controlled trial of nimodipine in patients with subarachnoid hemorrhage. *N. Engl. J. Med.* 1983;308(11):619–624.

89. Kassell NF, Torner JC, Haley EC Jr, Jane JA, Adams HP, Kongable GL. The International Cooperative Study on the Timing of Aneurysm Surgery. Part 1: Overall management results. *J. Neurosurg.* 1990;73(1):18–36.

90. Nilsson BW. Cerebral blood flow in patients with subarachnoid haemorrhage studied with an intravenous isotope technique. Its clinical significance in the timing of surgery of cerebral arterial aneurysm. *Acta. Neurochir.* 1977;37(1–2):33–48.

91. Ishii R. Regional cerebral blood flow in patients with ruptured intracranial aneurysms. *J. Neurosurg.* 1979;50(5):587–594.

92. Ingvar DH, Lassen NA. Cerebral function, metabolism and blood flow. News and trends from the VIIIth international CBF symposium in Copenhagen, June 1977. *Acta. Neurol. Scand.* 1978;57(3):262–269.

93. Voldby B, Enevoldsen EM, Jensen FT. Regional CBF, intraventricular pressure, and cerebral metabolism in patients with ruptured intracranial aneurysms. *J. Neurosurg.* 1985;62(1):48–58.

94. Jakobsen M, Skjodt T, Enevoldsen E. Cerebral blood flow and metabolism following subarachnoid haemorrhage: effect of subarachnoid blood. *Acta. Neurol. Scand.* 1991;83(4):226–233.

95. Medlock MD, Dulebohn SC, Elwood PW. Prophylactic hypervolemia without calcium channel blockers in early aneurysm surgery. *Neurosurgery* 1992;30(1):12–16.

96. Awad IA, Carter LP, Spetzler RF, Medina M, Williams FC Jr. Clinical vasospasm after subarachnoid hemorrhage: response to hypervolemic hemodilution and arterial hypertension. *Stroke* 1987;18(2):365–372.

97. Shimoda M, Oda S, Tsugane R, Sato O. Intracranial complications of hypervolemic therapy in patients with a delayed ischemic deficit attributed to vasospasm. *J. Neurosurg.* 1993;78(3):423–429.

98. Baron J. Positron emission tomography (PET) in acute ischemic stroke. In Caplan L, ed. *Brain Ischemia: Basic Concepts and Clinical Relevance.* Berlin: Springer-Verlag, 1994, pp. 19–27.

99. Marchal G, Beaudouin V, Rioux P, et al. Prolonged persistence of substantial volumes of potentially viable brain tissue after stroke: A correlative PET-CT study with voxel-based data analysis. *Stroke* 1996;27(4):599–606.

100. Furlan M, Marchal G, Viader F, Derlon JM, Baron JC. Spontaneous neurological recovery after stroke and the fate of the ischemic penumbra. *Ann. Neurol.* 1996;40(2):216–226.

101. Astrup J, Symon L, Branston NM, Lassen NA. Cortical evoked potential and extracellular K+ and H+ at critical levels of brain ischemia. *Stroke* 1977;8(1):51–57.

102. Olsen TS, Bruhn P, Oberg RG. Cortical hypoperfusion as a possible cause of 'subcortical aphasia.' *Brain* 1986;109(Pt 3):393–410.

103. Olsen TS, Larsen B, Herning M, Skriver EB, Lassen NA. Blood flow and vascular reactivity in collaterally perfused brain tissue. Evidence of an ischemic penumbra in patients with acute stroke. *Stroke* 1983;14(3):332–341.

104. Rordorf G, Cramer SC, Efird JT, Schwamm LH, Buonanno F, Koroshetz WJ. Pharmacological elevation of blood pressure in acute stroke. Clinical effects and safety. *Stroke* 1997;28(11):2133–2138.
105. Rordorf G, Koroshetz WJ, Ezzeddine MA, Segal AZ, Buonanno FS. A pilot study of drug-induced hypertension for treatment of acute stroke. *Neurology* 2001;56(9):1210–1213.
106. Wise G, Sutter R, Burkholder J. The treatment of brain ischemia with vasopressor drugs. Stroke 1972;3(2):135-40.
107. Fagan SC, Bowes MP, Lyden PD, Zivin JA. Acute hypertension promotes hemorrhagic transformation in a rabbit embolic stroke model: Effect of labetalol. *Exp. Neurol.* 1998;150(1):153–158.
108. Ropper AH, Zervas NT. Cerebral blood flow after experimental basal ganglia hemorrhage. *Ann. Neurol.* 1982;11(3):266–271.
109. Yang GY, Betz AL, Chenevert TL, Brunberg JA, Hoff JT. Experimental intracerebral hemorrhage: relationship between brain edema, blood flow, and blood-brain barrier permeability in rats. *J. Neurosurg.* 1994;81(1):93–102.
110. Qureshi AI, Wilson DA, Hanley DF, Traystman RJ. No evidence for an ischemic penumbra in massive experimental intracerebral hemorrhage. *Neurology* 1999;52(2):266–272.
111. Mayer SA, Lignelli A, Fink ME, et al. Perilesional blood flow and edema formation in acute intracerebral hemorrhage: A SPECT study. *Stroke* 1998;29(9):1791–1798.
112. Videen TO, Perlmutter JS, Herscovitch P, Raichle ME. Brain blood volume, flow, and oxygen utilization measured with 15O radiotracers and positron emission tomography: Revised metabolic computations. *J. Cereb. Blood Flow Metab.* 1987;7(4):513–516.
113. Zazulia AR, Diringer MN, Videen TO, et al. Hypoperfusion without ischemia surrounding acute intracerebral hemorrhage. *J. Cereb. Blood Flow Metab.* 2001;21(7):804–810.
114. Britton M, Carlsson A, de Faire U. Blood pressure course in patients with acute stroke and matched controls. *Stroke* 1986;17(5):861–864.
115. Carlberg B, Asplund K, Hagg E. The prognostic value of admission blood pressure in patients with acute stroke. *Stroke* 1993;24(9):1372–1375.
116. Broderick JP, Adams HP Jr, Barsan W, et al. Guidelines for the management of spontaneous intracerebral hemorrhage: A statement for healthcare professionals from a special writing group of the Stroke Council, American Heart Association. *Stroke* 1999;30(4):905–915.
117. Powers WJ. Acute hypertension after stroke: The scientific basis for treatment decisions. *Neurology* 1993;43(3 Pt 1):461–467.
118. Powers WJ, Zazulia AR, Videen TO, et al. Autoregulation of cerebral blood flow surrounding acute (6 to 22 hours) intracerebral hemorrhage. *Neurology* 2001;57(1):18–24.
119. Kuwata N, Kuroda K, Funayama M, Sato N, Kubo N, Ogawa A. Dysautoregulation in patients with hypertensive intracerebral hemorrhage. A SPECT study. *Neurosurg. Rev.* 1995;18(4):237–245.
120. von Helden A, Schneider GH, Unterberg A, Lanksch WR. Monitoring of jugular venous oxygen saturation in comatose patients with subarachnoid haemorrhage and intracerebral haematomas. *Acta. Neurochir. Suppl.* 1993;59:102–106.

4

Cerebral Metabolism

Implications for Neurocritically Ill Patients

Maria Briones-Galang and Claudia Robertson

INTRODUCTION

An understanding of normal cerebral metabolism and of the response of metabolism to pathological derangements is helpful in the management of the critically ill patient with neurological disorders. This article reviews the basic principles of cerebral metabolism, especially the relationship between cerebral metabolism and cerebral blood flow (CBF) in normal physiology and in the pathological states associated with traumatic brain injury (TBI), cerebral ischemia, cerebral edema, and intracranial hypertension. Management of secondary brain insults and the methods available for monitoring cerebral metabolism will also be discussed as a practical review of how cerebral metabolic derangements are managed in the neurosciences critical care unit (NSU).

BASIC PRINCIPLES OF CEREBRAL METABOLISM

Cerebral metabolism is determined by the energy required to maintain cellular integrity and to generate electrophysiological signals. The normal brain, which weighs 1200–1400 g (2–3 % of total body weight), has a high metabolic demand relative to many other tissues. The brain consumes 20% of the total oxygen consumption, 25% of total glucose consumption, and receives 15–20% of the cardiac output in the resting state *(1,2)*. Energy expenditure by the brain can be classified into two broad categories: (1) "activation energy" is the energy expended by the brain in the work of generating electric signals and consumes 55% of the total cerebral energy consumption; (2) basal metabolic processes consume the remaining 45% of the brain's energy production. These processes include membrane stabilization, ion pumping to preserve membrane ion gradients, and synthesis of structural and functional molecules *(3)*. To generate the necessary energy for these processes, the brain has the capacity to metabolize a number of energy substrates, including glucose, ketone bodies, lactate, glycerol, fatty acids, and amino acids but glucose is the preferred substrate in the normal adult brain.

At the whole organ level, the brain depends almost exclusively on the aerobic consumption of glucose for energy production. Glucose is primarily transported into brain cells via a carrier-mediated mechanism; 4% enters by simple diffusion. Glucose is metabolized in two sequential pathways: glycolysis and oxidative phosphorylation. Together these reactions generate a total of 38 molecules of adenosine triphosphate (ATP) per molecule of glucose consumed. When oxygen is unavailable or whenever transient increases in energy are required, the glycolytic pathway alone can produce a smaller amount of energy, consisting of two molecules of ATP and lactate per molecule of glucose. More than 99% of ATP production in resting cerebral tissue is via the more efficient process of

From: *Current Clinical Neurology*
Critical Care Neurology and Neurosurgery
Edited by: J. I. Suarez © Humana Press Inc., Totowa, NJ

glucose oxidation *(3)*. During functional activation, most of the increase in glucose metabolism above resting levels is associated with an increase in glycolysis *(4,5)*.

Indices have been described to quantify relative contribution of these two pathways of glucose metabolism to overall brain energy consumption—the aerobic and anaerobic indices. These indices quantify the percentage of the total cerebral glucose uptake by the brain that is metabolized aerobically and anaerobically, respectively (Table 1). The oxygen-glucose ratio (or aerobic index) has been measured as 5.5 in the resting adult, indicating that more than 90% of all resting state glucose consumption is oxidative and with less than or equal to 5% being metabolized to lactate *(6)*. Ketone bodies and other substrates normally account for less than 1% of the brain's total energy expenditure. Under certain physiological conditions, such as fasting or ketosis, ketone bodies (acetoacetate and B-hydroxybutyrate) can be used as an energy source *(7,8)*. With prolonged fasting, ketone bodies can provide as much as 60% of the brain's total energy metabolism.

These indices indicate only net uptake or production of metabolic substrates by the brain as a whole organ. It has been assumed from these global findings that both neurons and glia metabolize glucose as their sole energy substrate. Some recent evidence, however, suggests that there is cellular compartmentalization of bioenergetics, and that glucose transported into the brain from the circulation is consumed anaerobically primarily in astrocytes *(9)*. Lactate that is released into the extracellular space from astrocyte metabolism is subsequently consumed aerobically by neurons. Astrocytes and neurons are functionally coupled and increased neuronal activity leads to release of potassium and glutamate (and other neurotransmitters) into the extracellular space. Potassium and glutamate are taken up by astrocytes restoring the composition of the cerebral cortical microenvironment. The uptake of potassium and glutamate is an energy dependent process that requires increased astrocyte glycolysis and production of lactate. The lactate provides the energy substrate for the neuronal activity. It is the coupling of neuronal activity to astrocytic glycolysis that permits 2-deoxyglucose studies to reflect local functionality.

Under physiological conditions, this coupled astrocytic-neuronal unit leads to the several important consequences on measurements of tissue level metabolism. Increased neuronal activity leads to increased astrocytic glycolysis, which is measured as the cerebral metabolic rate of glucose (CMRG) and 2-deoxyglucose phosphorylation. The lactate produced by the astrocytes is then consumed aerobically by neurons; this metabolic activity is reflected by cerebral metabolic rate of oxygen ($CMRO_2$). The lactate consumed by the neurons is not derived from the blood and will not be reflected in arteriovenous differences of lactate, and will not be measured by conventional cerebral metabolic rate of lactate (CMRL) determinations. Microdialysis studies in experimental animals show the astrocytic neuronal metabolic coupling by demonstrating increased extracellular lactate following neuronal activation. Thus, the astrocyte compensates for increased neuronal activity by increasing its own glycolysis and release of lactate. This compensatory glycolysis is not associated with depletion of glucose from the extracellular space.

Although this concept of compartmentalization of bioenergetics in the brain remains controversial *(10)*, the consequence of the high metabolic expenditure of the brain is indisputable. The brain is completely dependent on the circulation to continuously supply metabolic substrates. Cerebral blood flow is normally tightly coupled to local metabolic expenditure and increases or decreases depending on local cerebral metabolic demands. This regulatory mechanism can be impaired by injury or disease, causing the brain to be vulnerable to secondary ischemic insults.

CEREBRAL METABOLISM IN THE HEAD-INJURED PATIENT

TBI induces pathological changes in both the cerebral vasculature and also in cerebral metabolism. In addition, because of the dependence of cerebral metabolism on substrates delivered by cerebral vessels, there may be interactions of the two systems. If the vascular derangements cause a sufficient reduction in cerebral blood, then ischemia can contribute to the damage to the brain caused

Table 1
Formulas for Calculating Cerebral Metabolic Parameters

Parameter (units)	Formula	Normal values[a] (n = 14)	Normal values[b] (n = 50)	Normal values[c] (n = 8)
CBF(mL/100 g/min)		54 + 12		52 + 12
CaO_2(mL/dL)	$1.34 \times Hgb \times SaO_2 + 0.0031 \times paO_2$		9.6 ± 1.2	$16.9 + 1.5$
$CjvO_2$(mL/dL)	$1.34 \times Hgb \times SjvO_2 + 0.0031 \times pjvO_2$		12.9 ± 1.3	
$AVDO_2$(mL/dL)	$CaO_2 \, (mL/dL) - CjvO_2 \, (mL/dL)$	6.3 ± 1.2	6.7 ± 0.8	6.5 ± 1.8
$CMRO_2$(mL/100 g/min)	$\dfrac{AVDO_2 \, (mL/dL) \times CBF \, (mL/100 \, g/min)}{100}$	3.3 ± 0.4		3.3 ± 0.6
$O_2ER(\%)$	$\dfrac{AVDO_2 \, (mL/dL) \times 100\%}{CaO_2 \, (mL/dL)}$		34 ± 4	
AVDG(mL/dL)	$ArtGluc \, (mL/dL) - JVGluc \, (mL/dL)$		9.6 ± 1.7	11.0 ± 2.3
CMRG(mL/100 g/min)	$\dfrac{AVDG \, (mL/dL) \times CBF \, (mL/100 \, g/min)}{100}$			5.5 ± 1.1
AVDL(mL/dL)	$ArtLact \, (mL/dL) - JVLact \, (mL/dL)$		-1.7 ± 0.9	-0.5 ± 0.9
CMRL(mL/100 g/min)	$\dfrac{AVDL \, (mL/dL) \times CBF \, (mL/100 \, g/min)}{100}$			-0.23 ± 0.37
AI	$AI(\%) = \dfrac{AVDO_2 \, (\mu mol/mL) \times 100\%}{6 \times AVDG \, (\mu mol/mL)}$			
ANI	$ANI(\%) = \dfrac{AVDL \, (\mu mol/mL) \times 100\%}{2 \times AVDG \, (\mu mol/mL)}$			

[a]From ref. 43.
[b]From ref. 55.
[c]From ref. 22.

39

by trauma. Finally, if the vascular derangements result in impairment in the ability of the brain to regulate CBF, then the brain may be more susceptible to systemic insults, such as hypotension or hypoxia. Both of these interactions occur in these critically ill patients, presenting a challenge to their management.

In experimental studies, a brief period of hypermetabolism (primarily because of glycolysis) has been observed immediately after brain trauma, followed then by a state of reduced metabolism *(11– 13)*. It has been thought that the initial increased metabolism represents a burst of energy expended by the brain to regain ionic gradients following widespread depolarization caused by the injury. Excitotoxic amino acids may also play a role *(14)*. The subsequent low cerebral metabolic rate is the result of the reduced need to expend energy to generate electrical signals in the comatose brain.

This phenomenon of increased metabolism has also been observed in a few patients who have been studied early after trauma, but usually a reduction in glucose metabolism is found *(15,16)*. Hypermetabolism of glucose is also observed in remote areas from injury such as the hippocampus, and has been observed with seizure activity after trauma. Hyperglycolysis may also be in part a compensatory response to a compromised oxidative energy pathway, as evidenced by persistent depression of $CMRO_2$ postinjury. In most TBI patients, however, the characteristic early metabolic derangements include a decrease in the aerobic metabolism of glucose and oxygen and an increase in anaerobic metabolism of glucose to the end product lactic acid *(16–20)*.

As in the normal brain, the major energy source for the injured brain is glucose, and other potential energy substrates, such as ketone bodies, are present in low concentrations because of the systemic stress response to the trauma *(21,22)*. When CBF is reduced sufficiently to limit delivery of oxygen, the observed reduction in $CMRO_2$ can be due to ischemia *(23)*. In this circumstance, an increase in CMRG and cerebral lactate production is characteristically found unless CBF is so low that glucose delivery is rate-limiting *(24)*. More commonly after TBI, however, CBF is not rate-limiting and the reduction in metabolism is because of the decreased need for energy associated with coma and/or to disturbances in oxidative capacity of cerebral mitochondria.

The degree of reduction in $CMRO_2$ after trauma is proportional to the level of consciousness as reflected by the Glasgow Coma Scale Score *(17–20)*. The more profound the coma, the less energy is expended in generating electrical activity. As a patient awakens from coma, and electrical activity in the brain increases, $CMRO_2$ increases. These studies have demonstrated that metabolic rate also predicts the outcome from head injury. Patients with low $CMRO_2$ values are either consistently severely disabled, in persistent vegetative state or dead; whereas in those who regained consciousness, $CMRO_2$ increases as functional status improves.

Although $CMRO_2$ is related to outcome and to level of consciousness, these same relationships have not been observed with CMRG *(25)*. Likely this is because CMRG can be increased as a consequence of both anaerobic metabolism and with aerobic metabolism. An increase in anaerobic metabolism of glucose would be a poor prognostic sign, while an increase in aerobic metabolism would more likely be associated with a favorable outcome. These two situations cannot be distinguished by measuring only CMRG, and the overall effect is that there is no clear relationship between global CMRG and neurological outcome.

Cerebrospinal fluid (CSF) acidosis detected after TBI is related to an elevation in cerebral lactate production and is proportional to the severity of injury. Increase in CSF lactate and CMRL is observed in the first few days after injury and decreases as patient improves. The highest levels of cerebral lactate are observed in patients who die *(26,27)*.

CBF is normally closely coupled to $CMRO_2$, and would be expected to decrease with the typical metabolic changes that occur in the brain after trauma. However, trauma also interrupts the cerebral vasculature's normal regulatory mechanisms, and CBF can become uncoupled from metabolism. Martin et al. *(28)* defined three characteristic hemodynamic phases during the first 2 wk after injury, namely, hypoperfusion (phase 1: d 0), hyperemia (phase 2: d 1–3), and vasospasm (phase 3: d 4–15). All phases are not observed in all patients, but this is a good description of the overall average response to brain injury. Experimental studies suggest that there may be a brief period of increased blood pressure and cerebral blood flow immediately after the trauma, however this has not been observed in human TBI perhaps because it is so transient. The first phase, the initial hours after injury, is marked by the lowest CBF, falling on average to approx 50% of normal. During the second phase, beginning 12 h after injury, there is a rise in CBF that approaches or exceeds normal values in some patients and persists for the next 4–5 d. This is then followed by a period of low CBF that remains low until the patient's level of consciousness improves.

Although the relationship of CBF and cerebral metabolism to outcome are interrelated in the ways discussed, each factor can be demonstrated to have a contribution to neurological outcome. When adjusted for multiple confounding factors such as age, initial GCS score, cerebral perfusion pressure (CPP), hemoglobin and $CMRO_2$, CBF significantly correlates with outcome, with a decreased CBF predicting poor outcome. A strong association was found between the level of CBF and neurological outcome—at each CBF level, neurological outcome was significantly better when $CMRO_2$ was higher *(19)*.

METABOLIC PATTERNS OF CEREBRAL ISCHEMIA

Cerebral ischemia occurs when cerebral metabolic requirements for oxygen exceed the delivery of oxygen to the brain, and energy failure develops. Cerebral ischemia can be global, involving the entire brain, or regional. Cerebral ischemia can be complete, such as occurs with cardiac arrest, or it can be incomplete with a variable degree of residual or collateral blood flow continuing to supply some metabolic substrates.

The functional and metabolic effects of ischemia depend on the severity of the reduction in CBF and the duration of the reduction in CBF. When CBF decreases below 58% of normal, or below 25–30 mL/100 g/min, alteration in the EEG and consciousness develop *(29)*. The EEG becomes isoelectric at a CBF less than 33% of normal, or below 18 mL/100 g/min *(30)*. Evoked potentials disappear at a CBF less than 10% of normal. Below this critical threshold, cellular ionic homeostasis is altered, resulting in an increase in extracellular K^+ and an increase in intracellular Na^+ and Ca^{2+}.

The duration of the CBF reduction is also crucial in determining whether irreversible injury occurs. For example, flow distal to a middle cerebral artery occlusion must remain less than 12 mL/100 g/min for at least 2 h before infarction develops *(31)*. In general, the lower the CBF, the shorter the time required for irreversible injury to develop.

As CBF decreases, the arterial-venous oxygen difference ($AVDO_2$) will proportionally increase as the brain compensates for reduced flow by extracting a greater amount of oxygen *(19)*. As long as increased extraction of oxygen completely compensates for reduced CBF, $CMRO_2$ remains unchanged (compensated hypoperfusion pattern). However, a point will be reached at which further decrease in CBF cannot be compensated for by increased oxygen extraction and at which ischemia follows, manifested by a fall in $CMRO_2$ and a rise in cerebral lactate production (ischemia/infarction pattern). Initially, these changes of ischemia may be reversible. However, as time passes, irreversible ischemic injury or infarction may develop. Other characteristic findings indicating cellular membrane failure, such as massive release of glutamate and potassium into the extracellular space, can be measured in CSF or with a microdialysis probe implanted in the brain. Figure 1 shows a typical example of the changes in some of these metabolic substrates during global ischemia caused by increased intracranial pressure.

With regional ischemia, these characteristic changes in cerebral metabolism cannot be detected with global monitors, such as $AVDO_2$ or even CSF. Local monitors, such as brain tissue pO_2 probes and microdialysis probes, can be placed in tissues to provide this information about different regions of the brain *(32,33)*.

For many years, most studies of CBF in patients with TBI demonstrated levels of CBF that appeared appropriate for the reduced metabolic requirements of coma, and it was often thought that ischemia did not play a prominent role in the pathophysiology of brain trauma. However, with the development of

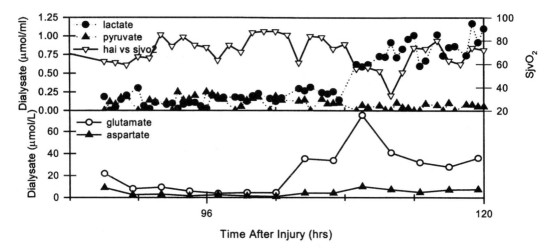

Fig. 1. Example of changes in metabolic substrates measured with microdialysis in a patient with severe global ischemia caused by intracranial hypertension. As the jugular venous oxygen saturation ($SjvO_2$) decreases, indicating a reduction in cerebral blood flow, the dialysate concentrations of lactate, glutamate, and aspartate markedly increase.

stable xenon-CT scanning, which allowed very early assessment of CBF *(23)*, and with development of continuous methods for monitoring cerebral oxygenation (jugular bulb oximetry and tissue pO_2), it has become clear that ischemia commonly complicates traumatic brain injury *(32–34)*.

METABOLIC PATTERNS OF BRAIN SWELLING/BRAIN EDEMA AND INTRACRANIAL HYPERTENSION

Brain swelling is an acute reaction of the brain parenchyma to any type of insult. Brain edema and vascular engorgement are often used interchangeably to describe brain swelling associated with severe brain trauma and the relative contribution of these compartments to the swelling process has been controversial. In the past, traumatic brain swelling was thought to be the result of vascular engorgement. Several investigators have observed a relationship between an elevated CBF, and the occurrence of increased intracranial pressure (ICP) *(35,36)*. Especially in children, hyperemia has been thought to be the primary cause of raised ICP following trauma, and treatments have been directed primarily at lowering CBF to control ICP *(37)*.

Recent magnetic resonance imaging (MRI) techniques, however, have allowed determination of the relative contributions of increased brain water content (edema) and hyperemia, as well as discrimination of the different types of edema. Studies in both experimental models of trauma and in human traumatic brain injury show that edema, and not vascular engorgement, is the major cause of brain swelling and therefore increased ICP *(38,39)*. Serial MRI studies suggest that there is a predominantly vasogenic edema formation immediately after injury and later a more widespread and slower edema formation due to a predominantly cellular swelling *(40,41)*.

The normal range for ICP is 0–10 mmHg. As a general rule, an ICP of 20–25 mmHg is the upper limit at which treatment should be initiated, but there may be some exceptions to this rule. ICP thresholds must be considered within the context of the nature of the brain injury, and may also be dependent on the level of the systemic blood pressure. With diffuse brain injuries, the primary adverse effect of intracranial hypertension is to decrease cerebral perfusion pressure and therefore CBF. With focal injuries, however, increasing brain edema can cause shift of intracranial structures and compress the brainstem. Because patients with focal, especially temporal, mass lesions can herniate with ICP levels less than 20 mmHg, it may be necessary to treat ICP at a lower threshold *(42)*.

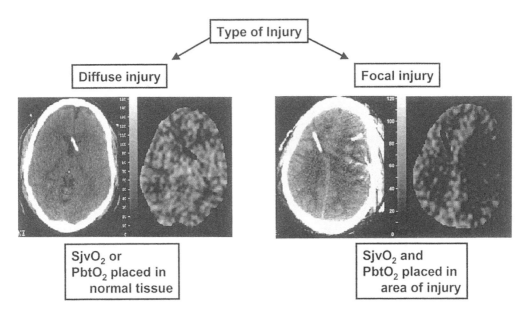

Fig. 2. One strategy to monitor patients for secondary ischemic insults uses the type of injury, based on either the CT scan (left image) or a measurement of CBF (right image). For those patients with a diffuse injury, either jugular venous oxygen saturation ($SjvO_2$) or brain tissue pO_2 with the probe placed in relatively normal brain is recommended. For those patients with a focal lesion, both a brain tissue pO_2 placed in the area of injury and $SjvO_2$ are needed to give a clear picture of the findings.

METHODS FOR MONITORING CEREBRAL METABOLISM IN THE NSU

Recent technological advancements have greatly expanded the scope of physiological and biochemical monitoring of the brain that are available for critically ill patients. The classical measurements of cerebral metabolism require measurement of global CBF and the arterial-venous difference of the substrate of interest, usually oxygen, glucose, or lactate. Then the cerebral metabolic rate of that substrate is calculated by multiplying the CBF by the arterial venous difference.

Procedures for the determination of global CBF and metabolism have been reported since the early 1940s, and are also discussed in Chapter 3. Kety and Schmidt *(43)* were the first to describe the use of an inert diffusible gas, nitrous oxide, to determine CBF and metabolism of oxygen in humans. This technique can be directly adapted to a bedside method for measuring CBF, but it is quite labor-intensive *(44,45)*. Modern imaging techniques, such as stable xenon CT scanning or perfusion CT scanning, can be used to provide the global CBF value to calculate the cerebral metabolic rate of substrate. However, these techniques require transport of critically ill patients to radiology and have limited capability for repeated measurements. These imaging techniques do have the ability to identify regional differences in blood flow, but cannot provide the same regional information about cerebral metabolism. Positron emission tomography (PET) scanning is capable of providing regional metabolic information. For research purposes, PET scanning has provided extremely valuable information about changes in cerebral metabolism after injury; however, this type of imaging is currently not widely available for clinical use.

All of these techniques for measuring cerebral metabolism have the limitation of being only a single point in time. Critically ill patients can have rapidly changing hemodynamics, and a single measurement may not truly reflect the whole picture of the patient. For continuous monitoring of metabolism in the ICU, indirect measures are usually applied. Jugular venous oxygen saturation ($SjvO_2$) monitoring provides continuous information about the global adequacy of CBF relative to the

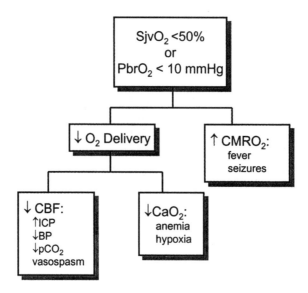

Fig. 3. The causes of an ischemic episode can be divided into two categories: those problems that decrease oxygen delivery and those that increase oxygen requirements.

metabolic requirements of the brain. This type of monitoring is simple, widely available, and has been successfully used to identify and follow treatment of secondary ischemic insults in brain injured patients *(34)*. The major limitation of $SjvO_2$ monitoring is the global nature of the information. A large area of the brain can become ischemic without significantly altering $SjvO_2$. When it is desirable to monitor oxygenation in a focal lesion, a brain tissue pO_2 probe can be placed into the tissue of interest *(32,46–48)*. These pO_2 probes give highly local measurements of tissue oxygenation, and values of tissue pO_2 of 8–10 mmHg indicate hypoperfusion. Figure 2 outlines a reasonable strategy for monitoring patients with TBI. In Chapter 6, there is further discussion on these monitoring techniques.

IDENTIFICATION AND TREATMENT OF SECONDARY INSULTS

The major clinical usefulness of monitoring cerebral metabolism has been in the early identification and treatment of secondary ischemic insults. Traumatic injury causes brain to be extremely vulnerable to secondary ischemic insults *(49)*. Numerous studies have emphasized the importance of secondary insults in determining the outcome following traumatic brain injury *(50–54)*. As shown in Fig. 3, the typical causes of these insults include hypotension, intracranial hypertension, hypoxia, hypocarbia, and anemia. All of these complications will ultimately result in a reduction in brain oxygenation. Therefore, $SjvO_2$ or brain tissue pO_2, are very useful in identifying these complications early. A reduction in $SjvO_2$ or tissue pO_2 should then initiate a search for a treatable cause, and treatment should be directed at the underlying cause.

REFERENCES

1. Wade OL, Bishop JM. *Cardiac output and Regional Blood Flow*. Oxford: Blackwell Scientific Publications, 1962.
2. Go KG. The cerebral blood supply. Energy metabolism of the brain. In: Go KG, ed. *Cerebral Pathophysiology* Amsterdam: Elsevier, 1991, pp. 66–172.
3. Astrup J. Energy requiring cell functions in the ischemic brain. Their critical supply and possible inhibition in protective therapy. *J. Neurosurg.* 1982;56:482–97.
4. Fox PT, Raichle ME, Mintun MA, Dence C. Nonoxidative glucose consumption during focal physiological neural activity. *Science* 1988;241:462–464.
5. Prichard J, Rothman D, Norothy E, et al. Lactate rise detected by HNMR in visual cortex during physiologic stimulation. *Proc. Natl. Acad. Sci. USA* 1991;88:5829–5831.

6. Hatazawa J, Matsuzawa T, Ido T, Watanuki S. Measurement of the ratio of cerebral oxygen consumption to glucose utilization by positron emission tomography: Its consistency with values determined by Kety Schmidt method in normal volunteers. *J. Cereb. Blood Flow Metab.* 1988;8:426–432.

7. Hasselbalch SG, Knudsen GM, Jakobsen J, Hageman lP, Holm S, Paulsen OB. Brain metabolism during short-term starvation in humans. *J. Cereb. Blood Flow Metab.* 1994;14:125–131.

8. Hasselbalch SG, Madsen PL, Hageman LP, Olsen KS, Justesen N, Holm S, Paulsen OB. Changes in cerebral blood flow and carbohydrate metabolism during acute hyperketonemia. *Am. J. Physiol.* 1996;270:E746–E751.

9. Tsacopoulos M, Magiestretti PJ. Metabolic coupling between glia and neurons. *J. Neuroscience* 1996;16:877–885.

10. Chih C-P, Lipton P, Roberts EL Jr. Do active cerebral neurons really use lactate rather than glucose? *Trends Neurosci.* 2001;24:573–578.

11. Andersen BJ, Marmarou A. Post-traumatic selective stimulation of glycolysis. *Brain Res.* 1992;585:184–189.

12. Yoshino A, Hovda DA, Kawamata T, et al. Dynamic changes in local cerebral glucose utilization following cerebral concussion in rats: Evidence of a hyper- and subsequent hypometabolic state. *Brain Res.* 1991;561:106–119.

13. Yang M, De Witt D, Becker D, et al. Regional brain metabolite levels following mild experimental head injury in cat. *J. Neurosurg.* 1985;63:617.

14. Kawamata T, Katayama Y, Hovda DA, et al. Administration of excitatory amino acid antagonists via microdialysis attenuates the increase in glucose utilization seen following concussive brain injury. *J Cereb. Blood Flow Metab.* 1992;12:12–24.

15. Hovda DA, Lee SM, Smith ML, et al. The neurochemical and metabolic cascade following brain injury: moving from animal models to man. *J. Neurotrauma* 1995;12:903–906.

16. Bergsneider M, Hovda DA, Shalmon E, et al. Cerebral hyperglycolysis following severe human traumatic brain injury in humans: A positron emission tomography study. *J. Neurosurg.* 1997;86:241–245.

17. Obrist WD, Langfitt TW, Jaggi JL, et al. Cerebral blood flow and metabolism in comatose patients with acute head injury. Relationship to intracranial hypertension. *J. Neurosurg.* 1984;61:241–253.

18. Jaggi JL, Obrist WD, Genarelli TA, et al. Relationship of early cerebral blood flow and metabolism to outcome in acute head injury. *J. Neurosurg.* 1990;72:176–182.

19. Robertson CS, Contant CF, Gokaslan ZL, et al. Cerebral blood flow, arteriovenous oxygen difference and outcome in head injured patients. *J. Neurol. Neurosurg. Psych.* 1992;55:594–603.

20. Muizelaar JP, Marmarou A, De Salles AA, et al. Cerebral blood flow and metabolism in severely head injured children. Part 1: Relationship with GCS score, outcome, ICP, and PVI. *J. Neurosurg.* 1989;71:63–71.

21. Robertson CS, Clifton GL, Grossman RG, et al. Alterations in cerebral availability of metabolic substrates after severe head injury. *J. Trauma* 1988;28:1523–1532.

22. Robertson CS, Goodman JC, Narayan RK, et al. Effect of glucose administration on carbohydrate metabolism after head injury. *J. Neurosurg.* 1991;74:43–50

23. Bouma GJ, Muizelaar JP, et al. Cerebral circulation and metabolism after severe traumatic brain injury: the elusive role of ischemia. *J. Neurosurg.* 1991;75:685–693.

24. Robertson CS, Grossman R, Goodman C, et al. The predictive value of cerebral anaerobic metabolism with cerebral infarction after head injury. *J. Neurosurg.* 1987;67:361–368.

25. Bergsneider M, Hovda DA, Lee SM, et al. Dissociation of cerebral glucose metabolism and level of consciousness during the period of metabolic depression following human traumatic brain injury. *J. Neurotrauma* 2000;17:389–401.

26. Inao S, Mamarou A, Clarke G, et al. Production and clearance of lactate from brain tissue, cerebrospinal fluid, serum following experimental brain injury. *J. Neurosurg.* 1988;69:736.

27. De Salles A, Muizelaar J, Young H. Hyperglycemia, cerebrospinal fluid lactic acidosis, and cerebral blood flow in severely head injured patients. *Neurosurgery* 1987;21:45–50.

28. Martin NA, Patwardhan RV, Alexander MJ, et al. Characterization of cerebral hemodynamic phases following severe head trauma: Hypoperfusion, hyperemia, and vasospasm. *J. Neurosurg.* 1997;87:9–19.

29. Morawetz RB, Krowell RH, DeGirolami U, et al. Regional cerebral blood flow thresholds during cerebral ischemia. *Fed. Proc.* 1979;38:2493–2494.

30. Astrup J, Symon L, Branston NM, et al. Cortical evoked potential and extracellular K^+ and H^+ at critical levels of brain ischemia. *Stroke* 1977;8:51–57.

31. Morawetz RB, DeGirolami U, Ojemann RG, et al. Cerebral blood flow determined by hydrogen clearance during middle cerebral artery occluion in unanesthetized monkeys. *Stroke* 1978;9:143–149.

32. Gopinath SP, Valadka AB, Uzura M, Robertson CS. Comparison of jugular venous O2 saturation and brain tissue pO2 as monitors of cerebral ischemia after head injury. *Crit. Care Med.* 1999;27: 2337–2345.

33. Hegstad E, Berg-Johnsen J, Haugstad TS, Hauglie-Hanssen E, Langmoen IA. Amino acid release from human cerebral cortex during simulated ischemia in vitro. *Acto Neurochir* (Wien) 1996;138:234–241.

34. Gopinath SP, Robertson CS, Contant CF, et al. Jugular venous desaturation and outcome after head injury. *J. Neurol. Neurosurg. Psych.* 1994;57:712–723.

35. Obrist WD, Langfitt TW, Jaggi JL, et al. Cerebral blood flow and metabolism in comatose patients with acute head injury. Relationship to intracranial hypertension. *J. Neurosurg.* 1984;61:241–253.

36. Kelly DF, Kordestani RK, Martin NA, et al. Hyperemia following traumatic brain injury: relation to intracranial hypertension and outcome. *J. Neurosurg.* 1996;85:762–771.

37. Bruce DA, Alavi A, Bilaniuk L, Dolinskas C, Obrist W, Uzzell B. Diffuse cerebral swelling following head injuries in children: the syndrome of "malignant brain edema." *J. Neurosurg.* 1981;54:170–178.

38. Kita H, Marmarou A. The cause of acute brain swelling after the closed head injury in rats. *Acta. Neurochir. Suppl. (Wien)* 1994;60:452–455.

39. Marmarou A, Barzo P, Fatouros P, Yamamoto T, Bullock R, Young H, Traumatic brain swelling in head injured patients: brain edema or vascular engorgement? *Acta. Neurochir. Suppl. (Wien)* 1997;70:68–70.

40. Barzo P, Marmarou A, Fatouros P, Hayasaki K, Corwin F. Biphasic pathophysiological response of vasogenic and cellular edema in traumatic brain swelling. *Acta. Neurochir. Suppl. (Wien)* 1997;70:119–122.

41. Ito J, Marmarou A, Barzo P, Fatouros P, Corwin F. Characterization of edema by diffusion-weighted imaging in experimental traumatic brain injury. *J. Neurosurg.* 1996;84:97–103.

42. Andrews BT, Chiles BW III, Oslen WL, et al. The effect of intracerebral hematoma location on the risk of brain stem compression and on clinical outcome. *J. Neurosurg.* 1988;69:518–522.

43. Kety SS, Schmidt CF. The nitrous oxide method for quantitative determination of CBF in man: Theory, procedure, and normal values. *J. Clin. Invest.* 1948;27:476–483.

44. Robertson CS. Measurement of CBF and measurement of metabolism in severe head injury using Kety-Schmidt technique. *Acta. Neurochir. (Wien)* 1993;59(Suppl):25–27.

45. Sharples PM, Stuart AG, Aynsley-Green A, et al. A practical method of serial bedside measurement of CBF and metabolism during neurointensive care. *Arch. Dis. Child.* 1991;66:1326–1332.

46. van Santbrink H, Mass AIR, Avezaat CJJ. Continuous monitoring of partial pressure of brain tissue oxygen in patients with severe head injury. *Neurosurgery* 1996;38:21–31.

47. Zauner A, Doppenberg E, Woodward JJ, et al. Multiparametric continuous monitoring of brain metabolism and substrate delivery in neurosurgical patients. *Neurol. Res.* 1997;19:265–273.

48. Kiening KL, Unterberg AW, Bardt TF, et al. Monitoring of cerebral oxygenation in patients with severe head injuries: Brain tissue PO$_2$ versus jugular vein oxygen saturation. *J. Neurosurg.* 1996;85:751–757.

49. De Witt DS, Jenkins LW, Prough DS. Enhanced vulnerability to secondary ischemic insults after experimental TBI. *New Horizon* 1995;3:372–383.

50. Signorini DF, Andrews PJ, Jones PA, Wardlaw J, Miller JD. Adding insult to injury: The prognostic value of early secondary insult for survival after traumatic brain injury. *J. Neurol. Neurosurg. Psych.* 1999;66(1):26–31.

51. Miller JD, Sweet RC, Narayan RK, et al. Early insults to the injured brain. *JAMA* 1978;240:439–442.

52. Chestnut RM, Marshall LF, Klauber MR, et al. The role of secondary brain injury in determining outcome for severe head injury. *J. Trauma* 1993;34:216–222.

53. Chambers IR, Treadwell L, Mendelow AD. The cause and incidence of secondary insults in severe head injury—adults and children. *Br. J. Neurosurg.* 2000;14:424–431.

54. Sarrafzadeh AS, Peltonen EE, Kaisers U, Kuchler I, Lanksch WR, Unterberg AW. Secondary insults in severe head injury. *Crit. Care Med.* 2001;29:1116–1123.

55. Rowe GG, Maxwell GM, Castillo CA, Freeman DJ, Crumpton CW. A study in man of cerebral blood flow and cerebral glucose, lactate and pyruvate metabolism before and after eating. *J. Clin. Invest.* 1959; 38: 2154–2158.

5

Cerebral Edema and Intracranial Dynamics

Monitoring and Management of Intracranial Pressure

Matthew Eccher and Jose I. Suarez

INTRODUCTION

Elevated intracranial pressure (ICP) is a relatively common clinical problem, potentially encountered daily in any neurocritical care unit. Intracranial hypertension can be a hyperacute emergency that must be reversed if profound morbidity or death are to be avoided. The astute clinician can improve patients' outcomes if judicious steps are taken at the right time (1). There have been many advances in our understanding of the physiology of intracranial dynamics. Although our armamentarium remains fairly limited, we may begin to envision its use on a rational, pathophysiologically grounded basis. Unfortunately, too little is yet known to predict exactly which interventions will be effective in exactly which disease states exactly when. Owing in part to the limits of our current technology, but also to a regrettable dearth of clinical trials in the field, current clinical practice is based on a conceptual understanding of underlying pathophysiology but backed by insufficient systematic research with patients. Practice is inevitably the product of the idiosyncratic experience of each individual intensivist. There are insufficient hard data to guide those in the process of gaining that experience.

The goal of this chapter is to first provide an overview of our models of pathophysiology, then to highlight their application in the management of deranged intracranial dynamics. Those few circumstances in which we have objective clinical trial data to guide patient management will be highlighted.

PATHOPHYSIOLOGY

Intracranial Elastance

In all normal humans whose cranial fontanelles have closed, the intracranial contents—brain, blood, and cerebrospinal fluid (CSF)—are encased in a rigid skull; in infants and others with incomplete closure of the calvaria, cerebral expansion is limited by the fibrous dura. In the average adult male, the skull encloses a volume of approx 1450 mL: 1300 mL of brain, 65 mL of CSF, and 110 mL of blood (2).

The Monro-Kellie doctrine dictates these anatomists' observation that the volume of the cranial vault is unchangeable—any process which adds volume to this system must therefore displace volume from elsewhere in the system. Which of the above components is displaced to accommodate extra volume will be considered below. Initially, there is minimal resistance to this displacement. When the limits of displaceability are reached, however, further addition encounters resistance, and this addition must be "squeezed" into the rigid container. This quickly results in an increase in the

From: *Current Clinical Neurology*
Critical Care Neurology and Neurosurgery
Edited by: J. I. Suarez © Humana Press Inc., Totowa, NJ

pressure within the system, i.e., raised ICP, which normally ranges between 5 and 15 mmHg (7.5 and 20 cm H_2O). This relationship of ICP to increasing volume of intracranial contents (in one experimental paradigm, an expanding subdural balloon) *(3)* can be expressed as a graph (Fig. 1). This model is just a model, and the pressure-volume curve it generates differs in some respects from that produced by other pathophysiological processes *(4)*, but the basic shape of the curve assumes an increasingly upsloping form in all cases. The slope represents the change in pressure produced by a given change in volume: $\Delta P/\Delta V$, termed "elastance." Initially, with low added volumes, CSF and venous blood are highly displaceable, and pressure rises little; elastance is low. With sufficient added volume, however, compensatory fluid shifts meet with increasing resistance, and pressure rises more and more precipitously—elastance rises. A simple analogy can be made to an elastic band: initial stretch on the band elicits little tensile resistance, but with increasing displacement (stretch), the elastic exerts greater and greater resistance. Likewise, with increasing addition of intracranial displacement (volume), the intracranial contents exert greater force (pressure), resisting further addition.

For semantic and historical reasons, most clinicians describe the status of the intracranial system in terms of $\Delta V/\Delta P$, "compliance," the inverse of elastance: a system which will accommodate significant changes in volume with little increase in pressure has high compliance (because it exerts little elastic resistance, i.e., has low elastance), whereas a system which has exhausted its compensating mechanisms can accommodate little additional volume without large changes in pressure has low compliance (increased elastance).

The Brain

The brain is a viscoelastic solid. It can be displaced to moderate degrees to accommodate an expanding mass. Slowly expanding masses can reach substantial sizes before becoming symptomatic, provided they are not primarily destructive of brain parenchyma, even if they encroach on structurally susceptible locations, such as the tentorial incisura or the foramen magnum *(5)*. The brain's inherent elastic properties generate pressure gradients in such situations *(6,7)*—gradients of up to 20 mmHg across as little as 2 cm of white matter have been reported *(8)*, and ICP is therefore not always uniform *(9)*. Brain is thus one source of intracranial elastance. Its inherent elastic properties can be modulated by changes in brain composition (*see* Brain Water/Brain Edema section) or by the addition of mass effect to the brain parenchyma (e.g., tumor, abscess).

While the glycoproteolipid matrix of the brain produces its structural integrity and elastic properties, the brain remains approx 80% water *(10,11)*, in two compartments. The extracellular compartment represents approx 15% of brain water *(10,11)*, and is in communication with the CSF space (as evidenced by edema bulk flow); the intracellular space comprises the other 85%. It is commonly held that neither of these spaces is appreciably compressible, with moderate direct evidence at best *(11)*. It is clear that either or both these spaces can expand in different disease states (*see* Brain Water/Brain Edema section). Such expansion leads, in effect, to an expansion of the volume of the brain. If such expansion overwhelms volume-compensatory mechanisms, ICP rises.

Brain, then, is minimally compressible, minimally displaceable, and can in some circumstances expand. Venous blood and CSF, by contrast, are much more displaceable, and represent the compensatory mechanisms for increased intracranial volume.

CSF

CSF buoys the brain and cushions it. It is produced as a modulated ultrafiltrate of plasma, with tight control of electrolyte and protein content. Most (80–90%) of its production is at the choroid plexus, with the remainder at the brain capillaries as brain interstitial fluid *(10–12)*. Roughly 500 cc is produced and resorbed each day *(13)*. Resorption occurs at the arachnoid villi into the cerebral venous sinuses (superior sagittal and transverse) by a mechanism that remains poorly understood *(14)*. Produc-

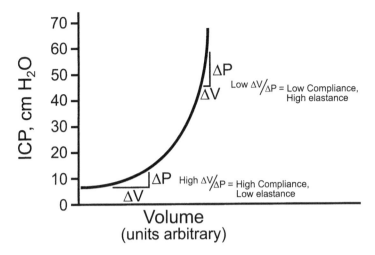

Fig. 1. Intracranial pressure-volume curve. An idealized graph of ICP vs an increasing volume of added mass effect. With increasing added volumes, compensatory mechanisms of the intracranial system are overwhelmed, and ICP becomes increasingly elevated. When compliance is low, small changes in the volume of intracranial tissue (e.g., blood) can precipitate large changes in ICP.

tion is virtually linear, falling off by a trivial amount with increasing ICP *(15)*. The rate at which CSF is resorbed, however, is tightly yoked to ICP: resorption is negligible below an ICP of 6.8 mmHg, and linear above that *(13)*. CSF overproduction, therefore, is very rarely a source of raised ICP.

A pressure gradient is consistently found from the subarachnoid space to cerebral sinus lumina, regardless of the organism's position (upright, supine, Trendelenberg), with a slightly lower pressure in the venous sinuses *(16)*. Venous obstruction, leading to increased venous pressure, increases subarachnoid pressure and thence ICP *(16)*. This has led to the presumption that impaired CSF absorption frequently plays a role in elevated ICP (a presumption with some conceptual justification, discussed in Fig. 4 and The Intracranial System section); however, because the mechanism of CSF absorption is not yet understood, this cannot be considered proven.

In contrast to brain, CSF is readily displaceable from the intracranial compartment, through the foramen magnum and into the lumbar cistern, in compensation for addition of volume elsewhere *(7)*. ICP compensation is profoundly compromised if this route is blocked—in one experimental model by an epidural balloon *(7)*, in some pathological states by tonsillar herniation *(3)*, or in cervical spondylosis by spinal epidural block *(17,18)*.

Of the three states of matter, fluid conveys pressure most effectively. CSF conveys pressure throughout the intracranial and spinal intradural space, as hydrostatic pressure. CSF conveys fluid pressure throughout the intracranial space, moderating the degree to which the brain parenchyma can produce compartmental gradients. Upright posture, by shifting fluid out of the head through the foramen magnum, decreases intracranial pressure and increases lumbar; Trendelenberg does vice versa *(17)*.

CSF, then, is of crucial consequence in states of ICP derangement. Unimpaired resorption likely plays a crucial role in ICP regulation. Maintenance of normal spinal shunting routes is vital to the normal ICP buffering mechanism. Head-up positioning (discussed in the Patient Positioning section) takes advantage of this principle. Direct drainage of CSF (discussed in the CSF Drainage section) can substantially reduce ICP.

Blood

Arterial Blood Flow

Regulation of arterial blood flow in the brain is accomplished by adjustment of the caliber of arterioles—narrow arteries and arterioles admit less blood. Arterial caliber adjusts spontaneously in response to several parameters: systemic arterial pressure, partial pressure of oxygen (pO_2), and partial pressure of carbon dioxide (pCO_2), among others.

At a fixed mean arterial pressure (MAP), cerebral blood flow (CBF) varies nearly linearly with pCO_2 values between 20 and 80 mmHg; this variation produces a change in cerebral blood volume (CBV) of 0.04 mL/100 g brain/mmHgCO$_2$. With a change in pCO_2 from 40 to 30, a 1200-g brain would see a 4.8-cc decrease in arterial blood volume. Through the normal physiologic range of pO_2, by contrast, CBF is constant. However, with a fall in pO_2 below 50 mmHg, CBF (and hence, CBV) increases rapidly.

Responses to pO_2 and pCO_2 are independent of ICP. Hence, either hypercarbia or hypoxia can dramatically exacerbate intracranial hypertension by further adding arterial blood volume to the intracranial compartment *(3)*. The 4.8-cc change in cerebral volume mentioned above can produce a change in ICP from 20 to 40 mmHg in a patient with decreased compliance. By contrast, however, hypocarbia can be utilized to decrease CBV and hence decrease ICP—either by spontaneous or therapeutic hyperventilation (a technique with limitations, as discussed in the Hyperventilation section).

With gas pressures held constant, CBV remains steady through a wide range of systemic MAP, from approx 50 to 150 mmHg (*see also* Chapter 3). With MAPs above this range of "autoregulation," arterial regulatory mechanisms are overwhelmed and CBV "forcibly" increased (as occurs in malignant hypertension, discussed below); MAPs below this range produce ischemia. Autoregulation does not change in direct response to raised ICP—rather, autonomic responses raise MAP (with a reflex bradycardia, the Cushing response). In many neurologic disease processes (e.g., severe head trauma, ischemia, status epilepticus) the autoregulatory mechanism itself fails, and blood flow becomes roughly linear relative to MAP. Departure from normotension in these circumstances can have profound effects on brain perfusion and CBV.

Systemic blood pressure must be maintained at a sufficient level to provide adequate perfusion to the brain. This dependency is abstracted through the concept of "cerebral perfusion pressure" (CPP), which depends on intracranial pressure and systemic BP through a fundamental relationship:

$$CPP = MAP - ICP$$

where MAP = mean arterial pressure: $(1/3 \cdot \text{systolic BP}) + (2/3 \cdot \text{diastolic BP})$. With typical MAPs of 75–90 and ICPs of 5–15, cerebral perfusion is rarely threatened in health. Syncope results when systemic pressure falls to levels insufficient to maintain CPP. With elevation of ICP, MAP must increase to maintain CPP (the Cushing response). If the cardiovascular system cannot produce a sufficient increase in blood pressure, ischemia ensues.

Arterial blood flow and blood volume are thus tightly yoked to physiologic parameters *other* than ICP, and cerebrovascular autoregulatory responses therefore have the capacity to produce intracranial hypertension in conditions of reduced compliance. It is intuitively easy to picture the vicious spiral: if a pathologic process produces decreased intracranial compliance and also threatens CPP, arterial dilation to preserve CPP will also produce a further increase in CBV, which will thereby add to the volume of an intracranial system with decreased compliance, further increasing ICP, necessitating *further* vasodilation to preserve CPP... it is possible that such a mechanism underlies paroxysmal elevations in ICP known as plateau waves (*see* A Waves section). The parameters which control CBF (pO_2, pCO_2, and MAP) must therefore be carefully attended to in patients with deranged intracranial dynamics (*see* the General Cardiopulmonary and Metabolic Support section).

Capillary Blood Flow

Capillary blood volume is difficult to study, and little attention has been paid in the literature to its role in intracranial volume and pressure.

Venous Blood Flow

Cerebral veins are significantly distensible. Evacuation of cerebral and dural venous sinus blood is thought to represent another volume-shifting pressure compensatory mechanism, similar to CSF. The postulated mechanism is intuitively obvious: shunt out of head and into the central venous pool. Direct evidence, however, is less clear for the case of venous blood shift than for CSF shift. It is clear that increased resistance to venous drainage, with elevation of venous pressure, will raise ICP *(16)*; whether the mechanism is impaired CSF resorption or intracranial venous hypervolemia has not yet been clarified. Whether increasing the intrathoracic pressure by positive-pressure ventilation retards cerebral venous drainage is also as yet unclear *(16,19)*.

Venous blood shunting may thus represent the second compensatory mechanism for elevated ICP. What is clear is that venous drainage must not be obstructed in patients with deranged intracranial dynamics *(see* the Patient Positioning section).

Brain Water/Brain Edema

Intracranial fluid can be conceptualized as divided into the same three spaces as in any other tissue of the body—intravascular, interstitial, and intracellular—with the elaboration that the brain contains a specialized compartment of interstitial fluid, the CSF. Proper regulation of brain fluid requires preserved integrity of the barriers between each fluid space; the most crucial and best studied of these barriers is the blood–brain barrier.

Barrier to Intravascular–Interstitial Flow: The Blood–Brain Barrier

Somatic capillary walls can be divided into three main categories—continuous, fenestrated, and sinusoidal *(21,22)*. Sinusoidal capillaries, found in spleen and marrow, contain wide unobstructed openings between endothelial cells to foster maximal exchange of cellular and proteinaceous elements between blood and tissue. Fenestrated capillaries, found in kidney and intestine, have narrower interendothelial spaces that contain a membrane which more tightly controls the plasma constituents allowed out of the vessel. Continuous capillaries, found in brain, nerve, skeletal muscle, heart, and lung, have no spaces between endothelial cells. This permits maximal control over which plasma constituents are permitted into the abluminal tissue.

Brain vasculature is highly restrictive of transendothelial molecular passage. It is this restrictiveness that has been dubbed the blood–brain barrier (BBB). Interendothelial tight junctions in brain capillary are amongst the most highly redoubled in the body *(20)*. They bind adjacent endothelial cells extremely tightly, leaving virtually no space between the cell membranes *(20,22)*. Because of the lack of space between endothelia, passive diffusion across the capillary wall is limited to gases and highly lipophilic substances, which can dissolve directly across the plasmalemmal lipid bilayer. Unlike in virtually every other tissue of the body, there is little to no fluid phase transfer across the endothelium via pinocytotic vesicles *(22–24)*. The only remaining mechanism for traversing the capillary wall, then, is carrier proteins and channels, which in the brain are highly selective to specific metabolites and compounds *(25)*. Endothelial cells in brain capillary contain a very high number of mitochondria *(23)*, suggesting that the functions necessary to maintain the BBB are highly energy-dependent. This barrier, however, is susceptible to opening by various inflammatory mediators, as well as by mechanical, traumatic and pharmacologic mechanisms *(see* Vasogenic Edema and the Starling Equation section).

Barrier to Intravascular–CSF Flow: The Choroid

For reasons of brevity, the complex electrochemical function of the choroid epithelium will not be discussed here. As mentioned previously, the choroid produces approx 80–90% of the CSF, which totals approx 500 cc/d, and rarely is overproduction as source of deranged intracranial dynamics. As discussed in the Acetazolamide section, carbonic anhydrase inhibition can decrease the rate of CSF production at the choroid, but in few pathologic states is this sufficient to ameliorate the derangement in ICP.

Barrier to Interstitial–Intracellular Flow: The Glia

Regulation of brain intracellular space volume is largely the responsibility of glial cells, as they represent the bulk of brain volume. Glial cell processes extend from the ependyma to the subarachnoid glia limitans, and encircle brain capillaries at every level between. It is now appreciated that glia may serve to traffic brain water from each of these locations to others. Recent work has demonstrated that water crosses lipid bilayer membranes in all tissues via a class of membrane channels collectively termed "aquaporins" *(26)*. Only one isoform, AQP-4, is expressed in brain parenchyma. The protein is highly concentrated at astrocytic pericapillary endfeet, and astrocytic processes in contact with subarachnoid and ventricular CSF. The intuitively obvious conjecture is that astroglia play a role in fluid homeostasis that involves conveying water between each of these three surfaces. Manley et al. *(27)* have demonstrated that AQP-4 knockout mice, which demonstrate no neurologic disturbances at baseline, have a dramatically reduced rate of mortality in a systemic hyponatremia model, and have substantially less CNS dysfunction in an MCA stroke model. Other studies have shown differential expression of AQP-4 in models of cerebral ischemia *(28)* and traumatic brain injury *(29)*. Much work remains to be done to clarify the dynamics of water flux through glia, and whether this system might be amenable to pharmacologic intervention in states of deranged intracranial fluid dynamics.

Mechanisms of Brain Edema Formation

Brain edema can be defined as "an abnormal accumulation of fluid within the brain parenchyma producing a volumetric enlargement of the brain tissue" *(30)*. As mentioned previously, swelling of brain tissue alone, if of sufficient magnitude, can displace enough CSF and blood to produce elevated ICP. Alternatively, a mass lesion of modest size can produce dramatic effect on ICP if it produces sufficient surrounding edema.

Brain edema results from accumulation of excess water in either the interstitial compartment, the intracellular compartment, or both. Klatzo *(31)* first promulgated an explicit dichotomy between interstitial vs intracellular fluid accumulation. Arguing that interstitial fluid accumulation results from increased blood vessel wall permeability, Klatzo labeled extracellular edema "vasogenic type." By contrast, he argued, intracellular fluid accumulation resulted from injury to the brain parenchyma itself, with normal vascular permeability; he therefore termed intracellular edema "cytotoxic type." This conceptual dichotomy between cytotoxic and vasogenic edema has been widely adopted. As will be discussed, the putative underlying mechanisms of fluid accumulation in each compartment is not so simple as then thought. Factors other than increased vascular permeability or brain parenchymal injury can result in abnormal amounts of water in each tissue space. Many of the pathologic states leading to brain edema actually exhibit both forms of edema to varying degrees. For these reasons the terms "cytotoxic edema" and "vasogenic edema" are overly reductionistic; however, owing to their universal utilization, this chapter maintains the conventional terminology (Fig. 2).

Vasogenic Edema and the Starling Equation

Accumulation of fluid in the interstitial space can be produced by derangement of the BBB. Flow of water from the intravascular to interstitial space can be modeled in all tissues by the Starling equation:

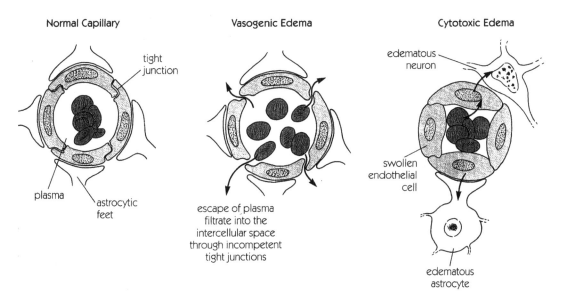

Fig. 2. Mechanisms of edema. This schematic illustrates the traditional conceptualization of brain edema mechanisms. At the capillary wall in normal brain, tight junctions retain protein-rich serum within the capillary. Vasogenic edema develops when tight junction maintenance is deranged, and protein-fluid leaks into the interstitium, drawing free water along with it. Cytotoxic edema develops when cellular energy metabolic failure leads to increased intracellular sodium, free water follows, and tissue swells as its cells take on water. Reprinted from Rengachary SS, Wilkins RA (eds.). Principles of Neurosurgery. London: Wolfe Pub Ltd., 1994, with permission.

$$\text{Fluid movement} = Lp(P_c - P_i) + \Sigma\sigma(\pi_i - \pi_c)$$

where:
L_p = capillary wall hydraulic conductivity;
P_c = hydrostatic pressure in the capillary;
P_i = hydrostatic pressure in the interstitium;
σ = reflection coefficient of the capillary wall for each solute;
π_c = oncotic pressure for each solute within the capillary; and
π_i = oncotic pressure for each solute in the interstitium *(30,32)*.

The first term, $Lp(P_c - P_i)$, reflects the contribution of hydrostatic pressure—that which one usually thinks of when referring to "blood pressure." Virtually always higher in vasculature than tissue, this hydraulic pressure will favor flow of water into tissue. In the brain, this gradient is held in check by the endothelial wall's impermeability to water—a very low Lp. Elevation of intravascular pressure (P_c), decrease in tissue pressure (P_i), or increased conductance of water through the vessel wall (Lp) will all favor increased accumulation of interstitial water—vasogenic edema *(30)*.

Multiple inflammatory mediator—have been implicated in increasing Lp—among them bradykinin, serotonin, histamine, adenine nucleotides (ATP, ADP and AMP), platelet aggregating factor, arachidonic acid, prostaglandins, leukotrienes, IL-1α, IL-1β, IL-2, macrophage inflammatory proteins MIP-1 and MIP-2, complement-derived C3a-desArg, nitric oxide, free radicals *(20,22,23)*, and thrombin *(33)*. The specific role of each of these systems in specific pathological processes is not yet known *(21)*. It is thought that the final common pathway is opening of endothelial tight junctions *(24)*, putatively through calcium-modulated endothelial cell contraction *(21)*, with a resulting profound increase in Lp. There does not appear to be an increase in pinocytosis across endothelium *(21,24)* underlying increased Lp. The role of inflammatory mediators such as nitric oxide and leukotrienes (metabolites of arachidonic acid) is controversial—it is unclear whether they are mediators of opening, or markers of a process that leads to opening *(21)*. Opening of tight junctions may also be provoked by intravascular osmolarity derangement (π_c) *(24)*, or acute elevation of intravascular pressure (P_c) *(34)*.

The second term in the above equation, $\Sigma\sigma(\pi_i - \pi_c)$, represents the contribution of oncotic (i.e., osmotic) pressure. Due to the normally low Lp of the brain capillary, therefore, most fluid shifts in health are a result of oncotic forces *(10,11)*. Only solutes that have an appreciable concentration gradient ($\pi_i - \pi_c$) across the capillary wall have the potential to create an osmotic gradient; whether they do depends on the capillary wall's permeability to each solute. A solute to which the wall is freely permeable will cross the wall along its gradient and produce no osmotic pressure; this is represented by a σ near zero. A solute with a σ near 1, by contrast (for example, sodium and mannitol), will produce a substantial osmotic gradient if its π_i and π_c are unequal. The net osmotic gradient is the sum (Σ) of the gradient of each individual solute.

Vasogenic edema, then, can be understood in terms of the different constituents of the Starling equation. If tight junctions open, Lp increases, and the magnitude of the first term increases substantially, favoring flow into interstitium. If gap junctions remain open long enough for plasma proteins such as albumin to leak into the interstitium, π_i will be increased by elevated interstitial protein load, further favoring water accumulation. If interstitial edema is to be avoided, the BBB must remain intact.

Once formed, vasogenic edema clears by "sinking" into the CSF *(35,36)*, following a pressure gradient from the edematous brain to CSF space *(37)*. It has been suggested without evidence that that flow takes place along perivascular spaces *(11,35)*; the degree of resistance (at pial-glial interface and at ependymal surface) to that movement is unclear *(11)*.

Obstructive Hydrocephalus

One other mechanism exists by which excess fluid can accumulate in the interstitial space. CSF normally proceeds from the choroid, where it is produced, to the subarachnoid space, where it is resorbed, via the ventricular system. With obstruction of the ventricular system anywhere between the lateral ventricle and the foramina of the fourth ventricle, the only alternate route for CSF to flow is across the brain parenchyma. When this occurs, flow is through the same space that vasogenic edema utilizes in its route from parenchyma into the CSF. This source of excess interstitial fluid differs pathophysiologically from that described above, leading many authors to use the term *interstitial edema* to make the pathophysiologic distinction *(38,39)*. The pressure gradient necessary to force the full volume of ventricular CSF flow across brain parenchyma instead of through the cerebral aqueduct produces profound derangements in brain function; sudden and complete obstruction of the system, as in the ball-valve mechanism of a foramen of Monro colloid cyst, produce a sufficient pressure gradient that cerebral circulatory arrest and death can occur. CSF diversion procedures are done to prevent this gradient of CSF pressure across the brain (*see* CSF Drainage section).

Cytotoxic Edema, Cell Energy Metabolism, and Cellular Fluid Balance

Most discussions of cytotoxic edema cite failure of the Na-K ATPase pump due to shortage of ATP, the putative mechanism being accumulation of intracellular sodium with resulting cell swelling. The name was initially chosen to highlight the presumption that disruption of cellular metabolism was the underlying cause *(31)*. Ischemic stroke is the typical prototype offered.

Brain parenchyma is capable of resisting intravascular osmotic pressure changes; this is largely a function of glia *(11)*. Evidence indicates that mammalian cells utilize small organic molecules, collectively known as organic osmolytes, to regulate the transmembrane osmotic gradient *(40)*. These include polyols such as sorbitol, amino acids such as alanine and taurine, and methylamines such as glycerophosphoral choline. Drop in interstitial osmotic pressure (P_i) results in a flux of these osmolytes out of the cell to drop intracellular osmolarity and maintain water balance. Outward flux of these osmolytes to prevent cell swelling requires expression of an ATP-dependent membrane channel. This provides a conceptual explanation for cell swelling in circumstances of impaired cellular energy metabolism—cell protein manufacture is impaired in conditions of inadequate ATP, and the function of those channels which are present is impaired by the absence of ATP. Direct evidence for this mechanism in vivo, however, is as yet lacking.

Unlike vasogenic edema, excess intracellular water cannot "sink" into the CSF. Resolution of cytotoxic edema depends upon resolution of the inciting factor. Cells not irreversibly injured will revert to their premorbid state.

Osmotic Edema

Systemic hyponatremia of sufficient severity can also bring about the accumulation of intracellular water by overwhelming cells' capability to accommodate to the hypotonic extracellular environment. In Klatzo's original dichotomy, this is cellular swelling, and hence "cytotoxic" edema. Finding the implication that water is a "toxin" problematic, some authors *(39)* have labeled hyponatremia-induced intracellular edema "osmotic edema" to distinguish it from cytotoxic edema.

Dynamics of ICP

Many processes that lead to accumulation of excess brain water can produce sufficient mass effect that intracranial hypertension ensues. ICP is not monolithic, however; in both pathology and health, ICP is highly variable. Some particular patterns of change, however, are characteristic of pathology.

Cardiac Waves

Intracranial pressure pulses with each pressure wave from the heart—as any neurosurgeon can attest, the brain pulsates. The normal cardiac pressure wave contains three consecutive peaks, in descending order of magnitude: P1 (percussion wave), P2 (tidal wave), and P3 (dicrotic wave) *(10)*. With increased ICP or decreased intracranial compliance, P2 increases in magnitude and P1 becomes blunted; merging of P1 into P2 is one clinical means of detecting declining compliance *(10)*.

Pulmonary Waves

A low-amplitude variation in ICP can also be detected in response to the cycle of intrathoracic pressure (Fig. 3).

A Waves

First demonstrated by Lundberg *(41)*, plateau waves (now commonly referred to as Lundberg A waves) are considered essentially pathognomonic of intracranial hypertension. A waves are sustained (5–20 min), high amplitude (50–100 mmHg) increases in ICP (*see* Fig. 3). Typically exhibited in patients with decreased intracranial compliance, they have however been observed in healthy individuals. Provoked by mental or physical activity, pain, or sleep, they often produce headache, restlessness, confusion, nausea, vomiting, or hyperventilation, but they may be asymptomatic *(41)*. The danger of a plateau wave is the potential for abolishment of the CPP (as previously discussed); sustained A waves can produce global ischemic injury or death. The likely (but unproven) *(42,43)* pathophysiology is arterial vasodilation to compensate for a drop in systemic arterial pressure, with a resulting increase in CBV causing a further increase in ICP—the vicious spiral previously alluded to in the section on Arterial blood flow. Plateau waves of sufficient severity and duration to produce global cerebral ischemia must be reversed, or "broken"—the usual steps undertaken to do so are CSF drainage, hyperventilation, and boluses of osmotic diuretics, to be discussed.

B and C Waves

Other periodic oscillations in ICP were also described by Lundberg, but are of much lesser pathologic consequence. B waves last 1–2 min, are of 20–50 mmHg in amplitude, and are frequently seen in normals, especially in sleep (*see* Fig. 3) *(41)*. C waves last 4–5 min, are less than 20 mmHg, are of no pathologic consequence, and likely represent ICP extension of Traube-Hering vasomotor waves, a poorly understood cyclic variation in systemic BP *(10)*.

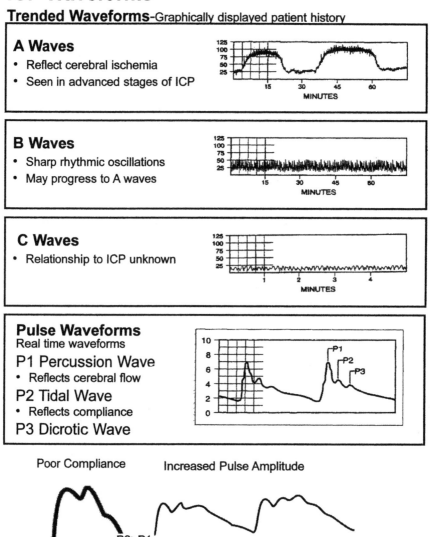

Fig. 3. Intracranial pressure monitoring. A waves are long-duration, sustained elevations of ICP of very high magnitude, sufficient to jeopardize CPP. B waves are of moderate magnitude, and C waves are of low magnitude; both are of short duration, and their pathologic significance is uncertain. CSF pressure monitors also transduce pulsations resulting from arterial blood pressure, and pulse waveforms can be studied for early signs of decreasing compliance—when the initial systolic wave (P1) is blunted and the tidal wave (P2) increased in amplitude, compliance is likely decreased, and the clinician should be alert for the development of A waves. Reprinted from ref. *10* and Integra Neurosciences with permission.

The Intracranial System

Intracranial pressure, then, is a function of the interaction between venous and arterial CBV and CBF, the production, resorption and redistributability of the CSF, the resistance of the brain to stretch, and the presence or absence of additional mass effect such as a tumor, hematoma or abscess. The exact shape of the P/V curve for a particular patient is a complex function of each of these variables. Computer models of the intracranial system *(44–46)* using differential equations to describe each of

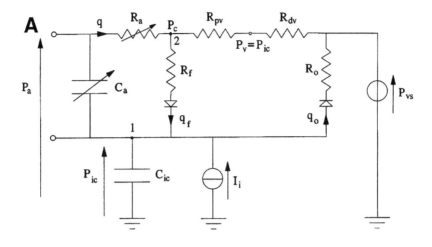

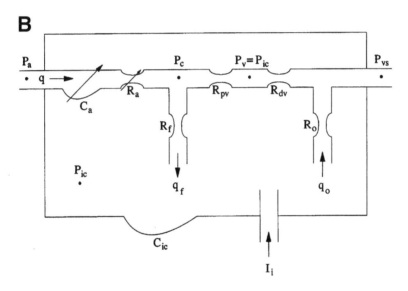

Fig. 4. Electrical (A) and mechanical (B) models of the intracranial system. Cerebral blood volume (q) enters the intracranial space under arterial pressure (P_a). Arterial tone regulates arterial blood volume (C_a) and resistance to its flow (R_a) into the capillaries (P_c). Capillary walls and choroids plexus maintain resistance to the filtration of CSF (Rf) from capillary blood, with a steady flow of CSF (q_f) resulting. Cerebral veins have an intrinsic resistance to blood flow both proximally (R_{pv}) and distally (R_{dv}) en route to the venous sinuses (P_{vs}). Rate of CSF resorption (q_o) depends on the resistance of the arachnoid granulations (R_o). Overall intracranial capacitance (C_{ic}) is an independent function of the fluid spaces; intracranial pressure (P_{ic}) is the net result and an interdependent function of all of the above. (The model also includes an inlet for experimental infusion of artificial CSF, Ii.) This model has a demonstrated ability to reproduce physiologic phenomena of deranged ICP, in particular A waves. Chief among its insights thus far are an increase in resistance to CSF resorption (R_o) in many states of elevated ICP, and the necessity of inclusion of the two separate venous resistances to accurately model ICP dynamics. Although this model has yet to be applied to real patients in real time, it provides conceptual support for the use of CSF drainage to overcome increased R_o, and its existence is reason to hope for rational approaches at some point in the future. Reprinted from ref. *45* with permission.

these factors, with parameters derived from clinical data and animal models, have achieved a remarkable ability to reproduce the behavior of the intracranial system—in particular, the most crucial clinical phenomenon of elevated ICP, A waves (Fig. 4). One of the most striking insights obtained from this model is its support of the association between increased resistance to CSF resorption (R_o) and elevations in ICP, a finding clinically confirmed by the utility of CSF drainage in controlling intracranial hypertension (*see* CSF Drainage section). It will likely be some time, unfortunately, before work on these models has proceeded to the point where they can predict ICP phenomena in individual patients.

ETIOLOGIES OF EDEMA AND RAISED ICP

Any process with the potential to affect one of the following can elevate ICP: (1) addition of sufficient intracranial volume to overwhelm compensatory mechanisms, (2) impairment of the normal regulation of intracranial blood flow in the arterial, capillary, or venous phase, or (3) impairment of normal CSF production and absorption. A list of conditions known to potentially elevate ICP can be found in Table 1. The underlying pathophysiologies as represented here are highly oversimplified. Many of the disease states listed provoke all effects to some extent, in changing proportions over the natural history of the disease; this table is introductory, not encyclopedic.

FINAL COMMON PATHWAYS OF BRAIN DAMAGE

Clinical Presentation

The clinical manifestations of the conditions mentioned in Table 1 are variegate because symptoms are a function both of ICP generally and any focal areas of brain dysfunction because of the pathologic process. The essential clinical manifestations of raised ICP are the same, regardless of the cause: headache, nausea, vomiting, blurred vision, and somnolence progressing to coma. Idiopathic intracranial hypertension, cerebral venous thrombosis, obstructive hydrocephalus, and high altitude cerebral edema, for example, typically present in this fashion. Acute expanding masses that have minimal direct effect on cortex or white matter tracts, such as an epidural hematoma, may produce no focal deficit before elevating ICP dramatically, and will therefore present clinically with the above nonspecific symptoms. By contrast, highly destructive lesions such as a cerebral metastasis will often produce highly focal neurologic deficits long before they reach sufficient size to elevate ICP. Less destructive lesions, such as a subdural hematoma, may only produce more widely distributed localized signs (e.g., mild weakness with impaired sensation over the contralateral body) before producing the nonspecific symptoms of intracranial hypertension. Impairment of consciousness is a final common expression of more than one mechanism, because patient series have demonstrated that mental status correlates moderately at best to ICP *(47)* and to the degree of midline shift *(48)*, demonstrating that other mechanisms must have been operative in each case. Clinical presentation of rising ICP is thus any combination of the essential symptoms of elevated ICP, the localizing signs from any causative or concurrent mass, and the consequences of deformation of brain that are called the herniation syndromes.

Impaction: The Herniation Syndromes

Herniation refers to passage of an organ or part thereof past a boundary or into a space where that organ should not be. Mass effect in the brain not infrequently results in placement of pressure on structurally susceptible areas, producing specific constellations of symptoms and signs.

Uncal (Lateral Transtentorial)

Uncal herniation refers to herniation of the medial temporal lobe (uncus) past the edge of the tentorium and downward, impacting on cranial nerve III. Caused by swelling or mass effect in the temporal lobe or temporoparietal junction. When of sufficient magnitude, pushes the midbrain to the

Table 1
Predominant Pathophysiology of Selected Disease States

Disease state	Increased CSF volume	Increased blood volume	Mass effect	Increased intracellular brain water	Increased extracellular brain water
Trauma	+/-	+/-	+/-	X	X
Hypoxia/ischemia (diffuse) (postcardiac arrest, near drowning)		+/-		X	+/-
Ischemic stroke (focal)			+/- (late)	X(early)	X(late)
Subarachnoid hemorrhage	X				X
Intracranial hemorrage			X		X*
Subdural hematoma			X		
Epidural hematoma			X		
Obstructive hydrocephalus	X				X
Cerebral venous sinus thrombosis	X	X			X
Idiopathic intracranial hypertension	X	X			X
Normal perfusion pressure breakthrough (postoperative phase of AVM repair, A–V fistula repair, or CEA)		X			X
Tumor			X		X*
Abscess			X		X*
Empyema			X		X*
Meningitis	+/-	X			X
Encephalitis		+/-		X	X
Malignant hypertension and eclampsia		X			X
Fulminant hepatic failure/Reye's synd.		+/-			+/-
H₂O intoxication				X	
Lead intoxication				X	
High-altitude cerebral edema (HACE)				+/-(?)	X
Hypercarbia (COPD, Pickwickian synd., permissive hypercapnia)		X			
Tension pneumocephalus			X		

*Adjacent edema produces this effect.

X, present; +/–, may be present; AVM, arteriovenous malformation; A-V, arteriovenous; CEA, carotid endarterectomy; COPD, chronic obstructive pulmonary disease; CSF, cerebrospinal fluid.

opposite side, impacting the contralateral cerebral peduncle on the contralateral tentorial edge, with resulting pyramidal weakness; this "Kernohan's notch" phenomenon is a false lateralizing sign because the weakness is ipsilateral to the causative mass effect.

Tonsillar (Foraminal Impaction, Cerebellar Cone)

Tonsillar herniation refers to mass effect from above shifting the pontomedullary junction down through the foramen magnum. With impaction of the cerebellar tonsils therein, the medulla is compressed, resulting in dysregulation, then collapse, of respiratory and cardiovascular systems. This impaction also precludes further CSF flow out of the cranium into the spinal cisterns, with subsequent dissociation of intracranial CSF pressure (which often thence exhibits a profound further increase) from lumbar CSF pressure (which may return to normal).

Subfalcine (Cingulate, Supracallosal)

Subfalcine herniation refers to mass effect in the high lateral frontal or parietal lobe forcing the cingulate gyrus up against and then under and past the falx cerebri. This produces personality change and mild contralateral leg weakness, which becomes more pronounced if the herniation is of sufficient magnitude to compress the anterior cerebral artery (ACA) against the falx and cause an ACA infarct.

Central Transtentorial

Central transtentorial herniation refers to diffuse bilateral hemispheric swelling with progressive decline in mental status and decompensation of respiratory function, correlating somewhat with the degree of downward displacement of the midbrain through the tentorial hiatus. When of sufficient degree, the mesial temporal lobes impact in the tentorial incisura, creating a CSF block at that level. This results in the same compartmental CSF pressure dissociation effect as produced by tonsillar impaction, except with the dissociation arising between the supratentorial and infratentorial compartments.

Upward Transtentorial (Reversed Tentorial)

Upward transtentorial refers to mass effect in the posterior fossa displacing the midbrain upward. This may produce diffuse symptoms of obstructive hydrocephalus if the cerebral aqueduct or fourth ventricle is occluded, or homonymous hemianopsia if the posterior cerebral artery (PCA) impacts on the tentorial edge, or variegate neurologic deficits if the great vein of Galen impacts on the tentorium, producing infarcts in the deep venous territory (thalami, internal capsules and basal ganglia).

Transcalvarial (External)

Transcalvarial herniation refers to focal cortical signs because of herniation of cortex through a defect in the skull. Seen rarely, as patients with such defects are usually unconscious, as a result of diffuse injury if the defect is traumatic or general anesthesia if it is surgical.

Abducens Nerve Palsy

While its dysfunction is not classically considered a herniation syndrome per se, the structurally susceptible position of the cranial nerve VI is of note with regards to the symptoms of elevated ICP. With substantial displacement of the pontomedullary junction downward or to the side, one or both of the sixth cranial nerves can be stretched sufficiently to produce dysfunction of the nerve and failure of abduction of the ispilateral eye. Most commonly seen in association with central transtentorial herniation, it can be seen in isolation or with any of the other herniation syndromes.

Ischemia

Herniations produce focal tissue damage by impacting brain or vasculature against rigid structures. The other fundamental process by which intracranial swelling or mass effect can produce brain damage is by raising the intracranial pressure to the point that cerebral perfusion pressure, MAP-ICP, is compromised. If ICP encroaches on CPP, cerebral arteries will dilate in an effort to preserve blood flow, CBV will increase, and ICP will further increase—the vicious spiral of mutually worsening ICP and ischemia. At its most pathologic extreme, this process proceeds until ICP equals MAP, CPP is abolished altogether, intracranial blood flow ceases, and the brain dies. Intermediate degrees of CPP impairment produce ischemic brain damage, resulting in neurologic deficits upon recovery. In an attempt to allow a safety margin above impending ischemia, CPP should be maintained at 70 mmHg if possible. This safety margin permits for the development of unappreciated pressure gradients within the brain, decreasing the chance that critically depressed CPP will develop at some point distant from the point at which ICP is being assessed. Attempting to maintain a target CPP, however, requires direct assessment of ICP-ICP monitoring, the means for which will now be discussed.

MONITORING THE PATIENT WITH POTENTIALLY ELEVATED INTRACRANIAL PRESSURE

The neurointensive care clinician must be attentive to all potential evidence of cerebral edema or intracranial hypertension. Currently, ICP can only be reliably assessed by invasive, neurosurgical means, which have relatively uncommon but potentially catastrophic complications. Many other noninvasive means of assessment must be used—to complement an invasive ICP monitor once one is in place, and during all phases of care when an ICP monitor is not in place. These will be discussed first.

Indirect Monitoring Techniques

Monitoring Clinical Status

The foremost noninvasive variable that must be followed, of course, is the clinical examination. The components of the neurological examination which we believe should be fully assessed and documented in the chart on at least a daily basis are presented in Table 2. Frequent and consistent documentation of these few variables permits dependable comparison between examiners of vital aspects of the patient's clinical status. Obviously, neither list even begins to approximate a complete neurologic examination; we wish to highlight here a select few items on the examination that are of high importance in assessing for a pathologic change in the nervous system, and can be done efficiently with a high degree of reproducibility between examiners. In patients with potential for elevated ICP, assessment of gag or cough and response to noxious stimuli may need to be omitted to avoid precipating plateau waves.

From the standpoint of assessing for the possibility of increased intracranial pressure, the paramount clinical findings to assess for are:

1. Level of alertness and GCS;
2. Pupillary examination;
3. Ocular motor examination (with special attention to the third and sixth cranial nerves);
4. Motor examination with special attention for hemiparesis;
5. Presence of nausea or vomiting;
6. Complaints of headache; and
7. Current vital signs and the recent course thereof.

Ophthalmoscopy, once of singularly central significance in the assessment for elevated intracranial pressure, has receded in importance in the era of modern neuroimaging. Papilledema does not develop until elevated ICP has been present for longer than 1 d. It should nonetheless be assessed for on initial evaluation, as its presence or absence (along with its sudden appearance in the context of previous absence) can provide useful information regarding the time course of the disease process.

Neuroimaging

Any patient in whom elevated ICP is suspected should at the very least receive an emergent noncontrast-enhanced head CT scan. Particular note should be made of any of the findings listed in Table 3, which suggest pathological states with the potential to cause intracranial hypertension. The

Table 2
**Essential Components of the Clinical Examination
in the Neurocritical Care Unit**

In the conscious patient
Language, to include at least comprehension, repetition, fluency, and
    dysarthria
Ocular motor examination (eye movements), including any subjective diplopia or
    nystagmus
Visual fields, to finger-counting, in all quadrants (or blink to visual threat
    if unable to comply)
Pupillary examination
Facial symmetry
Motor examination including proximal and distal strength in all limbs,
    and presence or absence of pronator drift of the arms

In the patient with impaired consciousness
GCS
Pupillary examination
Visual pursuit (eye tracking) of the examiner or another visual target
Blink to visual threat
Oculocephalic reflex ("doll's eyes" maneuver), if C-spine is not immobilized
Gag or cough
Nature of response to noxious stimuli (as outlined on motor scale of GCS),
    documented separately for all 4 limbs, especially with regard to symmetry

presence of more than one of these abnormalities is highly suggestive of elevated ICP *(49)*; the presence of any one suggests the potential for it. MRI or contrast-enhanced CT can be pursued if necessary to better characterize intracranial pathology (*see* Chapter 7); for initial decision making, although noncontrast-enhanced CT is often sufficient.

The essential decision which must be made in patients with potentially elevated ICP is whether a monitoring device should be placed (*see* Direct ICP Monitoring section). Neuroimaging is used to establish diagnoses that produce the risk of elevated ICP, supplementing information derived from the history and examination. Imaging cannot substitute for invasive ICP monitoring. Repeat CT scans can, however, be used beneficially when the patient's clinical status is just short of requiring placement of an ICP monitor. In these circumstances, repeat imaging whenever the patient's status changes can document the appearance of a new finding (e.g., delayed hematoma in head injury) *(50)*, which can then prompt monitor placement. This approach can be utilized to delay or avoid monitor placement in cases where the need for it is initially equivocal.

Neurosonology

Transcranial Doppler ultrasonography (TCD) has been proven a useful clinical tool for noninvasive assessment of basal arterial cerebral blood flow, and is now available from most tertiary hospital vascular sonography laboratories *(51,52; see also* Chapter 6*)*. All of the major intracranial arterial branches can usually be insonated—middle, anterior, and posterior cranial arteries across the temporal bone (except in 10% of patients, in whom transtemporal insonation is impossible), ophthalmic artery and carotid siphon across the orbit, and vertebral and basilar across the foramen magnum from below. TCD reveals the velocity of blood flow, in centimeters per second, which typically ranges from 40 to 70. A second essential monitoring variable is derived from the waveform recording: the pulsatility index (PI), the ratio of the difference between systolic and diastolic flow to diastolic flow ([systolic flow – diastolic flow] / diastolic flow), typically approximately equal to 1.

Table 3
Neuroimaging Findings Suggestive of Deranged Intracranial Dynamics

Intracranial blood (epidural, subdural, subarachnoid, intraparenchymal, or intraventricular)
Obstructive hydrocephalus (dilated lateral ventricles or luncency of white matter near the anterior horns of
   the lateral ventricles consistent with transependymal flow)
Diffuse or focal cerebral edema (blurring of the interface between gray and white matter or effacement of sulci)
Midline shift (most readily discerned at the septum pellucidum, the pineal gland, and the fourth ventricle)
Compression of basal cisterns (especially the ambient and perimesencephalic)
Obliteration of the third ventricle

The most common clinical use of TCD is monitoring for vasospasm, especially after SAH. With narrowing of the arterial lumen, systolic flow increases and diastolic decreases (systolic flow of 120 is highly suggestive and 200 confirmatory of decreased luminal diameter), resulting in an increase in PI (values above 3 : 1 are highly suggestive of luminal narrowing) *(53)*. Frequent serial TCD assessments can detect the progressive changes in flow velocity and PI which SAH vasospasm produces *(54)*.

Luminal narrowing can be produced by intrinsic constriction of arteries themselves—by smooth muscle action, as in autoregulation and true vasospasm, or by intimal hyperplasia as in the "vasospasm" of SAH. Vasospasm can also, however, by produced by extrinsic compression of arteries—most notably, diffuse elevation of ICP produces a compressive force that causes the basal arteries to be narrowed. Generalized increases in flow velocity and PI can therefore indicate diffuse extrinsic compression of arteries owing to increased ICP *(55)*. Unfortunately, despite the ability to demonstrate such changes, TCD is insufficiently sensitive and specific to provide a noninvasive alternative to ICP monitoring. It cannot substitute for direct ICP monitoring. The clinician who is using TCD to monitor SAH patients for arterial narrowing should thus bear in mind that diffusely distributed changes indicative of luminal narrowing may indicate increasing ICP.

Some attempts have been made to utilize TCD to assess for loss of autoregulation and for the presence of a critical MAP below which CPP is compromised *(56)*. Unfortunately, these uses have proven too insensitive and cumbersome to gain widespread acceptance.

Direct ICP Monitoring

At present, no means of accurately assessing ICP has yet been developed that does not require surgical placement of an invasive device. All such devices have attendant risks, mostly of hemorrhagic and infectious complications (discussed below; *see also* Chapter 6). The decision as to when an ICP monitoring device should be placed is therefore delicate, as equipoise must be achieved between the benefits to be derived from knowing the ICP versus the potential for morbidity and mortality attendant on device placement. Data regarding complication rates are of middling quality at best. Although there is no question that in some circumstances ICP monitoring provides treatment-altering and life-saving information, it is a sad fact that no systematic data are available for any clinical condition to help guide clinicians in judging when the benefits of monitor placement outweigh the risks.

Decision making with regard to which patients stand to benefit from ICP monitor placement can be difficult indeed. Generally, a device should be placed if (1) the condition leading to ICP elevation is amenable to treatment, (2) ongoing direct assessment of ICP will be of consequence in decisions regarding treatment interventions, and (3) the risks of device placement do not outweigh the potential benefits. If ventricular CSF drainage will be of instrumental use in decreasing ICP, then (4) a device with the capacity to drain CSF should be placed, again provided that the risks are not prohibitive. Most recent reviews *(10,14,47,56)* agree that the threshold for ICP monitor placement in the moderately to severely head injured patient is a GCS of 7–8 or less, or the presence of sufficient injury to other organ systems that either (a) aggressive treatment for hypotension or (b) endotracheal intubation are necessary *(10,14)*. There is general agreement that in the patient with subarachnoid hemorrhage, the development of hydrocephalus should prompt intraventricular catheter placement *(57,58)*. Few reviews offer good guidance regarding ICP monitor placement for any other condition listed in Table 1. In general, recommendations are offered by some that patients with a disease that is amenable to treatment have a monitor placed if the GCS is 7–8 or less *(10,57)*. In the end, the clinician must attempt to weigh considerations (a–d) for each patient. It is likely that with the further evolution of neurologic critical care, collective experience will permit the development of guidelines for other conditions.

Intraventricular Catheter (IVC)

The gold standard device for monitoring of ICP is a hollow catheter inserted through a burr hole, across the meninges and the brain, and into the cerebral ventricle *(14,56)*. A pressure transducer at the extracranial end of the device measures the pressure exerted through the catheter by the CSF. Because fluids convey pressure well, the CSF pressure thus measured can be regarded as representing the average pressure of the intracranial contents. The inherent accuracy of this arrangement makes the intraventricular catheter the "gold standard" of ICP monitoring devices. Its other chief advantage is the capability to drain CSF. As will be discussed, CSF drainage can be a potent means of decreasing ICP. However, there are several disadvantages to the IVC. If the lateral ventricle is collapsed, it cannot be placed. At 1–6%, it has the highest risk of hemorrhage of any of the devices; hemorrhage typically occurs at the time of insertion but can be delayed, and it can occur in subdural, intraparenchymal or ventricular spaces *(56)*. Lastly, infection can occur in any of the spaces through which the catheter passes—skin wound infection, calvarial osteomyelitis, subdural empyema, meningitis, parenchymal abscess, or ventriculitis *(56)*. Infection rates of 2–22% have been reported for intraventricular catheters *(59–61)*. The available literature is equivocal with regards to whether the prophylactic use of antibiotics–in usual clinical practice an antistaphylococcal penicillin (e.g., nafcillin)—consistently reduces the chances of infection *(60–62)*. Prophylactic antibiotics nonetheless remain standard practice for many clinicians. Most patient series consistently show few infections earlier than 3 d after catheter insertion, with most occurring after 5 d or later *(59, 60, 63)*. This led to the recommendation that any catheter required for longer than 5 d be replaced *(56,60)*. More recent data, however, do not indicate any decrease in the infection rate resulting from such "prophylactic" catheter exchange *(64)*, and also appear to show that while infection rates continue to rise from d 5 through d 10, infection after d 10 is rare. The most prudent course of action therefore is to maintain scrupulously sterile technique with intraventricular catheters, and to remove them as soon as possible, with no exchanges of new catheters for old. Flushing of catheters increases the risk of infection, and should be avoided *(60,61)*.

Parenchymal Catheters

The commercially available Camino catheter, also inserted through a burr hole and then the meninges, can be passed into either brain parenchyma or the lateral ventricle *(65)*. A fiberoptic transducer measures the pressure at the tip of the catheter. A similar parenchymally placed catheter with a strain-gauge transducer in the tip is also available *(66)*. The chief disadvantage of these devices is the inability to withdraw CSF. Other disadvantages are a tendency for pressure readings to "drift" over time; susceptibility to pressure gradients across brain tissue, when inserted into parenchyma; and risks of hemorrhage and infection similar to those of the IVC, with the exception that when passed only into parenchyma there is no risk of ventricular hemorrhage or ventriculitis. The chief potential advantage of these devices over the other non-IVC devices is a higher degree of accuracy of pressure measurements, but there are not enough data to substantiate this.

Subarachnoid Bolt

This device consists of a hollow saline-filled bolt which is screwed into a burr hole until its leading edges are flush to the dura *(67,68)*. With an incision in the dura at the opening of the lumen, the saline in the lumen is continuous with the CSF in the subarachnoid space; the fluid pressure in the bolt lumen is then taken to be equal to ICP. The chief advantages of this device are ease of insertion, much lower rates of hemorrhagic complication, and infectious complications in the range of only 2–7% *(59,61,69)*. Along with the inability to withdraw CSF, and questionable accuracy, an important limitation of this device in conditions of increased ICP is the possibility for swollen brain to herniate through the calvarial defect and occlude the lumen of the device. There is also a greater propensity to device occlusion than with intraventricular catheters *(70)*, necessitating device flushing, which increases the risk of infection *(61)*. Although this can be avoided by leaving the dura intact and thus assessing epidural and not subarachnoid pressure, this modification further decreases the accuracy of the device.

Epidural Device

Fiberoptic- and the strain-gauge–tipped catheters can also be placed into a pocket between the dura and the calvarium *(65,66)*. The chief advantage of such placement is a very low rate of hemorrhage and infection *(65,66)*; this comes at the cost of further tendency toward inaccuracy, and once again does not permit CSF drainage *(14)*.

Clinical Use of ICP Monitors

The simplest and most common use of ICP monitor data is assessment of the ICP itself, with titration of treatment to the concurrently measured pressure. Ideally, however, it would be preferable to anticipate ICP elevations before they happen, so that measures can be taken to prevent them. At any given time, the clinician would therefore prefer to know not only the instantaneous value of ICP, but also whether the intracranial system is in a state of normal or altered compliance (i.e., one would like to know not only the ICP, but the slope of the pressure-volume curve at that time).

The most straightforward means to assess concurrent intracranial compliance is visual examination of the ICP waveform, as discussed in Fig. 3. Merging of the P1 and P2 waves is highly suggestive of decreased compliance, and the potential for increases in ICP. Currently, visual inspection of waveforms may be the most widely utilized means of compliance assessment.

Efforts have been made at direct assessment of compliance. Miller and colleagues *(71–74)* demonstrated that the response of ICP to injection or withdrawal of a set amount of fluid through an intraventricular catheter could be used to assess compliance, and termed this change the volume-pressure response (VPR). In this paradigm, the greater the pressure change in response to a set change in volume, the lesser the intracranial compliance. This means of assessment has been standardized by means of the pressure-volume index (PVI), which is calculated as:

$$PVI_i = V_i / \log(P_p/P_0)$$

where: V_i = injected volume;
          P_p = peak ICP after injection; and
          P_0 = initial ICP before injection *(56)*.

PVI_w can also be defined as the equivalent value when a volume of fluid is withdrawn to derive it, and tends to be a lower and hence less accurate assessment of the true value *(56)*. Based as it is on logarithmic values, the PVI expresses the volume that must be injected into (or withdrawn from) the system in order to change the ICP by one log (a factor of 10), and hence it is not intuitively appealing. However, it does permit standardization for different values of injected or withdrawn fluid, and it permits establishment of normal ranges—PVI values greater than 20 mL indicate normal compliance, between 20 and 15 mL decreasing compliance, and less than 15 mL significantly decreased compliance. The PVI itself has subsequently been modified into a direct expression of compliance: $C = 0.4343(PVI/P_0)$ *(75)*. For various reasons, however, these means to assess compliance have not become standard practice—the degree of accuracy and reproducibility is disappointingly low, and the necessary manipulation of CSF through the intraventricular catheter increases risk of infection and entails a risk of precipitation of plateau waves *(56,60,61)*. One modification involves the use of extremely small volumes (0.5 mL), with a square-wave injection-withdrawal method, the short pulse response (SPR) *(76)*; another involves the use of a double-lumen device with similarly small volumes of injection *(77)*. Although no such direct assessment has yet been proven both reproducible and safe, there is no doubt that such a clinical tool would be highly useful; it is to be hoped that continued research in this area will bear fruit.

CBF MONITORING: BRIEF OVERVIEW

As discussed previously, the predominant final common pathway of brain injury in states of altered intracranial dynamics is ischemia. The ideal parameter to monitor to prevent such damage, then, would be regional CBF. A variety of means are available for such assessment *(78)*. Each available means of assessment, however, has significant limitations. The only currently available technique that provides information about the adequacy of specific regional blood flow is PET scanning, which is only available at a few academic centers. As discussed previously, TCD can be used to follow the velocity of blood flow in the basal intracranial arteries; the other commonly used techniques, Xenon clearance/Xenon CT and jugular venous oxygen saturation ($SjvO_2$) monitoring, are discussed in Chapters 3 and 6, respectively.

INTERVENTIONS

This section will review the various therapeutic interventions at the clinician's disposal in treating the patient with potential or realized cerebral edema and/or intracranial hypertension. Two fundamental questions must be kept in mind at every phase of care of a patient with potential brain edema or elevated ICP—whether an invasive ICP monitor is necessary and if the patient should be taken to the operating room for craniotomy. Surgical treatments will therefore be discussed first in this chapter. They are on occasion definitive, dramatically decreasing the need for further medical interventions; there are many circumstances in which no amount of medical management will achieve normalization of ICP while a space-occupying mass remains in place; and a consideration of surgical treatment can be much briefer than a discussion of the many medical measures available to the clinician. Lest this secondary placement of medical treatment be misconstrued, it must be reinforced that in most patients who have a lesion excised to control ICP, the principles of general medical management outlined here must be scrupulously followed in the perioperative and postoperative period if the full benefits of surgery are to be realized.

Surgical Interventions

Resection of Source of Mass Effect

If ICP is elevated because of a space-occupying lesion, no amount of medical intervention will satisfactorily normalize it; intracranial masses producing elevated ICP must be resected. Epidural hematoma, with bleeding into the epidural space under arterial pressure, has the potential to compromise CPP profoundly and precipitously, and evacuation is a hyperacute surgical emergency *(79)*. Acute subdural hematoma collects less rapidly and under less pressure, but what data are available are highly suggestive that surgical evacuation within 4 h improves outcome *(80)*. Brain abscess must be drained or resected to relieve mass effect *(81–84)*. Pneumocephalus must be evacuated if it is under sufficient tension to increase ICP. Spontaneous intracerebral hemorrhage is controversial; while most surgeons will elect for surgical drainage, it is far from clear from the available literature that this approach improves outcomes *(85,86; see* Chapter 19 for further discussion). Decision making regarding brain tumors is complex, taking into account the number and location of space-occupying lesions, and the expected response of the tumor type to chemotherapy and radiation; for reasons of space, this issue will not be discussed further.

CSF Drainage

It has been known for some time that extrinsic drainage of CSF can be a highly potent means to control elevated ICP. As discussed previously, an increase in the resistance to resorption of CSF (R_o) is probably, to a greater or lesser degree, part of the pathophysiology in most conditions that increase ICP *(45,46)*. Direct CSF drainage in effect decreases R_o.

INTRAVENTRICULAR CSF DRAINAGE

In standard clinical practice, CSF drainage has generally been accomplished via intraventricular catheter. This approach permits the conceptually and technically straightforward approach of draining CSF at any set pressure "above head level"—i.e., the threshold of CSF drainage is set manometrically (usually 20–25 cm CSF above the approximate level of the foramen of Monro), such that so long as catheter pressure exceeds this threshold and the system remains patent, CSF continues to drain. An intraventicular catheter is also the only appropriate intervention if obstructive hydrocephalus is present. As discussed previously, however, intraventricular catheters have a higher complication rate than other available ICP monitoring devices. Moreover, in some cases of ICP elevation, particularly those owing to head trauma, collapse of the ventricle due to parenchymal swelling may render catheter placement impossible.

LUMBAR CSF DRAINAGE

Several recent publications have drawn attention to an alternate means of CSF drainage, the lumbar drain *(87–89)*. Commonly utilized to produce a below-normal CSF pressure in order to decrease the incidence of CSF fistulae in cranial base surgeries *(90,91)*, these reports have focused instead on normalizing elevated CSF pressure. From the conceptual standpoint of decreasing R_o, the location from which CSF is drained matters little, and lumbar cistern catheter placement does not carry with it the same intracranial hemorrhagic risks as does intracranial catheter placement.

The most obvious potential adverse result of draining CSF from the spinal cistern is the precipitation of foraminal impaction of the cerebellar tonsils, uncal herniation over the tentorium, or the induction of severe spinal cord compression at an area of spondylotic narrowing with previously mild compression ("spinal coning"). While the total number of patients in these reports is low, such an effect did not occur in any of the reports, which drew on a population of head-injured and post-SAH patients *(87–89)*. The authors universally minimized the chances of such an event by using drainage only for patients in whom the basal cisterns were present and open on head CT. No cases of herniation were reported in the two reported series of patients treated with continuous lumbar CSF drainage *(91,92)*; however, of the 91 total patients so treated, a minority had conditions potentially consistent with elevation of ICP, and no ICP data are reported. Noteworthy complications in these reports include two cases of reversible vocal cord paralysis attributed to vagus nerve rootlet traction, a PCA distribution stroke attributed to PCA impaction on the tentorial edge, and a partial cauda equina syndrome with urinary retention that resolved after CSF catheter removal. It is also noteworthy that collectively, these series report 12 cases of meningitis complicating lumbar drains; in both series, prophylactic antibiotics were not utilized. Two patients died: aspiration pneumonia developed in 1 patient with vocal cord paralysis, and hepatic failure developed in 1 patient with meningitis. Minor complications were quite common: headache (26/91) and radicular pain (7/91), in particular. Lumbar CSF drainage would therefore appear to be fairly safe, in these series; however, few of the patients reported likely had elevated ICP, and two deaths did occur. To our knowledge, there is only one series available reporting simultaneous intraventricular and lumbar CSF pressures, recorded both before and after lumbar CSF drainage in patients with subarachnoid hemorrhage (SAH) *(93)*. These authors found that in 13 of 14 patients so evaluated, ventricular and lumbar CSF pressures were nearly equal both before and after lumbar CSF withdrawal. In the fourteenth patient, however, ventricular pressure after lumbar withdrawal was unchanged vs before, despite lumbar pressure having decreased by

19 cm H_2O. This report sounds a note of caution—when utilizing lumbar CSF drainage, careful attention should be paid that intracranial pressure is comparable to lumbar pressure or appropriately responsive to drainage from the lumbar cistern. Whether because of intracranial herniation at the tentorial hiatus or foramen magnum, spondyloarthropathic compression of the thecal sac in the spinal canal, or inflammatory obstruction of the subarachnoid space, subarachnoid block does occur, and its presence must be ruled out if lumbar CSF drainage is to be utilized safely and effectively.

Other reports of this approach to patients with ICP elevation are few. Two patient series do report the use of lumbar CSF drainage for cryptococcal meningitis with signs of ICP elevation *(94,95)*, and found the technique safe and effective. A cautionary note was sounded by another report of SAH patients, in which continuous CSF drainage was associated with an increased incidence of delayed ischemic deficits and shunt-dependent hydrocephalus. The technique in this series involved deliberate induction of CSF hypotension by overdrainage of CSF, and it thus seems likely that drainage to maintain CSF normotension should not be considered contraindicated for SAH patients on the basis of this report; induction of hypotension, in contrast, should be carefully avoided. Regarding to the laboratory evaluation of CSF so obtained, it has recently been demonstrated that CSF obtained from the lumbar space yields nearly the same erythrocyte and leukocyte count and differential when compared to simultaneous samples from the intraventricular space; glucose is only one-fifth lower in the lumbar than in the ventricular CSF *(96)*. Lumbar CSF can thus be regarded as interchangeable with ventricular CSF when assessing for meningitis.

At this time, pending publication of a sizable series of patients so treated, lumbar CSF drainage remains an attractive alternative whose relative risks and benefits remain ill-characterized. However, it is worth noting that the very same criticism can be justly made of ventricular catheters. A cautious approach to its use is appropriate, given the catastrophic consequences should herniation be induced. Spinal block should be carefully evaluated for and ruled out, and drainage should be titrated if possible to directly measured ICP, to avoid overdrainage and the induction of CSF hypotension. Provided these precautions are kept in mind, lumbar CSF drainage can be a useful tool in control of ICP.

Craniectomy

Possibly the most radical intervention for intracranial hypertension, the surgical removal of part of the calvarium creates a window in the cranial vault, negating the Monro-Kellie doctrine of fixed intracranial volume and allowing for herniation of swollen brain through the window to relieve pressure. Although described at least as early as the first decade of the twentieth century *(97)*, consistently poor outcomes led to its being regarded as a futile exercise *(98)*. A large number of reports since 1990 have revisited this issue, studying its use for treatment-refractory intracranial hypertension in head injury *(99–105)* and for large, space-occupying hemispheric stroke *(106–109)*. The approach in these trials has been the removal of a calvarial bone flap extending from above the orbit anteriorly to a few centimeters from the occipital pole posteriorly, and from near the midline medially to the vicinity of the floor of the middle cranial fossa near the origin of the zygoma laterally, thus creating a very large fenestration. The head-injury series have reported outcomes similar to or slightly better than historical norms, and outcomes in the stroke series appear similarly optimistic. To date, however, no trial has yet been reported for either condition which has randomized similar patients to either receive surgery or not. It is therefore impossible to know with certainty that this risky and highly expensive measure actually improves outcomes. Until such publication, it could be argued that hemicraniectomy should remain an experimental procedure; in some centers, however, sufficient experience has accrued that hemicraniectomy is beginning to become standard practice. Unfortunately for those patients and physicians not in these centers, insufficient formal evaluation of this technique has yet been published to offer good guidelines for its use.

Medical Interventions

General Cardiopulmonary and Metabolic Support

There are several principles of general patient care that should be scrupulously applied in all cases of manifest or impending intracranial hypertension. These measures are undertaken with the intent to avoid precipitating or exacerbating increased ICP, and should be followed fastidiously; in any patient with decompensated ICP requiring acute intervention, it is also worthwhile reviewing to these general principles of medical support to ensure that none have been overlooked. These guidelines are largely based on an understanding of the pathophysiology of deranged intracranial dynamics as discussed previously, but many are supported by patient data as well.

HEMODYNAMICS

Understanding of cerebral autoregulation dictates a few general guidelines that should be followed with regard to volume status and blood pressure management. In any patient with deranged intracranial dynamics, systemic hypotension must be avoided if at all possible. In a patient with elevated ICP and intact autoregulation, the vasodilatory response to decreased MAP will increase CBV and possibly precipitate a plateau wave *(42)*. In a patient with regional or global failure of autoregulation, hypotension will produce decreased CBF and ischemia. Some *(39,56)* have recommended pharmacologic elevation of MAP in all patients with elevated ICP, reasoning that elevated MAP will provoke vasoconstriction, decreased CBV, and a resulting drop in ICP. There is one head injury trial that appears to lend some support to such an approach *(110)*. There is a theoretical risk, however, that elevating intravascular pressure will exacerbate edema formation if the BBB is ruptured. It seems prudent, therefore, to use pharmacologic elevation of MAP only if an ICP monitor demonstrates a favorable response to a trial of a vasopressor.

Hypertension should only be pharmacologically lowered if there is reasonable clinical suspicion that it is directly responsible for deleterious consequences (hypertensive encephalopathy, retinal damage or renal damage), and then only if the lowering does not produce cerebral ischemia. Whenever possible, the vasodilating agents (nitroglycerin, nitroprusside and hydralazine) should be avoided because they directly dilate cerebral vasculature, potentially exacerbating cerebral hyperemia; labetolol is typically considered the agent of first choice for lowering blood pressure *(39)*.

Maintenance of normal to slightly elevated blood pressure dictates maintenance of normal to slightly expanded intravascular volume. This should be accomplished with isotonic fluids only, preferably 0.9% normal saline. Hypotonic fluids should be strictly avoided because the free water fraction of any such fluid is free to pass out of the intravascular space into the brain and thus contribute to cerebral edema. The only exception to this rule is the case of reversal of hypernatremia, which should be undertaken only when cerebral edema and intracranial hypertension are sufficiently controlled to permit it, and then in a slow gradual fashion with a few hundred milliliters of free water in each day's total fluids.

These are the general principles of fluid management that should be applied to all patients with or at risk of increased ICP. The deliberate use of hypertonic solutions is a separate matter, discussed in the Hypertonic Saline section.

GLUCOSE

In ischemic stroke patients, hyperglycemia has been associated with a three times greater likelihood of poor outcome (regardless of whether the patient was previously diabetic or not) *(111–113)*, is correlated with larger stroke size *(114)*, and is an independent predictor of intracranial hemorrhage complicating intra-arterial thrombolysis *(115)*. It is an independent predictor of poor outcome in subarachnoid hemorrhage *(116)*, and meningitis *(117)*. Hyperglycemia is also correlated with worse outcomes in head-injured patients *(118–120)*. Investigation in intracranial hemorrhage has yielded conflicting results *(110,121)*.

These observational data have been taken as evidence that control of hyperglycemia is advisable in cerebrovascular patients particularly in the neurocritically ill. Data to support an improvement in outcome with an aggressive treatment approach to control serum glucose, however, are weak. A recent trial has reported significantly improved outcome in unselected intensive care patients who received an insulin drip titrated to maintain euglycemia *(122)*. Unfortunately, whereas 20% of the patient sample consisted of neurologically ill patients (mostly head injury and postcraniotomy), results were not independently reported for this subset. We are unaware of any similar trial of aggressive control of serum glucose in the neurocritically ill. Although it is reasonable to surmise that controlling serum glucose is highly likely to improve outcomes, this cannot be considered proven, and it is unclear what treatment approach (insulin drip, scheduled insulin, oral hypoglycemics, and so on) offers the best risk-benefit ratio. If an aggressive treatment approach is pursued, the clinician must take special care not to induce hypoglycemia, which could be disastrous to an already diseased brain.

TEMPERATURE

Fever is an expected feature of infectious conditions of the central nervous system (CNS). In other etiologies of deranged intracranial dynamics, systemic responses to infection or inflammation elsewhere in the body can have a significantly deleterious effect on the intracranial process. Patient data indicate larger stroke size and a worse outcome with fever in patients with ischemic stroke *(123,124)*, and worse outcomes in SAH *(125)*, diffuse anoxic injury *(126)*, and intracerebral hemorrhage *(121)*.

With fever as with hyperglycemia, these observational data, coupled with animal model data *(127,128)*, have been interpreted as supporting an imperative to treat. Far and away, the most frequently utilized means in the United States is acetaminophen; typical usage is 325–650 mg by mouth or rectum q4h as needed for fever. The high degree of safety of acetaminophen in routine clinical use would likely render unethical any placebo-controlled trial to demonstrate an improved outcome with its use for fever. Unfortunately, little study has yet been given to what constitutes optimal use of this agent, and whether other approaches would produce better outcomes. A single pilot study in patients with acute stroke has shown that patients randomized to 1 g of acetaminophen scheduled four times daily enterically or rectally had a substantially lower risk of developing fever over the ensuing 5 d than did patients given placebo *(129)*. In those who remain febrile despite acetaminophen, a small number may respond to an air-circulating cooling blanket *(130)*. Currently, further measures in such patients, whether other antipyretic agents might be of greater efficacy, and whether any approach to antipyresis actually produces improved patient outcome are all subjects still in need of clarification.

The therapeutic use of induced hypothermia is another matter entirely, and shall be discussed in the section that follows.

NUTRITION

Prompt institution and maintenance of nutritional support is obligatory in patients with critical neurological illnesses; this is amply covered in Chapter 14 and is not further discussed here. However, it must be reiterated that special care should be taken to ensure that the osmotic content of all nutritional fluids should be such that there is no net administration of free water between enteral feedings, parenteral feedings and other intravenous fluids.

VENTILATORY SUPPORT

Many patients with serious intracranial diseases require intubation (*see also* Chapter 9). Any patient with a GCS score less than 8 should be intubated for airway protection, as should any patient requiring general anesthesia for control of ICP. Intubation should also be pursued in any patient with intercurrent pulmonary disease—(e.g., acute respiratory distress syndrome (ARDS) or pulmonary contusion acquired concurrently with head trauma, pneumococcal pneumonia intercurrent with meningitis, aspiration pneumonia subsequent to depressed level of consciousness or impaired pharyngeal control, etc.). Given the potential for hypercarbia and hypoxia to precipitate intracranial hypertension in patients with decreased compliance (or exacerbate it when already established), any patient at risk for elevated ICP should be intubated expectantly when the development of respiratory distress is anticipated.

Optimal ventilatory management in these patients has not been evaluated prospectively. However, on the basis of physiologic understanding and a few key observations that have been reported fairly consistently by multiple observers, a few guidelines can be offered.

The chief concern regarding to endotracheally delivered positive-pressure ventilation is the potential for elevation of central venous pressure with resulting inhibition of cerebral venous drainage, thus increasing ICP. After an initial report of just such a result in severely head-injured patients receiving positive end-expiratory pressure (PEEP) more than 10 cm H_2O *(19)*, subsequent reports in both head-injured *(131)* and SAH patients *(132)* have verified a slight increase in ICP with PEEP greater than 5 but have shown no clinical deterioration or other apparent deleterious consequences from this effect. Both of these studies documented an increase in MAP paralleling ICP, thus maintaining CPP greater than 60. It is therefore likely safe to use PEEP of up to 10 cm H_2O routinely when necessary to optimize oxygenation, and it may be safe up to 15 cm H_2O with careful direct observation to verify no adverse consequences. The guidelines offered are based on results reported from a total of 78 patients, all but 9 of whom had head trauma as the underlying disease process. In any individual patient, therefore, the effect of PEEP on ICP and CPP should be titrated on the basis of direct observation via pressure monitor, if possible.

Another source of concern in ventilated patients is the potential for coughing (spontaneous or induced by endotracheal suctioning) to produce spikes in ICP. Presuctioning endobronchial lidocaine *(56)* or increased sedation may be effective if such surges in ICP are encountered. If these measures prove ineffective, pharmacologic paralysis is an option *(39)*. These suggestions are entirely untested and empiric.

The deliberate use of hyperventilation as a specific therapeutic modality is discussed in the section that follows.

PATIENT POSITIONING

Elevation of the head, by decreasing CSF hydrostatic pressure and facilitating venous blood drainage, decreases ICP in normal humans *(17)* and in patients with head injury *(113)*. The robustness of the finding has led most practitioners to generalize its use, and recommend that patients with decreased intracranial compliance be positioned with the head elevated 30 degrees *(39,47,56)*. There is a single report of a few patients in whom such positioning actually increased ICP *(134)*. In this report, however, there were no patients whose ICP was observed to increase from below 20 cm H_2O supine to above 20 cm H_2O at an inclination of 60 degrees (that used by the authors). It is therefore likely safe to recommend the following approach: patients with some degree of suspected impairment of intracranial compliance but with insufficient indications for placement of an ICP monitoring device should be positioned at 30 degrees head elevation empirically; in patients with a monitoring device in place, the response of ICP to head elevation can be directly observed, and those few who have a higher ICP with head up can be positioned wherever ICP is the lowest.

Also of importance is that if at all possible no constricting garments or devices should encircle the neck (endotracheal tube tape, for example), as such items have the potential to compress the internal jugular veins and retard cerebral venous drainage. By the same token, the patient should be positioned with the head facing straight forward, as the head when turned to one side with the neck flexed can compress the internal jugular vein on that side. Although not prospectively evaluated, these measures are easily undertaken and we have seen them produce significant effects on ICP in a few patients.

ANTICONVULSANTS

The systemic hypoxia, hemodynamic alterations and cerebral autoregulatory derangements that accompany seizures can produce real harm in some patients with increased ICP. Many practitioners therefore use prophylactic phenytoin therapy, particularly in patients with head trauma *(135)*, SAH *(136)*, intracranial hemorrhage *(85)*, and other conditions. Data are available to validate prophylactic anticonvulsant therapy only in the case of traumatic brain injury, for the first 2 wk after injury only *(135)*; when such prophylaxis should be discontinued in the head-injured is a matter of great controversy *(137)*. Prophylactic use of phenytoin in patients with brain tumors does produce a decreased risk of seizures, but at an unacceptable cost in adverse effects *(138)*. There are no good data to support the prophylactic use of anticonvulsants for any other condition. Current clinical practice in many centers is to use anticonvulsants prophylactically regardless of the lack of supporting data.

ANTIBIOTICS

Empiric antibiotics are frequently used in trauma patients when there is an appreciable clinical risk of wound infections from the initial injury. Their use for patients with intracranial ICP monitoring devices is discussed in the Direct ICP Monitoring section.

Specific Interventions

In patients with elevations of ICP sufficient to produce or threaten ischemia or herniation, there are a limited number of medical interventions which can sufficiently reduce intracranial volume to lower ICP and prevent or ameliorate tissue damage. Their proper use depends on the clinical context and an understanding of the time frame over which they have their effect and how large that effect can be.

HYPERVENTILATION

As discussed previously, decreased carbon dioxide tension is a potent constricting stimulus to cerebral arteries. Decrease in CO_2 tension by 10 mmHg can produce sufficient reduction in CBV to effect a profound decrease in ICP. Unfortunately, this effect has several limitations. It may produce sufficient decrease in CBF to induce ischemia *(139)*. The constrictive effect on cerebral arterioles lasts a matter of 10–20 h, over which time cerebral arterioles redilate, possibly to a larger caliber than at baseline *(140)*; the initial reduction in CBV from hyperventilation thus comes at the cost of a possible rebound phase with *increased* ICP. Maintenance of deliberate respiratory alkalosis for a sustained time has been convincingly shown to worsen outcome in head injury patients *(141)*; even repeated serial episodes of hyperventilation may have deleterious consequences *(110)*. Although these results have not been replicated in other disease states, recognition of the temporary efficacy of this measure and its demonstrated potential adverse effects suggest that its use be limited to emergent situations in which there is an expectation of more definitive treatment to supercede in the near future. That is, hyperventilation is likely best used as a short-term measure, as a "bridge" to more definitive therapy *(142,143)*, never as a sustained therapy to be maintained for longer than a few hours at most. The best example of this use would be in a patient with an intracranial mass (hematoma, abscess) and signs of herniation, with use of hyperventilation during the time from recognition of the emergency to surgical evacuation of the mass; another example would be hyperventilation at the onset of a plateau wave while mannitol and barbiturates are being obtained and then administered. This approach, however, is not universal; despite the adverse outcomes demonstrated by Muizelaar and associates *(141)* with sustained hyperventilation, many practitioners still use it, even in head injury patients *(144,145)*. We recommend strongly against it.

Most authors agree that when hyperventilation is instituted, the goal should be lowering the pCO_2 by 10 mmHg, to approx 30 mmHg *(39,56,146)*. The best means by which to accomplish this is not known. Bingaman and Frank suggest tidal volumes of 12–15 cc/kg with a rate of 12–14/min *(47)*; Marshall and Mayer suggest rates of 16–20/min without specifying tidal volume *(146)*. All agree that hypocarbia once induced should be reversed slowly, with recommendations ranging from 6–24 h *(39,47,146)*, to minimize the rebound hyperemia of re-equilibration.

OSMOTHERAPY AND DIURETICS

Mannitol. Mannitol is the most widely used of a class of compounds intended to act as osmotic diuretics. The mechanism of action of the class is to increase serum osmolarity with a compound that has a high coefficient of reflection at the BBB, producing an osmotic gradient from the interstitial to the intravascular compartment, and thus pulling water out of the tissue. There is little doubt that brain dehydration, mainly from normal brain, is the predominant effect by which mannitol lowers ICP *(147,148)*. In the kidney, mannitol is filtered by the nephron, but unabsorbed by renal tubules; it then acts as an osmole in the lumen of the collecting duct, preventing resorption of water, producing a diuresis, and passing unmetabolized out of the body. Mannitol can therefore be conceptualized as a direct conveyer of free water from the diseased or injured brain through the kidneys and out of the body.

Mannitol has other mechanisms of action, however. It appears that mannitol reduces blood viscosity, perhaps by rendering erythrocyte membranes more flexible *(149)*. It appears that this produces a transient increase in cerebral blood flow and cerebral blood volume, and a compensatory vasoconstriction with a net reduction in CBV *(150,151)*. Mannitol may also decrease the rate of CSF formation *(148)*. By multiple mechanisms, then, mannitol removes volume from the intracranial compartment, lowering ICP.

Mannitol is generally utilized in boluses of 0.5–1.5 g/kg to lower elevated ICP, or when ICP elevation is suspected, but emergent evaluations (e.g., head CT) are yet pending. Several precautions should be taken in its administration. A urinary catheter must be in place to prevent bladder distention. Rapid administration of a bolus can produce immediate hypotension *(152)*, so isotonic fluid and a vasopressor agent should be immediately at hand *(39)*. A robust diuretic response can produce intravascular hypovolemia with resulting hypotension and even renal failure. Unless the patient is hypervolemic and a diuresis is desired, isotonic volume replacement should be maintained on an ongoing basis. Mannitol depletes body potassium, magnesium, and phosphorus *(153)*, rapid diuresis can produce an acute hyperkalemia *(10)*, and long-term use can produce sufficient derangement of renal medullary concentration gradients that nephrogenic diabetes insipidus results *(21,56)*. ICP typically responds briskly to mannitol administration, but may rebound again in a few patients, typically after 30–120 min *(154)*, requiring a repeat dose or some other intervention. Lastly, mannitol will pass out of the intravascular compartment and into the interstitium in areas of BBB damage, and thus may have the capacity to exacerbate vasogenic edema if used over a sustained time *(155)*. The demonstration of this phenomenon in an animal model *(155)* has led many to recommend that mannitol be used only in periodic boluses, not in frequent small doses to maintain a constant hyperosmolar state *(156)*. However, the model in question has a possible methodological confound (a net positive fluid balance in the animals given multiple boluses), and this potential adverse effect has not been convincingly demonstrated in human patients. Many practitioners therefore still use repeated doses of mannitol to maintain a "steady state" serum osmolality of 300–310 mOsm when a sustained effect of brain dehydration is desired. Whether this approach achieves its desired ends cannot be answered with certainty.

Which disease states mannitol is likely to treat with the greatest efficacy is not an issue which is well-established in the literature. Prospective evaluations of the use of mannitol in specific disease states are almost nonexistent. Conceptually, the osmotic diuretic mechanism would be predicted to have the greatest efficacy in conditions wherein the BBB is uniformly intact, the entire brain retains its blood flow, all areas of mass effect also maintain intact capillary wall integrity and blood flow, and all excess fluid resides in the interstitial space. No such conditions exist. In the absence of hard data for guidance, the most judicious use of mannitol for intracranial hypertension would seem to be as follows: (1) Initiation of treatment only once elevated ICP is demonstrated or highly suspected (no "prophylactic" or expectant usage). (2) Fastidious avoidance of hypovolemia, hypotension, and electrolyte depletion via careful volume status monitoring, ongoing isotonic fluid replacement, continuous blood pressure monitoring, and frequent (every 6 h) electrolyte assessments with ongoing repletion. (3) Frequent (every 6 h) assessment of serum osmolarity when repeated doses used, with repeat doses adjusted to a target osmolarity of 300–310 mOsm with an upper limit of 320. (4) The clinician can be reasonably justified in trying mannitol for virtually any etiology of elevated ICP.

Also ill-addressed is whether mannitol has the potential to worsen outcomes in some conditions. In massive hemispheric ischemic stroke, for example, mannitol, which dehydrates vascularized tissue, might worsen herniation by dehydrating non-infarcted brain more than the infarct and causing greater tissue shift *(157,158)*; however, this effect has not been found when sought *(159)*. Until randomized prospective trials are undertaken of specific osmotic regimens for specific intracranial conditions, this issue will remain unresolved.

Other Osmotic Compounds. Other osmotic agents have been used to the same effect, but have in large part have been abandoned in clinical practice, at least in the United States. Glycerol, a simple triol, can be administered either orally or intravenously, and does produce a decrease in ICP similar in magnitude to that of mannitol; however, it is inferior to mannitol in several respects: it has a much more frequent and severe rebound effect, it frequently produces hyperglycemia, and it causes hemolysis when used in the clinically effective range *(154,160)*. Despite these drawbacks, there is a possibility it may after further study find use as a complement to mannitol *(161)*. Sorbitol, like mannitol, can only be administered intravenously, also produces hyperglycemia, and has a duration of action of only 1–2 h (vs mannitol's 4–6 h) *(160)*. Urea is only of historical interest; it has a profound rebound effect, it produces nausea, vomiting, and diarrhea, it can generate a significant coagulopathy, and extravasation produces tissue necrosis *(162)*.

Hypertonic Saline. Hypertonic saline has received considerable attention recently for its capacity to reduce elevated ICP. Hypertonic saline (HS) began being studied in the late 1980s as a resuscitation fluid for hemorrhagic shock, with the rationale that relative to fluid resuscitation with a given volume of isotonic fluid, the same volume of hypertonic fluid results in a much greater increase in intravascular volume by drawing water from tissue *(163,164)*. It became apparent that patients in early traumatic shock trials who also had head injury fared better when given HS *(165)*. While successful hemodynamic resuscitation is critical to survival and optimization of outcome in traumatic brain injury *(166)*, it appears that there is an effect independent of successful resuscitation *(165)*. The most obvious interpretation has been that HS dehydrates brain via the same osmotic mechanism attributed to mannitol; offered in support of this argument is that the reflection coefficient of brain capillaries for sodium is 1.0 (vs mannitol's 0.9) *(163,164)*. This has led to study of hypertonic saline for the full range of patients with intracranial hypertension and cerebral edema, not merely head injured ones.

While animal model experience is now relatively extensive and shows great promise *(164)*, publication of human subject trials is unfortunately quite limited. Several case series *(156,167–169)* have consistently reported that in patients with severe traumatic brain injury and ICP more than 25 mmHg refractory to standard supportive care, mannitol, and (in most patients) barbiturate coma, hypertonic saline boluses reduced ICP to within normal range. Whereas in the 24 brain-injured patients reported in these works the response rate was 100%, publication bias precludes assessment of true response rate in such circumstances. Two case series have reported the use of HS as a maintenance fluid to produce a constant hypertonic state. One reported experience with 8 head injured, 5 postcraniotomy, 8 intracerebral hemorrhage, and 6 ischemic stroke patients *(170)*, suggested that continuous infusion of HS to maintain serum sodium of 145–155 mmol/L is safe and effective at lowering ICP, although more so for TBI and post-op patients than for the two stroke groups. The second reported a case series of 68 selected pediatric head injury patients who received HS infusion titrated to whatever serum sodium was necessary to produce ICP less than 20 mmHg, as part of a protocol including head elevation, sedation, hyperventilation, mannitol, and barbiturates. The authors concluded that hypertonic saline appeared safe and effective in their patients. Only two clinical trials have been reported. The first reported in-the-field resuscitation of 34 adult head trauma patients randomized to either lactated Ringer's solution (LR) or hypertonic saline *(171)*. No differences in outcome were detected between the groups, and the HS treated patients required more treatment interventions; the study was confounded, however, by more severe degree of injury in the treatment group than the LR-treated placebo group, and the data did suggest efficacy against elevated ICP despite showing no improved outcome. The second trial reported 35 pediatric head trauma patients randomized to either LR or HS maintenance fluids over the first 72 h in hospital *(145)*; whereas no differences in ICP and no differences in mortality were detected, the HS-treated patients had shorter ICU stays, lower rates of infectious and metabolic complications and a lower rate of development of ARDS.

Hypertonic saline is not without potential adverse effects. Although the specter of central pontine myelinolysis occurs to many neurologic clinicians, this appears to be related to antecedent hyponatremia and has yet to be reported in traumatic shock or intracranial hypertension patients treated with HS. Subdural hemorrhage and seizures are also theoretical complications of sudden electrolyte shifts *(164)*, but also have not been reported; nor has a rebound effect on intracranial hypertension yet been observed. Theoretical systemic adverse effects include volume overload, renal failure, coagulopathy, hypokalemia, and hyperchloremic metabolic acidosis *(164)*; of these, only the first two have been observed in the reports discussed previously, but whether they were deliberately sought cannot be assessed with confidence.

In summary, hypertonic saline is a treatment modality which appears to show great promise for treatment of intracranial hypertension, but is likely "not quite ready for prime time." Although it appears that judicious approaches to its use, such as careful titration of the serum sodium to a slight degree of hypernatremia (e.g., 145–150 mmol/L), may produce salutary effects on ICP, even this use cannot yet be supported on the basis of the available literature. As has been observed elsewhere in this chapter, though, these same criticisms can be justly made of the accepted standard of care, to wit, mannitol. Given the robust response reported by several authors and the lack of reported complications, it does seem justifiable at this point to consider HS an option in patients with elevated ICP refractory to all other measures. Optimally, we would like to see trials that compare the use of NS to mannitol for various specific conditions.

Acetazolamide. Carbonic anhydrase inhibition at the choroid plexus, when accomplished with sufficiently high doses of acetazolamide, can produce greater than 99% reduction in the rate of production of CSF *(172)*; unfortunately, as the derangement in CSF dynamics (if any) in most instances is an increased resistance to resorption, acetazolamide produces little effect on increased ICP in most pathologic states *(13)*. The single exception appears to be pseudotumor cerebri, which is rarely life-threatening. Recent negative results of trials of acetazolamide and furosemide for hydrocephalus after intraventricular hemorrhage in infants reinforce this view *(173–175)*.

Loop Diuretics. Loop diuretics are considered to be a therapeutic option for intracranial hypertension by some *(47,56)*, but not by others *(10,14,21,175)*. All authorities agree that loop diuretics are of minimal use when used alone *(47,56,176)*. Furosemide when co-administered with mannitol certainly produces a more profound diuresis *(177)*; it may act as a carbonic anhydrase inhibitor at the choroid, potentially decreasing CSF production *(172)*. Whether these mechanisms produce a more effective dehydration of brain, and if so for what duration, is unknown *(176)*. It seems reasonable to consider loop diuretics an option in patients with impaired myocardial contractility, who may respond poorly to the increased myocardial work resulting from the increased intravascular volume of a bolus of mannitol or hypertonic saline; however, their use alone or as a routine adjunct to hypertonic agents cannot be recommended. When they are used, meticulous care must be taken to ensure that hypovolemia does not ensue.

STEROIDS

While their underlying physiologic mechanisms of action remain an area of unresolved inquiry *(178)*, it is a fact of clinical certainty that glucocorticoids have potent efficacy against the cerebral edema associated with tumors. Contrary to the therapeutic enthusiasm that followed that discovery, however, it appears that their use is minimally beneficial or actually harmful when used for most of the other diagnoses listed previously.

Glucocorticoids are clearly beneficial to patients with intracranial tumors, both primary and metastatic. Focal neurological signs and decreased mental status due to surrounding edema typically begin to improve within hours *(179)*; increased ICP, when present, decreases over the following 2–5 d, in some cases to normal *(180,181)*. The exact cellular mechanisms by which peritumoral vasogenic edema is reduced remain unknown. The most commonly utilized regimen is intravenous dexamethasone, 4 mg every 6 h, but methylprednisolone can be substituted. Dose is often titrated to response. Decision making with regard to timing of excision is beyond the purview of this book, and the interested reader is referred to textbooks of oncologic neurosurgery.

The nearest comparable condition to brain tumor is brain abscess, in which a mass lesion is surrounded by vasogenic edema; however, the therapeutic usefulness of steroids for abscess is unclear. Experimental results demonstrate no improved outcome, nor do they show alteration in parameters which would be expected to improve outcome *(182–184)*; though these studies have not assessed ICP. A single small but well-reasoned radiologic report does suggest that steroids can reduce the amount of edema surrounding the abscess capsule *(185)*; extrapolation from the literature would suggest that this could translate into decreased ICP, but data are lacking. No trials have been done. Some authors argue that reducing peri-abscess inflammation with steroids may worsen outcome by decreasing delivery of antibiotics to the infected area *(186,187)*. Many authors *(81–84)* therefore recommend that if steroids are to be used at all, they be reserved for cases in which mass effect is producing life-threatening herniation, and that they be weaned off as soon as possible. In all cases, steroids are most certainly a mere adjunct to definitive antibiotic and surgical management (*see* discussion in Chapter 29).

A similar state of affairs exists with neurocysticercosis: no trial data are available, and there are arguments to be made both for and against the use of glucocorticoids *(188)*. Given this state of affairs, it seems prudent to reserve steroid use to patients with a high lesion load in whom the pericystic edema is sufficient to produce elevated ICP or a dangerous degree of herniation. As with bacterial abscess, surgically remediable situations (particularly, obstructive hydrocephalus) should be treated appropriately, and definitive antiparasitic treatment initiated as soon as possible (*see* Chapter 29).

Postinfectious encephalitis has been reported to respond favorably to steroids in some cases *(189)*; more systematic evaluation is needed. Multiple reports of treatment of herpes simplex virus (HSV) encephalitis with high-dose corticosteroids were made in the early 1970s *(190–192)*, and arguments have been made both for and against conceptual grounds. The controlled trials to answer the issue have never been carried out. Multiple subsequent reports of HSV encephalitis precipitated by steroid treatment have quelled enthusiasm for their use in less severely affected patients, and most modern authors who advocate their use do so only for patients in whom ICP is thought to be critically elevated *(193–194)*. The best evidence available comes from Whitley and associates' trial comparing vidarabine to acyclovir for HSV encephalitis *(195)*. Approximately one-third of patients in each treatment group received steroids, and a regression model found that steroid treatment did not contribute significantly to outcome (i.e., steroids neither helped nor hurt). No analysis was done, however, on the subset of patients with low GCS, who were most likely to have a large degree of swelling and hence raised ICP; therefore, even these data do not bear on the question as to whether the sickest of the sick would have anything to gain from steroid treatment. The clinician is therefore left to make his or her best guess, with no data for guidance.

Extensive study has been given to the use of steroids for meningitis *(196–201)*. It is clear that they decrease the frequency of deafness and other neurologic deficits in children (and possibly also in adults, though this is less clear). For reasons of improved neurologic outcome, therefore, corticosteroids are now standard of care in pediatric meningitis patients, and an option in adults (*see* Chapter 29). However, it is important to note that mortality rates have been unchanged in studies to date.

The best evidence available strongly suggests that there is no benefit from glucocorticoids in traumatic brain injury *(202,203)*, intracerebral hemorrhage *(204)*, or ischemic stroke *(205–208)*. While there are reports of high-dose steroids preventing vasospasm in SAH *(209–211)*, this use can only be regarded as experimental until a properly conducted trial is published.

For some of the other conditions listed Table 1, the use of glucocorticoids is advocated by some authors with very little in the way of supportive evidence available (*see* the High-Altitude Cerebral Edema section). Until better studies are published, we advise extreme judiciousness in their use for conditions other than brain tumors and possibly the various infectious conditions already discussed. The potential deleterious consequences of their use—hyperglycemia, agitation, peptic ulcers, immunosuppression, wound breakdown—dictate that they be utilized only when there is confidence that they will produce an improvement in outcome. Steroids were used widely and confidently for both ischemic stroke and head injury until well-conducted trials demonstrated no benefit. This experience should dictate a skeptical view toward their use in other conditions for which supportive evidence is lacking.

ANESTHESIA

Barbiturates. Although it took years to gain in popularity from its introduction in the late 1960s, generalized anesthesia with "barbiturate coma" has become an accepted option in the treatment of intracranial hypertension. The putative mechanism behind the decrease in ICP induced by barbiturates is a reduction in cerebral metabolic activity, leading to reduced CBF and CBV *(212,213)*. There is little doubt that in most patients, induction of barbiturate anesthesia produces an immediate drop in ICP, sometimes profound. What is far less certain is in which patients are their ultimate outcome improved by the intervention.

The clinical circumstance for which barbiturate coma is most supportable is head trauma. Eisenberg and associates' 1988 trial of pentobarbital for severe head injury established with reasonable certainty that induction of barbiturate coma has the potential to improve outcomes in a selected subpopulation of these patients *(214)*. In light of the negative results of other trials *(215,216)* in which barbiturates were used on a prophylactic basis, together with reported experiences of nonrandomized patient series *(212,217)*, the best balance between benefit from lowered ICP and the adverse effects of barbiturates themselves (discussed in this section below) can be accomplished by selecting TBI patients with a GCS score of less than 8 but more than 3, who have demonstrated sustained ICP greater than 20 despite excision of mass lesions (e.g., hematoma), head elevation, sedation, hypertonic therapy, and CSF drainage if possible. The only effective gauge of therapeutic response is continuous EEG monitoring, with titration of dose to a burst-suppression pattern; further dose increases to the point of electrocerebral silence appear to produce minimal further beneficial effect on ICP with added risk of adverse effects *(213,214)*.

There is little to be gained from barbiturate coma in circumstances of mass effect such as tumor, abscess or hematoma, which require excision or drainage. This surgical imperative has essentially precluded formal evaluation of barbiturates in these conditions. Massive hemispheric stroke, which produces a volume of devitalized swollen tissue, also appears to respond poorly to barbiturates *(212,218)*, which only decrease CBV of noninfarcted tissue. Fulminant hepatic failure, by contrast, may represent a pathology in which decreased cerebral metabolism has the potential to produce improved outcome (*see* Fulminant Hepatic Failure section). There is little available in the literature regarding the treatment of any other conditions with barbiturates, and defensible recommendations therefore cannot be made.

The adverse effects of barbiturate therapy are a significant limiting factor in their therapeutic use. Barbiturates produce an immediate and sustained depressive effect on systemic arterial blood pressure, which frequently necessitates vasopressor support if adverse consequences to CPP are to be avoided *(56,214)*; they also can produce myocardial suppression, which can be refractory to inotropes and pressors and potentially lethal. Barbiturates have a significant immunosuppressive effect, resulting in an increased risk of infection *(213,218)*. This is potentiated by the prolonged immobility and endotracheal intubation associated with induced coma. Barbiturates also tend to produce systemic hypothermia *(213)*, which may mask signs of infection *(56)*. Lastly, all barbiturate agents accumulate with prolonged exposure, and patients may remain comatose for days after cessation of therapy. Adverse consequences due to these effects must be minimized if the potential gains which barbiturate coma has to offer are to be realized. Detailed and fastidious care must be taken to optimize hemodynamic status as outlined elsewhere in this chapter; given the profound myocardial suppressive effect of these agents, many authorities *(47,56)* recommend the placement of a Swan-Ganz pulmonary artery catheter with frequent assessment of volume status and myocardial function, and titration of vasopressors and inotropic agents (e.g., dopamine and dobutamine) as necessary. Nursing must also aggressively monitor for any possible supervening infections and the development of decubitus ulcers, and deep venous thrombosis prophylaxis should be scrupulously applied.

There is a fair degree of concensus among recent reviewers regarding preferable regimen for the induction of barbiturate coma *(10,14,39,56,176,219)*: pentobarbital, administered as a bolus, followed by a continuous infusion of 0.5–3.0 mg/kg/h titrated to a burst-suppression pattern on EEG or normalization of ICP, whichever is achieved first. These effects are generally achieved at serum levels of approx 3 mg/dL *(10,176)*. Recommendations regarding the initial bolus itself vary somewhat, from 3–10 mg/kg over 30–180 min *(10)* to 5–30 mg/kg at 1 mg/kg/min *(39)*. Although there is no evidence that either thiopental or phenobarbital is less effective at suppressing cerebral activity and hence decreasing ICP, both of these agents have a longer physiologic half life than pentobarbital when given in repeated doses *(213)*; pentobarbital is therefore the preferred agent, because prolonged sedation is one of the identified drawbacks of this technique.

Barbiturate coma, when used, should be maintained for at least 48 h, or until the pathologic state underlying ICP elevation is likely to have reversed, as long as cardiovascular function permits this. Withdrawal of barbiturate coverage should be stepwise, not sudden; one reasonable approach is to decrease the hourly infusion rate by 50% each day *(56)*. (Regarding cardiovascular monitoring and the use of EEG patterns in continuous neurophysiologic monitoring, *see* Chapter 6.)

Propofol. Considerable attention has been given in the past few years to the utilization of propofol in neurointensive care, due to its brief duration of action and short washout period *(220,221)*. These features contrast to benzodiazepines and barbiturates, whose washout period is much longer, significantly complicating attempts to periodically discontinue sedation to assess neurologic functioning. Propofol has therefore seen use in neurointensive care as a sedative agent when frequent neurologic assessment is desired.

This application may also extend to the control of intracranial hypertension. Propofol produces a significant drop in ICP in patients with normal intracranial dynamics, with preserved CPP *(222,223)*, apparently because of the same fall in cerebral metabolic rate and, hence, CBF produced by barbiturates *(224)*. This effect is preserved in patients with increased ICP after head trauma *(225)*. The therapeutic use of this effect has been assessed in a single trial of propofol sedation of patients with head injury *(226)*. The chief achievement of this trial was to demonstrate the safety of prolonged use of propofol (mean time on propofol 95 h) in these patients. Propofol-treated patients required less CSF drainage, had lower ICP on day 3 of the study, and required less use of other pharmacologic interventions than did controls; these encouraging findings and equivalent outcome were despite a higher prevalence in the treatment group of negative predictive variables (greater age, lower GCS, more likely to have had early hypoxia or hypotension). However, this single trial was small (42 total patients) and did not demonstrate any improvement in outcome. Unfortunately, there are even less systematic data available pertaining to the prolonged use of propofol for any other etiology of elevated ICP. The same criticism, however, can be legitimately made of barbiturates.

Propofol does have significant adverse effects that must be carefully accounted for if its potential benefits are to be realized (*see also* Chapter 12). It has a profound hypotensive effect, and vasopressors very frequently must be coadministered *(220)*. Although previous evaluation has demonstrated that concurrent decrease in ICP is sufficient to produce a preservation of CPP despite systemic hypotension, prudence dictates that strict measures be taken to maintain systemic blood pressure and that an ICP monitor be in place to verify that ICP is not unexpectedly increasing from intracranial vasodilation. One other prominent adverse effect is a predisposition to infection. Whereas early reports of Gram-negative sepsis appear to have been successfully countered by addition of the preservative EDTA to the vehicle, there nonetheless does appear to be an increased risk for nosocomial infection while maintained on propofol sedation *(220,226)*, and any patient so maintained must be carefully watched for any signs of infection. This increased tendency cannot be considered a contraindication to propofol's use in appropriate circumstances, as the same increased risk is present with barbiturate sedation. Comparison of the relative rates on each agent awaits clarification in future trials. Other adverse effects or propofol which must be borne in mind are due to the lipid emulsification vehicle, and include hypertriglyceridemia, more likely in the elderly, and increased CO_2 production *(220)*. Serum lipids may be monitored periodically, any indication of pancreatitis watched for, and nutritional supplementation should be adjusted downward to account for the lipid and calorie content of the vehicle. Rare cases of metabolic acidosis, apparently idiosyncratic, have been reported, some of them fatal *(227)*. Lastly, a recent review has called into question whether propofol has the potential for epileptogenicity in some patients *(228)*; we are skeptical of such an association, as we have not seen it in many patients treated with propofol, but pending the publication of better data, this possibility must be borne in mind if a patient started on propofol begins to seize, and continuous EEG monitoring should be seriously considered if propofol anesthesia is to be used safely.

At this time, therefore, the use of prolonged propofol sedation for amelioration of intracranial hypertension can be considered a legitimate practice option, provided that the possibilities of acidosis and seizure are borne in mind and monitored for. Propofol sedation should be undertaken in the same circumstances in which barbiturate coma is pursued: intracranial hypertension refractory to general supportive management as outlined previously, surgical evacuation of mass lesions, and hyperosmotic therapy; additionally, in certain circumstances, its short duration of action may render it a legitimate short-term therapeutic option while definitive surgery is being arranged, provided that systemic blood pressure is scrupulously maintained and ideally with an ICP monitor already in place.

Other Anesthetic Agents. Other sedative-hypnotic agents bear mention only in passing. The routine use of benzodiazepines and opiates in the neuroscience intensive care unit is considered in Chapter 12; these agents' only role in the control of intracranial hypertension is to maintain quiet sedation, avoiding surges in ICP owing to agitated motor activity and "bucking" the ventilator. Etomidate is effective at reducing cerebral metabolic rate and cerebral blood volume, but is a potent inhibitor of steroidogenesis, producing adrenal insufficiency with repeated dosing, and its use is therefore contraindicated in any context other than rapid-sequence intubation or anesthetic induction. Anesthetic gasses (nitrous oxide and the halothanes) have the potential to increase cerebral blood flow profoundly, increasing ICP, and therefore can only be used safely if at all during craniotomy, not in the ICU.

Ketamine deserves special mention as an agent with the potential for future use. Formerly considered absolutely contraindicated in patients with the potential for elevated ICP *(221)*, ketamine has been demonstrated in two recent reports *(229,230)* to have no significant effect on ICP in head injured patients who were under sedation (with propofol in one report and midazolam or fentanyl in the other). In the one study with a control group, ketamine's sympathomimetic properties were found to decrease the need for vasopressors, resulted in a higher average CPP, and promoted intestinal motility in patients on opiates *(230)*. As a result of the small numbers studied (43 total) in these reports, it is too early to advocate ketamine's use, but with further study, it may come to play a role in the support of patients requiring heavy sedation for critical intracranial illnesses.

PHARMACOLOGIC PARALYSIS

The use of neuromuscular blockade paralysis has been advocated by some in the treatment of patients with dangerously elevated ICP, generally for the stated purpose of abolishing surges in ICP (especially plateau waves) that are induced by coughing or other such Valsalva equivalents *(39)*. At one time, this measure was considered routine, standard feature or the treatment of patients with severe head injury at many centers; however, recent retrospective analyses have demonstrated *higher* likelihood of elevated ICP *(231)* and worse rates of disability *(232)* in traumatic brain injury patients treated with neuromuscular blockade. No prospective trial has ever been conducted in any condition. There is no doubt that this technique can be successful in blunting surges in ICP provoked by endo-bronchial suctioning *(233)*. The wisest course of action therefore seems to be that if neuromuscular blockade is used at all, it be used only in patients who have a demonstrated propensity to surges of ICP associated with specific situations such as bronchial suctioning, and then only for limited periods of time. Nondepolarizing agents must be used, as succinylcholine has the potential to directly increase ICP through the muscle contraction it produces *(234)*. Unless absolutely necessary, use should probably be avoided altogether in any patient on glucocorticoids, given the potential of paralytic agents and steroids together to potentiate critical illness myopathy *(235)*.

INDOMETHACIN

There have been several reports since 1991 of a possible ICP-lowering effect of intravenous indomethacin. Aside from a single case report in a patient with fulminant hepatic failure and renal failure (who later died despite the observed effect) *(236)*, the patients have all had traumatic brain injury *(237–239)*. Animal data have suggested that indomethacin can produce a fall in CBF *(240)*. Those reports that permitted observation support a similar effect in traumatic brain injury patients *(237,239)*. Another possible mechanism in injured patients is reduction or prevention of fever, which was definitely seen in one patient series *(237)*, and possibly in another *(238)*. Until a larger trial is published, especially given the potential for indomethacin (like all high-dose nonsteroidal anti-inflammatory agents) to produce peptic ulcers, indomethacin must remain an agent with promise whose use cannot yet be recommended.

HYPOTHERMIA

The induction of systemic hypothermia has been shown to produce multiple salutary chemical and histologic effects in animal models of various acute intracranial processes. For the most part, unfortunately, these findings have not been translatable into improved outcomes in human trials.

The single exception to this is in the treatment of diffuse ischemic brain injury after cardiac arrest. Two simultaneously reported trials *(241,242)* recently investigated the effect of systemic hypothermia induced by external cooling in adults who suffered out-of-hospital cardiac arrest, with ventricular fibrillation as the first recorded rhythm, in whom spontaneous circulation was restored, who were comatose initially after return of circulation. Hypothermia to a temperature of about 32°C was accomplished within 8 h in both trials, maintained for 12 h in one study and 24 h in the other, and followed by passive rewarming. Overall survival was improved in the larger study, and survival to independence was improved in both. The chief limitation of these studies is the narrowly defined patient group: all patients had ventricular fibrillation arrest, almost all of cardiac origin; bystander CPR was performed in the majority; and time from collapse to return of spontaneous circulation was less than 25 min in the majority. It is estimated that less than 20% of patients with out-of-hospital arrest fit the inclusion criteria of these studies *(243)*. It is also important to note from the standpoint of treatment for intracranial hypertension that none of these patients had ICP monitors; therefore, it is unclear how many if any had sufficient brain swelling to increase ICP. Pending publication of any "negative" trials, however, it appears that induced systemic hypothermia improves outcome in a limited subset of patients with postarrest diffuse ischemic brain injury.

The role of hypothermia in the treatment of head injury is less clear. The recent completion of the National Brain Injury Study: Hypothermia trial *(244)* appears to emphatically confirm smaller trials' findings *(245,246)* that induced hypothermia for unselected patients with severe head injury does not improve long-term outcome. However, this finding is at odds with a large volume of animal literature *(244)*, as well as findings of at least one other trial of size *(247)*. Moreover, it remains possible that hypothermia may be beneficial when instituted only for those head-injured patients with demonstrated intracranial hypertension *(248)*. At present, the conservative interpretation of the available data is that the adverse effects of systemic hypothermia outweigh the benefits on intracranial dynamics, and that this treatment does not benefit unselected patients with severe head injury *(249)*. However, the large body of work suggesting potential benefits to some patients (particularly those with established tendency toward elevated ICP) is sufficiently compelling that some practitioners continue to utilize this measure *(250)*. The clarification of which subgroups of patients would benefit from hypothermia awaits the publication of further trials. Preliminary trials of hypothermia in acute ischemic stroke have been encouraging *(251–253)*, but this must be regarded as an experimental therapy until larger trials are published.

To date, all trials of systemic hypothermia have utilized external cooling (endovascular devices may have a future role, but are currently experimental *[254]*). Most trials have used water-circulating *(245,246,248,251–253)* or air-circulating *(241)* cooling blankets to achieve hypothermia; other means have included surface ice packs *(241,242,244)* and iced gastric lavage *(244,245)*. It appears that water-circulating blankets have slightly greater speed and efficacy vs other techniques, and are certainly the most convenient; however, surface ice packs and iced gastric lavage depress temperature only slightly less rapidly, and are readily available in all medical centers. Current concensus regarding the target body temperature is 32–34°C. Most trialists agree on the use of urinary bladder catheter thermistors for measurement of core body temperature. In most trials, shivering has been controlled with neuromuscular blockers *(241,242,244,245,251–253)*. As noted, the trials for postarrest coma maintained hypothermia for between 12 and 24 h after initiation; guidelines regarding duration of cooling for head trauma and stroke cannot be offered. There is no concensus regarding whether rewarming should be active (induced with an external device) or passive (spontaneous metabolic reequilibration on the patient's part).

Several potential complications of hypothermia must be actively guarded against if any therapeutic utility is to be realized. The absence of statistical significance in the postarrest trials *(241,242)* notwithstanding, the aggregate experience across human trials is highly suggestive of an elevated rate of infection, especially pneumonia *(249)*. Any patient in whom hypothermia is induced must therefore be monitored fastidiously for infection. Given that fever cannot be assessed, and given the high rates with which infection has been seen in some trials *(246)*, the prophylactic administration of broad-spectrum antibiotics is likely a defensible course of action, though this intervention has not itself been subjected to a trial. The second metabolic derangement classically associated with hypothermia, coagulopathy *(255,256)*, has remained more consistently nonevident in trials of therapeutic hypothermia, suggesting that it is less a primary effect of hypothermia itself than of other associated conditions, such as trauma, in whose company it has been seen. Nevertheless, careful attention to coagulation times and monitoring for hemorrhagic complications is warranted. Serum electrolytes, particularly potassium, magnesium, calcium and phosphate, can drop rapidly and significantly during the cooling phase *(257)*; electrolyte levels should be frequently assessed and repleted, and prophylactic administration may be of utility. The necessity of neuromuscular blockade to prevent shivering represents a significant potential source of iatrogenic complications (*see* Pharmacologic Paralysis section). A pharmacologic alternative to paralysis has been reported: coadministration of buspirone 30 mg enterally with moderate-dose (target serum level 0.4 μg/mL) meperidine parenterally was demonstrated to lower the shivering threshold to 33.4°C, 2.3°C below normal and significantly lower than either drug alone (*258*). This approach has advocates in the field (S. A. Mayer, personal communication), but we are hesitant to recommend it until reports of its safe use in neurocritically ill patients are published.

Currently, then, induced systemic hypothermia is a measure appropriately utilized for selected patients initially comatose after cardiac arrest. Other uses await further trial evaluation before they can be considered proven.

HYPERBARIC OXYGEN

A single English-language trial (*259*) reported increased survival in head-injured patients treated with hyperbaric oxygen (100% oxygen at 1.5 atm) for 1 h every 8 h, but survival with good outcome was identical between treated and nontreated patients (i.e., the margin of increased survival between treated and nontreated patients was entirely composed of patients with dependent or vegetative outcome). Fraught with potential complications as this therapy may be (*260*), further investigation may nonetheless prove fruitful (*261,262*).

THAM

Tris-hydroxymethyl-aminomethane (trometamol, tromethamine, THAM) is a buffer with a pKa of 7.8; after parenteral administration, it distributes rapidly into the extracellular fluid spaces of the body, then slowly into most intracellular spaces, including the brain, and acts as a proton acceptor, buffering acidotic states—both generalized (e.g., diabetic ketoacidosis) and focal (e.g., ischemic lactic acidosis) (*263*). Originally introduced in the early 1960s, its use for generalized acidoses was negatively received (*264*), and it has seen little use in the United States since. Elsewhere, particularly in northern continental Europe, it has been considered a standard therapeutic intervention for elevated ICP. By maintaining pH near physiologic, even in areas of profound oxygen depletion and cytotoxic edema, THAM can ameliorate secondary cellular damage. It has been shown to decrease the water content (and thus, presumably, swelling) of traumatized brain in patients (*265*), and to decrease both size of infarct and swelling thereof in animal models (*266,267*). In the one English-language randomized controlled trial of THAM for head injury, THAM-treated patients had significantly lower ICP at some stages of treatment, and were significantly less likely to require barbiturate anesthesia to control ICP; the outcomes in this trial, however, appeared to favor patients who did not receive THAM, though this did *not* achieve statistical significance (*268*). (This is a sobering realization vis-a-vis the many other treatments already discussed whose effects on ICP are known with confidence, but that have never been proven to improve outcomes in a randomized trial.) On the basis of the evidence currently available in the English-language literature, therefore, the use of THAM cannot be recommended; it remains possible, however, that future publications may necessitate reversal of this stance.

NEUROPROTECTION

Despite multiple therapeutic agents having shown promise in animal models, to date all trials of agents intended to protect nervous tissue from the consequences of ischemia or the harmful secondary sequelae of CNS trauma have shown no benefit in humans (*269,270*). The robustness of treatment effects in some animal paradigms renders the failure of crossover into clinical trials all the more frustrating. It is to be hoped that future evaluations may yet bear fruit.

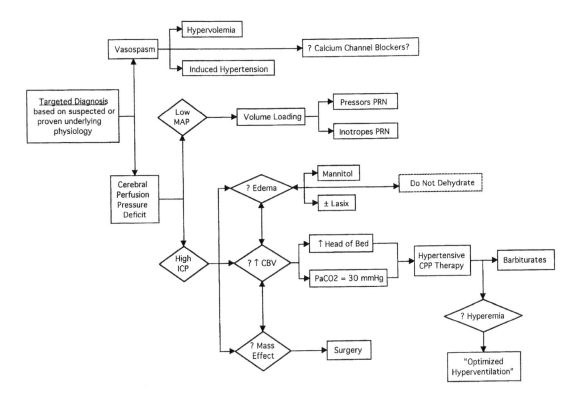

Fig. 5. ICP treatment algorithm. Developed for treating elated ICP resulting from head injury, this algorithm is derived from the physiologic principles discussed earlier in this chapter, and the "cerebral perfusion pressure deficit" arm can be conceptually applied to most pathologic states. Low arterial pressure (MAP) will produce intracranial vasodilation and potentiate A waves, and thus should be addressed with iso- or hyper-osmotic volume loading. Tissue edema may respond to mannitol or hypertonic saline. Mass effect that is surgically remediable must be addressed. Cerebral venous distention (venous CBV) must be avoided by positioning the head up 30°C; arterial CBV will respond transiently to hyperventilation. Although far from perfect, this algorithm offers a first attempt at rationalizing the use of interventions for specific pathophysiologies. Reprinted from ref. *56* with permission.

Summary

The range of therapeutic options available to the clinician dealing with a patient with brain edema or the potential for elevated ICP is thus at once both terribly narrow and dizzyingly broad. The work has yet to be done that permits clinicians to utilize them in specific disease states on a rational basis. For some clinical problems, collective clinical experience has provided enough knowledge that specific physiologically based protocols for intervention can be ventured—Fig. 5 offers an example suggested for use in severe traumatic brain injury. Hopefully, such protocols will be constructed for other disease states in the future.

This ends the review of specific interventions for brain edema and elevated intracranial pressure. The application of these interventions for most of the specific disease states already mentioned is covered in dedicated chapters elsewhere in this book; this chapter concludes with brief consideration of a few conditions not discussed elsewhere. Before concluding this section, however, it is appropriate to again note the dearth of good scientific evaluation of our therapeutic armamentarium for most

Table 4
Stages of Hepatic Encephalopathy

0 Normal function or minimal subtle neuropsychological impairment, with preserved attention span
I   Euphoria, anxiety, or depression; mild confusion; shortened attention span
II Lethargy; disorientation; moderate confusion, impaired cognition, and inappropriate behavior
III Somnolence or semistupor, with preserved arousability; profound confusion; purposeful response
      to noxious stimuli
IV Coma, with nonpurposeful or absent response to noxious stimuli

Adapted from refs. *276* and *285*.

of the conditions we treat. Too many publications have reported on the results of particular interventions in a heterogeneous group of patients *(134,271)*. One implication of such reports is that the pathophysiology of intracranial hypertension is the same between different disease states. It is not. The field will only move forward with the publication of trials evaluating specific interventions for specific disease states, and focusing on real outcomes instead of physiologic markers presumed to be associated with outcome. There is much work to be done.

TREATMENT OF SELECT SPECIFIC ETIOLOGIES

Hepatic Failure

Defined by general concensus as progression from normal to critically impaired hepatic function within less than 8 wk, fulminant hepatic failure (FHF) once carried a dismal prognosis. With the advent of orthotopic liver transplantation, however, prospects for patients so affected are dramatically better than they once were. Because 80% of patients dying with FHF die of generalized cerebral edema and brainstem compression *(272,273)*, optimization of outcome in FHF and proper timing of liver transplantation require fastidious management of the deranged intracranial dynamics that result from profound impairment of hepatic function. Although these patients are generally cared for in medical or surgical ICUs, neurologists and neurosurgeons may be consulted to aid in the management of ICP during the acute phase of illness. Those who participate in the care of such patients frequently will wish to reference other reviews as well *(272,274–276)*.

Clinical Manifestations and Diagnosis

The manifestations of hepatic encephalopathy are in most respects those of any toxic-metabolic encephalopathy. Many patients with hepatic disease will have milder degrees of encephalopathy as their initial presenting complaint. A clinical grading system has been devised (Table 4) to permit ease of communication between clinicians caring for these patients, and as part of a broader grading of severity of disease, the Child-Turcotte-Pugh score (Table 5) *(277)*. The diagnosis of hepatic encephalopathy is straightforward in any patient presenting with cognitive impairment in the setting of clinical manifestations of hepatic disease (e.g., visible jaundice, diffuse itching, abdominal pain) and can be considered established with the demonstration of impaired hepatic function on standard laboratory liver function tests (Table 6) without clinical or laboratory evidence of other causes of encephalopathy. The presence of asterixis, an intermittent loss of muscle tone in any muscle group engaged in sustained antigravity exertion *(278)*, is supportive; however, asterixis is not specific to hepatic encephalopathy *(279)*, and care must be taken to exclude the presence of uremia and hypercarbia. The presence of triphasic waves on EEG is likewise supportive, although this finding also can be present in other encephalopathies, may be demonstrable in only 25% of patients with confirmed hepatic encephalopathy, and may degrade to nonspecific delta coma with progression to stage IV encephalopathy *(280)*.

A distinction is generally made between patients with chronic, mild- to moderate-severity hepatic impairment, and those with severe, rapidly advancing, FHF. In general, chronic states are far better tolerated by the brain than is FHF. Even in patients with longstanding cirrhosis, however, sudden

Table 5
Child-Turcotte-Pugh Score

Points	1	2	3
Encephalopathy	None	Stage I–II	Stage III–IV
Ascites	Absent	Slight	Moderate–severe
Bilirubin (mg/dL)	<2.0	2.0–3.0	>3.0
Albumin (g/dL)	>3.5	2.8–3.5	<2.8
Prothrombin time (s)	<15	15–17	>17

decompensation of hepatic function has the potential to induce sufficient derangement of brain metabolism that diffuse brain edema develops *(281)*.

Establishing the diagnosis of FHF-associated brain edema is as simple as demonstrating characteristic findings on neuroimaging (diffuse gyral swelling, increased water content of white matter, abolishment of CSF spaces) in the appropriate clinical context. Seventy percent to 80% of patients who progress to stage IV hepatic coma will have such brain swelling *(272)*.

Pathophysiology

The cellular metabolic substrates of elevated ICP in hepatic failure remain a subject of controversy. Much attention has been paid to the role of hyperammonemia in hepatic failure *(282)*, and the argument has been advanced that resulting increases in intraglial glutamine induce cytotoxic edema *(275,283)*. One difficulty with this theory is that chronic hepatic impairment can result in the same apparent degree of ammonia-glutamine elevations, without inducing the same degree of cerebral edema *(275)*. Other factors appear to be at play as well, including impaired sodium-potassium AT-Pase function *(284)*.

Whatever the underlying biochemical substrate, the end result of FHF to the brain is diffuse cerebral edema, predominantly due to cellular swelling *(274,275)*. This can reach sufficient degree to produce tonsillar impaction, or diffuse elevation of ICP, abolishment of CPP, and devastating diffuse ischemic injury *(274,275)*. A tenuous intracranial system may be further destabilized by other systemic metabolic derangements which result from hepatic failure; specifically, failure of hepatic gluconeogenesis can lead to neurotoxic hypoglycemia, and the development of pulmonary arteriovenous shunting (hepatopulmonary syndrome) can produce systemic hypoxia *(285)*. These patients also often develop renal failure, which, while not necessarily directly neurotoxic, can significantly complicate management.

Treatment

Definitive treatment of FHF depends on identification and reversal of the inciting hepatic injury with restoration of function, and failing that goal, liver transplantation. Liver transplantation eligibility is a complex and evolving decision-making process; as this is the province of hepatologists and transplant surgeons, interested readers are referred elsewhere for discussion *(277)*.

In every patient with stage III or IV hepatic encephalopathy, all standard medical measures for intracranial hypertension should be taken (positioning, temperature, avoidance of hypotonic fluids, avoidance of agitation or Valsalva, volume repletion and BP support). Serum glucose must be frequently, vigilantly monitored, and intravenous dextrose administered when necessary, in as hypertonic a solution as possible. Any significant decrement in neurologic status should prompt head CT to evaluate for intracranial bleeding, which if detected should prompt redoubled efforts at reversal of coagulopathy, and appropriate surgical intervention. Steroids appear to have no salutary effect, and may possibly be detrimental *(39)*. Sedative use should be judicious, given the prolonged clearance that hepatic impairment produces, but should nonetheless be instituted in agitated, combative patients. Most published accounts report proceeding with elective intubation once patients progress to

Table 6
Laboratory Abnormalities Suggestive of Hepatic Impairment

Elevated bilirubin
Elevated ammonia
Elevated transaminases (AST [SGOT], ALT [SGPT])
Elevated prothrombin time
Decreased albumin

ALT [SGPT], alanine transaminase; AST [SGOT]; aspartate transaminase.

stage III encephalopathy (272,286). Other medical measures for ICP control should likely be utilized only in titration to directly measured ICP, and are discussed below in this section.

Authorities disagree about the issue of invasive ICP measurement. The impressive experience reported by Lidofsky and colleagues (272), using a standardized CPP-targeted approach including invasive monitoring in every patient, has proven convincing to many (274,275). Others (247), however, report that in their hands invasive monitoring yielded insufficient treatment-altering information to justify the risks of monitor placement. It must be admitted that invasive ICP monitoring has not been conclusively demonstrated to change patient outcome. A pessimistic reading of previous patient series' findings of universally poor outcome in patients who developed elevated ICP (287,288) would be to conclude that once ICP elevation is documented, poor outcome is highly likely, and transplantation should no longer be offered. The current climate of organ shortage encourages such pessimism. One goal of ICP monitoring, then, could be formulated as avoidance of intracranial hypertension and neurological injury in patients whose ICP has almost but not quite yet destabilized. Another definite indication for ICP monitoring is detection and reversal of ICP surges in the perioperative context; cumulative experience (272,289) strongly suggests that fastidious control of ICP during transplant surgery may significantly contribute to optimizing ultimate neurologic recovery from FHF requiring liver transplantation.

If invasive monitoring is elected, coagulopathy should be reversed with FFP and platelets before device insertion, to greater than 3 s prolongation of the prothrombin time and a platelet count of greater than 50,000/mm³ (274). Choice of device is a matter of argument. Most practitioners utilize the subarachnoid bolt or an epidural device, due to their lower risks of hemorrhagic complications. Ventricular catheter use seems unwise, given the substantially higher hemorrhagic and infectious risks, especially considering that diffuse cerebral edema of FHF often leads to ventricular effacement or even abolishment, rendering IVC placement more than usually risky. Whether the increased accuracy of the Camino catheter justifies the higher hemorrhagic risks must remain a case-by-case decision.

The optimal medical means by which to treat ICP in these patients cannot be known with any degree of confidence due to a complete lack of data, and therapeutic choices thus remain empiric. Those with experience (39,272,290) report that mannitol retains some efficacy against the diffuse edema of FHF; while its use may induce or exacerbate renal failure, hemodialysis can be utilized to counter this (272,291), permitting the osmotic dehydration of brain that is desired. (If hemodialysis is necessary, continuous venovenous dialysis is advisable, in the interests of minimizing the severity of fluid and electrolyte shifts.) The induction of barbiturate coma has been convincingly demonstrated (212,272,292) to reduce cerebral metabolic rate and decrease ICP in these patients. Short-term bolus administration of barbiturates can be potently useful for blunting ICP surges during surgery (272,293). The best use of these agents for pretransplant ICU patients is less clear, for the simple reason that induction of barbiturate coma confounds the grading of hepatic encephalopathy. If progression to refractory stage IV is regarded as the "point of no return" beyond which transplantation is not pursued because of a high likelihood of poor neurologic outcome, then barbiturate coma should only be induced in pretransplant patients for whom an organ has been identified to minimize the chance of ICP surges during the preoperative and perioperative period. The last means of medical ICP control that has received attention in the literature is induction of systemic hypothermia; recent reports *(294–296)* suggest that this technique is relatively safe and modestly effective at preventing or blunting ICP elevations. The relative benefits and adverse effects of hypothermia vs barbiturate administration cannot be known with any degree of confidence, and await publication.

Lastly, a note must be made regarding the subject of deliberate hyperventilation. As discussed previously, there is reason to believe both on conceptual grounds (vasoconstrictive effect is short-lived, comes at the expense of producing a rebound hyperemia, and can produce areas of focal ischemia) and patient data (demonstrating worse outcome in head-injured patients) that sustained hyperventilation is an inappropriate therapeutic modality for intracranial hypertension, and should be used only as a bridge to definitive therapy or when all other means have failed. A survey of recent publications on treatment of cerebral edema in FHF *(286,289,297)* indicates that institution and maintenance of sustained hyperventilation remains a standard component of therapy in many surgical centers. It seems unlikely that any trial of size will be undertaken to address whether sustained hyperventilation is advantageous or detrimental to FHF patients.

Outcome

Before the advent of orthotopic liver transplantation, the outcome for patients with fulminant hepatic failure was universally dismal. Contemporary patient series *(272,293,298)*; however, report survival rates ranging up to 74%. Of course, such rates depend fundamentally on how FHF is defined, and comparison of these rates for the current era vs the pretransplant era are further confounded by interim improvements in best medical management without transplantation. There can be little doubt, however, that orthotopic liver transplantation has afforded survival to some FHF patients that previously would have died. Future improvements in outcome will likely be based on (a) improving the availability of donor organs or substitutes thereto, and (b) improving the management of cerebral edema—the cause of death in 80% of those dying with FHF *(273)*.

High-Altitude Cerebral Edema

Commonly abbreviated HACE, cerebral edema in the context of recent ascent to high altitude is considered by many to be an extreme form of acute mountain sickness (AMS) *(299)*.

Clinical Manifestations

AMS, characterized by headache, fatigue, anorexia, nausea, and sleeplessness, characteristically affects those who have ascended from near sea level to 2500 m or higher, resolving over 1–3 d. Approximately 20% of those making such an ascent may be affected. HACE, by contrast, is much more severe, and much rarer. Both appear to correlate with rapidity and magnitude of ascent. HACE typically manifests first as AMS, with progression within 12–72 h of ascent to ataxia, confusion, lethargy and eventually coma; vomiting, hallucinations, and seizures have also been seen *(300)*.

Pathophysiology

Pathophysiology is incompletely understood. The diagnosis was initially appreciated on the basis of autopsy demonstration of diffuse brain swelling in those dying with the syndrome. Recent MRI data, showing that edema is limited to white matter only, have been interpreted as favoring a vasogenic mechanism *(301)*. Physiologic studies have demonstrated increased brain water and decreased brain compliance at altitude *(299)*. Awaiting clarification are why ascent to low oxygen tension environments should induce endothelial or other cellular dysfunction and what factors determine which few develop HACE while others are negligibly to merely mildly affected.

It is vital to the appropriate care of patients with HACE to also recognize the syndrome of high-altitude pulmonary edema (HAPE), which is coincident in a very high percentage of patients *(299,300)*. HAPE is characterized by a diffuse alveolar edema of high protein content, which has been taken as evidence of an underlying derangement of lung capillary permeability—(i.e., vasogenic edema in a different vessel bed; *300*). It shares the same risk factors as HACE, and is also rare.

Symptoms are dyspnea, fatigue, and a dry cough; clinical and laboratory examination reveal hypoxia, tachypnea with a respiratory alkalosis, fluffy radiographic infiltrates, and not uncommonly, a pyrexia of up to 38.5°C *(300)*.

Diagnosis

Diagnosis rests simply on recognition of characteristic clinical features in the context of ascent to altitude. MRI demonstration of edema is of interest, and may be of use in ruling out other conditions, but is otherwise not necessary for clinical management. Lumbar puncture is better avoided unless absolutely necessary to rule out meningitis, and should be done with standard measures to minimize risks of herniation—small-bore needle, slow removal of the minimal diagnostically necessary volume of CSF, and assurance of the ability to treat emergently in the event that herniation is induced (previously secured intravenous access, at-hand mannitol, and respiratory equipment for the institution of hyperventilation).

Treatment

As with other syndromes discussed in this chapter, the sine qua non of HACE treatment is reversal of the underlying pathophysiology, via either rapid descent to lower altitude or use of some mechanical means (e.g., barometric chamber) to increase the patient's experienced barometric pressure (rarely a practical possibility) *(299,300)*. Climbers and skiers must monitor themselves and their companions for signs of altered alertness or mentation, ataxia, and increasing lethargy, and hasten descent if they occur. Patients with pulmonary edema should be intubated. Moderate levels of PEEP (up to 10 cm H_2O) and high but nontoxic FiO_2s (up to 0.60) should be utilized to reverse hypoxemia. Nifedipine 10 mg orally every 4 h may be beneficial to pulmonary physiology *(302)*, but has not been evaluated as an acute treatment in intubated patients. Dexamethasone 10 mg IV followed by 4 mg every 6 h is advocated as highly efficacious by those in the field *(299,300)*; we are skeptical, because formal published evaluations to date have been insufficient to conclusively establish the efficacy of steroids. It is clear that they are no substitute for return to higher barometric pressure *(303)*. Clinical wisdom is that earlier descent and treatment favor good outcome *(300)*.

Prophylaxis

In this as in every disease, an ounce of prevention is worth a pound of cure. Optimally, a traveler from altitudes near sea level should acclimate in areas near 2500 m for 2 d before ascending to peak areas. Acetazolamide taken prophylactically before travel, starting the day before departure from home altitudes, has been shown to be effective at reducing the incidence of AMS *(304,305)*; this has been taken as indicating a probable decrease in the risk for HACE, but without strong data. Nifedipine 20 mg orally every 8 h *(302)* or salmeterol 125 µg by metered-dose inhaler every 12 h *(306)* are of demonstrated efficacy in decreasing the risk of developing HAPE.

Lead Intoxication

Chronic exposure to lead produces well-known syndromes of neurobehavioral impairment in children and sensorimotor neuropathy in adults. With extremely high levels, a syndrome of impaired brain function referred to as lead encephalopathy ensues. Far more common in the pediatric than the adult population, the recognition of the adverse health and cognitive effects of lead have produced such successful attention to its eradication that this complication is uncommonly seen in the United States any longer. Nevertheless, cases do continue to occur *(307,308)*.

Clinical Manifestations

The symptoms of lead encephalopathy are nonspecific: headache; ataxia and dysarthria; abdominal pain, anorexia, nausea, and vomiting; fatigue and lethargy progressing to stupor and coma; and seizures *(307,309,310)*. Untreated, it is often fatal; in such cases, the brain is found to be diffusely congested and edematous. Judging from the clinical phenomenology, it is likely that the pathophysiology is toxicity to cellular metabolism producing a diffuse cytotoxic edema. Susceptibility to this toxicity appears to be greater in the young *(311)*.

Diagnosis

The most crucial step in appropriate treatment of a patient with lead encephalopathy is diagnosis. The clinical presentation, given its nonspecific nature, is very frequently misattributed to systemic infection. The presence in the patient's history of any potential risk of lead exposure must raise the index of suspicion, as must the incidental detection of any of the laboratory abnormalities that commonly accompany longstanding toxicity (*see* below). The greatest risk factor is youth; children under the age of 6 yr are at particular risk of voluntary ingestion of lead-containing materials. Potential sources include peeling house paint (interior or exterior), water from inappropriately plumbed pipes, soil from around old houses or other painted structures, batteries, solder, fishing weights, folk medicines (azarcon and Greta from Mexico, Pay-loo-ah amongst Chinese and Hmong), cosmetics (surma, ceruse, and kohl, from Asia), and many other materials *(312,313)*. Parents of young children should be carefully interrogated for a history of pica *(307,308)*. Adults are typically exposed in industrial environments, such as smelting, soldering, battery manufacture, demolition and remodeling in old buildings, ships and bridges *(309)*, and the consumption of illegally distilled alcohol ("moonshine") *(314,315)*. Illegal alcohol represents a particularly insidious source, as it could be clinically tempting to attribute the symptoms and signs of lead toxicity to a combination of acute alcohol intoxication with coexistent effects of chronic alcohol abuse *(314)*.

In a few cases, there may be evidence on the clinical examination to suggest the diagnosis: wrist or foot drop may have developed if peripheral neuropathy is advanced, and visible bluish discoloration of the teeth at the gum line may be evident *(312,316)*. These features are much more frequently absent, however, especially in children *(316)*, and their absence should not be taken as evidence against lead toxicity.

Laboratory diagnosis is straightforward: demonstration of a severely elevated serum lead level—higher than 60 μg/dL, often in the hundreds in cases with encephalopathy *(307)*. Unfortunately, not all clinical laboratories have the capacity to run a lead level on an emergent basis, and other biomarkers may need to be used as supportive evidence while the definitive test is pending. The most specific of these is erythrocyte protoporphyrin, commonly elevated due to lead's interference with the heme synthesis pathway *(310)*. This biochemical disturbance produces the characteristic hematologic manifestation, of great clinical utility given the place of the complete blood cell count in standard laboratory evaluations: a normochromic, normocytic anemia. On microscopy, some erythrocytes may exhibit basophilic stippling. Serum uric acid may be elevated. At serum concentrations of lead sufficient to produce cerebral edema, there is often also an interstitial nephritis producing increased blood urea nitrogen and creatinine. Bands of density ("lead lines") may be seen on skeletal radiographs due to lead deposition in bone *(307,308,317)*. Most of these biochemical abnormalities require at least several weeks of biologic exposure to develop *(310)*; however, an acute exposure to a quantity of lead is more likely to produce encephalopathy if the patient already had an elevated lead level, and a search for evidence of preexisting lead toxicity may pay dividends if one is forced to wait for a lead level. In a patient without preexisting toxicity exposed to a catastrophic amount of lead, one may be left to depend on the clinical history and serum lead level alone. CSF examination in a patient with lead encephalopathy may reveal elevated protein and mild cellularity, usually monocytic, potentially misleading the clinician into a diagnosis of meningitis *(318)*.

Treatment

The sine qua non of optimal management is chelation therapy to emergently lower lead levels. Commonly used agents are calcium disodium edetate (CaNa$_2$EDTA), dimercaprol (BAL), and succimer (DMSA); D-penicillamine may also be used, although it is generally considered appropriate only if the other agents are unavailable *(310,312)*. Recommended dosages depend on the source, and consultation with the pharmacy is advised. It is generally agreed that a combination of BAL and CaNa$_2$EDTA is the first-line regimen, producing a rapid fall in serum lead level *(319)*. There is a report *(307)* of the safe use of EDTA, BAL, and DMSA concurrently in a 3-yr-old patient with a serum lead concentration of 550 mcg/dL.

The cerebral edema of lead encephalopathy must only be managed while the underlying toxin is removed. Fortunately for society, such cases are sufficiently rare today that no one has accrued any appreciable case series in the modern era of ICP management. Optimal management is therefore a matter of conjecture. Given that multiple-chelator regimens appear to return serum lead levels to less than 50 µg/dL within one and at the most 3 d after initiation of therapy, avoidance of the iatrogenic risks of ICP monitor placement is defensible *(307,319)*. Standard measures of positioning, ventilatory support, temperature control and cardiovascular and metabolic stabilization should be scrupulously applied; the judicious use of mannitol or barbiturates in those patients with severe encephalopathy are conceptually justifiable, but no data exist to guide their appropriate use. As an almost historical note, decompressive craniectomy has been tried in the past *(320,321)*, and although not subjected to a controlled trial, subsequent publications reported an increase in mortality *(322)*. Seizures complicating lead encephalopathy should be managed very aggressively, from the complete reversibility of the underlying pathophysiology. If seizures do not respond to aggressive doses of lorazepam (0.2 mg/kg), rapid progression to barbiturates or propofol might be considered preferable to waiting for the completion of a phenytoin load.

The majority of potential exposures to lead are by ingestion. In any patient with lead encephalopathy, therefore, a flat abdominal radiograph should be obtained to assess for radiopaque material in the gastrointestinal tract. Any material so detected represents a potential source of further absorption of lead, and should be evacuated to prevent further increases in the serum lead level. The effective use of whole bowel irrigation with polyethylene glycol solution has been reported *(323)*, and should be quite safe provided no contraindications to its use are present (bowel perforation or obstruction, ileus, uncontrolled gastrointestinal hemorrhage, uncontrollable vomiting, unsecured compromised airway, hemodynamic instability) *(324)*. The recommended regimen is 1500–2000 mL/h by nasogastric tube in adults (500 mL/h in children 9 mo–6 yr, 1000 mL/h in children 6–12 yr), with a drop to half-rate if emesis occurs; this should be continued until the rectal effluent is clear—generally anywhere from 3–12 h *(324)*.

Outcome

In the modern era of multiple-chelator regimens, even extraordinarily high lead levels are survivable *(307)*. Reports from before the establishment of combinations of chelators as the preferred treatment suggest a mortality rate of approx 30% among children comatose from lead poisoning *(322,325)*. Within a few years of these reports, series using EDTA and BAL in combination reported mortality rates of 0–5% in similar children *(317,319)*. With timely recognition and immediate institution of appropriate therapy, lead encephalopathy would appear to be an eminently survivable disease.

REFERENCES

1. Qureshi AI, Geocadin RG, Suarez JI, Ulatowski JA. Long-term outcome after medical reversal of transtentorial herniation in patients with supratentorial mass lesions. *Crit. Care Med.* 2000;28:1556–1564.
2. Manz HJ. Pathophysiology and pathology of elevated intracranial pressure. *Pathobiol. Ann.* 1979;9:359–381.
3. Langfitt TW, Weinstein JD, Kassell NF. Cerebral vasomotor paralysis produced by intracranial hypertension. *Neurology* 1965;15:622–641.
4. Miller JD, Sullivan HG. Severe intracranial hypertension. *Int. Anesth. Clin.* 1979;17:19–75.
5. Reich JB, Sierra J, Camp W, Zanzonico P, Deck MDF, Plum F. Magnetic resonance imaging measurements and clinical changes accompanying transtentorial and foramen magnum brain herniation. *Ann. Neurol.* 1993;33:159–170.
6. Wolfla CE, Luerssen TG, Bowman RM. Regional brain tissue pressure gradients created by expanding extradural temporal mass lesion. *J. Neurosurg.* 1997;86:505–510.

7. Wolfla CE, Luerssen TG. Brain tissue pressure gradients are dependent upon a normal spinal subarachnoid space. *Acta Neurochir.* 1998;71(Suppl):310–312.

8. Piek J, Plewe P, Bock WJ. Intrahemispheric gradients of brain tissue pressure in patients with brain tumors. *Acta Neurochir.* 1988;93:129–132.

9. Langfitt TW, Weinstein JD, Kassell NF, et al. Transmission of increased intracranial pressure: I. Within the craniospinal axis. *J. Neurosurg.* 1964;21:989–997.

10. Lee KR, Hoff JT. Intracranial pressure. In: Youmans JR, ed. *Neurological Surgery*, vol. 1. Philadelphia: Saunders, 1996, pp. 491–518.

11. Doczi T. Volume regulation of the brain tissue: a survey. *Acta Neurochir.* 1993;121:1–8.

12. McComb GJ. Recent research into the nature of cerebrospinal fluid formation and absorption. *J. Neurosurg.* 1983;59:369–383.

13. Cutler RWP, Page L, Galicich J, Watters GV. Formation and absorption of cerebrospinal fluid in man. *Brain* 1968;91:707–720.

14. Lyons MK, Meyer FB. Cerebrospinal fluid physiology and the management of increased intracranial pressure. *Mayo Clin. Proc.* 1990;65:684–707.

15. Gjerris F, Borgesen SE. Pathophysiology of cerebrospinal fluid circulation. In: Crockard A, Hayward R, Hoff JT, eds. *Neurosurgery: The Scientific Basis of Clinical Practice*, 3rd ed. Oxford: Blackwell Science, 2000, pp. 147–168.

16. Potts DG, Deonarine V. Effect of postural changes and jugular vein compression on the pressure gradient across the arachnoid villi granulations of the dog. *J. Neurosurg.* 1973;38:722–728.

17. Magnaes B. Body position and cerebrospinal fluid pressure: I. Clinical studies on the effect of rapid postural changes. *J. Neurosurg.* 1976;44:687–697.

18. Magnaes B. Clinical studies of cranial and spinal compliance and the craniospinal flow of cerebrospinal fluid. *Br. J. Neurosurg.* 1989;3:659–668.

19. Apuzzo MLJ, Weiss MH, Petersons V, Small RB, Kurze T, Heiden JS. Effect of positive end expiratory pressure ventilation on intracranial pressure in man. *J. Neurosurg.* 1977;46:227–232.

20. Abbott NJ, Revest PA. Control of brain endothelial permeability. *Cerebrovasc. Brain Metab. Rev.* 1991;3:39–72.

21. Hariri RJ. Cerebral edema. *Neurosurg. Clin. North Am.* 1994;5:687–706.

22. Abbott NJ. Inflammatory mediators and modulation of blood-brain barrier permeability. *Cell. Molec. Neurobiol.* 2000;20:131–147.

23. Schilling L, Wahl M. Mediators of cerebral edema. In: Roach RC, et al., eds. *Hypoxia: Into the Next Millenium.* New York: Kluwer Academic/Plenum Publishing, 1999, pp. 123–141.

24. Rapoport SI, Robinson PJ. Tight junctional modification as the basis of osmotic opening of the blood-brain barrier. *Ann. NY Acad. Sci.* 1986;481:250–266.

25. Drewes LR. What is the blood-brain barrier? A molecular perspective. In: Roach RC, Wagner PD, Hackett PH, eds. *Hypoxia: Into the Next Millenium.* New York: Kluwer Academic/Plenum Publishing 1999, pp. 111–122.

26. Venero JL, Vizuete ML, Machado A, Cano J. Aquaporins in the central nervous system. *Prog. Neurobiol.* 2000;63:321–336.

27. Manley GT, Fujimara M, Ma T, Noshita N, Filiz F, Bollen AW, Chan P, Verkman AS. Aquaporin-4 deletion in mice reduces brain edema after acute water intoxication and ischemic stroke. *Nat. Med.* 2000; 6:159–163.

28. Taniguchi M, Yamashita T, Kumura E, et al. Induction of aquaporin-4 water channel mRNA after focal cerebral ischemia in rat. *Mol. Brain Res.* 2000;78:131–137.

29. Ke C, Poon WS, Ng HK, Pang JCS, Chan Y. Heterogeneous responses of aquaporin-4 in oedema formation in a replicated severe traumatic brain injury model in rats. *Neurosci. Lett.* 2001;301:21–24.

30. Klatzo I. Evolution of brain edema concepts. *Acta Neurochir.* 1994;60(Suppl):3–6.

31. Klatzo I. Presidential address: Neuropathological aspects of brain edema. *J. Neuropath. Exp. Neurol.* 1967;26:1–14.

32. Nagashima T, Horwitz B, Rapaport SI. A mathematical model for vasogenic brain edema. In: Long DM, ed. *Brain Edema: Pathogenesis, Imaging and Therapy.* Advances in Neurology, volume 52. New York: Raven Press, 1990, pp. 317–326.

33. Lee KR, Betz AL, Keep RF, Chenevert TL, Kim S, Hoff JT. Intracerebral infusion of thrombin as a cause of brain edema. *J. Neurosurg.* 1995;83:1045–1050.

34. Rapoport SI. Opening of the blood-brain barrier by acute hypertension. *Exp. Neurol.* 1976;52:467–479.

35. Ohata K, Marmarou A. Clearance of brain edema and macromolecules through the cortical extracellular space. *J. Neurosurg.* 1992;77:387–396.

36. Wrba E, Nehring V, Chang RCC, Baethmann A, Reulen HJ, Uhl E. Quantitative analysis of brain edema resolution into the cerebral ventricles and subarachnoid space. *Acta Neurochir.* 1997;70(Suppl):288–290.

37. Reulen HJ, Graham R, Spatz M, Klatzo I. Role of pressure gradients and bulk flow in dynamics of vasogenic brain edema. *J. Neurosurg.* 1977;46:24–35.

38. Black K. Blood-brain barrier. In: Youmans JR, ed. *Neurological Surgery*, vol. 1. Philadelphia: Saunders, 1995, pp. 482–490.

39. Frank JI. Management of intracranial hypertension. *Med. Clin. North Am.* 1993;77:61–76.
40. Jackson PS, Madsen JR. Cerebral edema cell volume regulation and the role of ion channels in organic osmolyte transport. *Pediatr. Neurosurg.* 1997;27:279–285.
41. Lundberg N. Continuous recording and control of ventricular fluid pressure in neurosurgical practice. *Acta Psychiatr. Neurol. Scand.* 1960;36(Suppl 149):1–193.
42. Rosner MJ, Becker DP. Origin and evolution of plateau waves: experimental observations and a theoretical model. *J. Neurosurg.* 1984;60:312–324.
43. Hayashi M, Kobayashi H, Handa Y, Kawano H, Kabuto M. Brain blood volume and blood flow in patients with plateau waves. *J. Neurosurg.* 1985;63:556–561.
44. Giulioni M, Ursino M. Impact of cerebral perfusion pressure and autoregulation on intracranial dynamics: A modeling study. *Neurosurgery* 1996;39:1005–1015.
45. Ursino M, Lodi CA. A simple mathematical model of the interaction between intracranial pressure and cerbral hemo-dynamics. *J. Appl. Physiol.* 1997;82:1256–1269.
46. Ursino M, Lodi CA, Rossi S, Stocchetti N. Intracranial pressure dynamics in patients with acute brain damage. *J. Appl. Physiol.* 1997;82:1270–1282.
47. Bingaman WE, Frank JI. Malignant cerebral edema and intracranial hypertension. *Neurol. Clin. North Am.* 1995;13:479-509.
48. Ropper AH. Lateral displacement of the brain and level of consciousness in patients with an acute hemispheral mass. *N. Engl. J. Med.* 1986;314:953–958.
49. Teasdale E, Cardoso E, Galbraith S, Teasdale G. CT scan in severe diffuse head injury: physiological and clinical correlations. *J. Neurol. Neurosurg. Psychiatr.* 1984;47:600–603.
50. Roberson FC, Kishore PRS, Miller JD, Lipper MH, Becker DP. The value of serial computerized tomography in the management of severe head injury. *Surg. Neurol.* 1979;12:161–167.
51. Manno EM. Transcranial doppler ultrasonography in the neurocritical care unit. *Crit. Care Clin.* 1997;13:79–104.
52. Newell DW. Transcranial doppler ultrasonography. *Neurosurg. Clin. North Am.* 1994;5:619–631.
53. Homburg A-M, Jakobsen M, Enevoldsen E. Transcranial doppler recordings in raised intracranial pressure. *Acta Neurol. Scand.* 1993;87:488–493.
54. Suarez JI, Qureshi AI, Yahia AB, et al. Symptomatic vasospasm diagnosis after subarachnoid hemorrhage: evaluation of transcranial Doppler ultrasound and cerebral angiography as related to compromised vascular distribution. *Crit. Care Med.* 2002;30:1348–1355.
55. Chan K-H, Miller JD, Dearden NM, et al. The effect of changes in cerebral perfusion pressure upon middle cerebral artery blood flow velocty and jugular bulb venous oxygen saturation after severe brain injury. *J. Neurosurg.* 1992;77:55–61.
56. Lang EW, Chesnut RM. Intracranial pressure: monitoring and management. *Neurosurg. Clin. North Am.* 1994;5:573–605.
57. Jordan KG. Neurophysiologic monitoring in the neuroscience intensive care unit. *Neurol. Clin. North Am.* 1995;13:579–626.
58. King WA, Martin NA. Critical care of patients with subarachnoid hemorrhage. *Neurosurg. Clin. North Am.* 1994;5:767–787.
59. Narayan RK, Kishore PRS, Becker DP, et al. Intracranial pressure: To monitor or not to monitor? A review of our experience with severe head injury. *J. Neurosurg.* 1982;56:650–659.
60. Mayhall CG, Archer NH, Lamb VA, et al. Ventriculostomy-related infections: a prospective epidemiologic study. *N. Engl. J. Med.* 1984;310:553–559.
61. Aucoin PJ, Kotilainen HR, Gantz NM, Davidson R, Kellogg P, Stone B. Intracranial pressure monitors: epidemiologic study of risk factors and infections. *Am. J. Med.* 1986;80:369–376.
62. Wyler AR, Kelly WA. Use of antibiotics with external ventriculostomies. *J. Neurosurg.* 1972;37:185–187.
63. Paramore CG, Turner DA. Relative risks of ventriculostomy infection and morbidity. *Acta Neurochir.* 1994;127:79–84.
64. Holloway KL, Barnes T, Choi S, et al. Ventriculostomy infections: the effect of monitoring duration and catheter exchange in 584 patients. *J. Neurosurg.* 1996;85:419–424.
65. Crutchfield JS, Narayan RK, Robertson CS, Michael LH. Evaluation of a fiberoptic intracranial pressure monitor. *J. Neurosurg.* 1990;72:482–487.
66. Gray WP, Palmer JD, Gill J, Gardner M, Iannotti F. A clinical study of parenchymal and subdural miniature strain-guage transducers for monitoring intracranial pressure. *Neurosurgery* 1996;39:927–932.
67. Vries JK, Becker DP, Young HF. A subarachnoid screw for monitoring intracranial pressure: technical note. *J. Neurosurg.* 1973;39:416–419.
68. Swann KW, Cosman ER. Modification of the Richmond subarachnoid screw for monitoring intracranial pressure: technical note. *J. Neurosurg.* 1984;60:1102–1103.
69. Winn HR, Dacey RG, Jane JA. Intracranial subarachnoid pressure recording: experience with 650 patients. *Surg. Neurol.* 1977;8:41–47.
70. North B, Reilly P. Comparison among three methods of intracranial pressure recording. *Neurosurgery* 1986:18:730–732.
71. Leech P, Miller JD. Intracranial volume/pressure relationships during experimental brain compression in primates: 1. Pressure responses to changes inventricular volume. *J. Neurol. Neurosurg. Psychiatry* 1974;37:1093–1098.

72. Leech P, Miller JD. Intracranial volume/pressure relationships during experimental brain compression in primates: 2. Effect of induced changes in systemic arterial pressure and cerebral blood flow. *J. Neurol. Neurosurg. Psychiatry* 1974;37:1099–1104.

73. Leech P, Miller JD. Intracranial volume/pressure relationships during experimental brain compression in primates: 3. Effect of mannitol and hyperventilation. *J. Neurol. Neurosurg. Psychiatry* 1974;37:1105–1111.

74. Miller JD, Garibi J, Pickard JD. Induced changes of cerebrospinal fluid volume. *Arch. Neurol.* 1973;28:265–269.

75. Schettini A, Walsh EK. Contribution of brain distortion and displacement to CSF dynamics in experimental brain compression. *Am. J. Physiology* 1991;260:R172–R178.

76. Piper IR, Miller JD, Whittle IR, Lawson A. Automated time-averaged analysis of craniospinal compliance (short pulse response). *Acta Neurochir.* 1990;51(Suppl):387–390.

77. Piper I, Dunn L, Contant C, et al. Multi-center assessment of the Spiegelberg compliance monitor: preliminary results. *Acta Neurochir.* 2000;76(Suppl):491–494.

78. Martin NA, Doberstein C. Cerebral blood flow measurement in neurosurgical intensive care. *Neurosurg. Clin. North Am.* 1994;5:607–618.

79. Kelly DF, Nikas DL, Becker DP. Diagnosis and treatment of moderate and severe head injuries in adults. In: Youmans JR, ed. *Neurological Surgery*, vol. 3. Philadelphia: Saunders, 1996, pp. 1618–1718.

80. Seelig JM, Becker DP, Miller JD, Greenberg RP, Ward JD, Choi SC. Traumatic acute subdural hematoma: major mortality reduction in comatose patients treated within four hours. *N. Engl. J. Med.* 1981;304:1511–1518.

81. Osenbach RK, Loftus CM. Diagnosis and management of brain abscess. *Neurosurg. Clin. North Am.* 1992;3:403–420.

82. Mathisen GE, Johnson JP. Brain abscess. *Clin. Infect. Dis.* 1997;25:763–781.

83. Calfey DP, Wispelwey B. Brain abscess. *Semin. Neurol.* 2000;20:353–360.

84. Gormley WB, del Busto R, Saravolatz LD, Rosenblum ML. Cranial and intracranial bacterial infections. In: Youmans JR, ed. *Neurological Surgery*, 4th ed. Philadelphia: WB Saunders, 1996, pp. 3191–3220.

85. Broderick JP, Adams HP, Barsan W, et al. Guidelines for the management of spontaneous intracerebral hemorrhage. *Stroke* 1999;30:905–915.

86. Rabinstein AA, Atkinson JL, Wijdicks EFM. Emergency craniotomy in patients worsening due to expanded cerebral hematoma: To what purpose? *Neurology* 2002;58:1367–1372.

87. Munch EC, Bauhuf C, Horn P, Roth HR, Schmiedek P, Vajoczy P. Therapy of malignant intracranial hypertension by controlled lumbar cerebrospinal fluid drainage. *Crit. Care Med.* 2001;29:976–981.

88. Willemse RB, Egeler-Peerdeman SM. External lumbar drainage in uncontrollable intracranial pressure in adults with sever head injury: A report of 7 cases. *Acta Neurochir.* 1998;71(Suppl):37–39.

89. Levy DI, Rekate HL, Cherny WB, Manwaring K, Moss SD, Baldwin HZ. Controlled lumbar drainage in pediatric head injury. *J. Neurosurg.* 1995;83:453–460.

90. Hahn M, Murali R, Couldwell WT. Tunneled lumbar drain: Techical note. *J. Neurosurg.* 2002;96:1130–1131.

91. Roland PS, Marple BF, Meyerhoff WL, Mickey B. Complications of lumbar spinal fluid drainage. *Otolaryngol. Head Neck Surg.* 1992;107:564–569.

92. Acikbas SC, Akyuz M, Kazan S, Tuncer R. Complications of closed continuous lumbar drainage of cerebrospinal fluid. *Acta Neurochir.* 2002;144:475–480.

93. Kapadia FN, Jha AN. Simultaneous lumbar and intraventricular manometry to evaluate the role and safety of lumbar puncture in raised intracranial pressure following subarachnoid haemorrhage. *Br. J. Neurosurg.* 1996;10:585–587.

94. Fessler RD, Sobel J, Guyot L, et al. Management of elevated intracranial pressure in patients with cryptococcal meningitis. *J. Acq. Imm. Def. Synd. Hum. Retrovirol.* 1998;17:137–142.

95. Malessa R, Krams M, Hengge U, et al. Elevation of intracranial pressure in acute AIDS-related cryptococcal meningitis. *Clin. Invest.* 1994;72:1020–1026.

96. Sommer JB, Gaul C, Heckmann J, Neundorfer B, Erbguth FJ. Does Lumbar cerebrospinal fluid reflect ventricular cerebrospinal fluid? A prospective study in patients with external ventricular drainage. *Eur. Neurol.* 2002;47:224–232.

97. Spiller WG, Franzier CH. Cerebral decompression: palliative operations in the treatment of tumors of the brain, based on the observation of fourteen cases. *JAMA* 1906;47:679–683.

98. Kleist-Welch Guerra W, Piek J, Gaab MR. Decompressive craniectomy to treat intracranial hypertension in head injury patients. *Intensive Care Med.* 1999;25:1327–1329.

99. Gaab MR, Rittierodt M, Lorenz M, Heissler HE. Traumatic brain swelling and operative decompression: a prospective investigation. *Acta Neurochir.* 1990;51(Suppl):326–328.

100. Kunze E, Meixensberger J, Janka M, Sorensen N, Roosen K. Decompressive craniectomy in patients with uncontrollable intracranial hypertension. *Acta Neurochir.* 1998;71(Suppl):16–18.

101. Kleist-Welch Guerra W, Gaab MR, Dietz H, Mueller JU, Piek J, Fritsch MJ. Surgical decompression for traumatic brain swelling: indications and results. *J. Neurosurg.* 1999;90:187–196.

102. De Luca GP, Volpin L, Fornezza U, et al. The role of decompressive craniectomy in the treatment of uncontrollable intracranial hypertension. *Acta Neurochir.* 2000;76 (Suppl):401–404.
103. Meier U, Zeilinger FS, Henzka O. The use of decompressive craniectomy for the management of severe head injuries. *Acta Neurochir.* 2000;76(Suppl):475–478.
104. Munch EC, Horn P, Schurer L, Piepgras A, Paul T, Schmiedek P. Management of severe traumatic brain injury by decompressive craniectomy. *Neurosurgery* 2000;47:315–323.
105. Coplin WM, Cullen NK, Policherla PN, et al. Safety and feasibility of craniectomy with duraplasty as the initial surgical intervention for severe traumatic brain injury. *J. Trauma* 2001;50:1050–1059.
106. Delashaw JB, Broaddus WC, Kassell NF, et al. Treatment of right hemispheric cerebral infarction by hemicraniectomy. *Stroke* 1990;21:874–881.
107. Rieke K, Schwab S, Krieger D, et al. Decompressive surgery in space-occupying hemispheric infarction: results of an open, prospective trial. *Crit. Care Med.* 1995;23:1576–1587.
108. Schwab S, Steiner T, Aschoff A, et al. Early hemicraniectomy in patients with complete middle cerebral artery infarction. *Stroke* 1998;29:1888–1893.
109. Sakai K, Iwahashi K, Terada K, Gohda Y, Sakurai M, Matsumoto Y. Outcome after external decompression for massive cerebral infarction. *Neurol. Med. Chir. (Tokyo)* 1998;38:131–136.
110. Robertson CS, Valadka AB, Hannay HJ, et al. Prevention of secondary ischemic insults after severe head injury. *Crit. Care Med.* 1999;27:2086–2095.
111. Capes SE, Hunt D, Malmberg K, Pathak P, Gerstein HC. Stress hyperglycemia and prognosis of stroke in nondiabetic and diabetic patients: A systematic overview. *Stroke* 2001;32:2426–2432.
112. Pulsinelli W, Levy DE, Sigsbee B, Scherer P, Plum F. Increased damage after ischemic stroke in patients with hyperglycemia with or without established diabetes mellitus. *Am. J. Med.* 1983;74:540–544.
113. Parsons MW, Barber PA, Desmond PM, et al. Acute hyperglycemia adversely affects stroke outcome: a magnetic resonance imaging and spectroscopy study. *Ann. Neurol.* 2002;52:20–28.
114. Els T, Klisch J, Orszagh M, et al. Hyperglycemia in patients with focal cerebral ischemia after intravenous thrmbolysis: influcence of clinical outcome and infarct size. *Cerebrovasc. Dis.* 2002;13:89–94.
115. Kase CS, Furlan AJ, Wechsler LR, et al. Cerebral hemorrhage after intra-arterial thrombolysis for ischemic stroke: the PROACT-II trial. *Neurology* 2001;57:1603–1610.
116. Alberti O, Becker R, Benes L, Wallenfang T, Bertalanffy H. Initial hyperglycemia as an indicator of severity of the ictus in poor-grade patients with spontaneous subarachnoid hemorrhage. *Clin. Neurol. Neurosurg.* 2000;102:78–83.
117. Tang LM, Chen ST, Hsu WC, Lyu RK. Acute bacterial meningitis in adults: a hospital-based epidemiological study. *QJM* 1999;92:719–725.
118. Chiaretti A, Piastra M, Pulitano S, et al. Prognostic factors and outcome of children with severe head injury: An 8-year experience. *Child's Nerv. Sys.* 2002;18:129–136.
119. Rovlias A, Kotsou S. The influence of hyperglycemia on neurological outcome in patients with severe head injury. *Neurosurgery* 2000;46:335–342.
120. Yang SY, Zhang S, Wang ML. Clinical significance of admission hyperglycemia and factors related to it in patients with acute severe head injury. *Surg. Neurol.* 1995;44:373–377.
121. Schwartz S, Hafner K, Aschoff A, Schwab S. Incidence and prognostic significance of fever following intracerebral hemorrhage. *Neurology* 2000;54:354–361.
122. Van den Berghe G, Wouters P, Weekers F, et al. Intensive insulin therapy in critically ill patients. *N. Engl. J. Med.* 2001;345:1359–1367.
123. Castillo J, Davalos A, Marrugat J, Noya M. Timing for fever-related brain damage in acute ischemic stroke. *Stroke* 1998;29:2455–2460.
124. Hajat C, Hajat S, Sharma P. Effects of poststroke pyrexia on stroke outcome: A meta-analysis of studies in patients. *Stroke* 2000;31:410–414.
125. Oliveira-Filho J, Ezzeddine MA, Segal AZ, et al. Fever in subarachnoid hemorrhage: relationship to vasospasm and outcome. *Neurology* 2001;56:1299–1304.
126. Zeiner A, Holzer M, Sterz F, et al. Mild resuscitative hypothermia to improve neurological outcome after cardiac arrest: a clinical feasability trial. *Stroke* 2000;31:86–94.
127. Clasen RA, Pandolfi A, Laing I, et al. Experimental study of relation of fever to cerebral edema. *J. Neurosurg.* 1974;41:576–581.
128. Kim Y, Busto R, Dietrich WD, Karydieg S, Ginsberg MD. Delayed postischemic hyperthermia in awake rats worsens the histopathological outcome of transient focal cerebra ischemia. *Stroke* 1996;27:2274–2280.
129. Koennecke H-C, Leistner S. Prophylactic antipyretic treatment with acetaminophen in acute ischemic stroke: A pilot study. *Neurology* 2001;57:2301–3203.
130. Mayer W, Commichau C, Scarmeas N, Presciutti M, Bates J, Copeland D. Clinical trial of an air-circulating cooling blanket for fever control in critically ill neurologic patients. *Neurology* 2001;56:292–298.
131. Cooper KR, Boswell PA, Choi SC. Safe use of PEEP in patients with severe head injury. *J. Neurosurg.* 1985;63:552–555.

132. McGuire G, Crossley D, Richards J, Wong D. Effects of varying levels of positive end-expiratory pressure on intracranial pressure and cerebral perfusion pressure. *Crit. Care Med.* 1997;25:1059–1062.

133. Feldman Z, Kanter MJ, Robertson CS, et al. Effect of head elevation on intracranial pressure cerebral perfusion pressure and cerebral blood flow in head-injured patients. *J. Neurosurg.* 1992;76:207–211.

134. Ropper AH, O'Rourke D, Kennedy SK. Head position intracranial pressure and compliance. *Neurology* 1982;32:1288–1291.

135. Temkin NR, Dikmen SS, Wilensky AJ, Keihm J, Chabal S, Winn HR. A randomized, double-blind study of phenytoin for the prevention of post-traumatic seizures. *N. Engl. J. Med.* 1990;323:497–502.

136. Van Gijn J, Rinkel GJE. Subarachnoid hemorrhage: Diagnosis, causes and management. *Brain* 2001; 124:249–278.

137. Barry E. Posttraumatic epilepsy. In: Wyllie E, ed. *The Treatment of Epilepsy: Principles and Practice*, 3rd ed. Philadelphia: Lippincott Williams & Wilkins, 2001, pp. 609–614.

138. Glantz MJ, Cole BF, Forsyth PA, et al. Practice parameter: anticonvulsant prophylaxis in patients with newly diagnosed brain tumors. *Neurology* 2000;54:1886–1893.

139. Stringer WA, Hasso AN, Thompson JR, et al. Hyperventilation-induced cerebral ischemia in patients with acute brain lesions: Demonstration by xenon-enhanced CT. *AJNR* 1993;475–484.

140. Muizelaar HP, van der Poel HG, Zhongchao L, Lontos HA, Levasseur JE. Pial arteriolar vessel diameter and CO_2 reactivity during prolonged hyperventilation in the rabbit. *J. Neurosurg.* 1988;69:923–927.

141. Muizelaar JP, Marmarou A, Ward JD, et al. Adverse effects of prolonged hyperventilation in patients with severe head injury: a randomized controlled trial. *J. Neurosurg.* 1991;75:731–739.

142. Bullock RM, Chesnut RM, Clifton GL, et al. Hyperventilation. *J. Neurotrauma* 2000;17:513–520.

143. Yundt KD, Diringer MN. The use of hyperventilation and its impact on cerebral ischemia in the treatment of traumatic brain injury. *Crit. Care Clin.* 1997;13:163–184.

144. Peterson B, Khanna S, Fisher B, Marshall L. Prolonged hypernatremia controls elevated intracranial pressure in head-injured pediatric patients. *Crit. Care Med.* 2000;28:1136–1143.

145. Simma B, Burger R, Falk M, Sacher P, Fanconi S. A prospective, randomized, and controlled study of fluid management in children with severe head injury: lactated Ringer's solution versus hypertonic saline. *Crit. Care Med.* 1998;26:1265–1270.

146. Marshall RS, Mayer SA. *On Call Neurology*, 2nd ed. New York: WB Saunders, 2001.

147. Nath F, Galbraith S. The effect of mannitol on cerebral white matter water content. *J. Neurosurg.* 1986;65:41–43.

148. Donato T, Shapira Y, Artru A, Powers K. Effect of mannitol on cerebrospinal fluid dynamics and brain tissue edema. *Anesth. Analg.* 1994;78:58–66.

149. Burke AM, Quest DO, Chien S, Cerri C. The effects of mannitol on blood viscosity. *J. Neurosurg.* 1981;55:550–553.

150. Ravussin P, Abou-Madi M, Archer D, et al. Changes in CSF pressure after mannitol in patients with and without elevated CSF pressure. *J. Neurosurg.* 1988;69:869–876.

151. Mendelow AD, Teasdale GM, Russell T, Flood J, Patterson J, Murray GD. Effect of mannitol on cerebral blood flow and cerebral perfusion pressure in human head injury. *J. Neurosurg.* 1985;63:43–48.

152. Domaingue CM, Nye DH. Hypotensive effect of mannitol administered rapidly. *Anaesth. Intensive Care* 1985;13:134–136.

153. Paczynski RP. Osmotherapy: basic concepts and controversies. *Crit. Care Clin.* 1997;13:105–129.

154. Node Y, Nakazawa S. Clinical study of mannitol and glycerol on raised intracranial pressure and on their rebound phenomenon. In: Long DM (ed.) *Brain Edema: Pathogenesis, Imaging and Therapy. Advances in Neurology*, volume 52. New York: Raven Press, 1990, pp. 359–363.

155. Kaufmann AM, Cardoso ER. Aggravation of vasogenic cerebral edema by multiple-dose mannitol. *J. Neurosurg.* 1992;77:584–589.

156. Horn P, Munch E, Vajkoczy P, et al. Hypertonic saline solution for control of elevated intracranial pressure in patients with exhausted response to mannitol and barbiturates. *Neurol. Res.* 1999;21:758–764.

157. Frank JI. Large hemispheric infarction, deterioration and intracranial pressure. *Neurology* 1995;45:1286–1290.

158. Videen TO, Zazulia AR, Manno EM, et al. Mannitol bolus preferentially shrinks non-infarcted brain in patients with ischemic stroke. *Neurology* 2001;57:2120–2122.

159. Manno EM, Adams RE, Derdeyn CP, Powers WJ, Diringer MN. The effects of mannitol on cerebral edema after large hemispheric cerebral infarct. *Neurology* 1999;52:583–587.

160. Nau R. Osmotherapy for elevated intracranial pressure: A critical reappraisal. *Clin. Pharmacokinet.* 2000;38:23–40.

161. Righetti E, Celani MG, Cantisani T, Sterzi R, Boysen G, Ricci S. Glycerol for acute stroke (Cochrane Review). In: *The Cochrane Library*, issue 3, 2001. Oxford: Update Software.

162. De los Reyes RA, Ausman JI, Diaz FG. Agents for cerebral edema. *Clin. Neurosurg.* 1981;28:98–107.

163. Doyle JA, Davis DP, Hoyt DB. The use of hypertonic saline in the treatment of traumatic brain injury. *J. Trauma* 2001;50:367–383.

164. Qureshi AI, Suarez JI. Use of hypertonic saline solutions in treatment of cerebral edema and intracranial hypertension. *Crit. Care Med.* 2000;28:3301–3313.

165. Wade CE, Grady JJ, Kramer GC, Younes RN, Gehlsen K, Holcroft JW. Individual patient cohort analysis of the efficacy of hypertonic saline/dextran in patients with traumatic brain injury and hypotension. *J. Trauma* 1997;42(Suppl):S61–S65.

166. Chesnut RM. Avoidance of hypotension: conditio sine qua non of successful severe head-injury management. *J. Trauma* 1997;42(Suppl):S4–S9.
167. Worthley LIG, Cooper DJ, Jones N. Treatment of resistant intracranial hypertension with hypertonic saline: report of two cases. *J. Neurosurg.* 1988;68:478–481.
168. Schatzmann C, Heissler HE, Konig K, et al. Treatment of elevated intracranial pressure by infusions of 10% saline in severely head injured patients. *Acta Neurochir.* 1998;71(Suppl):31–33.
169. Khanna S, Davis D, Peterson B, et al. Use of hypertonic saline in the treatment of severe refractory posttraumatic intracranial hypertensions in pediatric traumatic brain injury. *Crit. Care Med.* 2000;28:1144–1151.
170. Qureshi AI, Suarez JI, Bhardwaj A, et al. Use of hypertonic (3%) saline/acetate infusion in the treatment of cerebral edema: Effect on intracranial pressure and lateral displacement of the brain. *Crit. Care Med.* 1998;26:440–446.
171. Shackford SR, Bourguignon PR, Wald SL, Rogers FB, Osler TM, Clark DE. Hypertonic saline resuscitation of patients with head injury: a prospective, randomized clinical trial. *J. Trauma* 1998;44:50–58.
172. McCarthy KD, Reed DJ. The effect of acetazolamide and furosemide on cerebrospinal fluid production and choroid plexus carbonic anhydrase activity. *J. Pharmacol. Ex. Ther.* 1974;189:194–201.
173. Kennedy CR, Ayers S, Campbell MJ, Elbourne D, Hope P, Johnson A. Randomized, controlled trial of acetazolamide and furosemide in posthemorrhagic ventricular dilation in infancy: follow-up at 1 year. *Pediatrics* 2001;108:597–607.
174. Libenson MH, Kaye EM, Rosman NP, Gilmore HE. Acetazolamide and furosemide for posthemorrhagic hydrocephalus of the newborn. *Pediatr. Neurol.* 1999;20:185–191.
175. Whitelaw A, Kennedy CR, Brion LP. Diuretic therapy for newborn infants with posthemorrhagic ventricular dilatation. In: *The Cochrane Library*, issue 1, 2002. Oxford: Update Software.
176. Allen CH, Ward JD. An evidence-based approach to management of increased intracranial pressure. *Crit. Care Clin.* 1998;14:485–495.
177. Roberts PA, Pollay M, Engles C, Pendleton B, Reynolds E, Stevens FA. Effect on intracranial pressure of furosemide combined with varying doses and administration rates of mannitol. *J. Neurosurg.* 1987;66:440–446.
178. Harkness KA, Adamson P, Sussman JD, et al. Dexamethasone regulation of matrix metalloproteinase expression in CNS vascular endothelium. *Brain* 2000;123:698–709.
179. Galicich JH, French LA. Use of dexamethasone in the treatment of cerebral edema resulting from brain tumors and brain surgery. *Am. Practit.* 1961;12:169–174.
180. Kullberg A, West KA. Influence of corticosteroids on the ventricular fluid pressure. *Acta Neurol. Scand.* 1965;41(Suppl 13, part II):445–452.
181. Miller JD, Sakalas R, Ward JD, et al. Methylprednisolone treatment in patients with brain tumors. *Neurosurgery* 1977;1:114–117.
182. Schroeder KA, McKeever PE, Schaberg DR, Hoff JT. Effect of dexamethasone on experimental brain abscess. *J. Neurosurg.* 1987;66:264–269.
183. Quartey GRC, Johnston JA, Rozdolisky B. Decadron in the treatment of cerebral abscess: an experimental study. *J. Neurosurg.* 1976;45:301–310.
184. Bohl I, Wallenfang T, Bothe H, et al. The effect of glucocorticoids in the combined treatment of experimental brain abscess in cats. *Adv. Neurosurg.* 1981;9:125–133.
185. Britt RH, Enzmann DR. Clinical stages of human brain abscesses on serial CT scans after contrast infusion: computerized tomographic, neuropathological, and clinical correlations. *J. Neurosurg.* 1983;59:972–989.
186. Wispelwey B, Dacey RG, Scheld WM. Brain abscess. In: Scheld WM, Whitley RJ, Durack DT, eds. *Infections of the Central Nervous System*, 2nd ed. Philadelphia: Lippincott-Raven, 1997, pp. 463–493.
187. Davis LE, Baldwin NG. Brain abscess. *Curr. Treat. Opt. Neurol.* 1999;1:157–166.
188. White AC. Neurocysticercosis: Updates on epidemiology, pathogenesis, diagnosis, and management. *Ann. Rev. Med.* 2000;51:187–206.
189. Carpenter TC. Corticosteroids in the treatment of severe mycoplasma encephalitis in children. *Crit. Care Med.* 2002;30:925–927.
190. Upton ARM, Barwick DD, Foster JB. Dexamethasone treatment in herpes-simplex encephalitis. *Lancet* 1971;1:290–291.
191. Longson M, Juel-Jensen BE, Liversedge LA. Systemic corticosteroids in treatment of herpes simplex encephalitis. *BMJ* 1975;4:578.
192. Habel AH, Brown JK. Dexamethasone in herpes-simplex encephalitis. *Lancet* 1972;1:695.
193. Ling GSF, Hanley DF. Neurocritical care of CNS infections. In: Scheld WM, Whitley RJ, Durack DT, eds. *Infections of the Central Nervous System*, 2nd ed. Philadelphia: Lippincott-Raven, 1997, pp. 973–979.
194. Corboy JR, Tyler KL. Neurovirology. In: Bradley WG, Daroff RB, Fenichel GM, Marsden CD, eds. *Neurology in Clinical Practice*, 3rd ed. Boston: Butterworth-Heinemann, 2000, pp. 823–840.
195. Whitley RJ, Alford CA, Hirsch MS, et al. Vidarabine versus acyclovir therapy in herpes simplex encephalitis. *N. Engl. J. Med.* 1986;314:144–149.

196. Quagliarello VJ, Scheld VM. Treatment of bacterial meningitis. *N. Engl. J. Med.* 1997;336:708–716.
197. McIntyre PR, Berkey CS, King SM, et al. Dexamethasone as adjunctive therapy in bacterial meningitis: a meta-analysis of randomized clinical trails since 1988. *JAMA* 1997;278:925–931.
198. Lebel MH, Freij BJ, Syrogiannopoulos GA, et al. Dexamethasone therapy for bacterial meningitis: results of two double-blind, placebo-controlled trials. *N. Engl. J. Med.* 1988;319:964–971.
199. Odio CM, Faingezicht I, Paris M, et al. The beneficial effects of early dexamthasone administration in infants and children with bacterial meningitis. *N. Engl. J. Med.* 1991;324:1525–1531.
200. Wald ER, Kaplan SL, Mason EO, et al. Dexamethasone therapy for children with bacterial meningitis. *Pediatrics* 1995;95:21–28.
201. Schaad UB, Lips U, Gnehm HE, Blumberg A, Heinzer I, Wedgwood J. Dexamethasone therapy for bacterial meningitis in children. *Lancet* 1993;342:457–461.
202. Dearden NM, Gibson JS, McDowall DG, Gibson RM, Cameron MM. Effect of high-dose dexamethasone on outcome from severe head injury. *J. Neurosurg.* 1986;64:81–88.
203. Bullock RM, Chesnut RM, Clifton GL, et al. Role of steroids. *J. Neurotrauma* 2000;17:531–535.
204. Poungvarin N, Bhoopat W, Viriyavejakul A, et al. Effects of dexamethasone in primary supratentorial intracerebral hemorrhage. *N. Engl. J. Med.* 1987;316:1229–1233.
205. Qizilbash N, Lewington SL, Lopez-Arrieta JM. Corticosteroids for acute ischaemic stroke. In: *The Cochrane Library*, issue 3, 2001. Oxford: Update Software.
206. Norris JW, Hachinski VC. High dose steroid treatment in cerebral infarction. *BMJ* 1986;292:21–23.
207. Anderson DC, Cranford RE. Corticosteroids in ischemic stroke. *Stroke* 1979;10:68–71.
208. Bauer RB, Tellez H. Dexamethasone as treatment in cerebrovascular disease, 2: a controlled study in acute cerebral infarction. *Stroke* 1973;4:547–555.
209. Chen D, Nishizawa S, Yokota N, Ohta S, Yokoyama T, Namba H. High-dose methylprednisolone prevents vasospasm after subarachnoid hemorrhage through inhibition of protein kinase C activation. *Neurol. Res.* 2002;24:215–222.
210. Chyatte D, Fode NC, Nichols DA, Sundt TM. Preliminary report: Effects of high dose methylprednisolone on delayed cerebral ischemia in patients at high risk for vasospasm after aneurysmal subarachnoid hemorrhage. *Neurosurgery* 1987;21:157–160.
211. Yamakawa K, Sasaki T, Tsubnaki S, Nakagomi T, Saito I, Takakura K. Effect of high-dose methylprednisolone on vasospasm after subarachnoid hemorrhage. *Neurol. Med. Chir. (Tokyo)* 1991;31:24–31.
212. Rockoff MA, Marshall LF, Shapiro HM. High-dose barbiturate therapy in humans: a clinical review of 60 patients. *Ann. Neurol.* 1979;6:194–199.
213. Piatt JH, Schiff SJ. High dose barbiturate therapy in neurosurgery and intensive care. *Neurosurgery* 1984;15:427–444.
214. Eisenberg HM, Frankowski RF, Contant CG, Marshall LF, Walker MD, and the Comprehensive Central Nervous System Trauma Centers. High dose barbiturate control of elevated intracranial pressure in patients with severe head injury. *J. Neurosurg.* 1988;69:15–23.
215. Ward JD, Becker DP, Miller JD, et al. Failure of prophylactic barbiturate coma in the treatment of severe head injury. *J. Neurosurg.* 1985;62:383–388.
216. Schwartz ML, Tator CH, Rowed DW, et al. The University of Toronto Head Injury Treatment Study: a prospective, randomized comparison of pentobarbital and mannitol. *Can. J. Neurol. Sci.* 1984;11:434–440.
217. Rea GL, Rockswold GL. Barbiturate therapy in uncontrolled intracranial hypertension. *Neurosurgery* 1983;12:401–404.
218. Schwab S, Spranger M, Schwarz S, Hacke W. Barbiturate coma in severe hemispheric stroke: Useful or obsolete? *Neurology* 1997;48:1608–1613.
219. Bullock RM, Chesnut RM, Clifton GL, et al. Use of barbiturates in the control of intracranial hypertension. *J. Neurotrauma* 2000;17:527–530.
220. Angelini G, Ketzler JT, Coursin DB. Use of propofol and other nonbenzodiazepine sedatives in the intensive care unit. *Crit. Care Clin.* 2001;17:863–880.
221. Mirski MA, Muffelman B, Ulatowski JA, Hanley DF. Sedation for the critically ill neurologic patient. *Crit. Care Med.* 1995;23:2038–2053.
222. Ravussin P, Guinard JP, Ralley F, Thorin D. Effect of propofol on cerebrospinal fluid pressure and cerebral perfusion pressure in patients undergoing craniotomy. *Anaesthesia* 1988;43(Suppl):37–41.
223. Vandesteene A, Trempont V, Engelman E, et al. Effect of propofol on cerebral blood flow and metabolism in man. *Anaesthesia* 1988;43(Suppl):42–43.
224. Stephan H, Sonntag H, Schenk HD, Kohlhausen S. Effects of disoprivan on cerebral blood flow, cerebral oxygen consumption, and cerebral vascular reactivity. *Anaesthesist* 1987;36:60–65.
225. Herregods L, Verbeke J, Rolly G, Colardyn F. Effect of propofol on elevated intracranial pressure: preliminary results. *Anaesthesia* 1988;43(Suppl):107–109.
226. Kelly DF, Goodale DB, Williams J, et al. Propofol in the treatment of moderate and severe head injury: a randomized, prospective double-blinded pilot trial. *J. Neurosurg.* 1999;90:1042–1052.
227. Perrier ND, Baerga-Varela Y, Murray MJ. Death related to propofol use in an adult patient. *Crit. Care Med.* 2000;28:3071–3074.

228. Walder B, Tramer MR, Seeck M. Seizure-like phenomena and propofol: a systematic review. *Neurology* 2002;58:1327–1332.

229. Albanese J, Arnaud S, Rey M, Thomachot L, Alliez B, Martin C. Ketamine decreases intracranial pressure and electroencephalographic activity in traumatic brain injury patients during propofol sedation. *Anesthesiology* 1997;87:1328–1334.

230. Kolenda H, Gremmelt A, Rading S, Braun U, Markakis E. Ketamine for analgosedative therapy in intensive care treatment of head-injured patients. *Acta Neurochir.* 1996;138:1193–1199.

231. Juul N, Morris GF, Marshall SB, Marshall LF. Neuromuscular blocking agents in neurointensive care. *Acta Neurochir.* 2000;76(Suppl):467–470.

232. HsiangJK, Chesnut RM, Crisp CB, Klauber MR, Blunt BA, Marshall LF. Early, routine paralysis for intracranial pressure control in severe head injury: Is it necessary? *Crit. Care Med.* 1994;22:1471–1476.

233. Werba A, Weinstabi C, Petricek W, et al. Vecuronium prevents increases in intracranial pressure during routine tracheobronchial suctioning in neurosurgical patients. *Anaesthesist* 1991;40:328–331.

234. Murphy GS, Vender JS. Neuromuscular-blocking drugs: use and misuse in the intensive care unit. *Crit. Care Clin.* 2001;17:925–942.

235. Hirano M, Ott BR, Raps EC, et al. Acute quadriplegic myopathy: A complication of treatment with steroids, nondepolarizing blocking agents, or both. *Neurology* 1992;42:2082–2087.

236. Clemmesen JO, Hansen BA, Larsen FS. Indomethacin normalizes intracranial pressure in acute liver failure: A twenty-three-year-old woman treated with indomethacin. *Hepatology* 1997;26:1423–1425.

237. Jensen K, Ohrstrom J, Cold GE, Astrup J. The effects of indomethacin on intracranial pressure, cerebral blood flow and cerebral metabolism in patients with severe head injury and intracranial hypertension. *Acta Neurochir.* 1991;108:116–121.

238. Biestro AA, Alberti RA, Soca AE, Cancela M, Puppo CB, Borovich B. Use of indomethacin in brain-injured patients with cerebral perfusion pressure impairment: preliminary report. *J. Neurosurg.* 1995:83:627-630.

239. Dahl B, Bergholt B, Cold GE, et al. CO_2 and indomethacin vasoreactivity in patients with head injury. *Acta Neurochir.* 1996;138:265–273.

240. Slavik RS, Rhoney DH. Indomethacin: a review of its cerebral blood flow effects and potential use for controlling intracranial pressure in traumatic brain injury patients. *Neurol. Res.* 1999;21:491–499.

241. Hypothermia After Cardiac Arrest Study Group. Mild therapeutic hypothermia to improve the neurologic outcome after cardiac arrest. *N. Engl. J. Med.* 2002;346:549–556.

242. Bernard SA, Gray TW, Buist MD, et al. Treatment of comatose survivors of out-of-hospital cardiac arrest with induced hypothermia. *N. Engl. J. Med.* 2002;346:557–563.

243. Padosch SA, Kern KB, Bottiger BW. Letter to the editor. *N. Engl. J. Med.* 2002;347:63.

244. Clifton GL, Miller ER, Choi SC, et al. Lack of effect of induction of hypothermia after acute brain injury. *N. Engl. J. Med.* 2001;344:556–563.

245. Marion DW, Obrist WD, Carlier PM, Penrod LE, Darby JM. The use of moderate therapeutic hypothermia for patients with severe head injuries: A preliminary report. *J. Neurosurg.* 1993;79:354–362.

246. Shiozaki T, Kato A, Taneda M, et al. Little benefit from mild hypothermia therapy for severely head injured patients with low intracranial pressure. *J. Neurosurg.* 1999;91:185–191.

247. Marion DW, Penrod LE, Kelsey SF, et al. Treatment of traumatic brain injury with moderate hypothermia. *N. Engl. J. Med.* 1997;336:540–546.

248. Shiozaki T, Sugimoto H, Taneda M, et al. Effect of mild hypothermia on uncontrollable intracranial hypertension after severe head injury. *J. Neurosurg.* 1993;79:363–368.

249. Gadkary CS, Alderson P, Signorini DF. Therapeutic hypothermia for head injury. In: *The Cochrane Library*, issue 2, 2002. Oxford: Update Software.

250. Polderman KG, Girbes ARJ. Letter to the editor. *N. Engl. J. Med.* 2002;347:64.

251. Schwab S, Schwarz S, Spranger M, Keller E, Bertram M, Hacke W. Moderate hypothermia in the treatment of patients with severe middle cerebral artery infarction. *Stroke* 1998;29:2461–2466.

252. Schwab S, Georgiadis D, Berrouschot J, Schellinger PD, Graffagnino C, Mayer SA. Feasibility and safety of moderate hypothermia after massive hemispheric infarction. *Stroke* 2001;32:2033–2035.

253. Krieger DW, De Georgia MA, Abou-Chebl A, et al. Cooling for acute ischemic brain damage (cool aid): an open pilot study of induced hypothermia in acute ischemic stroke. *Stroke* 2001;32:1847–1854.

254. DeGeorgia M, Abou-Chebl A, Devlin T, Jauss M, Davis S, Krieger D. Endovascular cooling for patients with acute ischemic stroke. *Neurology* 2002;58(Suppl 3):A506.

255. Rohrer MJ, Natale AM. Effect of hypothermia on the coagulation cascade. *Crit. Care Med.* 1992;20:1402–1405.

256. Patt A, McCroskey BL, Moore EE. Hypothermia-induced coagulopathies in trauma. *Surg. Clin. North Am.* 1988;68:775–785.

257. Polderman KH, Peerdeman SM, Girbes ARJ. Hypophosphatemia and hypomagnesemia induced by cooling in patients with severe head injury. *J. Neurosurg.* 2001;94:697–705.

258. Mokhtarani M, Mahgoub AN, Morioka N, et al. Buspirone and meperidine synergistically reduce the shivering threshold. *Anesth. Analg.* 2001;93:1233–1239.

259. Rockswold GL, Ford SE, Anderson DC, Bergman TA, Sherman RE. Results of a prospective randomized trial for treatment of severely brain-injured patients with hyperbaric oxygen. *J. Neurosurg.* 1992;76:929–934.

260. Plafki C, Peters P, Almeling M, Welslau W, Busch R. Complications and side effects of hyperbaric oxygen therapy. *Aviation Space Enviror. Med.* 2000;71:119–124.

261. Ren H, Wang W, Ge Z. Glasgow coma scale, brain electric activity mapping and Glasgow outcome scale after hyperbaric oxygen treatment of severe brain injury. *Chin. J. Traumatol.* 2001;4:239–241.

262. Singhal AB, Dijkhuizen RM, Rosen BR, Lo EH. Normobaric hyperoxia reduces MRI diffusion abnormalities and infarct size in experimental stroke. *Neurology* 2002;58:945–952.

263. Holmdahl MH, Wiklund L, Wetterberg T, et al. The place of THAM in the management of acidemia in clinical practice. *Acta Anaesthesiol. Scand.* 2000;44:524–527.

264. Bleich H, Schwartz W. Tris buffer (THAM): an appraisal of its physiologic effects and clinical usefulness. *N. Engl. J. Med.* 1966;274:782–787.

265. Gaab MR, Seegers K, Smedema RJ, Heissler HE, Goetz CH. A comparative analysis of THAM (Tris-buffer) in traumatic brain edema. *Acta Neurochir.* 1990;51(Suppl):320–323.

266. Nagao S, Kitaoka T, Fujita K, Kuyama H, Motoomi O. Effect of tris-(hydroxymethyl)-aminomethane on experimental focal cerebral ischemia. *Exp. Brain Res.* 1996;111:51–56.

267. Kiening KL, Schneider GH, Unterberg AW, Lanksch WR. Effect of tromethamine (THAM) on infarct volume following permanent middle cerebral aftery occlusion in rats. *Acta Neurochir.* 1997;70(Suppl):188–190.

268. Wolf AL, Levi L, Marmarou A, et al. Effect of THAM upon outcome in severe head injury: a randomized prospective clinical trial. *J. Neurosurg.* 1993;78:54–59.

269. Morgenstern LB. What have we learned from clinical neuroprotective trials? *Neurology* 2001;57(Suppl 2):S45–S47.

270. Faden AI. Neuroprotection and traumatic brain injury: the search continues. *Arch. Neurol.* 2001;58:1553–1555.

271. Ropper AH, King RB. Intracranial pressure monitoring in comatose patients with cerebral hemorrhage. *Arch. Neurol.* 1984;41:725–728.

272. Lidofsky SD, Bass NM, Prager MC, et al. Intracranial pressure monitoring and liver transplantation for fulminant hepatic failure. *Hepatology* 1992;16:1–7.

273. Ede RJ, Williams R. Hepatic encephalopathy and cerebral edema. *Semin. Liver Dis.* 1986;6:107–118.

274. Jones EA, Weissenborn K. Neurology and the liver. *J. Neurol. Neurosurg. Psychiatry* 1997;63:279–293.

275. Cordoba J, Blei AT. Cerebral edema and intracranial pressure monitoring. *Liver Transpl. Surg.* 1995;1:187–194.

276. Lockwood AH. *Hepatic Encephalopathy*. Boston: Butterworth-Heinemann, 1992.

277. Dienstag JL. Liver transplantation. In: Braunwald E, Fauci AS, Kasper DL, Hauser SL, Longo DL, Jameson JL, eds. *Harrison's Principles of Internal Medicine*, 15th ed. New York: McGraw-Hill, 2001, pp. 1770–1776.

278. Adams RD, Foley JM. The neurological disorder associated with liver disease. *Res. Publ. Assoc. Res. Nerv. Ment. Dis.* 1953;32:198–212.

279. Haerer AF. *Dejong's The Neurologic Examination*, 5th ed. Philadelphia: Lippincott-Raven, 1992.

280. Niedermeyer E. Metabolic central nervous system disorders. In: Niedermeyer E, Lopes da Silva F, eds. *Electroencephalography: Basic Principles, Clinical Applications, and Related Fields*, 4th ed. Baltimore: Williams & Wilkins, 1999, pp. 416–431.

281. Donovan JP, Schafer DF, Shaw BW, Sorrell MF. Cerebral edema and increased intracranial pressure in chronic liver disease. *Lancet* 1998;351:719–721.

282. Clemmesen JO, Larsen FS, Kondrup J, Hansen BA, Ott P. Cerebral herniation in patients with acute liver failure is correlated with arterial ammonia concentration. *Hepatology* 1999;29:648–653.

283. Record CO, Buxton B, Chase RA, et al. Plasma and brain aminoacids in fulminant hepatic failure and their relationship to hepatic encephalopathy. *Eur. J. Clin. Invest.* 1976;6:387–394.

284. Seda HMW, Hughes RD, Gove CD, et al. Inhibition of brain ATPase activity by serum from patients with fulminant hepatic failure. *Hepatology* 1984;4:186–191.

285. Chung RT, Podolsky DK. Cirrhosis and its complications. In: Braunwald E, Fauci AS, Kasper DL, Hauser SL, Longo DL, Jameson JL, eds. *Harrison's Principles of Internal Medicine*, 15th ed. New York: McGraw-Hill, 2001, pp. 1754–1766.

286. Daas M, Plevak DJ, Wijdicks EFM, et al. Acute liver failure: results of a 5-year clinical protocol. *Liver Transpl. Surg.* 1995;1:210–219.

287. Alper B, Jarjour IT, Reyes JD, et al. Outcome of children with cerebral edema caused by fulminant hepatic failure. *Pediatr. Neurol.* 1998;18:299–304.

288. Schafer DF, Shaw BW. Fulminant hepatic failure and orthotopic liver transplantation. *Semin. Liver Dis.* 1989;9:189–194.

289. Detry O, Arkadopoulos N, Ting P, et al. Intracranial pressure during liver transplantation for fulminant hepatic failure. *Transplantation* 1999;67:767–770.

290. Canalese J, Gimson AES, Davis C, Mellon PJ, Davis M, Williams R. Controlled trial of dexamethasone and mannitol for the cerebral oedema of fulminant hepatic failure. *Gut* 1982;23:625–629.

291. Bathgate AJ, Hayes PC. Acute liver failure: complications and current management. *Hosp. Med.* 1998;59:195–199.

292. Forbes A, Alexander GJM, O'Grady JG, et al. Thiopental infusion in the treatment of intracranial hypertension complicating fulminant hepatic failure. *Hepatology* 1989;10:306–310.

293. Keays R, Potter D, O'Grady J, Peachey T, Alexander G, Williams R. Intracranial and cerebral perfusion pressure changes before, during, and immediately after orthotopic liver transplantation for fulminant hepatic failure. *Q. J. Med.* 1991;79:425–433.

294. Butterworth RF. Mild hypothermia prevents cerebral edema in acute liver failure. *J. Hepatobil. Pancreatr. Surg.* 2001;8:16–19.

295. Jalan R, Damink SWMO, Deutz NEP, Hayes PC. Moderate hypothermia for uncontrolled intracranial hypertension in acute liver failure. *Lancet* 1999;354:1164–1168.

296. Roberts DRD, Manas D. Induced hypothermia in the management of cerebral oedema secondary to fulminant liver failure. *Clin. Transpl.* 1999;13:545–547.

297. Sidi A, Mahla ME. Noninvasive monitoring of cerebral perfusion by transcranial doppler during fulminant hepatic failure and liver transplantation. *Anesth. Analges.* 1995;80:194–200.

298. O'Grady JG, Alexander GJM, Thick M, Potter D, Calne RY, Williams R. Outcome of orthotopic liver transplantation in the aetiological and clinical variants of acute liver failure. *Q. J. Med.* 1988;69:817–824.

299. Hackett PH. High altitude cerebral edema and acute mountain sickness: a pathophysiology update. In: Roach RC, Wagner PD, Hackett PH, eds. *Hypoxia: Into the Next Millenium.* New York: Kluwer Academic/Plenum Publishing, 1999, pp. 23–45.

300. Klocke DL, Decker WW, Stepanek J. Altitude-related illnesses. *Mayo Clin. Proc.* 1998;73:988–993.

301. Hackett PH, Yarnell PR, Hill R, et al. High-altitude cerebral edema evaluated with magnetic resonance imaging. *JAMA* 1998;280:1920–1925.

302. Bartsch P, Maggiorini M, Ritter M, Noti C, Vock P, Oelz O. Prevention of high-altitude pulmonary edema by nifedipine. *N. Engl. J. Med.* 1992;116:461–465.

303. Levine BD, Yoshimura K, Kobayashi T, Rukushima M, Toshishige S, Ueda G. Dexamethasone in the treatment of acute mountain sickness. *N. Engl. J. Med.* 1989;321:1707–1713.

304. Forwand SA, Landowne M, Follansbee JN, Hansen JE. Effect of acetazolamide on acute mountain sickness. *N. Engl. J. Med.* 1968;279:839–845.

305. Grissom CK, Roach RC, Sarnquist FH, Hackett PH. Acetazolamide in the treatment of acute mountain sickness: clinical efficacy and effect on gas exchange. *Ann. Intern. Med.* 1992;116:461–465.

306. S artori C, Allemann Y, Duplain H, et al. Salmeterol for the prevention of high-altitude pulmonary edema. *N. Engl. J. Med.* 2002;346:1631–1636.

307. Gordon RA, Roberts G, Amin Z, Williams RH, Paloucek FP. Aggressive approach in the treatment of acute lead encephalopathy with an extraordinarily high concentration of lead. *Arch. Pediatr. Adolesc. Med.* 1998;152:1100–1104.

308. Selbst SM, Henretig FM, Pearce J. Lead encephalopathy: a case report and review of management. *Clin. Pediatr.* 1984;24:280–285.

309. Rempel D. The lead-exposed worker. *JAMA* 1989;262:532–534.

310. Hu H. Heavy metal poisoning. In: Fauci AS, Braunwald E, Isselbacher KJ, et al, eds. *Harrison's Principles of Internal Medicine*, 14th ed. New York: McGraw-Hill, 1998:2564–2569.

311. Audesirk G. Effects of lead exposure on the physiology of neurons. *Progr. Neurobiol.* 1985;24:199–231.

312. Markowitz M. Lead poisoning: a disease for the next millennium. *Curr. Prob. Pediatr.* 2000;30:62–70.

313. Committee on Environmental Hazards, and Committee on Accident and Poison Prevention, American Academy of Pediatrics. Statement on childhood lead poisoning. *Pediatrics* 1987;79:457–465.

314. Whitfield CL, Ch'ien LT, Whitehead JD. Lead encephalopathy in adults. *Am. J. Med.* 1972;52:289–298.

315. Pegues DA, Hughes BJ, Woernle CH. Elevated blood lead levels associated with illegally distilled alcohol. *Arch. Intern. Med.* 1993;153:1501–1504.

316. Barltop D. Lead poisoning. *Arch. Dis. Child.* 1971;46:233–235.

317. Coffin R, Phillips JL, Staples WI, Spector S. Treatment of lead encephalopathy in children. *J. Pediatr.* 1966;69:198–206.

318. Fishman RA. *Cerebrospinal Fluid in Diseases of the Nervous System.* Philadelphia: Saunders, 1980.

319. Chisolm JJ. The use of chelating agents in the treatment of acute and chronic lead intoxication in childhood. *J. Pediatr.* 1968;73:1–38.

320. McLaurin RL, Nichols JB. Extensive cranial decompression in the treatment of severe lead encephalopathy. *Pediatrics* 1957;20:653–667.

321. Greengard J, Voris DC, Hayden R. The surgical therapy of acute lead encephalopathy. *JAMA* 1962;180:660–664.

322. Greengard J, Adams B, Berman E. Acute lead encephalopathy in young children: evaluation of therapy with a corticosteroid and moderate hypothermia. *J. Pediatr.* 1965;66:707–711.

323. Roberge RJ, Martin TG. Whole bowel irrigation in an acute oral lead intoxication. *Am. J. Emerg. Med.* 1992;10:577–583.

324. American Academy of Clinical Toxicology; European Association of Poisons Centers and Clinical Toxicologists. Position statement: whole bowel irrigation. *Clin. Toxicol.* 1997;35:753–762.

325. Chisolm JJ, Harrison HE. The treatment of acute lead encephalopathy in children. *Pediatrics* 1957;19:2–20.

6

Neurologic and Systemic Monitoring in the NSU

Daniel W. Miller and Jose I. Suarez

INTRODUCTION

Monitoring technologies assume particular importance in the neurosciences critical care unit (NSU). Beyond the cardiac and respiratory monitoring modalities common to other intensive care units (ICU), the NSU uses a wide array of technologies for both whole brain monitoring and regional or focal brain monitoring (Table 1). This chapter addresses these brain monitoring modalities and also considers recent advances in general ICU monitoring strategies that are equally important to the welfare of the NSU patient.

The first and simplest form of monitoring in the NSU is the serial neurologic examination, performed at frequent intervals by nursing staff and physicians. The role of the carefully performed neurologic exam in critical care should not be dismissed, and the intent of this chapter is not to promote reliance on machines to the exclusion of the patient–doctor interaction. Nevertheless, the limitations of neurochecks must be acknowledged. First, the examination is frequently constricted or obliterated altogether by pharmocologic interventions, such as neuromuscular blockade, propofol or midazolam sedation, or barbiturate coma. Second, there are a number of pathologic conditions which a careful bedside exam can miss entirely: nonconvulsive status epilepticus, vasospasm (particularly in the obtunded patient post-subarachnoid hemorrhage [SAH]), early increased intracranial pressure (ICP) or cerebral hyperemia. Third, the neurologic examination is quite operator-dependent, and patients in the NSU are typically examined by several nurses and doctors who may approach even a relatively standardized examination (e.g., determination of the Glasgow Coma Scale score) in several subtly different fashions, perhaps trying different degrees of noxiousness to achieve a motor response, using different light levels when assessing the pupils, and so forth. Fourth, even the most precise neurologic examination remains a qualitative rather than quantitative assessment; an impression of elevated ICP may be quite correct, yet it cannot quantify the severity of the elevation nor accurately monitor the effects of therapeutic interventions. Finally, it has been argued that neurochecks tend to recognize problems after the fact, whereas the monitoring technologies presented here may provide the advantage of detecting pathologic cerebral processes at a stage where interventions are more likely to prevent irreversible central nervous system (CNS) damage (1).

TECHNIQUES FOR BRAIN MONITORING IN THE NSU

Whole-Brain Monitoring

Intracranial Pressure Monitoring

Because ICP monitoring forms the cornerstone of the neurointensivist's technical armamentarium, not only in the head injury population but also in many other NSU patients, a brief review of ICP pressure physiology is in order (*see* Chapter 5 for a more detailed discussion of ICP). The Monro-

From: *Current Clinical Neurology*
Critical Care Neurology and Neurosurgery
Edited by: J. I. Suarez © Humana Press Inc., Totowa, NJ

Table 1
Monitoring Technologies Used in the NSU

Whole-brain monitoring	Regional/focal brain monitoring
Intracranial pressure devices	Transcranial Doppler ultrasonography
Jugular bulb catheters	Near-infrared spectroscopy
Electroencephalography	Xenon-133 clearance
Evoked potentials	Laser Doppler flowmetry
	Thermal diffusion flowmetry
	Microdialysis catheters
	Tissue probes (pO_2, pCO_2, pH)

Kellie Doctrine states that by nature of the rigid cranial container the intracranial space represents a fixed volume, and that an increase in the volume of any of its 3 constituent compartments (brain, cerebrospinal fluid [CSF], blood) must be met by a corresponding decrease in the volume of other compartment(s) or ICP will rise *(2)*. This is clinically evident in transtentorial herniation from a hemispheric mass and in the use of hyperventilation to reduce the volume of the blood compartment in elevated ICP states. Normal mean ICP is less than 10 mmHg and levels exceeding 15 mmHg are generally considered abnormally elevated. However, it has been suggested that levels greater than 20 mmHg for at least 2 min be used as a treatment threshold *(3)*.

Cerebral perfusion pressure (CPP) is related to ICP and to mean arterial pressure (MAP) by the equation: CPP = MAP – ICP. Thus, assuming a relatively constant MAP, an elevation of ICP will be paralleled by a reduction of CPP, and it might be argued that the main reason for ICP monitoring is actually to monitor CPP, because the latter is more directly related to secondary brain injury. In fact, CPP can be directly related to cerebral blood flow by Poiseuille's law:

$$CBF = 8(CPP)r^4/pi(n)(l)$$

where *r* is vessel radius, *n* is viscosity, and *l* is vessel length *(2)*. Thus, cerebral blood flow (CBF) is directly proportional to CPP and vessel radius, and indirectly proportional to blood viscosity and vessel length.

ICP, like arterial blood pressure, is pulsatile and has systolic and diastolic components, though the mean ICP is what is generally followed clinically. The normal ICP waveform consists of a three-peaked wave. P1, the first and generally the tallest peak, is also known as the percussion wave and corresponds to the transmitted systolic blood pressure. P2 (the tidal wave) and P3 (the dicrotic wave) are normally smaller peaks, and the notch between them corresponds to the dicrotic notch of the arterial waveform *(1)*. As ICP increases, P2 and P3 rise to the level of and then surpass P1, and ultimately with continued elevation of ICP the waveform loses distinct peaks and assumes a triangular morphology (Fig. 1) *(1)*. Although a thorough review of ICP waveform analysis is beyond the scope of this chapter, mention should be made of the most famous pathologic finding, the plateau wave (or A-wave) of Lundberg (*see* Fig. 1) *(4)*. These waves bear a plateau morphology that reflects a sudden dramatic elevation in ICP to levels of 50–100 mmHg, which are then sustained for several minutes, followed by an equally precipitous sudden drop back to normal ICP levels *(2)*. Plateau waves indicate critically low intracranial compliance, such that very minor variations in intracranial volume result in marked changes in ICP *(1)*.

Intraventricular catheters were the first invasive ICP monitoring devices and have been used since the 1950s *(5)*. Two decades later, less invasive devices monitoring ICP via the epidural, subdural, or subarachnoid spaces were introduced, and most recently an intraparenchymal fiberoptic monitor has been developed for clinical use *(6)*. The ventricular catheter still remains the gold standard ICP monitor at present. In Table 2, we compare the major types of invasive ICP monitors.

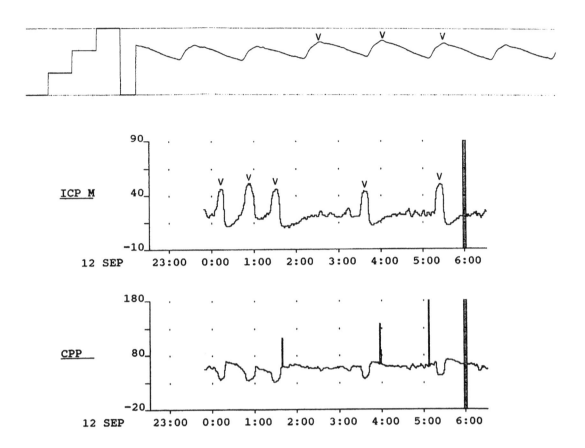

ICP   Scale (0/20.0/40.0/60)

Fig. 1. Continuous intracranial pressure (ICP) monitoring in a patient with poor intracranial compliance. Top figure shows a mean ICP of 36-mmHg (scale, 0, 20, 40, 60 mmHg) and abnormal P2 component (open arrowheads). The middle figure demonstrates A-waves in multiple occasions during the recording (open arrowhead), which are associated with decrements in the cerebral perfusion pressure (lower diagram).

Recent consensus indications for ICP monitoring in the context of head injury include: patient in coma (Glasgow Coma Scale score of 8 or less) with an abnormal head computed tomography (CT) scan; patient in coma with a normal head CT scan but at least two other risk factors for elevated ICP (age over 40 yr, posturing, systolic BP under 90 mmHg); and in other head injured patients at the physician's discretion (7). NSU patients with other intracranial processes are monitored on a less systematic basis; potential indications include hemispheric processes associated with midline shift and depressed consciousness (massive ischemic stroke or intracranial hemorrhage, tumors with significant vasogenic edema), nontraumatic processes leading to diffuse cerebral edema (fulminant hepatic failure, Reye's syndrome, encephalitis), and acute hydrocephalus (in which case the ventricular catheter would obviously be the device of choice) from SAH or other etiologies. Additional factors to consider include the presence of papilledema or any "soft" signs of elevated ICP (headache, nausea, vomiting, persistent hiccups, and sixth nerve palsies).

Table 2
Comparison of Invasive ICP Monitoring Devices

Type of device	Placement	Advantages	Disadvantages	Complications
Ventricular catheter	Burr hole→ nondominant Frontal lobe→ lateral ventricle	Global ICP Accuracy CSF drain Experience Potential recalibration	Maximally invasive Extremely high ICP may obliterate ventricles Calibration lost if detached	ICH ~ 1% Infection/ colonization ~ 4–7% Malfunction ~ 6%
Subarachnoid bolt	Through dura and arachnoid→ subarachnoid space	Brain is not breached Experience	Regional ICP Accuracy may drop with high ICP levels No CSF drain Clogs easily	ICH = low Infection/ colonization ~ 5% Malfunction ~16%
Subdural catheter	Through dura→subdural space	Penetrates dura only	Regional ICP Less accurate than ventricular No CSF drain	ICH = low Infection colonization ~ 5% Malfunction ~ 10%
Epidural monitor	Epidural space	Meninges not breached	Regional ICP Less accurate No CSF drain	ICH and infection rates appear to be low Malfunction=?
Parenchymal fiberoptic catheter	Burr hole→ through meninges into parenchyma of interest, to 13–14-mm depth	Accuracy Smaller than ventricular catheter	Regional ICP Generally no CSF drain Cannot be recalibrated Fragile Expensive	ICH ~ 3% Infection colonization ~ 14% (includes all parenchymal devices) Malfunction ranges 9–40%

Note: Overall incidence of intracranial hemorrhage (ICH) requiring surgical evacuation is 0.5% (3,5,69,74).

Jugular Bulb Oximetry

Jugular bulb oximetry is a well-established technique for continuous monitoring of the oxygen saturation of venous return from the brain, from which a number of useful parameters may be derived. Interest in sampling blood from the jugular system for this purpose began in the 1930s with serial direct venous punctures, and the investigations of Gibbs in the 1940s that compared simultaneous samples from the two jugular veins supported the notion that the two sides are similar enough to make unilateral measurements valid as a monitor of whole-brain oxygen balance *(8)*.

Indwelling fiberoptic jugular bulb catheters have since been developed to permit continuous monitoring. The fundamental goal of jugular venous oxygen saturation ($SjvO_2$) monitoring is to provide a continuous index of the changing (and frequently in the NSU population, deranged) balance between cerebral oxygen delivery and cerebral oxygen consumption or metabolic requirement. Determination of $SjvO_2$ using the jugular bulb catheter and simultaneous determination of the arterial oxygen saturation (SaO_2) allows one to calculate the arteriovenous oxygen difference ($AVDO_2$) (*see* Appendix).

From this parameter cerebral oxygen consumption (also referred to as cerebral metabolic rate) can be calculated as the product of $AVDO_2$ and cerebral blood flow (CBF). Cerebral oxygen extraction (O_2ER) can then be derived as the ratio of cerebral oxygen consumption to cerebral oxygen delivery. The equation involved in the calculation of these various physiologic parameters are given in Feldman's excellent review *(9)*, but several basic concepts bear mentioning here. First, CBF is normally closely coupled to cerebral metabolic rate, but this coupling is often lost in pathologic states, such as severe head injury. Second, cerebral metabolic rate itself is altered in many pathologic states *(9)*. Third, the NSU population by nature exhibits a high frequency of such pathologic processes. The jugular bulb catheter, admittedly reliant on the debatable premise that unilateral $SjvO_2$ is an accurate reflection of whole-brain oxygen utilization, offers potential insights into cerebral oxygen balance regardless of the severity of intracranial pathology.

The catheter used for continuous $SjvO_2$ monitoring employs fiberoptic technology to exploit the differential light-absorption characteristics of oxyhemoglobin and deoxyhemoglobin. It contains a light-transmitting fiber and a light-receiving fiber and is connected to a photosensor. The collected light-absorption data are used to derive $SjvO_2$ as the ratio of oxyhemoglobin to total hemoglobin. The catheter is designed so that a blood sample may be drawn directly from the jugular vein should there be a question as to the accuracy of the oximeter *(9)*. Technical issues frequently confound the practical application of jugular bulb oximetry. There is ongoing debate over the validity of unilateral $SjvO_2$ as an index of whole-brain oxygen utilization. Metz and associates, after studying 22 head injured patients with bilateral jugular catheters, concluded that in this population "even calculated unilateral jugular venous monitoring has an unpredictable risk for misleading or missing data" *(10)*. In a similar population reported by Lam and associates, sampling from the dominant jugular bulb accurately reflected global cerebral oxygenation (using measurements from the confluence of cerebral sinuses as the reference standard), whereas sampling of the nondominant jugular bulb was not as accurate *(11)*. Feldman has suggested that in diffuse head injury the dominant side should be catheterized, while noting that in patients with focal lesions debate exists as to whether the lesion side or the dominant side (regardless of lesion laterality) should be monitored. The dominant jugular bulb can be determined by observing the respective ICP elevations obtained with alternate compression of the two sides by direct CT visualization of the larger jugular foramen, or by ultrasonographic comparison of vein sizes *(9)*. A second technical consideration is catheter position, which may suffer from improper placement initially or from changes in the patient's head position; erroneous catheter position may give a false impression of jugular venous desaturations, which can also be verified radiographically.

Indications for $SjvO_2$ monitoring in the NSU have included head injury particularly, but also SAH, cerebral infarction, and perioperative monitoring for various intracranial procedures. Robertson and associates obtained reliable although qualitative estimates of CBF in patients in coma from various

Table 3
Troubleshooting Jugular Venous Desaturations

Cause of low SjvO$_2$ reading ($< 50\%$)	Intervention to Correct SjvO$_2$
Catheter malposition	Examine light intensity; if suboptimal, adjust head/catheter to achieve proper intensity
Improper calibration	Draw venous blood sample through catheter; if direct SjvO$_2$ > 50% catheter needs recalibration
Arterial hypoxia	Measure arterial oxygen saturation; correct if less than 90%
Anemia	Measure hemoglobin and correct if < 9 mg/dL
Inadequate cerebral blood flow	Measures to improve cerebral perfusion

Adapted from Sheinberg *(70)*.

causes, from the AVDO$_2$ and the arteriovenous lactate difference; using these two parameters, they could predict four different CBF patterns (ischemia/infarction, normal, hyperemia, and compensated hypoperfusion) *(12)*. Cruz and coworkers derived a new parameter, cerebral hemodynamic reserve (CHR), as the ratio of changes in global cerebral oxygen extraction to changes in cerebral perfusion pressure, and found that CHR trends correlated with ICP trends in their population of severe head injury patients *(13)*.

Advantages of the jugular bulb catheter as a monitoring modality include the practicality of continuous bedside monitoring, the capability to confirm the oximeter by drawing blood through the catheter, and the numerous physiologic parameters that can be derived from the SjvO$_2$ to arrive at a picture of cerebral oxygen balance. Robertson also suggests a potential role as a qualitative indicator of CBF trends. Disadvantages of the catheter include its susceptibility to artifacts of positioning and its invasiveness. SjvO$_2$ also seems frequently to show up poorly when evaluated in a multimodal context. Latronico and coworkers found in a population of head injured patients that SjvO$_2$ was frequently normal despite abnormalities of ICP or CPP and did not help management in 96% of observations *(14)*. Similarly, Kirkpatrick and associates found that of 38 patient events associated with clear linked changes in CPP, middle cerebral artery flow velocity, and laser Doppler flowmetry, near-infrared spectroscopy registered associated changes with 97% sensitivity whereas SjvO$_2$ showed only 53% sensitivity *(15)*. A recommended algorithm for troubleshooting jugular venous desaturations is presented in Table 3.

Complication of jugular bulb catheterization include carotid puncture, damage to other nearby structures (such as the cervical sympathetic trunk), simple bacterial colonization of the catheter (15% rate reported by Latronico) *(14)*, line sepsis (up to 5% incidence particularly with several days of monitoring) *(9)*, and venous thrombosis (particularly if medications are given through the catheter) *(9)*. The catheters do not significantly elevate ICP despite theoretical concerns about obstruction of venous return *(16)*.

Electrophysiologic Monitoring: Electroencephalography and Evoked Potentials

The movement of electroencephalography (EEG) into the ICU setting, first with portable but bulky analog machines and more recently with computerized digital systems, has dramatically affected patient care. Evoked potentials occupy a considerably smaller niche in the NSU but remain potentially valuable in the right clinical context.

An excellent review by Jordan delineates four major neurobiologic rationales for the use of EEG as a monitoring tool: its close relationship to cerebral metabolic rate, its sensitivity in detecting hypoxic-ischemic neuronal dysfunction at an early stage (based on selective vulnerability of the cortical layers that generate the EEG), its obvious primacy as a monitor of seizure activity, and its value in cerebral localization particularly when the patient is unstable for transport to neuroimaging *(1)*. Technical aspects of EEG application in the NSU do not differ greatly from the standard outpatient EEG: typically a 16-channel EEG and a channel for the heart rhythm are recorded; electrodes are placed in the usual fashion using the International 10-20 system (sometimes with modifications); and a variety of montages may be recorded (and retrospective montaging is possible with the digital machines). Some factors are relatively unique to the ICU setting, however, such as the sheer abundance of artifact sources (ventilators, drips, dialysis pumps, other electrical machinery, suctioning) and the inability of the patient to cooperate with the technician due to a combination of disease and pharmacologic sedation. Continuous EEG monitoring (hour after hour of real-time recording) is not always feasible for reasons of technician or machine availability, cost, or because the electrodes need to come off for CT or magnetic resonance imaging (MRI). Often the practical solution is frequent brief serial EEGs; with an analog machine at the bedside nursing staff can easily be taught to turn on at a predetermined time and record for a brief period. However, continuous EEG recording is strongly recommended.

Generalized convulsive status epilepticus (GCSE) is the most obvious indication for EEG monitoring, because clinical assessment of whether seizures are ongoing will be confounded by several factors: sedating anticonvulsants (benzodiazepines and barbiturates), intubation for various reasons (airway protection, pharmacologic respiratory depression, panic on the part of caregivers) accompanied by pharmacologic paralysis and further sedation, and ultimately obliteration of the neurologic exam by agents such as midazolam, propofol or pentobarbital. A progression through five EEG patterns has been noted to occur in GCSE (though not invariably): discrete electroclinical seizures, early merging of seizures into waxing and waning discharges, continuous electrographic seizure activity, interruption of the former by flat periods, and finally, periodic epileptiform activity on a flat background *(17)*. Once ongoing seizures are detected, the EEG becomes essential for monitoring the effects of therapeutic interventions, particularly when the decision is made to titrate medications to a burst-suppression EEG pattern, a frequent endpoint in management of refractory GCSE (Fig. 2).

Another major ICU indication for EEG monitoring is detection of nonconvulsive seizures and nonconvulsive status epilepticus (NCSE). Jordan applied continuous EEG to 124 consecutive NSU patients with various conditions and found seizures in 35%, 76% of which represented NCSE *(1)*. In patients with depressed sensorium—a large proportion of the NSU population—EEG is the only reliable method to rule out nonconvulsive seizures. Young and associates studied variables associated with mortality in 49 patients with NCSE and found in multivariate analysis that only seizure duration and delay to diagnosis were significantly associated with increased mortality *(18)*; continuous or serial EEG obviously has the potential to alter these variables and thereby reduce mortality from NCSE.

In the comatose NSU patient, EEG is valuable not only to detect nonconvulsive seizures but also to support a clinical impression of metabolic encephalopathy (in which it might show diffuse slowing and triphasic complexes), psychogenic unresponsiveness, locked-in state, and even focal mass lesions in the case of the patient who is unstable for transport to CT. When brain death is suggested by the clinical exam yet the diagnosis remains uncertain, EEG may serve as a confirmatory (not diagnostic) test, with the following stipulations: no electrical activity should be noted greater than 2 microvolts at a sensitivity of 2 microvolts/mm, filter setting of 0.1 or 0.3 s and 70 Hz, and at least 30 min of recording *(19)*. With lesser degrees of brain injury, the EEG has been used in a prognostic role; patterns, such as burst-suppression and alpha coma, have often been correlated with poor prognosis, as in a series of patients reported by Synck with postanoxic or traumatic coma *(20)*.

Finally EEG has been suggested as a monitor for cerebral ischemia in the NSU, an extension of its established role in the operating room during carotid endarterectomy. Jordan has reported the use of continuous EEG to detect acute cerebral ischemia (as from post-SAH vasospasm) and to guide hypertensive hypervolemic therapy, documenting the early appearance of focal or generalized EEG slowing or epileptiform activity and its resolution with therapy *(1)*.

Evoked potentials have a more restricted role in the NSU. While brainstem auditory-evoked potentials (BAEPs) and visual-evoked potentials (VEPs) are at the neurointensivist's disposal as

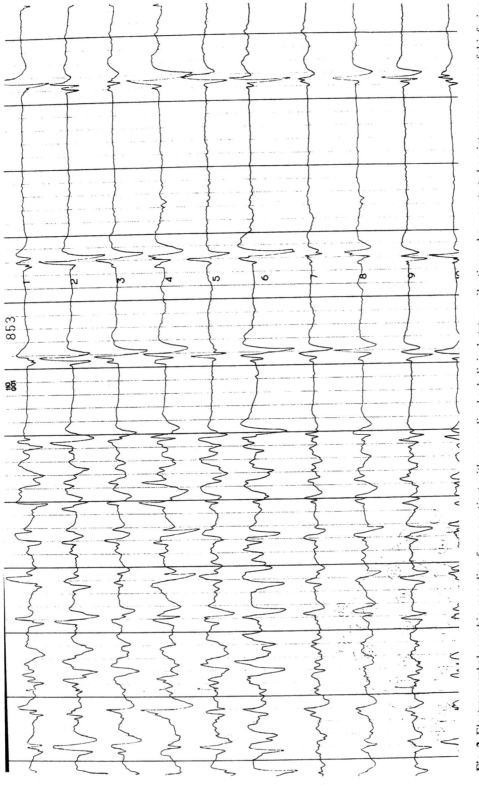

Fig. 2. Electroencephalographic recording from a patient with generalized subclinical status epilepticus who was started on intravenous propofol infusion to achieve burst suppression as seen to the right of the figure (speed 30 mm/s, amplitude 7.5 μV/mm, standard bipolar montage).

well, in practicality it is the median nerve somatosensory-evoked potential (SEP) that is most clearly useful and that comprises the bulk of evoked potential studies performed in the ICU setting. The median SEP entails peripheral electrical stimulation of the mixed median nerve with a stimulus just strong enough to produce a slight muscle twitch. The stimulus is repetitively delivered to the nerve at a frequency of around 5 Hz, which sends a volley of impulses up the neuraxis through the brachial plexus, brainstem, and ultimately to the cerebral cortex. Two components of the median SEP are of prime importance clinically, designated N20 (negative deflection of 20 ms latency) and P22 (positive deflection of 22 ms latency) and grouped together as the N20-P22 response. N20 is thought to be generated on the posterior bank of the rolandic sulcus, while P22 originates from motor cortex (area 4) *(21)*. Bilateral absence of the N20-P22 response has been associated with poor prognosis in coma in several studies *(1,22,23)*, generally indicating outcome no better than a persistent vegetative state. A recent meta-analysis of studies of poor predictors in hypoxic-ischemic coma identified three factors with 100% specificity for the poor outcome of death or vegetative state (no pupillary light reflexes on d 3, no motor response on d 3, and bilateral absence of N20-P22 within the first week) and concluded that of the 3, SEP is the most useful prognosticator because it is the least susceptible to toxicmetabolic effects; a caveat noted was that SEPs, like the other predictors, could on rare occasions be misleading if performed within 72 h of the hypoxic insult *(24)*. Moulton and associates found median SEPs useful for separating head-injured patients into outcome categories, particularly in patients without a reliable neurologic examination because of pharmacologic sedation and paralysis, whereas EEG power spectrum analysis could not reliably make such a distinction *(25)*. Finally, SEPs, like EEG, have also been proposed as a confirmatory test to support a clinical diagnosis of brain death, again based on bilateral absence of the N20-P22 response *(26)*.

Regional/Focal Brain Monitoring

Transcranial Doppler Ultrasonography

Transcranial Doppler ultrasonography (TCD) provides a noninvasive means of evaluating the large intracranial arteries at the bedside. TCD combines the principles of ultrasound (acoustic energy of high frequency, typically around 2 MHz, which can penetrate different biologic tissues to variable extents thus delineating body structures) and Doppler shift (the change in frequency of sound waves resulting from reflection by a moving object or particle) to image erythrocyte flow in the basal cerebral arteries. TCD can thus indicate presence or absence, velocity (systolic, diastolic, and mean), and direction of blood flow *(26)*. From these variables, conclusions may be reached regarding vessel patency, focal stenosis or vasospasm, intracranial pressure, autoregulatory function, and vasoreactivity *(27)*. TCD is also used as a confirmatory test supporting the clinical diagnosis of brain death.

Unlike ultrasonography of other body regions, TCD is subject to the constraints imposed by the cranium. Three probe approaches are routinely used to insonate the cerebral vessels: transtemporal, transorbital, and suboccipital. The transtemporal approach is used to insonate the proximal segments of the anterior and middle cerebral arteries (ACA and MCA), the ACA/MCA bifurcation, the posterior cerebral artery (PCA) and a portion of the carotid siphon; this approach cannot be used in 10% of individuals due to skull thickness. The transorbital approach insonates the ophthalmic artery and most of the carotid siphon. The suboccipital approach insonates the vertebrobasilar system *(27)*. Arteries are identified by the depth at which they are encountered: angle of the probe, direction of flow, and operator's experience and knowledge of intracranial vascular anatomy. The strongest signal (maximum velocity) is obtained when the angle of insonation, which corresponds to the long axis of the probe, is aligned with the arterial lumen *(28)*.

The ultrasound beam transmitted by the TCD probe encircles the artery of interest and is fed back through a receiver in the probe to generate a graphic waveform depicting erythrocyte velocities within the vessel, as well as a readout indicating depth of insonation, flow velocity, angle of insonation, and pulsatility index (which is calculated as peak systolic velocity—end-diastolic velocity/mean velocity, and indicates the degree of downstream resistance) *(27)*. This is depicted in Fig. 3. Another commonly followed parameter is the ratio of MCA to intracranial ICA flow velocities, termed the hemispheric index or Lindegaard ratio, which is used to distinguish vasospasm (ratio > 3) from hyperemia (ratio < 3) *(26)*.

The major indications for TCD in the NSU are listed in Table 4. TCD is noninvasive and safe. It does not pose the (generally small) risk of iatrogenic complications associated with several other NSU monitoring modalities, and it can be useful in monitoring the response to therapeutic measures. TCD does, however, require technical expertise in both the performance of the test and the interpretation of the data. The ultrasonographer must be aware of several patient variables that can affect TCD parameters; some of these are given in Table 5.

Near-Infrared Spectroscopy (Cerebral Oximetry)

Near-infrared spectroscopy (NIRS) is a modality somewhat analogous to the pulse oximetry devices routinely used to assess blood oxygenation rapidly and noninvasively. NIRS is based on the ability of incident light of 700–1000 nm wavelength to pass through tissues into all components of the vascular tree, indicating by its absorption characteristics trends in the oxygenation state of hemoglobin, thus providing a picture of the adequacy of tissue oxygenation. Jobsis in 1977 introduced the in vivo application of NIRS for cerebral oximetry *(29)*, although the technology is not yet in widespread use. NIRS potentially fills a significant void in the NSU by providing a noninvasive means of monitoring cerebral oxygen availability.

Cerebral oximeters such as the US Food and Drug Administration–approved INVOS3100A (Somanetics, Troy, MI) use a single-use sensor that is adhered to the patient's scalp and contains a near-infrared light source and two detectors. Thus, two elliptical paths from source to detector are described: a shallow path encompassing primarily scalp, skull, dura, and dural sinuses, and a deep path penetrating approx 2 cm into the underlying brain parenchyma *(30)*. The intent of such an arrangement is that the clinically irrelevant extracerebral contribution to the NIRS signal (the shallow path) will be subtracted out, yielding a signal that is primarily a reflection of cerebral oxygenation. Multiple oximeters can be applied to the scalp to increase the amount of brain being sampled. Once the oximeter is applied, the head may have to be wrapped in a light-proof drape because of the extreme sensitivity of the NIRS setup to extraneous light *(15)*. A readout of oxyhemoglobin and deoxyhemoglobin flux, as well as the redox state of cytochrome oxidase (cytox), is customarily obtained and can be correlated with other monitoring modalities *(15)*.

NIRS has been used for cerebral oximetry in head injury *(15)*, epilepsy *(30)*, cerebral venous thrombosis undergoing endovascular thrombolysis *(31)*, and ischemic stroke *(32)*. Kirkpatrick and associates reported a series of 14 ventilated patients with closed-head injury followed with multimodal monitoring (ICP, jugular venous saturation, TCD for MCA flow velocity, laser Doppler flowmetry, and NIRS). They identified 38 clinical events in 9 patients in which there were clear changes in cerebral perfusion pressure, MCA flow velocity, and cortical perfusion as assessed by laser Doppler flowmetry. NIRS recorded corresponding trend changes in 37 of the 38 events, whereas jugular venous sampling detected only 20 *(15)*. Adelson and associates used NIRS periictally in conjunction with continuous EEG monitoring in three patients; they found a preictal increase in cerebral oxygenation occurring up to several hours before the seizure, a progressive diminution of oxygen availability after even a single seizure, and different NIRS patterns associated with electrographic as opposed to electroclinical seizures *(30)*. A single patient monitored by NIRS during thrombolysis of extensive cerebral venous thromboses exhibited initially high levels of total hemoglobin as well as oxy- and deoxyhemoglobin, and correspondingly low cytox levels; these values normalized rapidly following the initiation of thrombolysis *(31)*. Nemoto and associates reported that NIRS appropriately indicated rapid oxyhemoglobin desaturation in a stroke patient who experienced cardiac arrest during monitoring, but that normal NIRS readings were obtained over an area of hemispheric infarction in a second patient *(32)*; others have also noted failure of the cerebral oximeter to indicate an abnormality

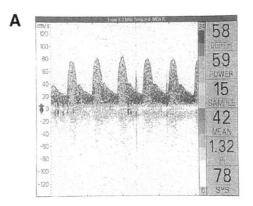

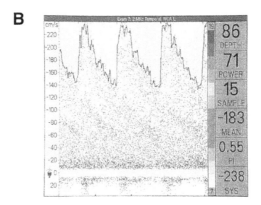

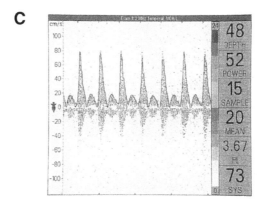

Fig. 3. Transcranial Doppler ultrasound recordings. **A**, normal middle cerebral artery mean blood flow velocities (MCBFVs); **B**, markedly elevated MCBFVs in right anterior cerebral artery indicating focal stenosis or vasospasm; **C**, MCBFVs of right middle cererbal artery in a clinically brain dead patient. Notice the absent diastolic pressure peak, to-and-fro pattern, and elevated pulsatility index.

even in the complete absence of flow *(33)*. The reliability of NIRS has also been called into question in severe closed-head injury *(34)* and increased ICP *(35)*. Clearly more investigation is needed into the appropriate applications of NIRS in the NSU.

Table 4
Indications for TCD Monitoring in the NSU

Process	Aneurysmal SAH	Head trauma	Brain death	Acute stroke
Complication(s) TCD may detect or prevent	Vasospasm Hyperemia	Elevated ICP SAH → vasospasm	Inaccuracy in diagnosis	Excessive thrombolytic use Reocclusion
Protocol	At least QOD exams during first 2–3 wk	Individualize to patient needs	Bilateral exam of MCA + VB or ophthalmic + VB	Monitor during thrombolysis, and thereafter if reocclusion is suspected
Key findings	MCA-FV 120–200 cm/s → 25–50% stenosis; > 200 cm/s → > 50% stenosis Lindegaard ratio >3 → vasospasm (severe if > 6)	*Rising ICP:* Increased PI Peaked waves Reversal of diastolic flow ("to-and-fro") Systolic spikes Absent signal *In general:* Low FV at admission→poor prognosis	Reverberating flow Absent flow in diastole Short systolic spikes *Absent TCD signal cannot not be used as a criterion*	Previously absent flow signal obtained (→recanalized) Loss of signal previously present→ reoccluded
Potential value	Early detection of vasospasm Guide hypervolemic therapy	Noninvasive ICP estimate Vasospasm detection	Confirmatory tests, supporting clinical diagnosis	Avoid excessive thrombolytics Safer than angiography
Disadvantages	Not as sensitive for spasm of vessels other than MCA Correlation of velocity with stenosis is inexact	Only qualitative estimate of ICP; cannot replace invasive monitors No CSF drainage potential	False positives and negatives Absent signal is not helpful	Need angio for IA thrombolysis Not therapeutic role, unlike angiography
Alternatives	Conventional angiography	Invasive ICP monitors	EEG, SEPs, angiography, technetium 99	Conventional angiography

SAH, subarachnoid hemorrhage; ICP, intracranial pressure; QOD, every other day; MCA, middle cerebral artery; VB, vertebrobasilar system; FV, flow velocity; PI, pulsatility index; CSF, cerebrospinal fluid; IA, intra-arterial; EEG, electroencephalogram; SEPs, somatosensory -evoked potentials. (*See* refs. *6,27,71,72*).

Table 5
Some Factors Affecting TCD Interpretation

Variable	Effect on TCD results
Hematocrit	Hematocrit is inversely proportional to flow velocity; thus severe anemia is associated with elevated velocities.
pCO_2	Flow velocity changes in direct proportion to pCO_2 (because of dilation and constriction of resistance vessels), assuming intact autoregulatory function.
Vessel diameter	Flow velocity is inversely proportional to vessel diameter. Normal vessel diameters vary considerably.
Age	Flow velocity declines with increasing age.
Blood pressure	Elevated blood pressure is associated with an elevated pulsatility index, due to a disproportionate effect on systolic velocity.
Nimodipine, nifedipine	These calcium channel blocking agents are associated with a decrease in flow velocities.
Fibrinogen	Flow velocity is inversely proportional to serum fibrinogen level, presumably due to effects on viscosity.

See refs. *26* and *27*.

Advantages of NIRS are that it is noninvasive, safe, can be performed at the bedside, and holds promise as a trend monitor particularly when used in conjunction with other monitoring modalities, as reported by Kirkpatrick. Much dissatisfaction exists over the limitations and technical difficulties associated with jugular venous sampling, the only other established technology for assessing cerebral oxygenation at the bedside.

Disadvantages of NIRS, in addition to the aforementioned uncertainty regarding its validity in certain patient populations, include its sensitivity to extraneous light, susceptibility to motion artifacts and signal drift, problems obtaining a signal through intracranial hematomas or through blood in the CSF, and its focality (though as noted earlier, more than one oximeter may be affixed to the scalp).

There have been no reports of any significant medical complications associated with NIRS. It is noninvasive, does not employ ionizing radiation and does not appear to alter the underlying brain tissue.

Regional Cerebral Blood Flow Techniques
XENON-133

Xenon-133 is a radioisotope chemically related to the inert elemental gas xenon and generated by fission of uranium-235. After administration by various routes, it is briefly taken up by the brain but does not undergo metabolism. It is then cleared by the venous system and exhaled with a 90% first-pass clearance from the body (*36*). Using multiple stationary scintillation detectors, the cerebral uptake and elimination of Xe133 can be measured and expressed as a two-dimensional regional cerebral blood flow (rCBF) map. Although both gray matter flow and white matter flow are evaluated by ^{133}Xe, the rCBF map generated emphasizes the former, that is cortical flow (*37*).

The clinical use of radioisotopes to determine cerebral blood flow was introduced by Ingvar and Lassen in 1961 (*38*), who used krypton-85 in the brain exposed at craniotomy. [133]Xe subsequently became established as the radioisotope of choice for rCBF determination because of several factors: it emits gamma rays detectable by extracranial scintillation counters, it has a short biologic half-life making it relatively safe, it can be administered via inhalation and intravenous routes as well as the original intracarotid method, it yields reproducible measurements, and it can be performed at the bedside, which naturally facilitates its application in the NSU (*37*). [133]Xe is the most well-established CBF monitoring modality employed in the NSU. (*See* Chapter 3 for a detailed discussion of CBF.)

Typically 5–8 scintillation detectors are used for ^{133}Xe evaluation in the ICU setting. Radiation exposure to patient and staff is relatively low, permitting multiple studies when indicated, and the short biologic half-life of ^{133}Xe allows the technologist to repeat the procedure as soon as 30 min later *(37)*. A preamplifier, amplifier, pulse height analyzer, count rate meter, and computer are required, as is the ^{133}Xe gas which is available dissolved in saline for injection *(36)*.

[133]Xe has been used extensively to determine rCBF in severe head injury and SAH *(37)*. It has been used intraoperatively during carotid endarterectomy and during carotid occlusion for aneurysm *(36)*. Halsey and associates found that ^{133}Xe can lateralize cerebral infarction with 85% sensitivity as judged against CT scan *(39)*.

The main advantages of the ^{133}Xe method are its long track record as reliable, reproducible gauge of rCBF; its minimally invasive nature and rapid clearance; and its portability, permitting bedside use in the NSU. Its major disadvantages include restricted range, measuring superficial CBF but not deep hemispheric or posterior circulation structures; the so-called "look through" phenomenon, referring to the obscuration of areas of very low flow by nearby areas of higher flow which contain more radioisotope; the approx 30-min wait required between serial measurements; and possible inaccuracy of the method in pathologic states that are associated with an abnormal blood-brain partition coefficient *(37)*. The method appears to be generally safe and involves little radiation exposure. One might intuitively predict a greater likelihood of morbidity with the intracarotid route of administration compared with the intravenous or inhalation routes.

LASER DOPPLER FLOWMETRY

Laser Doppler flowmetry (LDF) is a technology that indirectly estimates flow as a function of Doppler shift of monochromatic laser light. When laser light is imparted to a suspension of light-scattering particles (in practice, red blood cells within tissue capillaries), photons contact both stationary (tissue) cells and moving (blood) cells. In both cases the photons scatter as a result of the collision, but only those photons colliding with moving particles are Doppler frequency shifted. A proportion of the scattered photons (both shifted and unshifted) are then collected by a photodetector and an electrical signal is generated, which is analyzed to arrive at a qualitative estimate of blood flow as the product of blood velocity (a function of the magnitude of the frequency shift) and blood volume (a function of the power of the shifted light) *(40,41)*. Obviously LDF is not limited to brain monitoring, and it has been applied to various other organs as well, initially in 1977 for the measurement of cutaneous blood flow as described by Stern and coworkers *(42)*. It should be kept in mind that the flow that LDF directly assesses is microcirculatory (capillary) flow, and that inferences made about large-vessel or global CBF may be incorrect as a result.

The equipment required for LDF monitoring includes an infrared or helium-neon laser light source, a fiber optic probe containing a light delivery fiber and one or more light-collecting fibers (either on the tip or on the side of the probe), a photodetector where photons captured by the collecting fibers are heterodyned (mixed to produce an electrical signal), and a processor and display *(40,41)*. The LDF probe can be placed at the same time as an ICP probe via burr hole or craniotomy, but unlike the ICP probe, the LDF hardware is designed so that the probe tip typically sits only 2–3 mm deep to the cortical surface *(43)*. In this location, the tip is anchored which minimizes motion artifact because the entire probe moves with any head movement; also pial vessels are avoided, which is crucial since immediate proximity of the LDF probe to any vessels larger than capillaries will potentially yield an unreliable signal. The probe may also be placed such that it rests on the cortical surface, but this approach requires direct visualization to avoid pial vessels and increases the likelihood of motion artifact. In either case, the volume of tissue directly measured by LDF is only approx 1 mm^3, so as with some other brain monitoring methods (such as thermal diffusion flowmetry and NIRS) inferences about pathologic processes involving a significant volume of brain are made based on a small sample volume *(40)*. Although this is not necessarily invalid, it should be borne in mind as a potential limitation of these technologies.

LDF has been used intraoperatively and in the NSU to continuously monitor rCBF in a qualitative fashion with high temporal resolution. The probe can be directly applied to cortical areas of interest during craniotomy for aneurysm clipping or AVM procedures—similar to the thermal diffusion probe—where an impression of ischemia or hyperemia may importantly guide therapeutic interventions. Meyerson et al. report on the use of LDF monitoring in patients in coma from various etiologies, including severe head injury, aneurysmal SAH, and massive cerebral infarction with subsequent barbiturate coma. They simultaneously recorded ICP and noted that LDF patterns mirrored ICP patterns in inverted fashion when the patients' clinical status was poor, but that with improvement, patients developed regular 6–8 Hz LDF flow alterations independent of ICP waves, which disappeared upon full recovery in one patient *(44)*. These findings suggest a role for LDF in monitoring the status of such patients and possibly a role in prognostication as well. Kirkpatrick and coworkers reported a larger series of head-injured patients monitored continuously with LDF. In 16 of 22 patients, they were able to obtain reliable long-term LDF recordings. They generally found tight coupling between MCA flow velocities (as measured by TCD) and LDF recordings, suggesting a close relationship between large-vessel flow velocities and microvascular flux. This coupling was not invariably observed, however *(43)*.

LDF has several potential advantages as a means of monitoring rCBF. It provides the capability of continuous real-time bedside monitoring with high temporal resolution, permitting rapid recognition of changes in cerebral hemodynamics. The technology has been validated by comparison with other methods of measuring CBF and there is extensive experience with its application in various organs *(40)*. It shows a fairly tight correlation with large vessel flow velocities, yet unlike TCD, it also provides direct feedback from the cerebral microcirculation. There are also disadvantages to LDF. Results are not quantitative and are expressed in arbitrary units (unlike thermal diffusion flowmetry results, which can be expressed in flow units of mL/100 g/min) *(40)*. Questions arise about the accuracy of CBF estimations that are based on a 1 mm^3 sample of tissue. Hemodilution can lead to inaccurate readings *(40)*. LDF is also sensitive to motion artifact, respiration artifact, and distortion of the signal by blood vessels larger than capillaries. Finally, the technology is invasive, requiring either bur hole or craniectomy for probe placement.

Complications of LDF appear to be rare; Kirkpatrick and associates reported no complications—and specifically no CSF infections—in their series of 22 patients, other than probe malfunction requiring reinsertion in two patients *(43)*.

THERMAL DIFFUSION FLOWMETRY

Thermal diffusion flowmetry (TDF) provides an index of regional cortical blood flow by quantifying dissipation of heat per unit time from an implanted source. The technology dates to 1933 when Gibbs used a heated thermocouple placed in the internal jugular vein to determine CBF *(45)*. Since then, Carter and associates have described the application of TDF as an intracranial monitor of regional cortical blood flow (rCoBF), as it is currently employed in the neurosurgical and NSU settings *(46)*.

The conceptual basis for the use of TDF to monitor rCoBF is relatively straightforward. A thermocouple, comprised of a heat source maintained at a constant temperature and a nearby sensor, will express a known temperature gradient in the no-flow state because thermal conductivity in this state is constant. When the heated thermocouple is apposed to cortex it dissipates heat to the brain parenchyma. Because thermal conductivity in the no-flow state is constant, steepening of the baseline temperature gradient expressed by the thermocouple directly reflects cortical blood flow, and this flow can be quantified in mL/100 g tissue/min units *(46)*.

The TDF monitor consists of a thin silastic leaf containing 2 gold disks, one of which serves as the heat source and the other as the thermal sensor. The temperature difference between the 2 gold disks is continuously monitored and converted into flow units to express rCoBF. Both disks must rest directly on cortex, and this is achieved either during craniotomy or via burr hole. Blind placement of the TDF probe is not desirable because inaccurate CoBF readings may result if the device is placed in proximity to large blood vessels (similar to laser Doppler flowmetry), placed over sulci rather than on a gyrus, or placed on abnormal (tumor, infarct) tissue. This makes burr hole placement somewhat precarious compared to the direct visualization obtained with craniotomy *(47)*.

The TDF monitor appears to detect blood flow in the outermost 2–3 mm of cortex. It should be kept in mind that flow to this region (gray matter flow) normally approximates 70 mL/100 g tissue/min, although normal whole-brain flow is about 50 mL/100 g tissue/min *(46,47)*.

TDF has been used in the operating room to monitor for ischemia and vasospasm during aneurysm clipping, to monitor for normal perfusion pressure breakthrough during AVM procedures (in which setting it may also be used to guide the induction of barbiturate coma to control hyperemia), and to discriminate normal from pathologic brain during tumor resections and epilepsy surgeries.

Indications for TDF monitoring in the NSU include postoperatively after aneurysm clipping for SAH and after AVM procedures, severe head injury, and epilepsy. The patient postaneurysm clipping is at risk for vasospasm with resultant cerebral ischemia; this would be suspected in the context of low CoBF readings (roughly less than 40 mL/100 g/min). In the first few days after AVM procedures, the NSU patient is at risk for hyperemia (normal perfusion pressure breakthrough), which may precipitate critically elevated ICP or intracerebral hemorrhage. Hyperemia is suggested by CoBF readings greater than roughly 90 mL/100 g/min, and such values might prompt the institution of barbiturate therapy to reduce cerebral metabolism *(47)*. TDF has proven useful in the management of severe head injury. This population is routinely monitored invasively for ICP trends, but as Sioutos and associates have pointed out, management based on ICP changes alone can be incorrect at times. They found rCoBF trends, as determined by TDF, to be a valuable adjunct to ICP monitoring in differentiating ICP elevations associated with ischemia from those associated with hyperemia. The treatments for the two underlying pathologic processes are fundamentally different, yet ICP monitoring alone would have missed this distinction. They also found normalization of rCoBF to be predictive of better outcome, and markedly depressed rCoBF was associated with poor outcome *(48)*. Finally, TDF has been used in the localization of seizure foci in intractable epilepsy. Interictally the seizure focus may show markedly reduced rCoBF, while ictally rCoBF tends to rise dramatically *(46)*.

The advantages of TDF are several. It provides continuous, quantitative, real-time information about cortical blood flow in a region of interest, in a reproducible manner. It does not appear particularly susceptible to artifacts produced by the ICU setting, and it relies on a relatively simple physical principle. While invasive, TDF does not require penetration of the brain parenchyma and appears to pose a very small risk of infection *(46)*. It has been used to positive effect in a number of clinical settings as indicated previously. TDF may be compared favorably to laser Doppler flowmetry (which does not provide quantitative information) and jugular venous sampling, which is artifact-prone and does not directly measure CoBF *(48)*.

Disadvantages of TDF include its invasive nature; its susceptibility to signal distortion if the probe is placed over a vessel, sulcus or pathologic tissue or if both disks do not directly contact cortex; its regional nature as a monitor of the outermost 2–3 mm of cortex in a small patch of brain; and its lack of specificity as a monitor of vasospasm (that is, TDF cannot localize the vasospastic vessel in the sense that TCD can).

Complications of TDF appear to be few. Concern about the potential for thermal injury to the underlying cortex has been addressed with a feedback system that turns off the heat source at a predetermined temperature maximum. Prophylactic antibiotics may be given during monitoring but the risk of CNS infection appears to be low *(46,48)*.

Microdialysis

Microdialysis is a technique that has begun to move from the laboratory into the clinical arena in recent years. The basic concept involves the insertion of a fine catheter into a body tissue, perfusion of the catheter with a physiologic solution such as Ringer's solution, and thereby the facilitation of exchange of molecules between the perfusate and the extracellular fluid (ECF) across a dialysis membrane located within the catheter tip.

In this manner various dialyzable substances from the ECF may be sampled and analyzed in a relatively short time, providing a window into processes taking place at the cellular level. Microdialysis has been applied to diabetes mellitus as a means of continuous long-term ambulatory glucose monitoring, and subcutaneous microdialysis has also been tried in a series of ICU patients in whom it appeared to be useful primarily in the detection of periods of hypoglycemia not revealed by routine fingerstick checks *(49,50)*. This discussion will focus specifically on cerebral microdialysis—in which the tissue being monitored is the brain parenchyma—and its pertinence to the NSU patient population.

After exposure of the brain either at craniotomy or via burr hole, a fine flexible catheter is inserted into the area of interest to a variable depth (typically 10–20 mm) below the cortical surface. The catheter is then connected to a perfusion pump which introduces a physiologic perfusate that equilibrates with the ECF across the dialysis membrane. The fluid is pumped at a low flow rate, typically around 0.3 μL/min, which tends to optimize the recovery of molecules of interest from the ECF. The dialysate is sterilely sampled at hourly or other regular intervals in vials which are placed in a microdialysis analyzer at the bedside. In this manner, the clinician may monitor on-line pH, lactate and pyruvate, glucose, glycerol, glutatmate, urea, and potentially other soluble molecules of interest. Lactate and the lactate : pyruvate ratio have been used as indices of cerebral ischemia, as has the excitotoxic amino acid glutamate, while glycerol is felt most likely to reflect phospholipid breakdown as a result of cell membrane damage (Fig. 4) *(51)*.

Cerebral microdialysis has been employed in the NSU to monitor for cerebral vasospasm and delayed ischemic deterioration in SAH, to discern indicators of secondary brain insults in severe head injury, to follow severe hemispheric ischemic stroke, and to follow ECF glutamate levels periictally in epileptic patients *(51–55)*. The technique has also been used intraoperatively to monitor for ischemia during neurosurgical procedures *(56)*. Controversy exists regarding some aspects of microdialytic analysis, such as whether lactate alone or the lactate:pyruvate ratio is a better indicator of early cerebral ischemia, and the technology is not yet in widespread clinical use *(57)*.

There would seem to be several theoretical advantages to cerebral microdialysis as an NSU monitoring modality. It provides concrete, virtually real-time evidence of neurophysiologic and neuropathologic processes taking place on a molecular level. The technology is such that sampling and analysis of the ECF can take place on a regular basis at the patient's bedside or in the operating room. Software applications exist to integrate microdialysis trends with ICP and CPP trends, providing the NSU patient with multimodal monitoring. Yet microdialysis remains somewhat problematic for routine clinical application. Beyond mere technical considerations (invasiveness, variability in the data depending on catheter or tubing length or the flow rate), reliance on microdialysis to guide patient management raises additional concerns. From the literature cited herein it is clear that there remains some debate regarding not only which molecules (or ratios) should be monitored in particular pathologic conditions, but also regarding the reliability of these markers in comparison to other neuromonitoring techniques (such as transcranial Doppler for the detection of vasospasm) and hence the advisability of guiding treatment based on isolated microdialysis abnormalities. Nilsson and associates have raised another important technical question, in light of the fact that one of the areas of strongest clinical interest in cerebral microdialysis is in monitoring patients post-SAH for vasospasm and resultant ischemia: where should the catheter be placed?

They approached this conundrum by placing separate catheters in two locations; otherwise a certain amount of clairvoyance would seem to be required to assure that the catheter is properly placed to detect future regional ischemic changes *(51)*. Finally, further evaluation is required to determine whether microdialysis, as an index of ischemic amage that has already begun, will prove as useful to the clinician as monitoring modalities that might detect earlier changes (e.g., vasospasm itself or reductions in CBF).

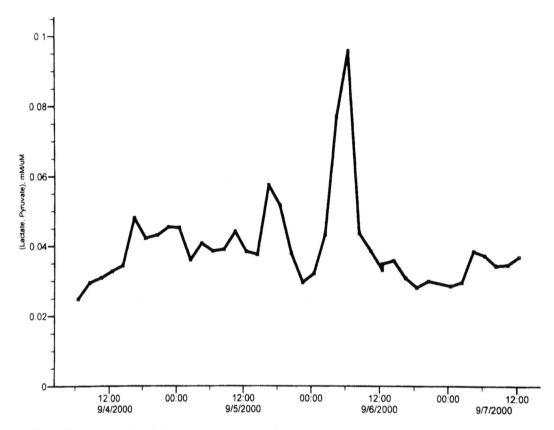

Fig. 4. Continuous microdialysis monitoring in a patient with subarachnoid hemorrhage. The highest lactate peak at around 00:00 hours corresponds to the time of aneurysm clipping in the right middle cerebral artery. The patient required partial clamping of the vessels due to intraoperative rupture of aneurysm. Lactate concentrations returned to normal and remained so for 6 more days. Left hemiparesis developed.

Complications associated with cerebral microdialysis catheters, as with any invasive probe, would potentially include damage to the brain parenchyma; however, as Landolt has noted, the volume of damaged tissue appears to be minimal (on the order of $0.75–1.5$ mm^3 in that study) and certainly much less than the volume of brain tissue affected by placement of a ventricular ICP catheter (57). The risk of infection also appears to be low, assuming sterile insertion and handling of the dialysis system.

Tissue Monitoring

Another recently introduced invasive cerebral monitor is the implantable microsensor catheter for the measurement of brain pO_2, pCO_2, pH, and temperature. Originally developed about a decade ago for continuous blood gas monitoring, the microsensor was approved as a brain parenchymal monitor in 1999. The 0.5-mm diameter probe contains separate sensors for oxygen, carbon dioxide and pH (hydrogen) that incorporate fluorescent dyes, as well as a temperature sensor *(58)*. One approach to probe insertion uses a special bolt with three entry ports, through two of which the parenchymal probe and an ICP catheter are introduced, typically into the nondominant frontal lobe to a variable depth *(59)*. Parameters may be monitored continuously or intermittently.

As with many other monitoring technologies described here, the tissue pO_2 probe has been applied most extensively in the head injury population. As a means of detecting cerebral ischemia in this setting, it has compared favorably to $SjvO_2$, and may aid prognostication *(60–62)*. A brain tissue pO_2 level below 15 mmHg has been suggested as a threshold for tissue damage *(63)*. Another potential indication for brain tissue pO_2 monitoring is subarachnoid hemorrhage *(64)*. The potential risks associated with tissue probes are those encountered with other invasive monitors, namely intracranial hemorrhage and infection, but the probe is of a fine caliber and the risk of these complications appears to be low.

NONBRAIN MONITORING IN THE NSU

Blood Pressure

The gold standard method of blood pressure monitoring in the ICU remains the indwelling arterial line. This method is more direct than an inflatable cuff and also allows continuous monitoring. The arterial waveform is displayed visually which allows caregivers to make the appropriate adjustments to correct an under- or overdampened waveform; the system may also be flushed to obtain a resonance frequency for a more accurate assessment than simple visual inspection of the waveform. The arterial line also facilitates blood gas sampling to guide ventilator management. Table 6 lists the major indications for continuous blood pressure monitoring in the NSU.

Blood Gases

Intermittent arterial blood gas sampling, like intermittent cuff blood pressure monitoring, is less than optimal in the ICU setting where patients can deteriorate rapidly requiring prompt recognition and intervention. Systems have been developed for continuous arterial blood gas monitoring. These rely primarily on fiberoptic technology.

Separate fibers associated with specific photochemical dyes for the measurement of pH, pO_2, and pCO_2 comprise the system, which can be inserted through a standard 20 gauge arterial catheter. Not yet in widespread use, these continuous blood gas monitors are described in detail in a recent review *(65)*.

Temperature

The goal of temperature monitoring in the ICU is to obtain accurate readings that closely reflect core temperature in both static and dynamic states, and regardless of whether the patient is normothermic, hypothermic, or febrile. In this respect, the pulmonary artery catheter (containing a thermistor) is considered the gold standard, but is not always practical and could hardly be justified for temperature monitoring alone.

Consequently several less direct routes of ascertaining body temperature have been explored. Regarding the literature comparing these various methods, the following conclusions may be drawn. First, the urinary bladder thermistor and (to a lesser extent) the rectal temperature are highly consistent with PA catheter core temperatures, but they are not ideal for monitoring during periods of rapid temperature change because they tend to lag behind such core changes *(67)*. Second, tympanic devices employing infrared technology tend to be quite operator-dependent, requiring proper placement and direction within the external ear canal, a tight seal, and a brief waiting period before repeat measurements from the cooling effect of the probe on the canal itself; oral thermometers have been found to exhibit less variability than tympanic probes *(66)*. Third, although a number of factors can bias oral temperatures (e.g., ingestion of cold liquids), the belief that oral endotracheal intubation yields inaccurate oral temperatures appears to be erroneous, provided that the probe is correctly placed in the posterior sublingual pocket *(67)*. In the intubated patient with no PA catheter, therefore, the oral route appears to be not only the simplest but probably also the most clinically helpful method of monitoring temperature.

CONCLUSION

The wide array of monitoring technologies available to the neurointensivist will likely continue to expand in the new millennium. With so many options, a number of factors (in addition to specific medical indications) will undoubtedly influence the choice of how best to follow patients in the NSU,

Table 6
Indications for Continuous Blood Pressure Monitoring in the NSU

Diagnosis	Value of continuous blood pressure (BP) monitoring
Acute ischemic stroke	Inadequate BP may exacerbate ischemic injury.
Post-thrombolysis	Excessive BP is associated with increased risk of ICH.
Intracerebral hemorrhage	Excessive BP may lead to hematoma expansion.
Subarachnoid hemorrhage	Monitoring guides induced hypertension for vasospasm.
Critical vascular stenosis	Induced hypertension may be employed here as well.
Guillain-Barre syndrome	Patients are at risk for autonomic instability.
Bacterial meningitis	Patients are at risk for septic shock (esp. meningococcus).
Status epilepticus	Autoregulation is lost; midazolam/propofol may drop BP.
Increased ICP	Adequate CPP, and control of ICP, require adequate MAP.

ICH, intracerebral hemorrhage; ICP, intracranial pressure; CPP, cerebral perfusion pressure; MAP, mean arterial pressure.

including clinician experience and philosophy, economics, and local practice standards. But it seems quite likely that the best results will be obtained not from reliance on a single (albeit familiar) modality, but rather from the judicious application of a multimodal monitoring approach, such as that described by Kirkpatrick and associates *(68)*. In this context, data that are corroborated by multiple technologies can be confidently acted on, whereas erroneous intelligence can be more readily detected and disregarded. Such a system holds great potential benefits for both patients and their caregivers.

REFERENCES

1. Jordan KG. Neurophysiologic monitoring in the neuroscience intensive care unit. *Neurol. Clin.* 1995;13:579–626.
2. Rosner MJ. Pathophysiology and management of increased intracranial pressure. In: Andrews BT, ed. *Neurosurgical Intensive Care*. New York: McGraw-Hill, 1993, pp. 57–112.
3. Lang EW, Chestnut RM. Intracranial pressure: Monitoring and management. *Neurosurg. Clin. North Am.* 1994;5:573–588.
4. Lundberg N. Continuous recording and control of ventricular fluid pressure in neurosurgical practice. *Acta Psychiatr. Scand.* 1960;36(Suppl 149):1.
5. Guyot LL, Dowling C, Diaz FG, Michael DB. Cerebral monitoring devices: Analysis of complications. *Acta Neurochir.* (Suppl)1998;71:47–49.
6. Ostrup RC, Luersssen TG, Marshall LF, Zornow MH. Continuous monitoring of intracranial pressure with a miniaturized fiberoptic device. *J. Neurosurg.* 1987;67:206–209.
7. The American Association of Neurological Surgeons, Joint Section on Neurotrauma and Critical Care. Indications for intracranial pressure monitoring. *J. Neurotrauma* 2000;17:479–491.
8. Gibbs EL, Lennox WG, Gibbs FA. Bilateral internal jugular blood: Comparison of A-V differences, oxygen-dextrose ratios and respiratory quotients. *Am. J. Psychiatry* 1945;102:184.
9. Feldman Z, Robertson CS. Monitoring of cerebral hemodynamics with jugular bulb catheters. *Crit. Care Clin.* 1997;13:51–77.
10. Metz C, Holzschuh M, Bein T, Woertgen C, et al. Monitoring of cerebral oxygen metabolism in the jugular bulb: Reliability of unilateral measurements in severe head injury. *J. Cereb. Blood Flow Metab.* 1998;18:332–343.
11. Lam JMK, Chan MSY, Poon WS. Cerebral venous oxygen saturation monitoring: Is dominant jugular bulb cannulation good enough? *Br. J. Neurosurg.* 1996;10:357–364.
12. Robertson CS, Narayan RK, Gokaslan ZL, Pahwa R, et al. Cerebral arteriovenous oxygen difference as an estimate of cerebral blood flow in comatose patients. *J. Neurosurg.* 1989;70:222–230.
13. Cruz J, Miner ME, Allen SJ, Alves WM, Gennarelli TA. Continuous monitoring of cerebral oxygenation in acute brain injury: Assessment of cerebral hemodynamic reserve. *Neurosurgery* 1991;29:743–749.
14. Latronico N, Beindorf AE, Rasulo FA, Febbrari P, et al. Limits of intermittent jugular bulb saturation monitoring in the management of severe head trauma patients. *Neurosurgery* 2000;46:1131–1138.
15. Kirkpatrick PJ, Smielewski P, Czosnyka M, Menon D, Pickard JD. Near-infrared spectroscopy use in patients with head injury. *J. Neurosurg.* 1995;83:963–970.
16. Goetting MG, Preston G. Jugular bulb catheterization does not increase intracranial pressure. *Intensive Care Med.* 1991;17:195–198.

17. Browne TR, Holmes GL. Status epilepticus. In: *Handbook of Epilepsy*, 2nd ed. Philadelphia: Lippincott Williams & Wilkins, 2000, pp. 197–214.

18. Young GB, Jordan KG, Doig GS. An assessment of nonconvulsive seizures in the intensive care unit using continuous EEG monitoring: An investigation of variables associated with mortality. *Neurology* 1996;47:83–89.

19. Wijdicks EFM. Determining brain death in adults. *Neurology* 1995;45:1003–1011.

20. Synek VM. Prognostically important EEG coma patterns in diffuse anoxic and traumatic encephalopathies in adults. *J. Clin. Neurophysiol.* 1988;5:161–174.

21. Aminoff MJ, Eisen AA. AAEM minimonograph 19: Somatosensory evoked potentials. *Muscle Nerve* 1998;21:277–290.

22. Diringer MN. Early prediction of outcome from coma. *Curr. Opin. Neurol. Neurosurg.* 1992;5:826.

23. Goldie WD, Chiappa KH, Young RR, et al. Brain stem auditory and short-latency somatosensory evoked responses in brain death. *Neurology* 1981;31:248–256.

24. Zandbergen EGL, de Haan RJ, Stoutenbeek CP, Koelman JHTM, Hijdra A. Systematic review of early prediction of poor outcome in anoxic-ischaemic coma. *Lancet* 1998;352:1808–1812.

25. Moulton RJ, Brown JIM, Konasiewicz SJ. Monitoring severe head injury: A comparison of EEG and somatosensory evoked potentials. *Can. J. Neurol. Sci.* 1998;25:S7–S11.

26. Tegeler CH, Babikian VL, Gomez CR. *Neurosonology*. St. Louis: Mosby, 1996.

27. Manno EM. Transcranial Doppler ultrasonography in the neurocritical care unit. *Crit. Care Clin.* 1997;13:79–104.

28. Aaslid R, Markwalder T, Nornes H. Noninvasive transcranial Doppler ultrasound recording of flow velocities in the basal cerebral arteries. *J. Neurosurg.* 1982;57:769–774.

29. Jobsis FF. Noninvasive, infrared monitoring of cerebral and myocardial oxygen sufficiency and circulatory parameters. *Science* 1977;198:1264–1267.

30. Adelson PD, Nemoto E, Scheuer M, Painter M, et al. Noninvasive continuous monitoring of cerebral oxygenation periictally using near-infrared spectroscopy: A preliminary report. *Epilepsia* 1999;40:1484–1489.

31. Witham TF, Nemoto EM, Jungreis CA, Kaufmann AM. Near-infrared spectroscopy monitored cerebral venous thrombolysis. *Can. J. Neurol. Sci.* 1999;26:48–52.

32. Nemoto EM, Yonas H, Kassam A. Clinical experience with cerebral oximetry in stroke and cardiac arrest. *Crit. Care Med.* 2000;28:1052–1054.

33. Gomersall CD, Joynt GM, Gin T, et al. Failure of the INVOS3100 cerebral oximeter to detect complete absence of cerebral blood flow. *Crit. Care Med.* 1997;25:1252–1254.

34. Lewis SB, Myburgh JA, Thornton EL, et al. Cerebral oxygenation monitoring by near-infrared spectroscopy is not clinically useful in patients with severe closed-head injury: A comparison with jugular venous bulb oximetry. *Crit. Care Med.* 1996;24:1334–1338.

35. Muellner T, Schramm W, Kwasny O, Vecsei V. Patients with increased intracranial pressure cannot be monitored using near infrared spectroscopy. *Br. J. Neurosurg.* 1998;12:136–139.

36. Anderson RE. Cerebral blood flow xenon-133. *Neurosurg. Clin. North Am.* 1996;7:703–708.

37. Martin NA, Doberstein C. Cerebral blood flow measurement in neurosurgical intensive care. *Neurosurg. Clin. North Am.* 1994;5:607–618.

38. Ingvar DH, Lassen NA. Quantitavie determination of cerebral blood flow in man. *Lancet* 1961;2:806–807.

39. Halsey JH, Nakai K, Wariyar B. Sensitivity of rCBF to focal lesion. *Stroke* 1981;12:631–635.

40. Arbit E, DiResta GR. Application of laser Doppler flowmetry in neurosurgery. *Neurosurg. Clin. North Am.* 1996;7:741–748.

41. Haberl PL, Villringer A, Dirnagl U. Applicability of laser-Doppler flowmetry for cerebral blood flow monitoring in neurological intensive care. *Acta Neurochir (Suppl)* 1993;59:64–68.

42. Stern MD, Lappe LD, Bowen PD, et al. Continuous measurement of tissue blood flow by laser-Doppler spectroscopy. *Am. J. Physiol.* 1977;232:H441–H448.

43. Kirkpatrick PJ, Smielewski P, Czosnyka M, Pickard JD. Continuous monitoring of cortical perfusion by laser Doppler flowmetry in ventilated patients with head injury. *J. Neurol. Neurosurg. Psych.* 1994;57:1382–1388.

44. Meyerson BA, Gunasekera L, Linderoth B, Gazelius B. Bedside monitoring of regional cortical blood flow in comatose patients using laser Doppler flowmetry. *Neurosurgery* 1991;29:750–755.

45. Gibbs FA. A thermoelectric blood flow recorder in the form of a needle. In: *Proceedings of the Society for Experimental Biology and Medicine*, San Francisco 1933, pp. 141–146.

46. Carter LP, Weinand ME, Oommen KJ. Cerebral blood flow (CBF) monitoring in intensive care by thermal diffusion. *Acta Neurochir.* 1993;(Suppl)59:43–46.

47. Carter LP. Thermal diffusion flowmetry. *Neurosurg. Clin. North Am.* 1996;7:749–754.

48. Sioutos PJ, Orozco JZ, Carter LP, Weinand ME, et al. Continuous regional cerebral cortical blood flow monitoring in head-injured patients. *Neurosurgery* 1995;36:943–950.

49. Bolinder J, Ungerstedt U, Arner P. Long-term continuous glucose monitoring with microdialysis in ambulatory insulin-dependent diabetic patients. *Lancet* 1993;342:1080–1085.

50. Hutchinson PJA, O'Connell MY, Maskell LB, Pickard JD. Monitoring by subcutaneous microdialysis in neurosurgical intensive care. *Acta Neurochir. (Suppl)* 1999;75:57–59.

51. Nilsson OG, Brandt L, Ungerstedt U, Saveland H. Bedside detection of brain ischemia using intracerebral microdialysis: Subarachnoid hemorrhage and delayed ischemic deterioration. *Neurosurgery* 1999;45:1176–1185.

52. Schulz MK, Wang LP Tange M, Bjerre P. Cerebral microdialysis monitoring: determination of normal and ischemic cerebral metabolisms in patients with aneurysmal subarachnoid hemorrhage. *J. Neurosurg.* 2000;93:808–814.

53. Vespa P, Prins M, Ronne-Engstrom E, Caron M, et al. Increase in extracellular glutamate caused by reduced cerebral perfusion and seizures after human traumatic brain injury: a microdialysis study. *J. Neurosurg.* 1998;89:971–982.

54. Berger C, Annecke A, Aschoff A, et al. Neurochemical monitoring of fatal middle cerebral artery infarction. *Stroke* 1999;30:460–463.

55. During MJ, Spencer DD. Extracellular hippocampal glutamate and spontaneous seizure in the conscious human brain. *Lancet* 1993;341:1607–1610.

56. Mendelowitsch A, Sekhar LN, Wright DC, et al. An increase in intracellular glutamate is a sensitive method of detecting ischaemic neuronal damage during cranial base and cerebrovascular surgery: An in vivo microdialysis study. *Acta Neurochir.* 1998;140:349–355.

57. Landolt H, Langemann H, Alessandri B. A concept for the introduction of cerebral microdialysis in neurointensive care. *Acta Neurochir.* 1996;(Suppl)67:31–36.

58. Andrews RJ. Monitoring for neuroprotection: New technologies for the new millennium. *Ann. NY Acad. Sci.* 2000:101–113.

59. van Santbrink H, Maas AIR, Avezaat CJJ. Continuous monitoring of partial pressure of brain tissue oxygen in patients with severe head injury. *Neurosurgery* 1996;38:21–31.

60. Kiening KL, Unterberg AW, Bardt TF, et al. Monitoring of cerebral oxygenation in patients with severe head injuries: brain tissue pO_2 versus jugular vein oxygen saturation. *J. Neurosurg.* 1996;85:751–757.

61. van den Brink WA, van Santbrink H, Steyerberg EW, et al. Brain oxygen tension in severe head injury. *Neurosurgery* 2000;46:868–878.

62. Valadka AB, Shankar SP, Contant CF, et al. Relationship of brain tissue pO_2 to outcome after severe head injury. *Crit. Care Med.* 1998;26:1576–1581.

63. Alvarez del Castillo M. Monitoring neurologic patients in intensive care. *Curr. Opin. Crit. Care* 2001;7:49–60.

64. Hoffman WE, Wheeler P, Edelman G. Hypoxic brain tissue following subarachnoid hemorrhage. *Anesthesiology* 2000;92:442–446.

65. Zimmerman JL, Dellinger RP. Blood gas monitoring. *Crit. Care Clin.* 1996;12:865–874.

66. Giuliano KK, Giuliano AJ, Scott SS, et al. Temperature measurement in critically ill adults: a comparison of tympanic and oral methods. *Am. J. Crit. Care* 2000;9:254–261.

67. Fallis WM. Oral measurement of temperature in orally intubated critical care patients: state-of-the-science review. *Am. J. Crit. Care* 2000;9:334–343.

68. Kirkpatrick PJ, Czosnyka M, Pickard JD. Multimodal monitoring in neurointensive care. *J. Neurol. Neurosurg. Psychiatry* 1996;60:131–139.

69. Khan SH, Kureshi IU, Mulgrew T, et al. Comparison of percutaneous ventriculostomies and intraparenchymal monitor: A retrospective evaluation of 156 patients. *Acta Neurochir. (Suppl)* 1998;71:50–52.

70. Sheinberg M, Kanter MJ, Robertson CS, et al. Continuous monitoring of jugular venous oxygen saturation in head-injured patients. *J. Neurosurg.* 1992;76:212–217.

71. Hassler W, Steinmetz H, Gawlowski J. Transcranial Doppler ultrasonography in raised intracranial pressure and in intracranial circulatory arrest. *J. Neurosurg.* 1988;68:745–751.

72. Wardlaw JM, Offin R, Teasdale GM, et al. Is routine transcranial Doppler ultrasound monitoring useful in the management of subarachnoid hemorrhage? *J. Neurosurg.* 1998;88:272–276.

73. Brass LM, Pavlakis SG, DeVivo D, et al. Transcranial Doppler measurements of the middle cerebral artery: Effect of hematocrit. *Stroke* 1988;19:1466–1469.

74. Recommendations for intracranial pressure monitoring technology. *J. Neurotrauma* 2000;17:497–505.

7

Neuroimaging in Neuroemergencies

Jeffrey L. Sunshine and Robert W. Tarr

INTRODUCTION

Imaging is a crucial component of management and therapeutic decision making for the neurosciences critical care unit (NSU) patient. The importance of imaging is especially pertinent for those patients in whom an accurate neurological examination is not possible. Imaging in this setting may provide the first clue to potentially treatable causes of neurologic deterioration.

Neurological deterioration in NSU patients may be secondary to hemorrhagic pathologies, ischemic changes, infectious processes, or other physiologic phenomenon such as hydrocephalus. To optimize the use of imaging techniques for decision-making purposes the appropriate technology and protocol must be chosen for each clinical situation. This chapter reviews indications for several basic neuroimaging techniques such as computed tomography (CT), magnetic resonance imaging (MRI), magnetic resonance angiography (MRA), computed tomographic angiography (CTA), and conventional digital subtraction angiography (DSA). Additionally, more advanced imaging techniques such as diffusion/perfusion MRI, and single photon emission tomography (SPECT) will also be discussed.

COMPUTED TOMOGRAPHY

CT is the mainstay for diagnosis in emergent neurologic situations. At most institutions CT is available 24 h/d and actual scan time on modern multidetector scanners is less than 1 min. CT is extremely sensitive to detect acute intracranial hemorrhage (ICH). The sensitivity of non–contrast-enhanced CT for the detection of subarachnoid hemorrhage (SAH) (Fig. 1A) is approx 90% in the first 24 h after ictus and falls to approx 50% 1 wk following the initial ictus (1–4). The sensitivity of detection for small amounts of SAH at the periphery of the brain, or for subdural hemorrhages (SDH) along the brain skull interface can be increased by viewing the scan at wider window settings, thus increasing the contrast between blood and the overlying bone.

The CT appearance of ICH varies with time. Pathologically, ICH can be divided into four stages: acute (1–3 d), subacute (4–8 d), capsule (9–13 d), and organization (> 13 d) (5,6). Acutely, noncontrast-enhanced CT scans demonstrate a well-marginated hyperdense mass resulting from the high protein content of intact red blood cells (Fig. 1B). There may be some low density in the surrounding brain from perivascular inflammation and edema. As erythrocytes lyse and progressively lose hemoglobin in the subacute stage, the hematoma becomes progressively isodense with brain parenchyma. In the early organizational stage the filling of the acellular hematoma with a vascularized matrix may cause the hematoma to again be slightly hyperdense when compared with brain parenchyma. Eventually, an area of encephalomalacia is seen as a low-density area with negative mass effect.

On postcontrast-enhanced CT, enhancement of the hematoma is first seen in the subacute stage and is related to perivascular inflammation. The enhancement pattern is initially a complete or almost complete ring around the periphery of the hematoma. The ring of enhancement gradually decreases

From: *Current Clinical Neurology*
Critical Care Neurology and Neurosurgery
Edited by: J. I. Suarez © Humana Press Inc., Totowa, NJ

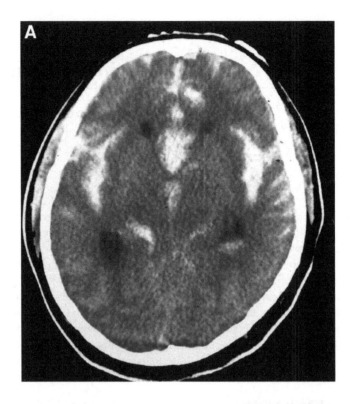

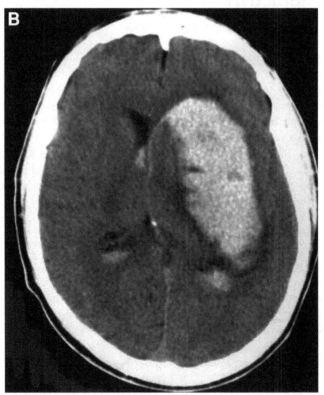

Fig.1. (*Continued on next page*)

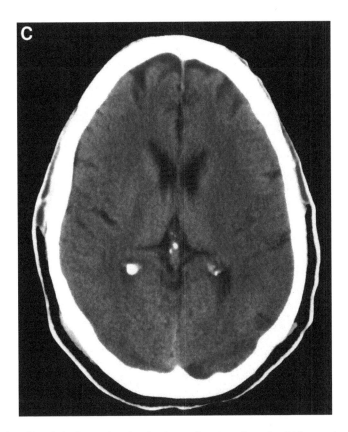

Fig. 1. CT imaging. Panel **A** shows the classic signs of acute subarachnoid hemorrhage with hyperdense fluid filling the basal cisterns, the Sylvian fissures, the anterior interhemispheric fissure and to a lesser degree the left atrium of the lateral ventricle. Panel **B** reveals an unfortunately typical large hyperdense hematoma centered in the parenchyma of the left basal ganglia that displaces surrounding tissues. Panel **C** demonstrates loss of the gray-white distinction among the left basal ganglia and the beginning loss of that definition along the parietal lobe in the posterior distribution of the left middle cerebral artery. Note also the early effacement of the thinner sulci of the upper left Sylvian fissure.

in diameter and becomes more irregular and more intense. Eventually the ring pattern of enhancement is replaced by a nodular pattern as a result of filling in the center of the hematoma by developing neovascularity.

In the setting of acute neurological deficit thought to be due to ischemic stroke, the main purpose of imaging with CT is to exclude a hemorrhagic etiology. However, noncontrast-enhanced CT may provide important clues to the ischemic nature of the deficit within 6 h of the initial ictus. Early CT signs of ischemic changes are subtle (Fig. 1C) and include slight hypodensity, minimal mass effect (often seen as asymmetry of sulci from one hemisphere to the other), and loss of distinction between the densities of gray and white matter *(7)*. One of the earliest signs on noncontrast-enhanced CT of middle cerebral artery infarction is loss of definition of the insular ribbon *(8)*. This sign refers to early loss of distinction between the Island of Reil, the extreme capsule, and the claustrum due to developing cytotoxic edema. Occasionally CT slices through the suprasellar cistern will demonstrate a hyperdense middle cerebral artery, indicative of thrombus within the artery. A hyperdense middle cerebral artery is seen in approx 35% of patients with symptoms of acute middle cerebral artery infarction and may be predictive of a larger volume of eventual infarct *(9,10)*.

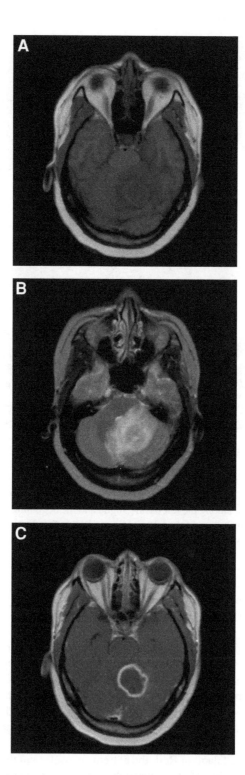

Fig. 2. Brain abscess. Panel **A** contains a T1-weighted axial image without contrast. This shows a slightly hyperintense collagenous ring around the area of abscess. Panel **B** has a T2-weighted age showing the hypointense rim, the central hyperintense fluid, and the surrounding edema. Panel **C**, a postcontrast-enhanced, T1-weighted image reveals the classic thin rim of enhancement without any focal nodules.

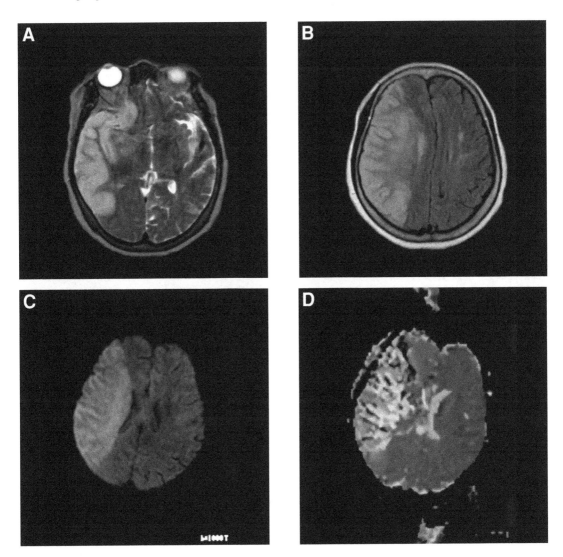

Fig. 3. Acute ischemic infarct. Panel **A** contains a T2-weighted axial image that shows a clearly demarcated area of hyperintense signal along the right temporal lobe consistent with acute ischemia. In addition note the mild early mass effect apparent as an effacement of the sulci in the involved territory. Panel **B** has a FLAIR image showing the expected suppression of the background spinal fluid signal. Yet the technique still allows the prominent display of abnormal T2 signal in the brain parenchyma of the right middle cerebral artery territory. Panel **C** shows a diffusion weighted axial image with the expected loss of parenchymal signal and gray-white differentiation of the unaffected tissue. In distinct contrast, the image reveals clear bright signal from water molecules trapped in the region of acute infarction. Panel **D** shows a perfusion time-to-peak effect parameter map that has been constructed from nearly 60 base images. This shows the delay in contrast material delivery from slowed perfusion throughout the right middle cerebral artery territory.

MAGNETIC RESONANCE IMAGING

The exquisite tissue contrast resolution, anatomic definition, and multiplanar capabilities of MRI make it an ideal tool for neurodiagnosis. In the NSU setting, the three main reasons to use MRI are the evaluation of patients with suspected intracranial or spinal infections, evaluation for suspected neoplasm, and evaluation of suspected ischemic events.

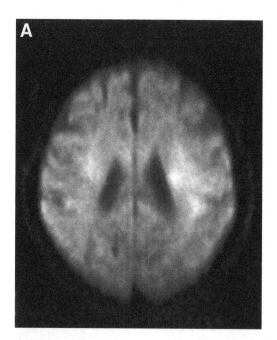 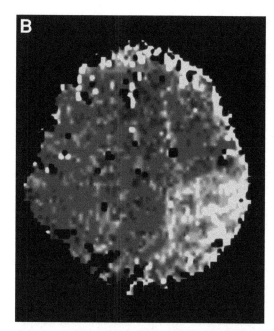

Fig. 4. Acute ischemic penumbra. Panel **A** shows a diffusion-weighted image with minimal areas of increased signal in the posterior left hemispheric white matter. At the same time, the time-to-peak effect parameter map in Panel **B** reveals a large wedge-shaped area of marked hypoperfusion in the posterior left middle cerebral artery territory. The difference between abnormal areas in **B** from those in **A** represent estimated salvageable brain tissue or penumbra.

MRI: Intracranial Infection

Intracranial infections can broadly be divided into those affecting lining structures (meningitis, ventriculitis) and those involving brain parenchyma (encephalitis, brain abcess).

Although gadolinium (Gd-DTPA)–enhanced MRI may detect meningitis by demonstrating diffuse meningeal enhancement, the literature states that it is only approx 50–70% sensitive in doing so *(11–13)*. Some authors feel that the addition of fluid attenuation inversion-recovery sequence (FLAIR) to the imaging paradigm increases the sensitivity of MRI to inflammatory meningeal disease *(14)*. Despite its limited sensitivity in diagnosing inflammatory meningeal disease, MRI plays a vital diagnostic role in detecting the sequela of inflammatory meningeal disease such as subdural/epidural empyema, parenchymal spread with cerebritis or discrete cerebral abscess, and central nervous system infarction secondary to venous thrombosis or arterial vasospasm. The ability to image the cerebral vasculature with MRA or magnetic resonance venography (MRV) techniques is particularly useful with regard to assessing the sequela of central nervous system infarction.

Although uncommon, ventriculitis is a potentially serious infectious process involving the cerebral ependyma. Often cerebrospinal fluid (CSF) analysis shows no evidence of abnormal cytology and culture results may remain normal *(15)*. Because of this, MRI can play a vital role in the diagnosis of ventriculitis. Usually, hydrocephalus is present. Additionally, there may be subependymal edema that is best detected on FLAIR imaging. Following Gad-DTPA administration, there is diffuse enhancement of the ependyma. Additionally, there may be enlargement of the choroid plexi due to inflammatory involvement of these structures.

The clinical presentation of brain abscesses is often protean. MRI is the technique of choice when brain abscess is a diagnostic possibility (Fig. 2). On noncontrast MRI the collagenous capsule of the abscess can be seen as a thin-walled ring that is isointense to slightly hyperintense to brain on T1-

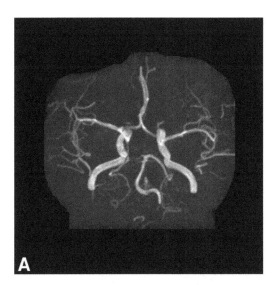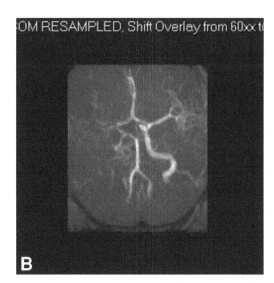

Fig. 5. Time-of-flight MRA. Panel **A** contains a maximum intensity projection from bright flow images obtained with suppression of venous flows. This clearly depicts the major vessels that supply the brain and comprise the Circle of Willis. Panel **B** has a similar projection that now demonstrates loss of flow signal from the right middle cerebral artery.

weighted images and is hypointense on T2-weighted images *(16,17)*. Following contrast material administration, brain abscesses classically demonstrate a thin ring of peripheral enhancement. The thinness of the rim of peripheral enhancement as well as the lack of nodularity can help to distinguish abscess from necrotic tumor. However, often this distinction is not absolutely clear. Diffusion-weighted MRI (DWI) can aid with this distinction. On DWI abscess cavities demonstrate increased signal intensity and are low signal intensity on apparent diffusion coefficient (ADC) maps because of abnormal diffusion of protons within the necrotic center. Necrotic tumors may show mildly increased signal on DWI due to T2 shine-through, but do not exhibit diminished signal intensity on ADC maps *(18,19)*.

MRI: Ischemia

In general, routine spin-echo (SE) MRI is more sensitive than CT for imaging the pathophysiologic changes occurring during an acute ischemic event *(20)*. The early changes related to ischemia that are seen on SE MRI are time-dependent and can be identified as morphologic changes caused by tissue swelling, such as enlargement and distortion of cortical gyri and narrowing of adjacent sulci *(21)*.

These changes are best seen on T1-weighted SE images and although they can be detected within 6 h post-ictus, they are not well appreciated until 1–3 d. Signal intensity changes on T2-weighted SE images are more conspicuous than the morphological changes described above (Fig. 3A). These changes can usually be detected between 8 and 24 h post-ictus. Increased gyral and subcortical signal intensity is seen on proton density and T2-weighted images due to increased intracellular free water caused by depleted adenosine triphosphate (ATP)-dependent pumps.

FLAIR pulse sequences have even more sensitivity for detecting early cortical ischemic changes compared to routine SE imaging (Fig. 3B). Although this sequence is heavily T2 weighted, CSF is turned dark, therefore increasing the contrast between a cortical ischemic lesion and adjacent CSF in sulci *(22)*.

DWI is the most sensitive imaging technique for detecting acute ischemic changes. In animal models signs of ischemic changes can be seen on DWI within the first 30 min after onset *(23)*. DWI scans are performed at multiple gradient strengths to allow calculation of ADC *(24)*. Areas in the brain where protons are least likely to have dephased through random phenomena, such as brownian

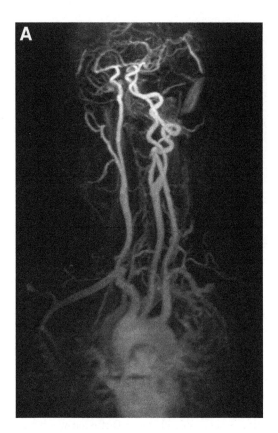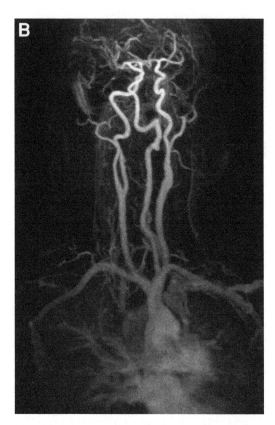

Fig. 6. Contrast-enhanced MRA. Panel **A** shows an MRA obtained during intravenous bolus administration of contrast. Notice the large field of view allows direct review of all arteries from the arch through the circle of Willis. Panel **B** shows the same data in a rotated reconstruction that allows better evaluation of the opposite carotid bifurcation. This rotation also reveals the left vertebral origin for review.

motion and microvascular perfusion, are depicted as areas of increased signal intensity. During an acute ischemic episode, there is abnormal trapping of free intracellular water from failure of the high-energy Na^+-K^+-ATPase pump, membrane breakdown, and the development of cytotoxic edema. Therefore, these areas have decreased diffusion coefficients and are visualized on DWI images as areas of increased signal intensity (Fig. 3C). ADC maps are often obtained with the DWI scans. These maps represent pixel-by-pixel analysis of tissue diffusion coefficients. Areas of diminished diffusion coefficient such as is seen with ischemic tissues are evident by decreased signal intensity regions on ADC maps.

Perfusion MRI (PWI) provides information related to the microcirculation of the brain in the form of mean transit times (MTT), time-to-peak (TTP) arrival of contrast material, and regional cerebral blood flow (rCBF) maps. Perfusion images are generated during the transit of a first-pass bolus of intravenous paramagnetic contrast agent through the cerebral circulation. The bolus is followed temporally during dynamic acquisition of sequences designed to accentuate magnetic susceptibility *(25)*. Areas of normal perfusion show a transient signal drop as the gadolinium first passes through. Areas of ischemia show delayed signal change, because the paramagnetic substance cannot be delivered in a normal phase. Therefore, areas of hypoperfusion are depicted as areas of bright signal intensity on the time-to-peak perfusion map (Fig. 3D).

An estimate of ischemic penumbra can be formed through the combined analysis of PWI and DWI data *(26–28)*. Areas of abnormal diffusion restriction represent an estimate of tissue already destined

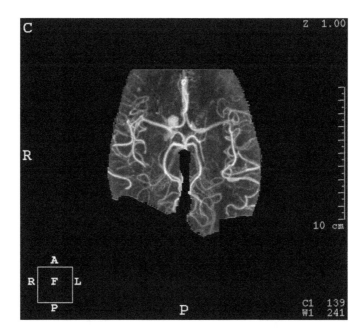

Fig. 7. CT angiogram. Prominent vasculature of the brain offset on a relatively black background after subtraction of bone and soft tissues. One then observes the underlying anatomy, including the right internal carotid artery aneurysm, without the surrounding noise in the image.

to perish, the infarct core. Meanwhile, all areas of decreased contrast delivery represent all the tissue under ischemic stress. Those areas with diminished perfusion but not with restricted diffusion then represent tissue at ischemic risk for infarct, or the penumbra (Fig. 4). These estimates can be extremely helpful in the decision matrix of various therapeutic choices in a patient with a new neurologic deficit *(29)* (*see also* Chapter 18).

Other Cerebral Perfusion Methods

The evaluation of cerebral perfusion can be obtained through many imaging modalities. In addition to PWI, rapid imaging on an NSU patient can occur with Tc99m SPECT imaging *(30,31)*, xenon-enhanced CT with the appropriate equipment, and with common iodinated contrast-enhanced CT perfusion studies. The latter uses similar postprocessing techniques to generate relative cerebral blood flow, MTT, or TTP parameter maps *(32)*. Any of these relative perfusion measures can be used to help determine the need and extent of therapeutic intervention for the NSU patient. In addition to obtaining useful information for cerebral ischemia and stroke patients these studies can be used in evaluating a patient in cerebral vasospasm following SAH. In conjunction with transcranial Doppler screening examinations, brain perfusion may be assessed to determine the need for aggressive hypervolemic and hypertensive therapy, angiography, or endovascular interventions (*see also* Chapters 3, 4, and 20).

Magnetic Resonance Angiography

Conventional MRA has consisted of so-called bright blood techniques acquired in 2D or 3D image formats *(33)*. These data are then projected in multiple planes through a maximum intensity projection technique that produces the commonly seen MRA images (Fig. 5). These techniques have proven excellent and reliable for evaluation of cervical, skull base, and intracranial arteries at least through the second order branches off the Circle of Willis. However, they have proven limited in the settings

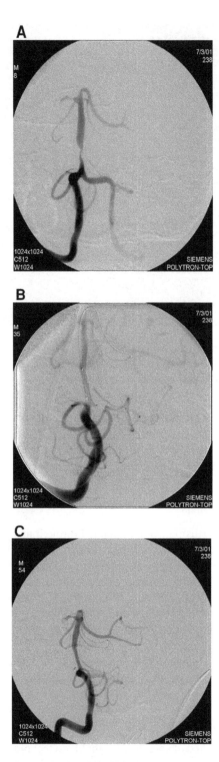

Fig. 8. Digital subtraction angiograms and stent. Panel **A** shows the basilar artery from a right vertebral injection with a high-grade stenosis along the proximal third of the vessel. Panel **B** reveals the stent delivery system in correct position centered on the stenosis. Panel **C** demonstrates the nearly normal lumen with no residual stenosis after placement of the metal stent and removal of the delivery devices.

of patient motion, the presence of susceptibility artifacts from sinuses or metal, and when marked tortuosity produces a vessel oriented in the cranial to caudal direction rather than flowing toward the head.

MRA has allowed screening of vessels without the need for an invasive procedure. This permits the NSU physician to assess the patency of the vessels once or serially as the clinical course may dictate. Specific diagnostic concerns, for example vessel dissection *(34)*, can be sensitively and specifically identified. Further the continued patency of the vessels can be observed after interventions ranging from medical such as anticoagulation, to surgical clipping *(35)* or coil embolization *(36)*, to endovascular stenting. Baseline images can be obtained toward the end of hospital care and then compared to repeat studies generated in the outpatient follow-up phases.

Recently MRA has been improved through the addition of a Gd-DTPA contrast bolus. This technique performed on a modern MR scanner can permit imaging, including the aortic arch through the Circle of Willis from a single acquisition *(37)*. This widened field of view can allow the physician to assess all of the relevant cerebral vasculature and exclude a majority of abnormalities in a single examination (Fig. 6). These contrast-enhanced MRA, however, can still be limited by areas of tortuosity or regions of artifact from nearby sinuses or metal implantation. Nevertheless in many patients these images add much additional information without requiring the risks of invasive imaging.

Similar techniques have also been applied with CT and common iodine based contrast. When coupled with modern advanced multislice CT scanners a wide range CTA of the neck, head or both may be obtained *(38)*. This has proven useful in screening acute stroke patients for vessel patency *(39)*. More specifically CTA has found great use in the pretreatment evaluation of an intracerebral aneurysm *(40)*. This technology allows the intracranial vasculature to be offset from the surrounding tissue and bone (Fig. 7). The vessels can then be viewed in isolation in either a maximum intensity projection similar to angiography or as shaded-surface 3D type representations. These complex image projections permit the evaluation of the vessel and the aneurysm from virtually any conceivable angle, which allows for far better assessment of associated vessel branches, anatomic structures, and parent anatomy *(41)*.

CONVENTIONAL DIGITAL SUBTRACTION ANGIOGRAPHY

Traditional catheter-based DSA can now be used as the final tool to assess cerebral vasculature. This test remains, barely for some, the gold standard for viewing the vessels to and from the brain. Thus, absent sufficient answers from any or all the preceding tests, an angiogram may reveal the subtle anatomy or distortions of dissection, aneurysm, vasculopathies, neoplasm, emboli or thrombus. This technique has taken on an especially enhanced role in serving as the base for endovascular interventions from the interventional neuroradiologists. In this setting, not only can the diseases be correctly diagnosed, but also they can then be treated. This can include stent placements for atherosclerosis (Fig. 8) or dissections *(42)*; embolizations of aneurysms, vascular malformations, or tumors *(43)*; and drug delivery to or mechanical removal of thrombo-emboli *(44)*.

CONCLUSION

As in all arenas of current medical care, imaging has taken on a central role in the diagnosis and management of critically ill neurological and neurosurgical patients. Almost all NSU patients will require a basic head CT, whereas many will require almost all of the techniques we have reviewed here. The additional guidance provided by image technology has added to the improved outcomes of these patients over the past decades. Better comprehension of the benefits of each technique will hopefully enable our optimal care of each and every patient.

REFERENCES

1. Ghoshhajra K, Scotti L, Marasco J, et al. CT detection of intracranial aneurysm in subarachnoid hemorrhage. *AJR* 1979;132:613–616.

2. Inoue Y, Saiwai S, Miyamoto T, et al. Post contrast computed tomography in subarachnoid hemorrhage from ruptured aneurysms. *J. Comput. Assist. Tomogr.* 1981;5:341–344.

3. Liliequist B, Lindquist m, Valdimarsson E. Computed tomography and subarachnoid hemorrhage. *Neuroradiology* 1977;14:21–26.

4. Lim ST, Sage DJ. Detection of subarachoid blood clot and other thin flat structures by computed tomography. *Radiology* 1977;123:79–84.

5. Enzmann DR, Britt RH, Lyons BE, et al. Natural history of experimental intracerebral hemorrhage: Sonography, computed tomography and neuropathology. *AJNR* 1981;2:517–526.

6. Lee YY, Moser R, Bruner JM, Van Tassel P. Organized intracerbral hematoma with acute hemorrhage: CT patterns and pathological correlations. *AJR* 1986;147:111–118.

7. Wall SD, Brant-Zawadzki M, Jeffrey RB, et al. High frequency CT findings within 24 hors after cerebral infarction. *AJR* 1982;138:307–311.

8. Truwit CL, Barkovich AJ, Gean-Marton A, et al. Loss of the insular ribbon: Another early sign of acute middle cerebral artery infarction. *Radiology* 1990;176:801–806.

9. Tomsick TA, Brott TG, Chambers AA, et al. Hyperdense middle cerebral artery: Incidence and quantitative significance. *Neuroradiololgy* 1989;31:312–315.

10. Tomsick T, Brott T, Barsan W, et al. Thrombus localization with emergency cerebral CT. *AJNR* 1992;13:257–263

11. Chang K, Han M, Roh JK, et al. Gd-DTPA enhanced MR imaging of the brain in patients with meningitis: Evaluation and comparison with CT. *AJNR* 1990;11:69–76.

12. Ginsberg L. Contrast enhancement in meningeal and extra-axial disease. *Neuroimaging Clin. North Am.* 1994;4:133–152.

13. Phillips M, Ryals T, Kambhu S, et al. Neoplastic vs inflammatory meningeal enhancement with Gd-DTPA. *J. Comput. Assist. Tomogr.* 1990;14:536–541.

14. Singer MB, Atlas SW, Drayer BP. Subarachnoid space disease: Diagnosis with fluid-attenuated inversion-recovery MR imaging and comparison with gadolinium-enhanced spin-echo MR imagingblinded reader study. *Radiology* 1998;208:417–422.

15. Katzman M, Ellner JL. Chronic meningitis. In Mandell GL, Douglas RG Jr, Bennett JE, eds. *Principles and Practice of Infectious Diseases*, 3rd ed. New York: Churchill Livingstone, 1990, pp. 771–786.

16. Haimes AB, Zimmerman RD, Morgello S, et al. MR imaging of brain abscesses. *AJR* 1989;152:1073–1085.

17. Sze G, Zimmerman RD. The magnetic resonance imaging of infections and inflammatory diseases. *Radiol. Clin. North Am.* 1988;26:839–859.

18. Despechins B, Stadnick T, Koerts G, et al. Use of diffusion-weighted MR imaging in differential diagnosis between intracerebral necrotic tumors and cerebral abscesses. *AJNR* 1999;20:1252–1257.

19. Kim YJ, Chang KH , Song IC, et al. Brain abcess and necrotic or cystic brain tumor: discrimination with signal intensity on diffusion weighted MR imaging. *AJR* 1998;171:1487–1490.

20. Yuh WTC, Crain MR Loes DJ, et al. MR imaging of cerebral ischemia: Findings in the first 24 hours. *AJNR* 1991;12:611–620.

21. Bryan RN, Levy LM, Whitlow WD, et al. Diagnosis of acute cerebral infarction: Comparison of CT and MR imaging. *AJNR* 1991;12:611–620.

22. Rydberg JN, Hammon CA, Grimm RC. Initial clinical experience in MR imaging of brain with a fast fluid attenuated inversion recovery pulse sequence. *Radiology* 1994;193:173–180.

23. Finelli DA, Hopkins AL, Selman WP, et al. Evaluation of experimental early acute cerebral ischemia before the development of edema: Use of dynamic contrast-enhanced and diffusion-weighted MR scanning. *Magn. Reson. Med.* 1992;27:189–197.

24. LeBihan D, Turner R, Dock P, et al. Diffusion MR imaging: Clinical applications. *AJR* 1992;159:591–599.

25. Rosen BR, Belliveau JW, Vevea JM, Brady TJ. Perfusion imaging with NMR contrast agents. *Magn. Reson. Med.* 1990;14:249–265.

26. Sorensen AG, Buonanno FS, Gonzalez RG, et al. Hyperacute stroke: evaluation with combined multisection diffusion-weighted and hemodynamically weighted echo-planar MR imaging. *Radiology* 1996;199:391–401.

27. Baird AE, Warach S. Magnetic resonance imaging of acute stroke [published erratum appears in *J. Cereb. Blood Flow Metab.* 1998;18:preceding 1047]. *J. Cereb. Blood Flow Metab.* 1998;18:583–609.

28. Fisher M, Albers GW. Applications of diffusion-perfusion magnetic resonance imaging in acute ischemic stroke [see comments]. *Neurology* 1999;52:1750–1756

29. Sunshine JL, Tarr RW, Lanzieri CF, Landis DM, Selman WR, Lewin JS. Hyperacute stroke: ultrafast MR imaging to triage patients prior to therapy. *Radiology* 1999; 212:325–332.

30. Nakano S, Iseda T, Ikeda T, Yoneyama T, Wakisaka S. Thresholds of ischemia salvageable with intravenous tissue plasminogen activator therapy: Evaluation with cerebral blood flow single-photon emission computed tomographic measurements. *Neurosurgery* 2000;47:68–71

31. Ueda T, Sakaki S, Yuh WT, Nochide I, Ohta S. Outcome in acute stroke with successful intra-arterial thrombolysis and predictive value of initial single-photon emission-computed tomography. *J. Cereb. Blood Flow Metab.* 1999;19:99–108.

32. Hamberg LM, Hunter GJ, Halpern EF, Hoop B, Gazelle GS, Wolf GL. Quantitative high-resolution measurement of cerebrovascular physiology with slip-ring CT. *AJNR* 1996;17:639–650.

33. Litt, AW. MR *Angiography of the Central Nervous System*. MRI Clinics of North America. Philadelphia: WB Saunders, 1995.

34. Mascalchi M, Bianchi MC, Mangiafico S, et al. MRI and MR angiography of vertebral artery dissection. *Neuroradiology* 1997;39:329–340.

35. Shellock FG, Kanal E. Yasargil aneurysm clips: evaluation of interactions with a 1.5-T MR system. *Radiology* 1998;207:587–591.

36. Gonner F, Heid O, Remonda L, et al. MR angiography with ultrashort echo time in cerebral aneurysms treated with Guglielmi detachable coils. *AJNR* 1998;19:1324–1328.

37. Leclerc X, Gauvrit JY, Nicol L, Pruvo JP. Contrast-enhanced MR angiography of the craniocervical vessels: A review. *Neuroradiology* 1999;41:867–874.

38. Lev MH, Farkas J, Rodriguez VR, et al. CT angiography in the rapid triage of patients with hyperacute stroke to intraarterial thrombolysis: Accuracy in the detection of large vessel thrombus. *J. Comput. Assist. Tomogr.* 2001;25:520–528.

39. Ezzeddine MA, Lev MH, McDonald CT, et al. CT angiography with whole brain perfused blood volume imaging: Added clinical value in the assessment of acute stroke. *Stroke* 2002;33:959–966.

40. Anderson GB, Steinke DE, Petruk KC, Ashforth R, Findlay JM. Computed tomographic angiography versus digital subtraction angiography for the diagnosis and early treatment of ruptured intracranial aneurysms. *Neurosurgery* 1999;45:1315–1320.

41. Villablanca JP, Jahan R, Hooshi P, et al. Detection and characterization of very small cerebral aneurysms by using 2D and 3D helical CT angiography. *AJNR* 2002;23:1187–1198.

42. Levy EI, Horowitz MB, Koebbe CJ, et al. Transluminal stent-assisted angioplasty of the intracranial vertebrobasilar system for medically refractory, posterior circulation ischemia: early results. *Neurosurgery* 2001;48:1215–1221.

43. The n-BCA Trail Investigators. N-butyl cyanoacrylate embolization of cerebral arteriovenous malformations: results of a prospective, randomized, multi-center trial. *AJNR* 2002;23:748–755.

44. Suarez JI, Zaidat OO, Sunshine JL, Tarr R, Selman WR, Landis DM. Endovascular administration after intravenous infusion of thrombolytic agents for the treatment of patients with acute ischemic strokes. *Neurosurgery* 2002;50:251–259.

8

Cardiac Monitoring in the Neurosciences Critical Care Unit

Dinesh Arab, Jawad F. Kirmani, Andrew R. Xavier, Abutaher M. Yahia, Jose I. Suarez, and Adnan I. Qureshi

INTRODUCTION

The cardiovascular and central nervous systems (CNS) are closely related. Coronary artery disease and ischemic stroke share similar risk factors, including age, gender, hypertension, diabetes, hyperlipidemia, and cigarette smoking *(1,2)*. In addition, structural heart disease, such as atrial fibrillation, decreased left ventricular function, patent foramen ovale, and atrial septal aneurysm, are independent risk factors for stroke *(3–6)*. The cardiovascular system in turn is closely regulated by the nervous system, which helps modulate cardiovascular changes to demand during various physiological and pathologic states *(7,8)* (*see also* Chapter 10). Afferent fibers from the heart and arterial baroreceptors are carried to the nucleus tractus solitarius (NTS) and dorsal vagal nucleus (DVN), located in the brainstem via the glossopharyngeal and vagus nerves. The efferent parasympathetic fibers arise in the DVN, and the efferent sympathetic fibers arise in the intermediolateral column (IML) of the spinal cord. These nuclei are extensively connected to each other and in turn receive input from the hypothalamus and the cerebral cortex *(9–13)*. The CNS acts primarily by modulating the autonomic nervous system by excitatory or inhibitory impulses. The resultant changes in efferent sympathetic and parasympathetic activity allow for rapid changes in heart rate, blood pressure, vasomotor tone, cardiac metabolism and cardiac output *(14,15)*. Therefore lesions affecting the CNS can be caused by a primary cardiac problem or may cause cardiovascular dysfunction in a previously normal heart or may precipitate underlying cardiac disease. Cardiovascular diseases can be grouped under three clinical entities: arrhythmias, myocardial contractile dysfunction, and hemodynamic changes.

PATHOPHYSIOLOGY

Acute intracranial lesions cause an increase in intracranial pressure (ICP), which in turn causes an increased release of catecholamines, both in the systemic circulation and at neuronal synapses *(16,17)* (*see also* Chapter 5). In addition, experimental evidence has shown that stimulation of different areas of the brain; particularly the hypothalamus, amygdala, and insular cortex, are associated with an increase in catecholamine release *(18–21)*. Catecholamine excess is known to cause cardiac damage. Epinephrine infusion causes histological evidence of myocardial damage described as contraction band necrosis, myocytolysis or focal coagulative necrosis *(22,23)*. Histological examinations of myocardial tissue in patients who have had acute intracranial lesions have shown similar changes *(24)*. Catecholamines are thought to cause myocardial dysfunction and arrhythmias by a number of mechanisms, which include relative hypoxia from increased demand caused by hemodynamic changes,

From: *Current Clinical Neurology*
Critical Care Neurology and Neurosurgery
Edited by: J. I. Suarez © Humana Press Inc., Totowa, NJ

Table 1
Cardiovascular Manifestations Associated With Specific Neurologic Conditions

Disease entity	Cardiovascular manifestation
Guillian-Barré syndrome	Myocardial dysfunction, hypertension, hypotension, labile blood pressure, tachycardia, bradycardia, nonspecific T wave abnormality on EKG
Myasthenia gravis	Adverse effect of anticholinesterase drugs that cause sinus bradycardia, various degrees of AV block, paradoxical sinus tachycardia
Acute ischemic stroke	Sinus bradycardia, sinus tachycardia, atrial flutter, atrial fibrillation, premature ventricular complexes, ventricular tachycardia, sudden cardiac death
Subarachnoid and ICH	Deep symmetric T wave inversion, acute left ventricular failure, sinus bradycardia, sinus tachycardia, atrial tachycardias, ventricular tachycardia, hypertension, hypotension, cardiogenic shock
Spinal cord injury	Extreme sinus bradycardia, junctional rhythm, various degrees of AV block, sinus tachycardia, hypotension, labile hypertension

ICH, intracerebral hemorrhage; EKG, electrocradiography; AV, atrioventricular.

coronary vasospasm, and catecholamine oxidation products *(25,26)*. In addition, patients with cerebrovascular disease, may have coexistent coronary artery disease that is aggravated by the increased stress placed on the cardiovascular system *(see also* Chapter 18). Acute spinal cord injury (SCI), especially involving the cervical region, is associated with arrhythmias and hemodynamic instability *(see also* Chapter 23). This is the result of interruption of sympathetic fibers that exit the spinal cord and cause unopposed parasympathetic outflow. The most common arrhythmia seen is bradycardia, although tachyarrhythmias can also occur *(27)*. Arrhythmias occur most commonly during the first 14 d after the injury and are directly proportional to the extent and severity of neurologic damage.

Hypotension can occur because of loss of sympathetic tone, leading to vasodilation and subsequent pooling of blood in the peripheral vasculature and is seen with brainstem and spinal cord lesions *(28)*. Hypertension can occur because of the worsening of preexisting hypertension by increased sympathetic discharge, seizures, or as a protective response (Cushing's response) to preserve cerebral perfusion particularly in patients with brainstem compression *(29,30)*. In addition to the aforementioned changes in the cardiovascular system, certain disease states affect specific areas of the cardiovascular system (Table 1) *(see also* Chapters 18–20, 23, 26, and 27). Also various testing modalities are available to detect cardiovascular manifestations of neurologic illnesses (Table 2).

LABORATORY TESTING

Screening for evidence of myocardial ischemia can be routinely performed in the neurosciences critical care unit (NSU) by use of biochemical markers. The biochemical markers most commonly used in hospitals currently are creatine kinase (CK) and cardiac-specific troponins. Serum CK levels begin to rise within 4–8 h after the onset of myocardial injury and return to baseline within 2 to 3 d, with a peak occurring at approx 24 h *(31)*. Peak CK levels occur earlier in patients who have undergone reperfusion *(32)*. CK levels can, however, be elevated by a number of other causes, which include patients with muscle disease, skeletal muscle trauma, alcohol ingestion, seizures, diabetes mellitus, and pulmonary embolism *(33,34)*. To improve their specificity, CK isoenzymes and their isoforms are now being used. The MB isoenzyme is found in cardiac myocytes, accounting for 20% of the total CK level. The BB isoenzyme is found predominantly in the brain and kidney, whereas the

Table 2
Indications for the Testing Modalities in the Neurosciences Critical Care Unit

Test	Indication
EKG monitoring (1–3 lead)	All patients for continuous cardiac monitoring
EKG (12 lead)	All patients to establish a baseline and subsequently for cardiac events and changes
Spectrum analysis	Experimental-only specialized use
Pulmonary artery catheter	Multisystem disease, hypotension not related to fluid depletion
Transthoracic echocardiography	Pulmonary edema, hypotension not related to fluid depletion
Transesophageal echocardiography	Sources of emboli, looking for cardiac valvular vegetations and valvular dysfunction
	Aortic pathology, including dissection

EKG, electrocardiography.

MM isoenzyme is found predominantly in the skeletal muscle. The Biochemical Markers for Acute Myocardial Ischemia (BAMI) study demonstrated the specificity of CK-MB for the diagnosis of myocardial infarction to be 100%, its sensitivity within 3 h of onset of chest pain to be 30%, increasing to 70% between 6 and 9 h and greater than 97% at 9–12 h *(35)*. The isoforms of the MB isoenzyme have been used, to increase the sensitivity at earlier time intervals, for diagnosing myocardial damage. An absolute value of CK-MB2 isoform greater than 1.0 U/L or a ratio of CK-MB2/CK-MB1 greater than 2.5 has a sensitivity of 46% for diagnosing myocardial injury at 4 h and 91% at 6 h *(36)*.

The troponin complex that regulates the calcium mediated contractile properties of skeletal and cardiac muscle consists of three subunits. Troponin I (TnI), binds to actin and inhibits the actin-myosin interactions, troponin T (TnT), binds to tropomyosin and troponin C binds to calcium. Although TnI and TnT are found in both skeletal and cardiac muscle fibers, they have a different amino acid sequence, which permits the detection of cardiac muscle damage *(37)*. TnI and TnT begin to increase 3 h after the onset of chest pain in myocardial infarction and remain elevated for 7–14 d. Patients with reperfusion have a more rapid release of troponins *(38)*. Patients with elevated serum troponin have an increased risk for adverse clinical outcomes, which are independent of other risk factors, such as age, electrocardiographic (EKG) abnormalities, and elevated CK-MB levels *(39)*.

In addition to monitoring for evidence of myocardial damage, electrolytes should be routinely checked, and aggressively corrected as imbalances may precipitate cardiac arrhythmias. Moreover, diabetes insipidus is a common occurrence in patients with acute intracranial neurological insult, necessitating aggressive fluid resuscitation.

ELECTROCARDIOGRAPHY

The interpretation of the electrocardiogram (EKG) is challenging in patients with acute neurological injury, as dramatic changes in the EKG can occur in the absence of underlying cardiac abnormalities. EKG abnormalities simulating acute myocardial infarction have been reported to occur in 0.8–10.2% patients with subarachnoid (SAH) and intracerebral (ICH) hemorrhage *(40)*. The abnormalities seen on the EKG include ST segment elevation, depression, T wave inversion, pathologic Q waves, and prolongation of the QT interval. Although these changes have been shown to occur with increased frequency with SAH, they may also occur with ICH, acute stroke, hydrocephalus, and meningitis *(41,42)*. The presence of EKG abnormalities alone should not be used as a marker for myocardial ischemia or infarction. A comprehensive history, physical examination, and adjunctive tests such as cardiac enzymes and echocardiography should be used to evaluate for the presence of myocardial damage.

There is controversy over whether these electrocardiographic changes are indicators of underlying cardiac damage with initial studies showing a positive correlation *(43)*. However subsequent studies have shown a poor correlation between EKG and underlying histologic changes *(44)*. The two EKG manifestations that the physician should be aware of are the presence of a J wave (also called Osborn wave) and the QTc interval. The J wave is a deflection, which appears as a late delta wave at the end of the QRS complex. The J wave occurs with traumatic brain injury (TBI), SAH, hypothermia, and electrolyte disturbances. The J wave is caused by a difference in voltage gradient between the epicardium and endocardium. The presence of a J wave and prolonged QTc interval are predictors of malignant arrhythmias *(45–47)*.

In addition, the EKG provides clues to the etiology of the neurological event. Atrial fibrillation indicates a cardiac source of emboli. The presence of left ventricular hypertrophy indicates the presence of hypertension with end organ effects. Frequent premature ventricular complexes or nonsustained ventricular tachycardia may indicate the propensity for more malignant arrhythmias, and may be a cause of syncope in cases of TBI.

POWER SPECTRUM ANALYSIS

Power spectrum analysis (PSA), also referred to as frequency domain analysis has been used to asses heat rate variability, and has been shown to be a valuable tool in evaluating the prognosis of critically ill patients, in the NSU. PSA can be performed at high frequency on high-resolution signals, and heart rate variability can be assessed as a measure of autonomic activity *(47,48)*. Heart rate variability in the low frequency range results from both sympathetic and parasympathetic input, with a predominance of sympathetic input during stressful situations. The high frequency range represents parasympathetic input. Haji-Michael and associates *(49)* showed that a reduction of the total power variability of electrocardiograph R-R intervals, and a lowered low-frequency (LF)/high-frequency (HF) ratio of the electrocardiograph R-R interval predicts a poor outcome after neurosurgical illness. Patients with a raised normalized LF power in R-R interval variability had a greater likelihood of good quality recovery.

TRANSTHORACIC ECHOCARDIOGRAPHY

Transthoracic echocardiography (TTE) is indicated when a cardiac source of embolism is suspected in ischemic stroke. These patients should undergo TTE initially and transesophageal echo (TEE) if the image quality is unsatisfactory. TTE is useful for evaluating valvular heart disease, left ventricular function (LVF) and other structural abnormalities of the heart like cardiac tumors, which may be a cause for embolic stroke. TTE is less accurate in evaluating the left atrial appendage, the aortic arch and the interatrial septum *(50)*.

The frequency by which myocardial dysfunction occurs in previously normal hearts after an acute intracranial insult ranges from 10 to 30% *(51)*. Segmental wall motion abnormalities with relative sparing of the apex have been shown to occur in ICH and SAH. This occurs because of a relative lack of adrenergic innervation at the apex *(52)*. The optimum time for echocardiography remains uncertain. Animal studies have shown dysfunction to occur within the first 6 h *(53)*. A practical approach would be to perform echocardiography after the first 24 h to evaluate LVF or earlier if the patient develops symptoms or signs of congestive heart failure.

TRANSESOPHAGEAL ECHOCARDIOGRAPHY

Transesophageal echocardiography (TEE) offers the advantage of improved image quality when compared to the TTE images, particularly of the posterior structures such as the pulmonary veins, left atrium and the mitral valve. Also the visualization of the aorta and interatrial septum is superior with TEE. Image quality is improved both because of the decreased distance between the transducer and the structure of interest and because of the absence of intervening structures such as lungs and bones *(50)*.

With the advent of omni plane TEE probe, a higher incidence of cardiac source of embolism (CSE) has been identified in patients with embolic stroke *(54,55)*. The prevalence of CSE varies among studies. In pre-TEE era, its prevalence was much lower than recent studies. TEE is considered superior to TTE in detecting atrial septal aneurysm, patent foramen ovale (Fig. 1), left atrial spontaneous echo contrast and intracavitary thrombus (Fig. 2) *(55–57)*. Recently, using TEE, thoracic aortic atheroma (TAA) has been identified in a large number of patients with ischemic stroke and proven to be a potential source of embolus (Fig. 3) *(57–60)*. TAA is associated with poor prognosis *(61)*. Early identification and treatment of potential source of emboli reduces the risk of subsequent ischemic strokes. Special attention is given to evaluation of each segment of aortic arch for atheromas, especially for detection of mobile and ulcerated segments both in anterior and the posterior walls and for detection of possible aortic dissection.

TEE also demonstrates pathology of cardiac valves, a potential CSE, with better accuracy and reliability than TTE *(49)*. Segmental and global ventricular function abnormalities that may compromise cardiac output associated with intracranial pathology including SAH are readily identified with TEE *(51)*. A practical approach would be to perform TEE in all patients suspected of having CSE. Also, unstable patients suspected of having an aortic dissection associated with multiple traumas or secondary to other causes may undergo TEE in the NSU setting for rapid detection.

RIGHT HEART CATHETERIZATION

The bedside assessment of cardiac function and ventricular preload is difficult in the NSU setting *(62)*. According to the Frank-Starling principle, the force of cardiac contraction is directly proportional to the muscle fiber length at the end of diastole *(63)*. The presystolic fiber stretch in turn is directly proportional to the left ventricular end diastolic volume (LVEDV), which is a measure of preload. The preload is a major determinant of cardiac output.

The pulmonary artery catheter (PAC) is used to asses the preload and the cardiac output. In addition various other parameters, such as systemic vascular resistance, pulmonary vascular resistance and left ventricular stroke work, can be calculated (*see* Appendix). Pulmonary capillary wedge pressure should be measured at the end of expiration. The PAC is an accurate measure of preload only if there is a linear and predictable relationship between the left ventricular end diastolic pressure (LVEDP) and LVEDV and an accurate tracing of the pulmonary artery occlusion pressure (PAOP) is obtained. In addition problems arising from incorrect interpretation, interobserver variability, incorrect calibration and balancing the transducer and overdamping affect the accuracy of the PAOP *(64,65)*. To further complicate the issue, patients on positive pressure ventilation and positive end-expiratory pressure (PEEP), have an erroneously high PAOP. This is because of the fact that the distending pressure, which results in left ventricular diastolic filling, is the difference between simultaneous intracavitary pressure and juxtacardiac pressure. PEEP increases the juxtacardiac pressure that in turn causes the intracavitary pressure to increase, to achieve a similar presystolic volume. The formulas that subtract a portion of PEEP from the PAOP are inaccurate, from the difficulty in estimating the amount of PEEP that is transmitted to the heart *(66)*.

Over the past decade, there has been an extensive debate on the utility of the PAC. Connors et al. reported an observational study on the use of PAC in the critical care setting, which showed an increased mortality and utilization of resources, when compared to case-matched control patients who did not undergo PAC placement *(67)*. The use of PAC in the NSU has not been specifically evaluated. Despite these limitations the PAC is a valuable tool in the NSU, when used by appropriate personnel, who are trained in its use and interpretation of derived data.

Cardiac output can be calculated by either the thermodilution, or Fick's method. The thermodilution method is more commonly used in the NSU. The thermistor port of a PAC has a temperature sensitive wire at the catheter tip. Normal saline or dextrose is injected through the proximal port of the PAC. The cardiac output is determined by the magnitude of blood temperature change, from the

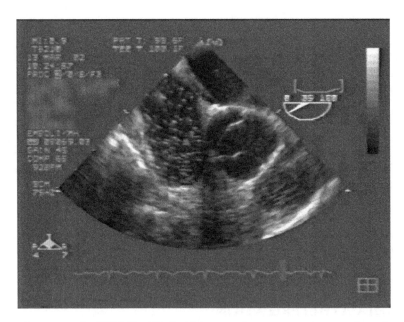

Fig. 1. Patent foramen ovale (PFO) identified with improved accuracy on transesophageal echocardiogram is a potential source of cardiac embolus. In the figure when the agitated saline is injected the bubbles are seen to cross from the right atrium to the left atrium confirming a PFO with right-to-left shunt.

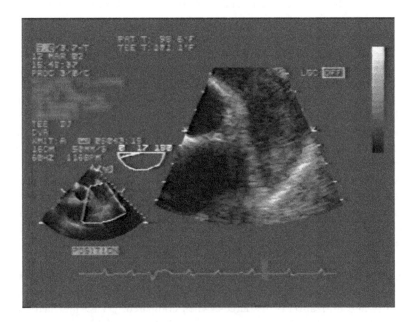

Fig. 2. Left atrial thrombus. In this patient, transesophgeal echocardiogram demonstrates a left atrial appendage thrombus as the only identifiable source of an embolic cerebral event. The left atrial appendage has been magnified to show the thrombus.

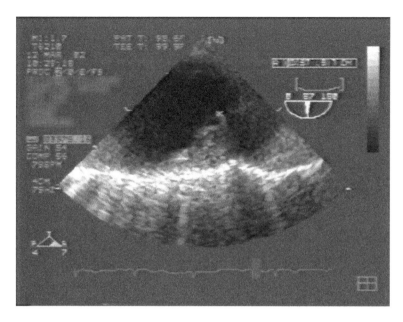

Fig. 3. Complex aortic arch plaque is seen here along the posterio-inferior wall of the aorta measuring well over 0.9 cm in diameter with a mobile segment on top. The transesophageal echocardiogram can reliably demonstrate aortic pathology, including dissections.

right atrium to the pulmonary artery over time, since in the absence of an intracardiac shunt, flow in the pulmonary circulation is equal to flow in the systemic circulation *(68)*. The thermodilution method is inaccurate in the presence of severe tricuspid regurgitation. The thermodilution method also tends to overestimate cardiac output in patients with low flow states, resulting from warming of blood by the walls of the cardiac chambers. In these cases the Fick's method is used, wherein the cardiac output is equal to oxygen consumption divided by the arteriovenous oxygen difference.

The PAC can be useful in distinguishing neurogenic pulmonary edema from pulmonary edema secondary to myocardial dysfunction, particularly in the patient with pre-existing myocardial dysfunction. Patients with cardiogenic pulmonary edema typically have an elevated wedge pressure, a decreased cardiac index and increased systemic vascular resistance. The patient with neurogenic pulmonary edema has a normal cardiac index and a normal to low wedge pressure. The PAC is also useful as a guide for fluid replacement and the use of hyperosmolar therapy for reducing elevated ICP.

The advent of the volumetric PAC, which consists of a rapid response thermistor and an EKG electrode measures the temperature drop between two successive beats allowing for calculation of the right ventricular ejection fraction (RVEF). The right ventricular end-systolic and end-diastolic volumes can then be calculated from the stroke volume. The RVEF obtained by thermodilution has been validated by comparing it to echocardiography and radionuclide imaging *(69,70)*. The right ventricular end diastolic volume index (RVEDI), has been shown to be a good predictor of recruitable cardiac output (i.e., the change of cardiac output in response to a fluid challenge). Additionally, the volumetric PAC is useful in determining the preload in patients who are being ventilated with PEEP *(71)*.

ESOPHAGEAL DOPPLER

The esophageal Doppler is a noninvasive test for monitoring cardiac function in the intensive care unit. It is particularly useful in the patient with bleeding diathesis in whom invasive procedures are relatively contraindicated. The principle for calculating cardiac output is similar to the doppler principle used in two-dimensional echocardiography. Cardiac output is derived by multiplying the measured velocity by the ejection time and by the cross-sectional area of the aorta. A correction factor is incorporated to transform the blood flow in the descending aorta, into a global cardiac output. Studies have shown the cardiac output correlates well when compared to thermodilution *(72)*. Unlike TEE, the probe can be left in the esophagus to provide continuous monitoring of cardiac output.

HYPOTENSION AND COMMON CARDIAC ARRHYTHMIAS

Hypotension

NSU patients frequently experience hypotension and shock as a result of either a primary neurogenic event or a systemic dysfunction. As mentioned previously, and also in Chapter 10, neurally mediated hypotension can result from injuries to sympathetic pathways leading to loss of vascular tone or cardiac muscle dysfunction from an adrenergic surge (stunt myocardium). However, other non-neurologic possibilities need to be considered because these patients, just as in other intensive care units, are also prone to developing systemic conditions such as dehydration, acute blood loss, sepsis, massive pulmonary embolism, or pericardial tamponade.

Although a detailed discussion of shock is beyond the scope of this chapter, it is important to remember that it is a life-threatening emergency. Shock is characterized by tachycardia (provided that sympathetic fibers are intact), tachypnea, oliguria, encephalopathy, and hypotension (systolic blood pressure < 90 mmHg or mean arterial pressure < 65 mmHg) *(73)*. Aggressive management and investigation to identify the underlying etiology should be undertaken. For instance, elevated white blood cell count and fever suggest infection, whereas a drop in hematocrit suggests acute blood loss. These patients require invasive and continuous monitoring of hemodynamic parameters including arterial pressure catheter, central venous catheter monitor, PAC, continuous EKG and echocardiography. Several imaging studies are useful at identifying sources of abnormalities such as pneumonia on a chest roentgenogram, retroperitoneal hematoma on body and pelvis CT scanning, or poor LVF on a TTE. Prompt and generous fluid resuscitation should be started immediately after the diagnosis is entertained. Concomitantly vasopressors are usually administered. A list of the most common vasopressive agents used in the NSU is presented in Table 3 *(73–78)*.

Cardiac Arrhythmias

Tachyarrhythmias and bradyarrhythmias are frequent conditions that neurointensivists are faced with and may be related to primary neurological disease in patients with no cardiac history or exacerbation of underlying cardiac dysfunction. One of the most important tests that will help determine the nature of the abnormal heart rhythm is a 12-lead EKG and should be obtained as soon as alterations are suspected. Tachyarrhythmias are usually divided into narrow complex (QRS < 0.12 s) and wide complex (QRS ≥ 0.12 s) tachycardias *(79)*. The latter include ventricular (VT) and supraventricular (SVT) tachycardias. VT can be monomorphic (each beat looks similar) or polymorphous (each beat varies). SVT, with or without conducted or retrograde P waves, can have aberrant or antegrade conduction via an accessory pathway. Narrow-complex tachycardias can be irregularly irregular (i.e., atrial fibrillation), irregular (i.e., multifocal atrial tachycardia), or regular (i.e., sinus tachycardia, atrial flutter, paroxysmal SVT, ectopic atrial, or junctional ectopic tachycardia). In those patients with VT, ventricular fibrillation, or atrial fibrillation with very rapid response associated with hemodynamic instability immediate direct-current cardioversion should be carried out. However, in those with hemodynamic stability medical management with various medications should be instituted (Table 4) *(79–85)*.

Bradyarrhythmias in NSU patients can result from the use of medication (e.g., digoxin, betablockers, calcium-channel blockers), acute myocardial infarction, or high vagal tone. The latter is a frequent finding in those patients with autonomic dysfunction *(see also* Chapter 10). Bradyarrhythmias are classified as sinus node dysfunction (SND) and atrioventricular nodal His-block (AV block) *(86)*. SND is characterized by profound sinus bradycardia, sinus arrest (pauses in sinus rhythm), sinoatrial block, or a combination of these. AV block can be of three major types: First-degree AV block (defined

Table 3
Inotropes and Vasopressors Commonly Used in the Neurosciences Critical Care Unit

Agent	Mechanism of action	Dose	Indication	Adverse effects
Norepinephrine	Inotrope (β1-agonist) Vasoconstrictor (α1-agonist)	2–20 μg/min (or 0.3–3 μg/kg/min)	Refractory hypotension in septic shock or for HHH therapy in SAH	Reduced cardiac forward flow, limb and gut ischemia
Phenylephrine	Vasoconstrictor (α1-agonist)	20–200 μg/min	Septic shock, HHH therapy in SAH, induced hypertension in stroke	Bradycardia, reduced cardiac forward flow
Dopamine	Vasodilator at "low dose": DA$_2$-agonist Inotrope at "medium dose": β1-agonist Vasoconstrictor at "high dose": α1-agonist	1–4 μg/kg/min 5–10 μg/kg/min 11–20 μg/kg/min	Maintenance of renal perfusion Low CO states All shock	Natriuresis Tachyarrhythmais Tachycardia and reduced forward cardiac flow, limb necrosis
Dobutamine	Inotrope α-agonist (β1-agonist) Vasodilator (β2-agonist)	1–20 μg/kg/min	Cardiogenic and septic shock, CHF, HHH therapy in SAH	Tachycardia, hypotension
Epinephrine	Inotrope (α-agonist, β1-agonist predominantly) Vasodilator (β2-agonist)	1–8 μg/min	Anaphylactic shock, refractory septic shock, HHH therapy in SAH	Impaired myocardial perfusion in CAD, ischemic renal failure
Amrinone	Inotrope: phosphodiesterase inhibition with increased cyclic AMP	0.75 mg/kg bolus (5 min) and 5–15 μ/kg/min	Cardiogenic shock, CHF	Hypotension, thrombocytopenia

SAH, subarachnoid hemorrhage; HHH, hyperdynamic, hypervolemic, hypertensive therapy; DA, dopamine; CO, cardiac output; CHF, congestive heart failure; CAD, coronary artery disease. *See* refs. 73–78.

145

Table 4
Medications Commonly Used for Management of Tachyarrhythmias

Drug	Dose	Indications	Side effects
Digoxin	0.5 mg IV followed by 0.25 mg q 2–6 h (total 0.75–1.5 mg)	Atrial fibrillation and atrial flutter (rate control). Avoid in WPW	Nausea, emesis, disturbed vision, atrial or ventricular arrhythmias
Diltiazem	0.25 mg/kg IV over 2–3 min, followed by 5–15 mg/h infusion	Atrial fibrillation and atrial flutter (rate control)	Hypotension, sinus node depression, AV block
Esmolol	0.5 mg/kg IV load followed by 50–300 μg/kg/min	Paroxysmal SVT	Bronchospasm, LVF depression, suppression of AV nodal function
Metoprolol	5 mg IV over 2 min, then repeat q 5 min (total 15 mg)	Atrial fibrillation and atrial flutter (rate control)	Suppression of AV nodal function, hypotension
Procainamide	10 mg/kg IV load (<25 mg/min) followed by 1–6 mg/min infusion	Atrial fibrillation with rapid rate due to WPW monomorphic VT	QT prolongation, transiently facilitates AV conduction, negative inotrope
Verapamil	0.075 mg/kg IV over 2 min, then 0.15 mg/kg IV in 15 min (if needed), then 5 μg/kg/min infusion	Atrial fibrillation and atrial flutter (rate control). Avoid in WPW	Hypotension, sinu node depression, AV block
Magnesium/electrolyte balance	2 g MSO₄ IV over 15 min, then 6 g infusion over 6 h (both diluted in normal saline)	Polymorphous VT	Muscle weakness, sedation
Adenosine	6 mg IV rapid injection (peripheral veins and flush with saline). Then 12 mg IV after 2 min. Then 12 mg IV can be repeated	Paroxysmal SVT	Facial flushing, sinus bradycardia, AV block, dyspnea, nausea, headache, anginal-type pain
Lidocaine	1–1.5 mg/kg IV bolus, followed by 2–4 mg/min infusion	Monomorphic VT	Seizures, respiratory arrest
Amiodarone	5 mg/kg IV 1.2 g/d for 10 d PO, then 200–400 mg/d	Monomorphic VT	Thyroid dysfunction, pulmonary fibrosis, corneal deposits, hepatic fibrosis

IV, intravenous; WPW, Wolff-Parkinson-White syndrome; AV, atrioventricular; SVT, supraventriuclar tachycardia; LVF, left ventricular function; VT, ventricular tachycardia.

See refs. 79–85.

146

as PR interval > 0.20 s on EKG); second-degree AV block (type I or Wenkebach is present when the conduction of atrial impulses to the ventricles is progressively delayed; type II is characterized by atrial impulses that fail to be transmitted without an increase in conduction delay and can be 2 : 1, 4 : 3, and so on); and high-degree AV block (where the AV conduction ratio is 3 : 1 or greater). Patients with SND may or may not respond to atropine. When bradyarrhythmias lead to cerebral hypoperfusion or hemodynamic instability temporary cardiac pacing (transcutaneous or transvenous) should be instituted. The transvenous route is preferred. Common indications for permanent cardiac pacemaker placement include the following *(87)*: SND with symptoms of cerebral hypoperfusion; high-grade AV block with symptoms or with asystolic pauses more than 3 s; second-degree AV block (type I or II) with symptoms; vasovagal syndromes with recurrent syncope; and carotid sinus hypersensitivity with symptoms or with asystolic pauses more than 3 s.

CONCLUSION

Cardiac disturbances are common in the NSU. Aggressive monitoring for early detection and management usually requires a combination of clinical evaluation as well as the use of noninvasive and invasive investigations. Symptomatic management of cardiac abnormalities along with treatment of underlying CNS diseases is required.

REFERENCES

1. Sacco, RL. Newer risk factors for stroke. *Neurology* 2001;57(Suppl 2):S31–S34.
2. Sacco RL, Benson RT, Kargman DE, et al. High-density lioprotein cholesterol and ischemic stroke in the elderly: the Northern manhattan Stroke Study. *JAMA* 2001;285:2729–2735.
3. Gorelick PB, Sacco RL, Smith D, et al. Prevention of a first stroke- A review of guidelines and a multidisciplinary consensus statement from the National Stroke Association. *JAMA* 1999;281:1112–1120.
4. Pullicino PM, Halperin JL, Thompson JL. Stroke in patients with heart failure and reduced left ventricular ejection fraction. *Neurology* 2000;54:288–294.
5. Atrial Fibrillation Investigators. Risk factors for stroke and efficacy of antithrombotic therapy in atrial fibrillation. *Arch. Intern. Med.* 1994;154:1449–1457.
6. Wolf PA, Abbott RD, Kannel WB. Atrial fibrillation, a major contributor to stroke in the elderly: the Framingham study. *Arch. Intern. Med.* 1987;147:1561–1564.
7. Kannel WB, Wolf PA, Verter J. Manifestations of coronary disease predisposing to stroke: the Framingham study. *JAMA* 1983;250:2942–2946.
8. Smith OA, Galosy RA, Weiss SM. *Circulation, Neurobiology and Behavior.* New York: Elsevier, 1982.
9. Natelson BH. Neurocardiology: an interdisciplinary area for the 80s. *Arch. Neurol.* 1985;42:178–184.
10. Dampney RAL. Functional organization of central cardiovascular pathways. *Clin. Exp. Pharmacol. Physiol.* 1981;8:241–259.
11. Loewy. Descending pathways to the sympathetic preganglionic neurons. *Prog. Brain Res.* 1982;57:267–277.
12. Loewy AD, Burton H. Nuclei of the solitary tract: efferent projections to the lower brainstem. and the spinal cord of the cat. *J. Comp. Neurol.* 1978;181:421–449.
13. Loewy AD, McKellar S, Saper CB. Direct projections from the A5 catecholamine cell group to the intermediolateral cell column. *Brain Res.* 1979;174:309–314.
14. Korner PI. Integrative neural cardiovascular control. *Physiol. Rev.* 1971;51:312–367.
15. Talman WT. Cardiovascular regulation and lesions of the central nervous system. *Ann. Neurol.* 1985;18:1–12.
16. Randall WC, Wechsler JS, Pace JB, Szentivanyi M : Alteration in myocardial contractility during stimulation of cardiac nerves. *Am. J. Physiol.* 1968;214:1205–1212.
17. Shivalkar B, Van Loon J, Wieland W, et al. Variable effects of explosive or gradual increase of intracranial pressure on myocardial structure and function. *Circulation* 1993;87:230–239.
18. Powner DJ, Hendrich A, Nyhuis A, Strate R. Changes in serum catecholamine levels in patients who are brain dead. *J. Heart Lung Transplant.* 1992;11:1046–1053.
19. Pitts RF, Bronk DW. Excitability cycle of the hypothalamus-sympathetic neurone system. *Am. J. Physiol.* 1941;135:504–522.
20. Reis DJ, Oliphant MC. Bradycardia and tachycardia following electrical stimulation of the amygdaloid region in the monkey. *J. Neurophysiol.* 1964;27:893–912.
21. Anand DK, Dua S. Circulatory and respiratory changes induced by electrical stimulation of the limbic system (visceral brain). *J. Neurophysiol.* 1956;19:393–400.

22. Tokgozoglu SL, Batur MF, Topcuoglu MA, et al. Effects of stroke localization on cardiac autonomic balance and sudden death. *Stroke* 1999;30:1307–1311.
23. Rona G. Catecholamine cardiotoxicity. *J. Mol. Cell Cardiol.* 1985;17:291–306.
24. Todd GL, Baroldi G, Pieper GM, et al. Experimental catecholamine-induced myocardial necrosis: Morphology, quantification and regional distribution of acute contraction band necrosis. *J. Mol. Cell. Cardiol.* 1985;17:317–338.
25. Benedict CR, Loach AB. Clinical significance of plasma adrenaline and noradrenaline concentrations in patients with subarachnoid hemorrhage. *J. Neurol. Neurosurg. Psychiatry* 1978;41:113–117.
26. Greenhoot JH, Reichenbach DD. Cardiac injury and subarachnoid hemorrhage: A clinical, pathological and physiological correlation. *J. Neurosurg.* 1969;30:521–531.
27. Samuels MA. Neurogenic heart disease: A unifying hypothesis. *Am. J. Cardiol.* 1987;60:15J–19J.
28. Lehmann KG, Lane JG, Piepmeier JM, et al. Cardiovascular abnormalities accompanying acute spinal cord injury in humans: incidence time course and severity. *J. Am. Coll. Cardiol.* 1987;10:46–52.
29. Ball PA. Critical care of spinal cord injury. *Spine* 2001;26:S27–S30.
30. Qureshi AI, Tuhrim S, Broderick JP, Batjer HH, Hondo H, Hanley DF. Spontaneous intracerebral hemorrhage. *N. Engl. J. Med.* 2001;344:1450–1460.
31. Qureshi AI. Geocadin RG. Suarez JI. Ulatowski JA. Long-term outcome after medical reversal of transtentorial herniation in patients with supratentorial mass lesions. *Crit. Care Med.* 2000;28:1556–1564.
32. Adams J, Abendschein D, Jaffe A. Biochemical markers of myocardial injury. Is MB creatine kinase the choice for the 1990s? *Circulation* 1993;88:750–763.
33. Lee TH, Goldman L. Serum enzyme assays in the diagnosis of myocardial infarction. *Ann. Intern. Med.* 1986;105:221–225.
34. Mair J, Dienstl J, Puschendorf B. Cardiac troponin T in the diagnosis of myocardial injury. *Crit. Rev. Clin. Lab. Sci.* 1992;29:31–57.
35. Wu AH, Apple FS, Gibler WB, et al. National Academy of Clinical Biochemistry Standards of Laboratory Practice: Recommendation for the use of cardiac markers in coronary artery disease. *Clin. Chem.* 1999;45:1104–1121.
36. Brogan GX Jr, Hollander JE, McCuskey CF, et al. Evaluation of a new assay for cardiac troponin I vs creatine kinase-MB for the diagnosis of acute myocardial infarction. Biochemical Markers for Acute Myocardial Ischemia (BAMI) Study Group. *Acad. Emerg. Med.* 1997;4:6–12.
37. Zimmerman J, Fromm R, Meyer D, et al. Diagnostic marker cooperative study for the diagnosis of myocardial infarction. *Circulation* 1999;1671–1677.
38. Hamm CW. New serum markers for acute myocardial infarction. *N. Engl. J. Med.* 1994;331:607–608.
39. Tanasijevic MJ, Cannon CP, Antman EM, et al. Myoglobin, creatine kinase-MB and cardiac troponin –I 60-minute ratios predict infarct related artery patency after thrombolysis for acute myocardial infarction: results from the Thrombolysis in Myocardial Infarction study (TIMI) 10B. *J. Am. Coll. Cardiol.* 1999;34:739–747.
40. Heeschen C, Hamm CW, Goldmann B, et al. Troponin concentrations for stratification of patients with acute coronary syndromes in relation to therapeutic efficacy of tirofiban. PRISM Study Investigators. *Lancet* 1999;354:1757–1762.
41. Kreus KE, Kemila SJ, Takala JK. Electrocardiographic changes in cerebrovascular accidents. *Acta. Med. Scand.* 1969;185:327–334.
42. Davis TP, Alexander J, Lesch M. Electrocardiographic changes associated with acute cerebrovascular disease: A clinical review. *Prog. Cardiovasc. Dis.* 1993;36:245–260.
43. Chua HC, Sen S, Cosgriff RF, Gerstenblith G, Beauchamp NJ Jr, Oppenheimer SM. Neurogenic ST depression in stroke. *Clin. Neurol. Neurosurg.* 1999;101:44–48.
44. Kono T, Morita H, Kuroiwa T, et al. Left ventricular wall motion abnormalities in patients with subarachnoid hemorrhage: Neurogenic stunned myocardium. *J. Am. Coll. Cardiol.* 1994;24:636–640.
45. Dujardin KS, McCully RB, Wijdicks EFM, et al. Myocardial dysfunction associated with brain death: Clinical, echocardiographic and pathologic features. *J. Heart Lung Transplant.* 2001;20:350–357.
46. Heckmann J, Lang CJ, Neundorfer B, et al. Should stroke caregivers recognize the J wave (Osborn Wave). *Stroke* 2001;32:1692–1694.
47. Daisuke Y, Testuya H, Kenichiro T, et al. An association between QTc prolongation and left ventricular hypokinesis during sequential episodes of subarachnoid hemorrhage. *Anesth. Analg.* 1999;89:962–966.
48. Winchell RJ, Hoyt DB. Analysis of heart rate variability: A noninvasive predictor of death and poor outcome in patients with severe head injury. *J. Trauma* 1997;43:927–933.
49. Haji-Michael PG, Vincent JL, Degaute JP, van de Borne P. Power spectral analysis of cardiovascular variability in critically ill neurosurgical patients. *Crit. Care Med.* 2000;28:2578–2583.
50. Channon KM, Banning AP. Echocardiography in stroke and thromboembolism: transoesophageal imaging for all? *QJM* 1999;92:619–621.
51. Gilbert EM, Kreuger SK, Murray JL, et al. Echocardiographic evaluation of potential cardiac transplant donors. *J. Thorac. Cardiovasc. Surg.* 1988;95:1003–1007.
52. Dae MW, O'Connell JW, Botvinick EH, et al. Scintigraphic assessment of regional cardiac adrenergic innervation. *Circulation* 1989;79:634–644.

53. Elrifai AM, Bailes JE, Shih SR, et al. Characterization of cardiac effects of acute subarachnoid hemorrhage in dogs. *Stroke* 1996;27:737–741.

54. Pearson AC. Transthoracic echocardiography versus transesophageal echocardiography in detecting cardiac sources of embolism. *Echocardiography* 1993;10:397–403.

55. Albers GW, Comess KA, DeRook FA, et al. Transesophageal echocardiographic findings in stroke subtypes. *Stroke* 1994;25:23–28.

56. Archer SL, James KE, Kvernen LR, Cohen IS, Ezekowitz MD, Gornick CC. Role of transesophageal echocardiography in the detection of left atrial thrombus in patients with chronic nonrheumatic atrial fibrillation. *Am. Heart J.* 1995;130:287–295.

57. Mahagney A, Sharif D, Weller B, Abineder E, Sharf B. [Diagnosis of cerebral embolism by transesophageal echocardiography]. *Harefuah* 1998;134:256–259, 336.

58. Tullio MR, Sacco RL, Savoia MT, Sciacca RR, Homma S. Aortic atheroma morphology and the risk of ischemic stroke in a multiethnic population. *Am. Heart J.* 2000;139(2 Pt 1):329–336.

59. Sen S, Wu K, McNamara R, Lima J, Piantadosi S, Oppenheimer SM. Distribution, severity and risk factors for aortic atherosclerosis in cerebral ischemia. *Cerebrovasc. Dis.* 2000;10:102–109.

60. Rundek T, Di Tullio MR, Sciacca RR, et al. Association between large aortic arch atheromas and high-intensity transient signals in elderly stroke patients. *Stroke* 1999;30:2683–2686.

61. Ferrari E,Vidal R, Chevallier T, Baudouy M. Atherosclerosis of the thoracic aorta and aortic debris as a marker of poor prognosis: benefit of oral anticoagulants. *J. Am. Coll. Cardiol.* 1999;33:1317–1322.

62. Connors AF, MCCaffree DR, Gray BA. Evaluation of right-heart catheterization in the critically ill patient without acute myocardial infarction. *N. Engl. J. Med.* 1983;308:263–267.

63. Starling EH. The Linacre Lecture on the Law of the Heart. London, UK: Longmans, Green, 1918.

64. Marik PE, Varon J, Heard SO. Interpretation of the pulmonary artery occlusion (wedge) pressure: physicians' knowledge versus the experts' knowledge. *Crit. Care Med.* 1998;26:1761–1763.

65. Morris AH, Chapman RH, Gardner RM. Frequency of technical problems encountered in the measurement of pulmonary artery wedge pressure. *Crit. Care Med.* 1984;12:164–170 .

66. Pinsky M, Vincent JL, De Smet JM. Estimating left ventricular filling pressure during positive end-expiratory pressure in humans. *Am. Rev. Respir. Dis.* 1991;143:25–31.

67. Connors AF, Speroff T, Dawson NV, et al. The effectiveness of right heart catheterization in the initial care of critically ill patients. *JAMA* 1996;276:889–897.

68. Weisel RD, Berger RL, Hechtman HB. Measurement of cardiac output by thermodilution. *N. Engl. J. Med.* 1975;292:682–85.

69. Jardin F, Brun-Ney D, Hardy A, et al. Combined thermodilution and two-dimensional echocardiographic evaluation of right ventricular function during respiratory support with PEEP. *Chest* 1991;99:162–168.

70. Dhainaut JF, Brunet F, Monsallier JF, et al. Bedside evaluation of right ventricular performance using a rapid computerized thermodilution method. *Crit. Care Med.* 1987;15:148–152.

71. Cheatham ML, Nelson LD, Chang MC, et al. Right ventricular end-diastolic volume index as a predictor of preload status in patients on positive end-expiratory pressure. *Crit. Care Med.* 1998;26:1801–1806.

72. Davies JN, Allen DR, Chant AD. Non-invasive Doppler-derived cardiac output: a validation study comparing this technique with thermodilution and Fick methods. *Eur. J. Vasc. Surg.* 1991;5:497–500.

73. Kumar A, Parrillo JE. Shock: classification, pathophysiology, and approach to management. In: Parrillo JE, Dellinger RP, eds. *Critical Care Medicine: Principles of Diagnosis and Management in the Adult*, 2nd ed. St Louis: Mosby, 2001, pp. 371–420.

74. Zaloga GP, Prielipp RC, Butterworth JF, Royster RL. Pharmacologic cardiovascular support. *Crit. Care Clin.* 1993;9:335–362.

75. Trujillo MH, Arai K, Bellorin-Font E. Practical guide for durg administration by intravenous infusion in intensive care units. *Crit. Care Med.* 1994;22:1049–1063.

76. Levy JH, Bailey JM. Amrinone: its effects on vascular resistance and capacitance in human subjects. *Chest* 1994;105:62–64.

77. Hollingsworth HM, Giansiracusa DF, Upchurch KS. Anaphylaxis. *J. Intensive Care Med.* 1991;6:55-70.

78. Desairs P, Pinaud M, Bugnon D, Tasseau F. Norepinephrine therapy has no deleterious renal effects in human septic shock. *Crit. Care Med.* 1989;17:426–429.

79. Scheinman MM. Recognition and management of patients with tachyarrhythmias. In: Goldman L, Braunwald E, eds. *Primary Cardiology*. Philadelphia: WB Saunders, 1998, pp. 330–352.

80. Collier WW, Holt SE, Wellford LA. Narrow complex tachycardias. *Emerg. Med. Clin. North Am.* 1995;13:925–954.

81. Dellbridge TR, Yealy DM. Wide complex tachycardia. *Emerg. Med. Clin. North Am.* 1995;13:903–924.

82. Marcus FI, Opie LH. Antiarrhythmic drugs. In: Opie LH, ed. *Drugs for the Heart*, 4th ed. Philadelphia: WB Saunders, 1995, pp. 207–246.

83. Chronister C. Clinical management of supraventricular tachycardia with adenosine. *Am. J. Crit. Care* 1993;2:41–47.
84. Slovis CM, Wrenn KD. The technique of managing ventricular tachycardia. *J. Crit. Illness* 1993;8:731–741.
85. Roden D. Magnesium treatment of ventricular arrhythmias. *Am. J. Cardiol.* 1989;63:43G–46G.
86. Goldschlager N. Recognition and mangement of patients with bradyarrhythmias. In: Goldman L, Braunwald E, eds. *Primary Cardiology*. Philadelphia: WB Saunders, 1998, pp. 353–369.
87. Kusumoto FM, Goldschlager N. Cardiac pacing. *N. Engl. J. Med.* 1996;334:89–97.

9

Ventilatory Management in the Neurosciences Critical Care Unit

David L. McDonagh and Cecil O. Borel

INTRODUCTION

Mechanical ventilation was developed a century ago but not put into clinical use to any significant extent until the 1950s. At that time it was needed for the management of neuromuscular disease, specifically the polio epidemics (1). Subsequently, this technology has been applied to a variety of diseases and used by multiple medical specialties. Nonetheless, a recent point prevalence study of over 1600 patients in 412 intensive care units around the world found that 20% were being mechanically ventilated for neurologic indications, specifically coma or neuromuscular disease (2). The evolution of specialty intensive care units (ICUs) lead to the evolution of neurointensive care units in the 1970s and 1980s to handle the unique problems found in critically ill neurology and neurosurgery patients (3). Specific ventilatory strategies have been applied to many illnesses seen in the neurologic intensive care units today. Respiratory compromise occurs in a variety of these diseases and demands efficient, aggressive airway and ventilatory management.

INDICATIONS FOR INTUBATION AND MECHANICAL VENTILATION IN NEUROLOGIC DISEASE

Endotracheal intubation is indicated to provide airway protection and ensure airway patency in patients with depressed levels of consciousness or bulbar dysfunction even in the absence of ventilatory dysfunction. A patient with a Glasgow Coma Scale (GCS) score less than 10 should be considered at high risk for airway compromise. Aspiration increases with a decline in the level of consciousness as measured by the GCS (4). Likewise, the patient with a depressed gag or cough reflex has limited ability to protect the airway and requires endotracheal intubation. Patients with head and neck trauma may have airway compromise secondary to mechanical obstruction or edema.

Mechanical ventilation, on the other hand, is indicated when neurological patients lose adequate ventilatory drive, or when they develop respiratory muscle weakness, inadequate lung compliance, or inefficient gas exchange.

Central nervous system injury can alter respiratory drive. Patients may hypoventilate or spontaneously hyperventilate. Resultant hypoxia or hypercapnea may require the use of mechanical ventilation. Ventilatory support is needed to prevent further neurologic or systemic injury from hypoxia, hypercapnea, or muscle fatigue.

In neuromuscular disease, clinical deterioration and a number of objective parameters herald ventilatory failure. Tachypnea, with a respiratory rate above 30 breaths/min, use of accessory muscles,

From: *Current Clinical Neurology*
Critical Care Neurology and Neurosurgery
Edited by: J. I. Suarez © Humana Press Inc., Totowa, NJ

and paradoxical breathing are signs of respiratory compromise. A vital capacity of 15 mL/kg or less or maximum inspiratory pressure (NIF) less than −30 mmHg foretell eminent respiratory collapse.

Mechanical ventilation for pulmonary complications is common in neurologically injured patients *(5)*. The aspiration of oropharyngeal secretions or gastric contents is a frequent problem in the neurosciences critical care unit (NSU). Subsequent pneumonitis, pneumonia, and/or acute respiratory distress syndrome can occur. Many patients have concomitant pre-existing/co-existing cardiopulmonary disease that impairs ventilatory capacity. Neurogenic pulmonary edema is occasionally seen following severe central nervous system injuries. Finally, patients with traumatic brain injury may also have accompanying thoracic injury with pulmonary contusions, pneumothoracies, or even flail chest syndrome.

Whatever the cause, a number of physiologic abnormalities warrant consideration of mechanical ventilation. Respiratory rate less than 6 or greater than 30; acidosis and/or hypercapnea (pH < 7.25, $PCO_2 > 50$); hypoxemia ($PO_2 < 60$ or $PaO_2/FiO_2 < 200$); or poor pulmonary compliance due to pulmonary edema or ARDS.

AIRWAY MANAGEMENT

Jaw Lift Maneuver and Bag-Mask Ventilation

Airway clearance and ventilation with adequate supplemental oxygen are of primary importance in preventing secondary organ injury and further neurologic injury in the setting of acute neurologic disease. Resting tension in the tongue (genioglossus muscle) is high in a normal awake person, and increases during inspiration *(6)*. This tone is lost under conditions such as coma, obstructive sleep apnea, and general anesthesia *(7)*. In these conditions, the tongue collapses against the posterior pharyngeal wall opposite the second and third cervical vertebrae, causing partial or total airway obstruction.

Initially, simple maneuvers can be employed to clear the tongue from the airway. In the comatose patient, a jaw lift maneuver can elevate the tongue off the posterior pharyngeal wall. This is performed by extension of the neck at the atlanto-occipital joint with simultaneous forward displacement of the mandible *(8)*. This will increase the distance between the tongue and the pharyngeal wall by approx 25%. This maneuver will usually clear the airway in an unconscious patient. However, the maneuver should be avoided in patients with the possibility of unstable cervical spine injuries. Although gravity causes the tongue to obstruct the airway in the supine position, repositioning the patient in lateral decubitus or prone position does not reliably relieve the obstruction *(7)*.

Ventilation is accomplished with a bag-mask apparatus connected to an oxygen supply that delivers 10–15 L/min of oxygen flow *(9)*. The airway is first secured by jaw lift/head tilt. The thumb and index finger are placed on the mask and the remaining fingers behind the body of the mandible followed by gentle lifting of the jaw upward to open the collapsed airway. Low airway pressures should be maintained to prevent passive insufflation of the stomach, with the associated risk of pulmonary aspiration of gastric contents. An assistant should apply cricoid pressure if the patient is suspected to have any gastric contents. Bag and mask ventilation without intubation can be used to ventilate the patient for up to 1 h if needed. This is well suited for the practitioner that is not highly experienced in intubation techniques.

Oral and Nasal Airways

An oropharyngeal airway is useful in maintaining airway patency by lifting the tongue off of the posterior pharynx. The oral airway device will also prevent tongue biting during seizures. An oral airway that is too long pushes the epiglottis down and compresses the larynx thereby partially obstructing the airway, and increases the risk of gastric insufflation. A short oral airway will push the tongue posteriorly with resultant airway compromise. Oral airway insertion can by facilitated by a tongue depressor to push aside the tongue. However, one may advance the device with its tip along the palate pushing the tongue downward and subsequently gradually turning the tip toward the base of the tongue. The cuffed oropharyngeal airway is an adjunctive airway management tool that may offer an adequate airway for ventilation during resuscitation by hospital staff unskilled in endotracheal intubation (10).

A nasal airway provides a passage between the nostril and nasopharynx. Nasal airways are particularly useful for managing the airway in patients with jaw clenching and subsequent airway obstruction. The tube should be lubricated and inserted gently to prevent injury and bleeding in the airway. Nasal airways are contraindicated in the setting of facial or basilar skull fractures to prevent intracranial intubation.

Laryngeal Mask Airway

The LMA was designed to provide a patent airway during general anesthesia without endotracheal intubation or need for laryngoscopy. It has been shown to be a good device for use by nonanesthetists in a variety of settings (11). Clinicians without expertise in endotracheal intubation have been successful using the device after a brief training period (12,13). The LMA does not prevent aspiration of gastric contents, but reduces gastric insufflation during positive pressure ventilation (peak airway pressures should be kept less than 20 cm H_2O). Thus the LMA is contraindicated in patients at risk for gastric aspiration. It should also be avoided in those with subglottic obstruction, low pulmonary compliance or elevated airway resistance, pharyngeal pathology, and/or small oral cavities (14).

Airway management is extremely challenging in patients with unstable cervical spines. The necessity of maintaining a patent airway is complicated by the risk of secondary cervical injury. In patients with depressed levels of consciousness, cervical spine injuries are difficult to assess. Head immobilization while holding the neck in a neutral position is the best approach (15). The LMA can be used in this setting without neck flexion or laryngoscopy. The LMA can serve as a guide for fiberoptic laryngoscopy or even blind tracheal intubation (16,17).

In the presence of intact airway reflexes, the LMA can only be inserted after adequate anesthesia of the oropharynx. Propofol or topical anesthesia may be adequate (18). The head is typically positioned in the sniffing position (in the absence of cervical injury) and the LMA is inserted blindly after deflation and flattening of the mask. The tip is pressed against the hard palate and advanced into the oropharynx and then the hypopharynx (18,19). The mask is then inflated and ventilation is attempted.

Intubating Laryngeal Mask Airway

The intubating laryngeal mask airway (ILMA) is a modified LMA that facilitates endotracheal intubation through the device. The LMA is not an optimal device for endotracheal tube placement. The ILMA is a curved, wide bore, stainless steel tube sheathed in silicone and bonded to a laryngeal mask and a metal handle. It has an adjustable epiglottic elevation bar, a guiding ramp, and can accommodate various sizes of silicone endotracheal tubes (not the traditional polyvinylchloride tubes) (20). Endotracheal tube placement does not require manipulation of the head and neck, or insertion of the fingers in the patient's mouth. The ILMA can be left in place or removed over the endotracheal tube. Blind tracheal intubation using a silicone endotracheal tube was performed in 149 of 150 patients in one study (21). This device improves the success rate and ease of intubation in normal patients with cervical stabilization using manual in-line cervical traction (22). The ILMA can be more problematic in the patient wearing a hard cervical collar (20). At this time, we suggest that the ILMA only be used by practitioners trained in its use and in advanced airway management (23).

Endotracheal Intubation

The standard of care for emergency airway management remains the placement of a cuffed endotracheal tube (Table 1). This tube is inserted through the larynx and into the trachea and is sealed by an inflatable distal cuff. Aspiration of gastric contents and gastric insufflation is prevented or markedly

Table 1
Endotracheal Intubation in Patients With Neurological Impairment

Impairment	Physiological confirmation	Indication	Considerations during intubation	Technique
Decreased level of consciousness	GCS < 10	Prevention of aspiration	Prevent passive regurgitation; Minimal sedation necessary	Oral tracheal intubation under direct laryngoscopy
Raised intracranial pressure	GCS < 9; CT scan	Prevention of hypoxia or hypercarbia; Hyperventilation	Block ↑ in ICP during laryngoscopy; Prevent aspiration; Avoid 2 degrees cervical or facial injury	"Rapid sequence" intubation with cervical stabilization
Posterior fossa injury not affecting consciousness	Positional airway obstruction; Decreased gag reflex; ↑ Resting PCO_2	Maintain patent airway; Prevent aspiration	Exaggerated ↑ or ↓ BP response; Minimal sedation necessary	Oral tracheal intubation under direct laryngoscopy
Medullary lesion	No response to inhaled CO_2	Loss of ventilatory drive	Exaggerated response to narcotics and sedatives	Oral tracheal intubation under direct laryngoscopy
High cervical spine injury	↓ Inspiratory muscle effort	Phrenic paralysis	Avoid 2 degrees cervical injury	Best possible cervical stabilization; Fiberoptic intubation; Oral intubation using LMA; Blind nasal
Lower cervical thoracic injury	↓ Inspiratory and expiratory function; ↓ PO_2 2 degrees to atelectasis, pneumonia	↓ Intercostal, abdominal strength	Avoid 2 degrees cervical injury; Rigid stabilization already present; ↑ K^+ response to succinylcholine	Fiberoptic intubation; Oral intubation using LMA; Blind nasal intubation

(continued on next page)

Disease	Physiologic derangements	Mechanical effects	Anesthetic considerations	Airway management
Acute polyneuropathy	↓ PO_2 2 degrees to aspiration, atelectasis, pneumonia ↑ PCO_2 2 degrees to ↓ ventilation Inspiratory force < 30 mmHg Vital capacity <10 mL/kg	↓ Ventilatory muscle strength Airway obstruction	Dysautonomia exaggerates ↓BP with sedation or anesthesia ↑K^+ response to succinylcholine	Topical local anesthesia Oral intubation technique of choice
Neuromuscular junction disease	↓ PO_2 2 degrees to aspiration, atelectasis, pneumonia ↑ PCO_2 2 degrees to ventilation Inspiratory force < 30 mmHg Vital capacity < 10 ML/kg	↓ Ventilatory muscle strength Airway obstruction	Exaggerated response to non-depolarizing muscle relaxants Unpredictable response to succinylcholine	Topical local anesthesia Light sedation Oral intubation technique of choice
Myopathy	↑ PCO_2 2 degrees to ventilation ↓ PO_2 2 degrees to aspiration, atelectasis, pneumonia Inspiratory force < 30 mmHg Vital capacity < 10 mL/kg	↓ Ventilatory muscle strength	Risk of malignant hyperthermia with some myopathies	Oral intubation technique of choice No succinylcholine

Reprinted by permission: Airway management and mechanical ventilation. In *Neurological Therapeutics: Principles and Practice*. Martin Dunitz Limited, Publishers, New York, 2003.

reduced. Endotracheal intubation should be performed efficiently with efforts to minimize the risk of injury from the procedure itself. A carbon dioxide detection device or other intubation detection device is extremely valuable in verifying endotracheal placement.

MECHANICAL VENTILATION

Modes of Mechanical Ventilation

Controlled Modes of Mechanical Ventilation

Controlled modes of mechanical ventilation maintain a set minimal minute ventilation by delivering air to either a given volume or inspiratory pressure. This mode is best suited for those patients who lack adequate ventilatory drive, either because of brainstem injury, sedation, or narcosis. The respiratory rate is selected to maintain adequate minute ventilation at the tidal volume anticipated by the pressure or volume setting. Controlled modes become problematic when ventilatory drive recovers, because of discoordinated breathing synchrony or "bucking" *(24)*.

Assisted Modes of Mechanical Ventilation

An assisted mode supplements the patient's ventilatory efforts by providing either pressure or volume support to the spontaneous breaths. Assisted modes of mechanical ventilation augment the patient's inspiratory efforts in order to reduce the work of breathing. The patient triggers the ventilator. The level of assistance is variable and depends on the patient's effort as well as the level of mechanical support *(24,25)*. This mode is useful for patients with respiratory muscle weakness but normal ventilatory drive. This can be in the form of synchronized intermittent mandatory ventilation (SIMV), with accompanying pressure support on breaths not controlled by the machine. Alternatively, it can be in the form of pressure support alone to augment tidal volumes and remove the added respiratory work related to the ventilator tubing and artificial airway.

Positive End-Expiratory Pressure

Positive end-expiratory pressure (PEEP) is used to improve airflow to collapsed portions of the lung. This effect is achieved through improved lung compliance, decreased pulmonary arteriovenous shunting, and/or improved arterial oxygenation (in alveolar injury). In the neurologic intensive care unit, the use of PEEP is controversial for patients with reduced intracranial compliance or raised intracranial pressure. Thoracic pressure is transmitted to central venous pressure and right atrial pressure as mean airway pressure is increased. Eventually, this pressure is transmitted to the jugular veins and impedes cerebral venous drainage. This increases cerebral blood volume and raises intracranial pressure.

The effect of PEEP on intracranial pressure (ICP) is not predictable for several reasons. Jugular venous collapse may prevent the transmission of right atrial pressure to cerebral venous pressure in an upright position *(26)*. One study reported that intrathoracic PEEP-induced venous hypertension was transmitted to the intracranial compartment, without intracranial hypertension, for patients in the supine position but not in the sitting position. Head flexion and rotation in the patient with increased ICP with the addition of PEEP can cause a significant increase in ICP, whereas supine or sitting *(27)*. PEEP tends not to increase ICP in patients with poor lung compliance but can increase ICP in patients with normal compliance *(28)*. It is our practice to use PEEP carefully in patients with raised ICP or increased intrapulmonary shunting. PEEP levels up to 12 cm H_2O are usually well tolerated *(29,30)*. In patients with elevated ICP or with suspected intracranial hypertension, PEEP should be used along with ICP monitoring and frequent neurologic examinations *(31)*.

Situation-Specific Ventilatory Strategies

Depressed Level of Consciousness

A reduced level of consciousness (GCS score < 10) correlates strongly with increased mortality in ischemic stroke and intracerebral hemorrhage *(32–35)*. The decreased level of consciousness is associated with tissue shifts secondary to edema with or without increased intracranial pressure *(36,37)*. Intubation and mechanical ventilation are used in this setting to support patients through the acute phase of their illness (Table 2). Some will require long-term airway management with a tracheotomy and or mechanical ventilation. Controlled ventilatory modes work well in the patient with minimal respiratory drive. As patients recover, assisted modes are superior.

Elevated Intracranial Pressure

Intubation and mechanical ventilation are used in the management of elevated intracranial pressure *(38)*. Correction of the hypoxemia, hypercarbia, and acidosis occurring in the setting of elevated ICP reduce secondary neurologic and systemic injury. Patients with elevated ICP often have depressed levels of consciousness, further necessitating intubation and ventilatory management. Herniation syndromes associated with increased ICP and brainstem injury impair airway reflexes and ventilatory drive *(39,40)*. Controlled hyperventilation is frequently employed as a therapeutic measure to reduce ICP as described later in this chapter.

The intubation procedure including laryngoscopy and the sympathetic response secondary to airway reflexes can increase ICP. Hypoventilation/hypercapnea preceding intubation can also increase the ICP. Succinylcholine can cause muscle fasciculation and a resultant rise in the ICP *(41)*. It should be used with a nondepolarizing neuromuscular blocking agent. The use of lidocaine, thiopental, or propofol may blunt the ICP response during intubation.

Cerebral Hemisphere and Brainstem Lesions

Central control of respiration is complex and emanates from a number of centers in the cerebral hemispheres and brainstem. Cortical regions including the insula, hippocampus, and temporal lobes influence respiration. Abnormal stimulation of these areas, such as during a seizure, can cause hypopnea or apnea. Unilateral lesions do not cause significant respiratory compromise *(42)*. Cheyne-Stokes breathing (alternating hypo- and hyperventilation) is seen with bihemispheric dysfunction as can occur in many metabolic encephalopathies *(43)*.

Brainstem damage can cause a variety of respiratory problems. The dorsolateral medulla is responsible for automatic respiratory drive and rhythmic breathing. Patients with more rostral brainstem infarction sparing the dorsolateral medulla may have normal respiratory drive *(44)*. Injury to the dorsolateral medulla, most commonly seen in the setting of a lateral medullary infarction (Wallenburg syndrome), can cause hypopnea or apnea *(45,46)*. Patients may suffer from mild hypoventilation while awake, which is voluntarily overcome by cortical centers. However, respirations may cease entirely during sleep (Ondine's Curse). Pontine damage can result in Cheyne-Stokes breathing, apneustic respirations, and ataxic respiratory excursions. Damage at the pontomesencephalic junction and some toxic-metabolic states can cause neurogenic hyperventilation *(47–50)*. Finally, central or obstructive sleep apnea can occur following brainstem stroke *(42)*. Controlled modes of ventilatory support with mild sedation work best in the initial management of these patients who have lost respiratory drive.

Spinal Cord Injury

Spinal immobilization must be maintained during airway management in any patient with a potential spinal cord injury. Air movement can be determined by feeling airflow at the mouth or nares. Patients who can speak without stridor or hoarseness usually have unobstructed airways. A jaw lift maneuver can be used while avoiding spine manipulation. Many patients will require at least temporary endotracheal intubation. Emergent tracheotomy may be needed in the event of severe head and neck injuries. A depressed level of consciousness because of concomitant head injury will necessitate intubation for airway protection. Gastrointestinal ileus often develops soon after spinal cord injury increasing the risk for regurgitation and aspiration *(51)*. Nasogastric suction should be used until resolution of the ileus *(52)*. Awake or rapid sequence intubation techniques can reduce the occurrence of aspiration. High cervical lesions (at or above C3) may result in loss of diaphragmatic function from the inability to activate the phrenic nerves, while lesions below this level will compromise

Table 2
Modes of Mechanical Ventilation in Patients With Neurological Impairment

Mode of mechanical ventilation	Effect on inspiration	Effect on breathing cycle	Indications	Risks
Controlled modes	Maintain minimum minute ventilation	Maintain minimum breathing frequency	Inefficient gas exchange	Barotrauma
			↓CO_2 response	↑Sedation or narcotic required
				Muscle paralysis may be required
Synchronized intermittent mandatory ventilation (SIMV)	Volume controlled pressure variable	Mandatory breath early in cycle	Weakness too profound to trigger the device "Safe" mode when ventilatory status unknown	↑ Peak airway pressures
	Each IMV breath fully supported	Spontaneous breathing allowed at end of cycle	Therapeutic coma, hypothermia, or hyperventilation	Wasted spontaneous breathing effort
	Each spontaneous breath unsupported			
"Assist controlled" mandatory ventilation	Volume controlled, pressure variable	Breathing rate set at acceptable minimum	Prevent hyperpnea in patients requiring increased ventilation	Ventilatory muscle atrophy with prolonged use
	Each breath volume controlled	Patient triggers volume cycled breath above minimum	Prevent nocturnal hypoventilation	
Pressure-assisted controlled ventilation	Pressure controlled, volume variable	Inspiratory time control limits high frequency	"Rest" patient Minimize airway pressure in patients with noncompliant lungs	Changes in lung compliance alter ventilation
	Each breath pressure controlled	Device set to maintain rate above minimum frequency	Optiminize phases of breathing cycle	

(continued on next page)

Assisted modes	Augment inspiratory airflow	Breathing frequency determined by patient	Normal CO$_2$ response	Minute ventilation altered by:
				↓CO$_2$ response
				↑Muscle weakness
				↑Airway resistance
Pressure-supported ventilation	Pressure cycled, volume variable	Frequency depends on adequacy of inspiratory support	Ventilatory muscle weakness	Changes in lung compliance may radically alter ventilation
	Minute ventilation depends on effort and inspiratory pressure		↑Airway resistance	
			Weaning from controlled ventilation	
			Patient requires artifical airway	
Inspiratory positive airway pressure	Inspiratory and expiratory pressure delivered via mask,	Frequency depends on adequacy of ventilation	Long-term, intermittent ventilatory assistance:	Changes in airway function or CO$_2$ sensitivity may radically alter ventilation
	Ventilation depends on airway patency, effort, and inspiratory pressure		Adequate bulbar function	

Reprinted by permission: Airway management and mechanical ventilation. In *Neurological Therapeutics: Principles and Practice*. Martin Dunitz Limited, Publishers, New York, 2003.

some or all accessory muscles of inspiration. Patients with adequate respiratory movements on 1admission should be watched carefully for delayed apnea. This can occur following cervical cord injury and has been reported up to 1 wk after the injury *(53)*.

The intubation technique used in patients with suspected cervical cord injuries should avoid further cord injury and prevent aspiration. Blind or fiberoptically guided nasotracheal intubation with local or topical anesthesia are appropriate approaches. Rapid sequence intubation techniques using a short-acting barbiturate and neuromuscular blocking agent (with simultaneous cricoid pressure) can also be used *(54)*. There is no conclusive evidence for or against the use of any particular technique *(55,56)*. Manual in-line neck traction has fallen out of favor from concerns about dislocation of an unstable cervical spine *(15)*. However, in-line head immobilization continues to be recommended *(55)*.

Patients with spinal cord injury will display hypersensitivity to depolarizing neuromuscular blockers (succinylcholine). If a depolarizing agent is used to facilitate intubation, it can be used within the first 48 h of the injury. Thereafter, massive release of skeletal muscle potassium can occur after succinylcholine administration, possibly leading to cardiac arrest *(57–59)*. This may be the result of an upregulation of acetylcholine receptors at the motor endplate. The phenomenon is thought to last at least 3–6 mo. This can be avoided by the use of a rapid-onset nondepolarizing neuromuscular blocker (rocuronium, vecuronium, or cis-atracurium) instead of succinylcholine.

Neuromuscular Ventilatory Failure

Neuromuscular ventilatory failure is a common yet complex problem in the NSU. Patients with diaphragmatic weakness will develop tachycardia and tachypnea *(60,61)*. Patients will also have dyspnea on minimal exertion and may be conversationally dyspneic. Tachypnea may become more severe while supine with significant orthopnea due to the weight of abdominal contents on the weakened diaphragm *(61)*. Palpation of the sternocleidomastoid muscles and careful observation for use of the accessory muscles of respiration are valuable parts of the bedside examination. A simple bedside test can be used to estimate the vital capacity. The patient should be asked to count out loud on a single breath. If the patient cannot count to 20, significant respiratory compromise is present.

Some quantitative parameters allow the clinician to predict/detect respiratory failure. Most of these tests are effort-dependent and require clear instruction to the patient. Forced vital capacity is defined as the volume of air that can be exhaled from the lungs after a full inhalation. The maximum inspiratory pressure and maximum expiratory pressure are also clinically useful. Transient oxygen desaturation detected by pulse oximetry also foretells respiratory embarrassment.

The normal physiologic response to maintain adequate minute ventilation is primarily an increase in tidal volume *(62)*. In the setting of neuromuscular ventilatory failure, the patient will breathe shallowly and quickly in an effort to maintain minute ventilation. Thus, serial measurements of vital capacity and resting breathing rate should be monitored. A 50% decline from baseline in Guillain-Barré syndrome (GBS) has been shown to predict the need for ventilatory support within 36 h and a decline to less than 1 L predicted ventilatory support within 18 h *(63)*.

Threshold values for intubation from clinical studies have included a vital capacity less than 10 mL/kg, PO_2 less than 70. Other triggers included respiratory fatigue and bulbar dysfunction *(64)*. Lawn et al. recently published a retrospective survey of 114 cases of severe GBS over a 20-yr period. They identified factors that predicted progression to mechanical ventilation. These included vital capacity less than 10 mL/kg, maximal inspiratory pressure less than 30 cm H_2O, maximal expiratory pressure less than 40 cm H_2O, and a reduction of more than 30% in the vital capacity, maximal inspiratory, or maximal expiratory force from baseline. Clinical factors included rapid disease progression, bulbar dysfunction, bilateral facial weakness, and dysautonomia *(65)*. The ultimate decision to intubate will be predicated upon the patients' disease process, clinical appearance, and ventilatory parameters. Early elective intubation is usually preferable to emergent intubation.

The airway management of patients with GBS is complicated by dysautonomia and potentially lethal hyperkalemia following succinylcholine administration *(66–69)*. Cardiac arrhythmias and arrest can result from the hyperkalemia. This is thought to be due to hypersensitivity to acetylcholine in the denervated muscle. Dysautonomia can be fatal in GBS *(70,71)*. Anesthetic agents including the barbiturates, benzodiazepines, and narcotics must be titrated carefully to prevent hypotension. Heart rate and rhythm should be monitored because of the possibility of bradycardia and other arrhythmias. Medications for cardiac resuscitation should be kept at the bedside.

Airway management in the patient with GBS must be performed in such a way so as to minimize the complications listed above. Topically anesthetizing the airway allows endotracheal intubation under short-acting benzodiazepine sedation and atropine, and decreases the risk of arrhythmia and hypotension. Blind nasal endotracheal intubation is advantageous in that laryngoscopy is avoided and remaining airway reflexes and breathing efforts can be preserved. If laryngoscopy and endotracheal intubation are required in a given situation, a rapid sequence intubation technique can be used (preoxygenation, cricoid pressure, atropine, lidocaine, and low dose thiopental). Short-acting nondepolarizing muscle relaxants can be used but are rarely needed. Mechanical ventilation with an SIMV (synchronized intermittent mandatory ventilation) mode and pressure support is usually the optimal approach. Noninvasive ventilation may be increasingly used in the future in neuromuscular ventilatory failure, but experience is limited.

PULMONARY COMPLICATIONS

Aspiration frequently causes impaired gas exchange in patients with neurological injury and is usually not witnessed by caregivers. There is a spectrum of possible injuries. Patients may have silent (asymptomatic) aspiration resulting in arterial desaturation and radiological abnormalities on chest radiographs. Others have mild symptoms such as coughing or wheezing *(72)*. Some go on to develop a fulminant aspiration pneumonitis (Mendelson's syndrome) with or without concomitant infection (aspiration pneumonia). The common radiographic findings in adults are right lower lobe infiltrates, atelectasis, and air bronchograms when a segmental infiltrate is present. In supine patients, the infiltrates will be posterior in the upper and lower lobes. Aspiration of large amounts of gastric acid may cause acute hypoxemia, cyanosis, and shock *(73)*. Occasionally, patients develop the acute respiratory distress syndrome, which carries a high mortality *(74)*.

Neurogenic pulmonary-edema has been often described in the setting of acute central nervous system injuries and is occasionally seen in daily practice *(75,76)*. Its clinical presentation is similar to that of adult respiratory distress syndrome. Clinically, neurogenic pulmonary edema is dramatic with tachypnea, diaphoresis, hypertension, and frothy sputum *(77–79)*. Diffuse pulmonary infiltrates (white out) are seen on chest radiography. Hypoxic respiratory failure (hypoxemia and markedly increased alveolar-arterial oxygen gradient) is present in the setting of a normal pulmonary artery wedge pressure. Mechanical ventilation with PEEP (usually 10–15 cm/H_2O titrated to maximize PO_2) is very effective in reversing the condition and radiographic improvement is seen in hours. This measure alone is usually sufficient to treat the condition, and weaning is usually uneventful *(80,81)*.

Traumatic lung injury should be suspected in patients with head injury. Pulmonary contusions may become apparent on chest X-ray usually within the first hours of admission. Patients with associated flail chest should be treated with mechanical ventilation. A widened alveolar-arterial oxygen gradient on an FIO_2 of 1.0, PaO_2/FIO_2 less than 200, or a PO_2 of less than 50 mmHg on face mask oxygen prompt ventilatory support.

TRACHEOTOMY

Coma and Vegetative States

In general, early tracheotomy is desirable for patients in whom prolonged ventilatory support is foreseen. Patients who remain comatose or in a vegetative state usually have a persistent inability to protect the airway and clear secretions. Those who recover the ability to ventilate may not recover the ability to maintain an airway because of positional airway obstruction, recurrent aspiration, or inadequate management of secretions. Intubated patients who do not open their eyes spontaneously or follow commands (GCS < 11) are candidates for long term airway management (around intubation d 14) *(82)*.

Bulbar Dysfunction

Bulbar or lower cranial nerve injury disables protective airway reflexes and may result in the need for long-term airway and ventilatory management with a tracheotomy.

Prolonged Mechanical Ventilation

Patients likely to be extubated within 2 wk from the time of intubation can be managed with an endotracheal tube. However, significant patient discomfort, facial injuries that would complicate reintubation, or upper airway edema/obstruction that would complicate reintubation may necessitate early tracheotomy in these patients. Any patient who fails to improve within 1 wk or who is expected to need artificial airway management beyond 2 wk should be given a tracheotomy *(83)*.

In patients with an evolving illness such as myasthenic crisis or Guillain-Barré, it is prudent to wait 14 d before placement of a tracheotomy. This gives the patient time to respond to immunotherapy or spontaneously recover. One third of patients may no longer need intubation after 2 wk.

THERAPEUTIC HYPERVENTILATION

Hyperventilation has long been used in the management of intracranial hypertension. Carbon dioxide is a potent cerebral vasodilator. The reduction in the arterial partial pressure of carbon dioxide ($PaCO_2$) achieved by hyperventilation acts to constrict the cerebral vasculature, thus reducing cerebral blood flow and intracranial pressure. The cerebral blood flow decreases by approx 1–2 mL/min per 1 mmHg drop in $PaCO_2$ *(84)*. However, the efficacy of hyperventilation is short-lived (lasting 4–6 h) and the resultant vasoconstriction can dangerously compromise cerebral blood flow.

Hyperventilation should be limited to a $PaCO_2$ of 30–35 mmHg unless the patient is not responding to combined efforts to reduce ICP *(84)*. This level reduces the risk of cerebral ischemia that can result from more aggressive hyperventilation *(85)*. Prolonged hyperventilation is no longer recommended in the management of elevated ICP given the deleterious effects on cerebral blood flow. Temporary hyperventilation, although not proven to improve clinical outcomes, is widely used in the acute control of elevated intracranial pressure in combination with other measures *(86)*. This is often an effective temporizing measure but should be used as a bridge to more definitive therapy for ICP reduction.

WEANING VENTILATORY SUPPORT AND EXTUBATION

Extubation can be considered when the patient is able to handle secretions, protect the airway, and spontaneously ventilate. A patient should not have significant hypoxemia, or hemodynamic instability, and should be on minimal positive end-expiratory pressure *(87)*. A patient breathing comfortably on minimal ventilatory support (i.e., a pressure support of 5 cm H_2O) can undergo a trial of extubation. The endotracheal tube cuff should be lowered before extubation to ensure air movement around the tube and the absence of significant laryngeal edema. Close monitoring is obviously important in the postextubation period and the patient should be kept NPO for at least a few hours.

For many patients, some period of weaning will be necessary. Some will require a prolonged wean or may remain ventilator dependent. Numerous weaning parameters and indices have been investigated for use as clinical predictors. In neuromuscular and postoperative patients, the negative inspiratory force and vital capacity can be useful in assessing respiratory pump function but in general univariate predictors such as these are suboptimal *(88,89)*. Multivariate indices tend to have greater predictive value. The rapid shallow breathing index (RSBI = RR/V_T ratio) is perhaps the most frequently used parameter. An RSBI (obtained while off ventilatory support) of less than 105 correlates with a successful weaning *(90)*, but should not be used in isolation.

Ventilatory drive and chemosensitivity are the first functions to be regained in a patient with respiratory failure secondary to neurologic injury. This allows for weaning from controlled to assisted modes of mechanical ventilation. The ventilatory response to hypercapnea may be altered with decreased levels of consciousness *(91)*, and patients may become hypercapneic at night. Therefore, a controlled mode may be required at night, with an assisted mode during the day. It is our practice to wean from controlled ventilatory modes to a pressure support mode, although an SIMV mode with pressure support is an acceptable alternative.

Respiratory muscle strength recovers after ventilatory drive and chemosensitivity in the neurologically injured patient. Patients usually require conditioning and training to maintain spontaneous ventilation. The pressure support ventilatory mode is ideal for this phase of weaning *(92)*. The inspiratory flow is not volume limited. Therefore, the tidal volume achieved is a result of the inspiratory effort as well as the inspiratory pressure assist by the ventilator. If the inspiratory pressure is inadequate, the patient will become progressively tachypneic in an effort to maintain minute ventilation at low tidal volumes. Patients with low respiratory rates and high tidal volumes can tolerate progressive lowering of inspiratory pressure support until the respiratory rate increases. Added airway resistance due to the ventilator circuitry will necessitate some level of inspiratory pressure support in all patients to avoid excessive respiratory work load *(93)*. For patients with persistent encephalopathy, weaning is facilitated by the use of a tracheotomy.

REFERENCES

1. Prien T, Meyer J, Lawin P. Development of intensive care medicine in Germany. *J. Clin. Anesth.* 1991;3:253–258.
2. Esteban A, and the Mechanical Ventilation International Study Group. How is mechanical ventilation employed in the intensive care unit? *Am. J. Respir. Crit. Care Med.* 2000;161:1450–1458.
3. Ropper AH, Ed. *Neurological and Neurosurgical Intensive Care*, 3rd ed. New York: Raven Press, 1993: 1–10.
4. Adnet F, Baud F. Relation between Glasgow Coma Scale and aspiration pneumonia. *Lancet* 1996;348:123–124.
5. Horner J, Massey EW, Brazer SR. Aspiration in bilateral stroke patients. *Neurology* 1990;40:1686–1688.
6. Remmers JE, deGroot WJ, Sauerland JE, Anch AM. Pathogenesis of upper airway occlusion during sleep. *J. Appl. Physiol.* 1978;44:931–938.
7. Nunn JF. *Applied Respiratory Physiology*, 3rd ed. Boston: Butterworths, 1987.
8. Safar P, Escarraga LA, Chang F. Upper airway obstruction in the unconscious patient. *J. Appl. Physiol.* 1959;14:760–764.
9. Heffner JE. Airway management in the critically ill patient. *Crit. Care Clin.* 1990;6:533–550.
10. Rees SG, Gabbott DA. Use of the cuffed oropharyngeal airway for manual ventilation by non-anaesthetists. *Anaesthesia* 1999;54:1089–1093.
11. Benumof JL. Laryngeal mask airway and the ASA difficult airway algorithm. *Anesthesiology* 1996;84(3):686–699.
12. Yardy N, Hancox D, Strang T. A comparison of two airway aids for emergency use by unskilled personnel. The Combitube and laryngeal mask. *Anaesthesia* 1999;54:181–183.
13. Rumball CJ, MacDonald D. The PTL, Combitube, laryngeal mask, and oral airway: a randomized prehospital comparative study of ventilatory device effectiveness and cost-effectiveness in 470 cases of cardiorespiratory arrest. *Prehosp. Emerg. Care* 1997;1:1–10.
14. Foley LJ, Ochroch EA. Bridges to establish an emergency airway and alternate intubating techniques. *Crit. Care Clin.* 2000;16:429–444.
15. Twiner LM. Cervical spine immobilization with axial traction: a practice to be discouraged. *J. Emerg. Med.* 1989;7:385–386.
16. Wong JK, Tongier WK, Armbruster SC, White PF. Use of the intubating laryngeal mask airway to facilitate awake orotracheal intubation in patients with cervical spine disorders. *J. Clin. Anesth.* 1999;11:346–348.
17. Kadota Y, et al. Application of a laryngeal mask to a fiberoptic bronchoscope-aided tracheal intubation. *J. Clin. Anesth.* 1992;4:503–504.
18. Ferson DZ. Laryngeal mask airway: preanesthetic evaluation and insertion technique in adults. *Int. Anesthesiol. Clin.* 1998;36:29–45.
19. Campo SL, Denman WT. The laryngeal mask airway: its role in the difficult airway. *Int. Anesthesiol. Clin.* 2000;38:29–45.
20. Wakeling HG, Nightingale J. The intubating laryngeal mask airway does not facilitate tracheal intubation in the presence of a neck collar in simulated trauma. *Br. J. Anaesth.* 2000;84:254–256.

21. Brain AI, Verghese C, Addy EV, Kapila A, Brimacombe J. The intubating laryngeal mask. II: A preliminary clinical report of a new means of intubating the trachea. *Br. J. Anaesth.* 1997;79:704–709.
22. Asai T, Murao K, Tsutsumi T, Shingu K. Ease of tracheal intubation through the intubating laryngeal mask during manual in-line head and neck stabilization. *Anaesthesia* 2000;55:82–85.
23. Avidan MS, Harvey A, Chitkara N, Ponte J. The intubating laryngeal mask airway compared with direct laryngoscopy. *Br. J. Anaesth.* 1999;83:615–617.
24. Tobin MJ. Advances in mechanical ventilation. *N. Engl. J. Med.* 2001;344:1986–1996.
25. MacIntyre NR. Respiratory function during pressure support ventilation. *Chest* 1986;89:677–683.
26. Toung TJ, Aizawa H, Traystman RJ. Effects of positive end-expiratory pressure ventilation on cerebral venous pressure with head elevation in dogs. *J. Appl. Physiol.* 2000;88:655–661.
27. Lodrini S, Montolivo M, Pluchino F, Borroni V. Positive end-expiratory pressure in supine and sitting positions: its effects on intrathoracic and intracranial pressures. *Neurosurgery* 1989;24:873–837.
28. Burchiel KJ, Steege TD, Wyler AR. Intracranial pressure changes in brain-injured patients requiring positive end-expiratory pressure ventilation. *Neurosurgery* 1981;8:443–439.
29. McGuire G, Crossley D, Richards J, Wong D. Effects of varying levels of positive end-expiratory pressure on intracranial pressure and cerebral perfusion pressure. *Crit. Care Med.* 1997;25:1059–1062.
30. Cooper KR, Boswell PA, Choi SC. Safe use of PEEP in patients with severe head injury. *J. Neurosurg.* 1993;63: 552–555.
31. Shapiro HM, Marshall LF. Intracranial pressure responses to PEEP in head-injured patients. *J. Trauma Injury Infection Crit. Care* 1978;18:254–256.
32. Bushnell CD, Phillips-Bute BG, Laskowitz DT, Lynch JR, Chilukuri V, Borel CO. Survival and outcome after endotracheal intubation for acute stroke. *Neurology* 1999;52:1374–1381.
33. Burtin P, Bollaert PE, Feldmann L, et al. Prognosis of stroke patients undergoing mechanical ventilation. *Intensive Care Med.* 1994;20:32–36.
34. Steiner T, Mendoza G, De Georgia M, Schellinger P, Holle R, Hacke W. Prognosis of stroke patients requiring mechanical ventilation in a neurological critical care unit. *Stroke* 1997;28:711–715.
35. Gujjar AR, Deibert E, Manno EM, Duff S, Diringer MN. Mechanical ventilation for ischemic stroke and intracerebral hemorrhage: indications, timing, and outcome [see comments]. *Neurology* 1998;51:447–451.
36. Frank JI. Large hemispheric infarction, deterioration, and intracranial pressure. *Neurology* 1995;45:1286–1290.
37. Schwab S, Aschoff A, Spranger M, Albert F, Hacke W. The value of intracranial pressure monitoring in acute hemispheric stroke. *Neurology* 1996;47:393–398.
38. O'Brien MJ, Van Eykern LA, Oetomo SB, Van Vught HAJ. Transcutaneous respiratory electromyographic monitoring. *Crit. Care Med.* 1987;15:294–299.
39. Silvestri S, Aronson S. Severe head injury: prehospital and emergency department management. *Mount Sinai J. Med.* 1997;64:329–338.
40. Ampel L, Hott KA, Sielaff GW, Sloan TB. An approach to airway management in the acutely head-injured. *J. Emerg. Med.* 1988;6:1–7.
41. Stirt JA, Grosslight KR, Bedford RF, Vollmer D. Defasciculation with metocurine prevents succinylcholine-induced increases in intracranial pressure. *Anesthesiology* 1987;67:50–53.
42. Laskowitz DT, Borel CO. Respiratory and bulbar dysfunction in neurologic disease. In Miller EH, Raps EC, (eds). *Critical Care Neurology.* Boston: Butterworth Heinemann, 1999.
43. Simon RP. Breathing and the nervous system. In Aminoff JM, (ed). *Neurology and General Medicine.* New York: Churchill Livingstone, 1989: 1–22.
44. Feldman MH. Physiological observations in a chronic case of "locked in" syndrome. *Neurology* 1971;21:459.
45. Devereaux MW, Keane JR, Davis RL. Automatic respiratory failure associated with infarction in the medulla. *Arch. Neurol.* 1973;29:46.
46. Levin BE, Margolis G. Acute failure of autonomic respirations secondary to unilateral brainstem infarct. *Ann. Neurol.* 1973;29:46.
47. Posner JB, Plum F. Toxic effects of carbon dioxide and acetazolamide in hepatic encephalopathy. *J. Clin. Investig.* 1980;39:1246.
48. Lane DJ, Rout MW, Williamson DH. Mechanism of hyperventilation in acute cerebrovascular accidents. *BMJ* 1971;3:9–12.
49. Froman C, Crampton Smith A. Hyperventilation associated with low pH of cerebrospinal fluid after intracranial hemorrhage. *Lancet* 1966;1:780–782.
50. Posner JB, Plum F. Toxic effects of carbon dioxide and acetazolamide in hepatic encephalopathy. *J. Clin. Investig.* 1980;39:1246.
51. Gore RM, Mintzer RA, Calenoff L. Gastrointestinal complications of spinal cord injury. *Spine* 1981;6:538–544.
52. Sutton VS, Macphail I, Bentley R, Nandy MK. Acute gastric dilatation as a relatively late complication of tetraplegia due to very high cervical cord injury. *Paraplegia* 1981;19:17–19.
53. Kang L, et al. Delayed apnea in patients with mid- to lower cervical spinal cord injury. *Spine* 2000;25:1332–1338.
54. Talucci RC, Shaikh KA, Schwab CW. Rapid sequence induction with oral endotracheal intubation in the multiply injured patient. *Am. Surg.* 1988;54:185–187.

55. Suderman VS, Crosby ET, Lui A. Elective oral tracheal intubation in the cervical spine-injured adult. *Can. J. Anaesth.* 1991;38:785–789.

56. Meschino A, Devitt JH, Kock JP, Schwartz ML. The safety of awake tracheal intubation in cervical spine injury. *Can. J. Anaesth.* 1992;39:114–117.

57. Stone WA, Beach TP, Hamburg W. Succinylcholine danger in the spinal cord injured patient. *Anesthesiology* 1970;32:168–169.

58. Cooperman LH, Strobel GE, Kennell EM. Massive hyperkalemia after administration of succinylcholine. *Anesthesiology* 1970;32:161–164.

59. Smith RB, Crenvik A. Cardiac arrest following succinylcholine administration in patients with central nervous system injuries. *Anesthesiology* 1970;33:558–560.

60. Borel CO, Tilford C, Nichols DG, Hanley DF, Traystman RJ. Diaphragmatic performance during recovery from acute ventilatory failure in Guillain-Barre' syndrome and myasthenia gravis. *Chest* 1991;99:444–451.

61. Borel CO, Teitelbaum JS, Hanley DF. Ventilatory drive and carbon dioxide response in ventilatory failure due to myasthenia gravis and Guillain-Barré syndrome. *Crit. Care Med.* 1993;21:1717–1726.

62. Caruana-Montaldo B, Gleeson K, Zwillich CW. The control of breathing in clinical practice. *Chest* 2000;117:205–225.

63. Chevrolet JC, Deleamont P. Repeated vital capacity measurments as predictive parameters for mechanical ventilation need and weaning success in Guillain-Barré syndrome. *Am. Rev. Respir. Dis.* 1991;144:814–818.

64. Ropper AH, Kehne SM. Guillain-Barré syndrome: management of respiratory failure. *Neurology* 1985;35:1662–1665.

65. Lawn ND, Dade DF, Henderson RD, Wolter TD, Wijdicks EFM. Anticipating mechanical ventilation in Guillain-Barré syndrome. *Arch. Neurol.* 2001;58:893–898.

66. Cooperman LH. Succinylcholine-induced hyperkalemia in neuromuscular disease. *JAMA* 1970;213:1867–1871.

67. Fergusson RJ, Wright DJ, Willey RF, Crompton GK, Grant IWB. Suxamethonium is dangerous in polyneuropathy. *BMJ* 1981;232:298–299.

68. Sunderrajan EV, Davenport J. The Guillian-Barre' syndrome: pulmonary neurologic correlations. *Medicine* 1985;64:333–341.

69. Beach TP, Stone WA, Hamelberg W. Circulatory collapse following succinylcholine: report of a patient with diffuse lower motor neuron disease. *Anesth. Analg.* 1971;50:431.

70. Lichtenfeld P. Autonomic dysfunction in the guillian-barre' syndrome. *Am. J. Med.* 1971;50:772–780.

71. Dalos NP, Borel C, Hanley DF. Cardiovascular autonomic dysfunction in Guillain-Barre syndrome. Therapeutic implications of Swan-Ganz monitoring. *Arch. Neurol.* 1988;45:115–117.

72. Marik PE. Aspiration pneumonitis and aspiration pneumonia. *N. Engl. J. Med.* 2001;344:665–671.

73. Gibbs CP, Modell JH. Pulmonary aspiration of gastric contents: pathophysiology, prevention, and management. In Miller RD, ed. *Anesthesia*, 4th ed, vol 2. New York: Churchill Livingstone, 1994:1437–1464.

74. Ware LB, Matthay MA. The acute respiratory distress syndrome. *N. Engl. J. Med.* 2000;342:1334–1349.

75. Colice GL, Matthay MA, Bass E, Matthay RA. Neurogenic pulmonary edema. *Am. Rev. Resp. Dis.* 1984;130:941–948.

76. Chen HI, Sun SC, Chai CY. Pulmonary edema and hemorrhage resulting from cerebral compression. *Am. J. Physiol.* 1973;224:223.

77. Carlson RW, Schaeffer RC, Michaels SG, Weil MH. Pulmonary edema following intracranial hemorrhage. *Chest* 1979;75:6.

78. Yabumoto M, Kuriyama T, Iwamota M, Kinoshita T. Neurogenic pulmonary edema associated with ruptured intracranial aneurysm: case report. *Neurosurgery* 1986;19:300.

79. Touho H, Karasawa J, Shishido H, Yamada K, Yamazaki Y. Neurogenic pulmonary edema in the acute stage of hemorrhagic cerebrovascular disease. *Neurosurgery* 1989;25:762–768.

80. Maron MB, Holcomb PH, Dawson CA, Rickaby DA, Clough AV, Linehan JH. Edema development and recovery in neurogenic pulmonary edema. *J. Appl. Physiol.* 1994;77:1155–1163.

81. Rogers FB, Shackford SR, Trevisani GT, Davis JW, Mackersie RC, Hoyt DB. Neurogenic pulmonary edema in fatal and nonfatal head injuries. *J. Trauma Inj. Infect. Crit. Care* 1995;39:860–868.

82. Plummer AL, Gracey DL. Consensus conference on artificial airways in patients receiving mechanical ventilation. *Chest* 1989;96:178–180.

83. Heffner JE, Casey K, Hoffman C. Care of the mechanically ventilated patient with a tracheotomy. In Tobin MJ, ed. *Principles and Practice of Mechanical Ventilation*. New York: McGraw-Hill, 1994:749–774.

84. Bendo AA, Luba K. Recent changes in the management of intracranial hypertension. *Int. Anesthesiol. Clin.* 2000;38:69–85.

85. Muizelaar JP, et al. Adverse effects of prolonged hyperventilation in patients with severe head injury: a randomized clinical trial. *J. Neurosurg.* 1991;75:731–739.

86. Allen CH, Ward JD. An evidence-based approach to management of increased intracranial pressure. *Crit. Care Clin.* 1998;14:485–495.

87. Hendra KP, Celli BR. Weaning from mechanical ventilation. *Int. Anesthesiol. Clin.* 1999;37:127–143.

88. Chao DC, Scheinhorn DJ. Weaning from mechanical ventilation. *Crit. Care Clin.* 1998;14:799–817.
89. Sahn SA, Lakshminarayan S. Bedside criteria for discontinuation of mechanical ventilation. *Chest* 1973;63:1002–1005.
90. Yang K, Tobin MJ. A prospective study of the indexes predicting outcome of trials of weaning from mechanical ventilation. *N. Engl. J. Med.* 1991;324:1445.
91. Kunitomo F, Kimura H, Tatsumi K, et al. Abnormal breathing during sleep and chemical control of breathing during wakefulness in patients with sleep apnea syndrome. *Am. Rev. Respir. Dis.* 1989;139:164–169.
92. Brochard L, Rauss A, Benito S, et al. Comparison of three methods of gradual withdrawal from ventilatory support during weaning from mechanical ventilation [see comments]. *Am. J. Respir. Crit. Care Med.* 1994;150:896–903.
93. Brochard L, Rua F, Lorino H, Harf A. Inspiratory pressure support compensates for the additional work of breathing caused by the endotracheal tube. *Anesthesiology* 1991;75:739–745.

10

Treatment of Autonomic Disorders Requiring Intensive Care Management

Marek Buczek, Jose I. Suarez, and Thomas C. Chelimsky

INTRODUCTION

A variety of autonomic nervous system (ANS) disorders are now being recognized with increasing frequency. They can range from autonomic disturbances associated with common medical problems, such as diabetes to various syndromes of acute, subacute, and chronic autonomic failure. Intracranial pathology is frequently associated with acute autonomic dysfunction which may result in life-threatening cardiac arrhythmias. Several neurological disorders such as subarachnoid hemorrhage (SAH), stroke, seizures, and traumatic brain injury (TBI) are frequently observed to be accompanied by electrocardiographic (ECG) changes and myocardial damage. Many other conditions, such as delirium, coma, and loss of consciousness in epilepsy and stroke are important autonomic crises. Clinical signs and symptoms of autonomic dysfunction are often overlooked by physicians or overshadowed by more prominent language, behavioral, motor and sensory findings. The increasing awareness of progressive autonomic dysfunction affecting the course of many human diseases is leading to more accurate and rapid diagnosis and proper management of autonomic failure (AF) (1,2).

Clinical autonomic disorders can be classified into major groups based on the part of the nervous system being involved. Those involving central nervous system (CNS) are properly named central, and those involving peripheral nervous system (PNS) are peripheral, with mixed autonomic problems involving both CNS and PNS. Another classification divides autonomic disorders into primary (pure autonomic failure [PAF]), in which no apparent cause can be determined, and secondary, which are the result of specific diseases (i.e., diabetes, amyloidosis). Subclassifications include more detailed etiologies, such as paroxysmal autonomic disorders, autonomic neuropathies, diseases with reduced orthostatic tolerance, and autonomic problems related to drugs and toxins, among others (1). In patients with secondary autonomic dysfunction, the overall prognosis depends largely on the severity of the associated illness. In central disorders (i.e., brain tumors, SAH), the primary pathological process often dominates the outcome, whereas in conditions, such as botulism or tetanus, the complications arising from autonomic impairment play a key role in determining morbidity and mortality. Also in diseases such as diabetes or amyloidosis, autonomic dysfunction worsens the overall long-term prognosis (1).

In this chapter, we aim to provide a review of the diagnosis and management of potentially life-threatening autonomic disorders that may require aggressive hospital treatment in a neurosciences critical care unit (NSU) setting.

From: *Current Clinical Neurology*
Critical Care Neurology and Neurosurgery
Edited by: J. I. Suarez © Humana Press Inc., Totowa, NJ

ANATOMY AND PHYSIOLOGY OF THE AUTONOMIC NERVOUS SYSTEM

The ANS was considered for a long time an anatomic subdivision of PNS. However, its central components and connections have been recognized quite recently. The division of the basic framework of ANS, as seen in the majority of neural systems, combines an afferent limb (an input), a central decision-making structure (an integrator), and an efferent limb (an output). The ANS contains visceral sensory (afferent) and visceral motor (efferent) pathways with visceral reflexes mediated mainly by local circuits in the brainstem and/or spinal cord. These reflexes are carefully coordinated and integrated into higher CNS circuitry, but they are generally not under voluntary control, making ANS an involuntary (visceral) part of the nervous system, in contrast to the voluntary (somatic) nervous system. Autonomic refers to independence and self-regulation, the unique hallmarks and qualities of the ANS, placing control of most vital body functions beyond the reach of conscious control. A major portion of the activity of ANS is reflex in nature with the afferent limb for such reflexes located in any somatic afferent nerve and transmitting information regarding the functional state of the particular autonomic end organ of interest. This portion of the circuit is often regarded as visceral afferent rather than truly autonomic. Both physiologic and pathologic stimuli arising from visceral or cutaneous receptors can induce reflex activity in autonomic nerves. Viewed in this framework, the ANS originates with the central autonomic network (CAN) and sends out efferent connections, classically divided into sympathetic and parasympathetic divisions *(3,4)*. The two branches have different sites of origin in the CNS for first-order preganglionic neurons. The sympathetic division is called thoraco-lumbar, and the parasympathetic division is craniosacral (*see* details below). The two divisions may function as physiological antagonists, or as complementary to each other. For instance, in the control of male sexual function complementary actions of the parasympathetic (erection) and sympathetic (ejaculation) divisions are needed *(2,5)*.

The autonomic nervous system innervates mainly three types of tissue—cardiac muscle, smooth muscle and exocrine gland. Autonomic pathways influence cardiovascular, metabolic, digestive, and genitourinary systems as well as pupillary and pilomotor sphincters. Maintenance of the internal homeostasis in the setting of ever changing external conditions requires the concerted intervention of both ANS and endocrine system. The former provides the fast neural component of this functional system. ANS is involved in visceromotor, neuroendocrine, circadian, behavioral, adaptive, and pain-modulating mechanisms.

Early on, the ANS was considered to have only two divisions: the sympathetic nervous system (SNS) and the parasympathetic nervous system (PSNS). However, the enteric nervous system (ENS) should be considered as the third division of the ANS because even though both sympathetic and parasympathetic fibers supply enteric neurons, ENS can perform many sensory-motor integrative functions independent of this extrinsic neural input. The enteric division is located entirely in the periphery and comprises a self-contained system with limited connections to the rest of the nervous system. It consists of sensory and motor neurons of the gastrointestinal (GI) tract in Auerbach's (myenteric) and Meissner's (submucosal) plexi and its primary role is to mediate digestive, motility, and peristaltic reflexes.

The innervation of the organs by ANS is fundamentally different in organization from innervation of skeletal musculature. While skeletal muscles have innervation mediated directly by motor neurons, autonomic innervated smooth muscles are linked to the CNS by two neurons. The cell body of the preganglionic neuron is located in the CNS and its axon follows various peripheral neural conduits synapsing on postganglionic neurons in peripheral ganglia.

Neuroanatomical localization of SNS and PSNS divisions has major differences. The sympathetic fibers originate in the functional nuclei of the hypothalamus, which give rise to neurons projecting to autonomic centers in the brainstem, the periaqueductal gray matter in the midbrain, the parabrachial region in the pons, and the intermediate reticular formation located in the ventrolateral medulla. Projections from these structures terminate in the spinal cord nuclei. The sympathetic preganglionic neurons originate in the intermediolateral cell column (nucleus) between the first thoracic and second lumbar segments (T1 to L2), therefore called thoraco-lumbar branch. They exit in 22 pairs of paravertebral sympathetic trunk ganglia located parallel and close to vertebral column. Sympathetic nerve fibers have more ramifications and are more widely distributed than the parasympathetic fibers. The main sympathetic ganglia include cervical and stellate ganglia located in the sympathetic trunk, and celiac ganglion, and superior and inferior mesenteric ganglia constituting prevertebral ganglia. Most of the postganglionic neurons originate in those structures and innervate target visceral organs. The adrenal medulla is the only exception by receiving only preganglionic fibers and being equivalent to a sympathetic ganglion. The SNS can be simplistically conceptualized as responsible for restoring homeostasis in the organism exposed to the external or internal challenges or stressors. SNS activation often leads to a "fight-or-flight" response, with mydriasis, bronchodilation, vasoconstriction and increased blood pressure, increased heart rate, and hyperglycemia.

The PSNS can be subdivided into cranial and sacral parts and for that reason is properly named craniosacral branch. The cranial subdivision originates from the brainstem nuclei of cranial nerves III, VII, IX, X, XI with major nuclei being the Edinger-Westphal nucleus, superior and inferior salivary nuclei, nucleus ambiguous, and dorsal motor nucleus of vagus. The cranial preganglionic neurons traveling along cranial nerves synapse in the parasympathetic ganglia, in the close vicinity or within the target organs. The main parasympathetic ganglia include ciliary, pterygopalatine, submandibular, otic, and visceral ganglion. Sacral subdivision originates in sacral spinal cord (segments S2–S4) forming the lateral intermediate gray zone (nucleus) where preganglionic autonomic neurons travel with the pelvic nerve to the inferior hypogastric plexus and synapse on parasympathetic ganglia within the target organs. Based on the traditional view, the PSNS is primarily responsible for maintenance of homeostasis in the resting organism. Parasympathetic activation leads to miosis, bronchial constriction, bradycardia, and increased salivation.

Both SNS and PSNS are integrated with CNS activity through the CAN that includes orbitofrontal and insular cortices, the limbic system with the amygdaloid complex, hypothalamus, reticular formation with periaqueductal gray and ventrolateral medulla with parabrachial nucleus and nucleus of tractus solitarius. CAN is an integral component of an internal regulation system through which the brain controls visceromotor, pain, neuroendocrine, and behavioral responses essential for our survival. Its complex neurocircuitry is characterized by interchangeable connections with parallel organization, and its activity is state-dependent *(4)*. The general organization is hierarchical, so that higher centers modulate the state of the next center under their control. Lower centers contain progressively more precise programs for the control of effector organs under different states of operation. Insular and orbitofrontal cortices mediate higher order autonomic control and their involvement in stroke may produce severe cardiac arrhythmias among other autonomic manifestations (*see also* Chapter 8). The limbic system and amygdaloid complex participate in mediating visceral consequences of emotions and behavior through both the ANS and the endocrine systems. The limbic system influences the ANS, especially the sympathetic division, through both direct and indirect connections with the hypothalamus (historically known as a "head ganglion" of the ANS). In turn, hypothalamic control of the ANS originates from posterior hypothalamus, lateral hypothalamic area, dorsomedial hypothalamic nucleus, and paraventricular nucleus. From these regions, two descending hypothalamic pathways (dorsal longitudinal fasciculus and medial forebrain bundle) transmit information to autonomic centers in the brainstem and spinal cord. Nucleus of tractus solitarius (NTS) and ventrolateral medulla contain a network of respiratory, cardiovagal, and vasomotor neurons. NTS receives visceral input from cranial nerves VII, IX, X, and XI and provides central link for multiple ANS sensorimotor reflexes such as carotid sinus baroreceptor reflex, and gastric receptive relaxation reflex. The parabrachial nucleus relay visceral sensory outflow from NTS to forebrain important in behavioral responses to visceral sensations. The reticular formation is considered to be the rostral extension of the intermediate zone of the spinal cord important in integrating visceral and somatic sensory and motor information *(4,6)*.

For decades, autonomic neurotransmitters have been thought to be confined exclusively to the well-characterized acetilcholine (ACh) and norepinephrine (NE) (noradrenaline [NA]). ACh is the neurotransmitter in all preganglionic neurons both, parasympathetic and sympathetic, and for the parasympathetic postganglionic neurons. NE is the transmitter in the postganglionic neurons in the SNS. One exception is the nerve fibers innervating the sweat glands, which are sympathetic but secrete ACh as a postganglionic neurotransmitter. Cholinergic sympathetic dilator nerves to skin vessels also exist. At present, many more substances have been identified as certain (or putative) neurotransmitters or neuromodulators that are responsible together with hormones for coordinated ANS activity, including; vasoactive intestinal peptide (VIP), glutamate, aspartate, glycine, GABA (γ-aminobutyric acid), dopamine, neuropeptide Y, serotonin, calcitonin gene-related peptide (CGRP), histamine, and substance P, just to name a few. These neurotransmitters also act as co-transmitters or modulate synaptic transmission at the autonomic ganglia. VIP, for example, is concentrated mainly in the sacral spinal cord and may be co-released with ACh at cholinergic muscarinic junctions, while neuropeptide Y is co-released with NE. On the other hand, substance P, believed to be one of the most important autonomic neuromediators, is found mainly in the GI system, where it plays a role in the myenteric reflex *(2,7,8)*.

CLINICAL EVALUATION OF PATIENTS WITH AUTONOMIC DYSFUNCTION IN THE NEUROSCIENCES CRITICAL CARE UNIT

In the patient with a suspected autonomic problem the major aim of investigation is to assess the degree of dysfunction with an emphasis on detecting the site of the lesion and the nature of functional deficit. This can be done by either qualitative ANS testing to determine whether autonomic dysfunction is present or absent, or quantitative ANS testing to measure or estimate the extent of autonomic deficit and to localize the site of the lesion within the ANS. It is also important to differentiate between primary ANS dysfunction (ischemic, degenerative, immune-mediated, infectious, etc.), and secondary autonomic response to other medical and/or neurological disorders (sepsis, hypoxia, GI bleeding, pulmonary embolus, disturbances in fluid or electrolyte status, and so on). The results of the ANS tests must be linked with the relevant clinical signs and symptoms in the given patient. Although most tests provide an indication of the overall integrity of a autonomic reflex structure, more complex testing allows for separate evaluation of isolated reflex arc's pathways; afferent, central, and efferent connections. Laboratory testing is an extension of the careful clinical evaluation. Many forms of ANS evaluation are simple and can be performed at the bedside, even in the NSU setting, whereas others require specialized equipment. Clinical investigations in the autonomic failure patient include testing cardiovascular, pupillary, gastrointestinal, respiratory, sweating, genitourinary and sexual functions (Table 1) *(1–3)*.

Cardiovascular Testing

Routine cardiovascular monitoring with intra-arterial blood pressure (BP) and continuous ECG tracing can detect most arrhythmias—common manifestation of ANS dysfunction. However, more specialized tests can assess ANS pathology in greater detail and suggest its influence on the clinical picture. The regulation of cardiac output is markedly affected by venomotor reflexes present during upright posture/tilt, Valsalva's maneuver (VM), deep breathing/hyperventilation, and physical exercise. Screening investigations help determine the site and extent of the cardiovascular autonomic abnormality, and aid significantly in planned therapy. Depending on the disorder, additional tests may be required, such as carotid sinus massage, meal challenge, pressor stimuli, or appropriate biochemical and pharmacological measurements.

Orthostatic (postural) hypotension is one of the major cardiovascular manifestations of autonomic failure and this can be often detected with routine "orthostatic vitals," where postural change can be induced simply by making patients stand up. Tilt-table test (45–90 degrees) can be used in patients

Table 1
Summary of the Most Common ANS Tests Suitable for NSU With Their Normative Values

Test	SNS	PSNS	Parameters measured/normal values
Cardiovascular			*HR, BP, ECG changes*
1. Response to standing (orthostatic vitals, head-up tilt table)	+	+	SBP < 20 mmHg, DBP < 10 mmHg, HR < 15 bpm
2. Valsalva's maneuver (forceful expiration)	+	+	Age and sex-dependent
3. Deep breathing	+		Inspiration/expiration ECG R-R intervals difference/ratio, difference between HRmax and HRmin > 15 indicates normal vagal cardiac control
4. Resting HR variability	+		Beat-to-beat changes of HR an R-R intervals
5. Sustained handgrip	+	+	Submaximal handgrip power, pressor response through muscle afferents
6. Cold pressor test	+		Evaluates sympathetic adrenergic function mediated by skin pain and temperature receptors
7. Baroreflex sensitivity	+		Utilizes medications to determine HR response to artificially increased BP
Thermoregulation/sweat			*Hyper- and/or hypohidriosis*
1. QSART	+		Postganglionic sudomotor fibers (cholinergic sympathetic), sweat output in response to ACh iontophoresis
2. TST	+		Pre- and postganglionic sudomotor fibers, sweat output in response to heat (whole body)
3. SSR	+	+ (?)	EDA in response to electrical stimulation of peripheral nerve afferents
Pupillometry			*Reflects sympathetic/parasympathetic balance*
	+	+	Dark-adapted pupil; sympathetic efferents, parasympathetic efferents (III CN); pupillary constriction
Chemical testing			*Supine/standing plasma catecholamines*
	+		Central vs peripheral stimulation of sympathetic postganglionic noradrenergic terminals, in the normal state, the baseline supine value doubles after 10 min of standing

SNS, sympathetic nervous system; PSNS, parasympathetic nervous system; HR, heart rate; RR, respiratory rate; BP, blood pressure; SBP, systolic BP; DBP, diastolic BP; bpm, beats per minute; ECG, electrocardiogram; ACh, acetylcholine; QSART, quantitative sudomotor axon reflex test; TST, thermoregulatory sweat test; SSR, sympathetic skin response; EDA, evoked electrodermal activity.

unable to sustain an erect posture and is more sensitive than a simple stand because it inactivates the venous muscle pump. Postural variations of heart rate (HR) and BP reflect the integrity of parasympathetic and sympathetic cardiovagal function. Postural hypotension is usually defined as a symptomatic fall in BP of at least 20 mmHg systolic or 10 mmHg diastolic within 3 min of standing or of head-up tilt of at least 60 degrees. There is normally a small-to-moderate rise in heart rate during postural change. In the presence of significant fall of BP, a lack of change in heart rate usually indicates baroreflex abnormality or cardiac sympathetic failure.

Cardiovascular response to VM provides additional assessment of the baroreflex pathways and consists of a precisely timed forced expiration against resistance. With the rise in intrathoracic pressure during VM, the venous return falls along with BP (phase II) and when intrathoracic pressure is released, BP overshoots because of slow speed of vasomotor sympathetic withdrawal. Baroreflex activation results in a secondary fall in heart rate to below baseline levels (phase IV). The Valsalva ratio (VR) is a compound of heart rate acceleration in phase II (sympathetic) to heart rate deceleration in phase IV (parasympathetic). VR reflects the integrity of the sympathetic adrenergic (similar to variations of BP alone), and the parasympathetic cholinergic cardiovagal functions. If the ratio is low, determination whether the predominant problem lies in phase II or IV helps to differentiate whether the PSNS or SNS is affected *(3)*. Lower body negative pressure (using lower body airtight chamber), which can mimic circulatory gravitational stress, can be used to stimulate baroreflex activity in the NSU patient unable to stand or perform VM.

HR response to respiratory change assesses vagal nerve function. Normally, with inspiration there is a rise and with expiration a fall in HR. This change in HR (respiratory sinus arrhythmia) depends on the integrity of efferent vagal neurons, and is triggered by stretch receptors in the chest and lungs. In several autonomic neuropathies, lesions to the longer vagus nerve occur prior to sympathetic impairment, and the HR responses to changes in respiration may be abnormal early in the course. Heart rate variability with deep breathing (HRDB) is one of the most commonly utilized tests to evaluate the autonomic innervation of the heart. During HRDB, inspiration-expiration differences and ratios, and ECG R-R changes are measured. Normal values are age-dependent and a reduced value indicates abnormal vagal cardiac control. Carotid sinus massage is used to test carotid baroreceptors sensitivity and assess integrity of parasympathetic efferent pathways activity. In normal subjects, it usually produces moderate HR slowing and a decrease in BP, but can result in prominent bradycardia or cardiac arrest, and hypotension (vasodilatation) in patients with carotid sinus hypersensitivity. This method should also be used with caution because strokes of the ipsilateral hemisphere have been reported. Resting HR variability during quiet supine rest, as measured by beat-to-beat changes in HR and R-R intervals, is another measure of parasympathetic cardiac outflow and can be quantified by power spectrum analysis. A "fixed" HR that does not significantly change with respirations during rest, exercise, stress or sleep indicates autonomic cardiac denervation. The sympathoexcitatory cold pressor test evaluates sympathetic adrenergic function most likely mediated by the afferent stimulus of skin cold and pain receptors. Sympathetic activation (α-adrenergic system) results in an increase in total peripheral resistance and subsequent pressor response. This method is especially useful to assess cardiovascular system function through an afferent structure that bypasses the baroreflex. Baroreflex sensitivity uses pharmacologic agents to determine HR response to artificially raised BP. Because this method is invasive, cumbersome, and caries some risks it has been replaced by various methods of spontaneous baroreflex measurement.

Transcranial Doppler ultrasound (TCD) has been employed in the evaluation of patients with ANS disorders, particularly orthostatic intolerance syndromes where continuous noninvasive monitoring of cerebral blood flow velocity shows reduced cerebral perfusion pressure (CPP) *(2)*. Continuous EEG monitoring during tilt-table testing also aides in detecting diffuse or focal cerebral hypoxia/ischemia, or seizure activity, especially in patients with unexplained loss of consciousness when the differential diagnosis between syncope and seizures is critical. The new concept of amplitude modulation of the EEG (AM-EEG) has been introduced, and refers to the slow rhythms superimposed on the baseline EEG activity. These rhythms are believed to reflect activity of CAN and propagate to the cerebral cortex from the brainstem autonomic centers *(9–11)*. Use of Swan-Ganz catheter monitoring may be beneficial in the NSU setting in patients with autonomic dysfunction where intravascular volume issues are critical.

Respiratory Tests

In addition to routine measurements of pulmonary function tests, including vital capacity (VC) and negative inspiratory force (NIF) useful in patients with respiratory compromise and facing possible ventilatory support, several tests are available to assess autonomic control of respiration. Arterial blood gas monitoring during sleep may be necessary to detect periods of nocturnal apnea in patients with structural CNS damage. Abnormalities in regulation of ventilation are present in certain primary cardiac and lung disorders, as well as a secondary perturbation in neurologic diseases. The magnitude of respiratory drive can directly contribute to the degree of apnea. Hypoxic ventilatory drive and single-breath carbon dioxide testing reflects functional integrity and responsiveness of peripheral chemoreceptors responsible for adequate ventilation.

Thermoregulation and Sweat Testing of Sudomotor Function

The regulation of body temperature reflects the careful balance between heat production and heat dissipation. A temperature setpoint is established by communication between the septal nuclei and the hypothalamic control center in the anterior nucleus. Sensors in this region compare blood temperature afferent information from skin and venous dermal sensors with the setpoint. When appropriate, body cooling signals arise directly from the anterior hypothalamus to efferent skin vasodilation and sweating, while heating signals are generated through communication with the posterior hypothalamus to produce skin vasoconstriction, piloerection, and (if needed) shivering via somatic motor activation.

Sweat secretion is under the control of sympathetic postganglionic fibers, with ACh as a principal terminal neurotransmitter. The quantitative sudomotor axon reflex test (Q-SART) evaluates the postganglionic sudomotor (cholinergic sympathetic) nerve fibers by stimulating the nerve in one location and recording the sweat response at a distance. Q-SART is a very sensitive test for the detection of a postganglionic neuropathy. Unfortunately, it is not always able to distinguish CNS from PNS disorders since it may also be abnormal in other conditions affecting the ANS, such as postural orthostatic tachycardia syndrome (POTS), and multiple system atrophy (MSA), and progressive pure autonomic failure (PAF).

The thermoregulatory sweat test (TST) evaluates the entire system through the sweating response to a strong heat stimulus to the entire body. It is performed in a specialized laboratory and is not practical for patients restricted to the neurosciences critical care unit (NSU). The sympathetic skin response (SSR) allows the assessment of the integrity of the peripheral sudomotor sympathetic nerve using standard (stationary or portable) electromyography. Like the Q-SART, SSR is reduced in diseases affecting distal small fibers, although it is probably less sensitive and specific than the Q-SART.

Testing Eye and Pupillary Abnormalities

The pupil is an important objective marker of both visual and autonomic pathways (*see* Chapter 30). Mydriasis (dilation of the pupil) is produced by sympathetic activation of the radial smooth muscle of the pupil and by parasympathetic inhibition mediated by the Edinger-Westphal nucleus, which houses the preganglionic neurons. Both are controlled by fibers projecting from the posterior hypothalamus and the superior colliculi. Postganglionic sympathetic neurons release NE at the α-adrenergic receptors within the dilator pupillae muscle resulting in pupillary dilation whereas parasympathetic postganglionic neurons release ACh and activate muscarinic receptors. Miosis (contraction of the pupil) occurs when the pupil is exposed to light or with accommodation to near vision. Both miotic reflexes are mediated by the activation of parasympathetic preganglionic neurons originating in the Edinger-Westphal nucleus and inhibition of the sympathetic pathways. Because afferent impulses are transmitted to these nuclei by crossing fibers on both sides, illumination of one eye produces constriction of both pupils. The constriction of the eye being stimulated is the direct response, whereas the constriction of the contralateral eye is the consensual response *(3,12,13)*. The pupil is involved in a number of autonomic disorders and a variety of pupillary abnormalities can be seen including dilated myotonic pupils in Holmes-Adie syndrome, a miotic pupil in Horner's syndrome, or irregular pupils in syphilitic Argyll-Robertson syndrome. In addition to routine testing of light and accommodation response during neurological examination, several more specialized physiological function tests and/or pharmacological approaches (supersensitivity, cholinomimetics, sympathomimetics) can refine the diagnosis, especially with the use of modern pupillometers. In localized disorders, like Horner's syndrome or oculomotor nerve lesions, localization of the ANS lesion can be achieved with brain and spine imaging.

Pupillary diameter depends on the balance between sympathetic activation and parasympathetic inhibition. A pupil cycle time is a simple bedside method of testing pupillary autonomic function with measurements of 100 subsequent light responses. Abnormally prolonged pupil cycle time signifies autonomic dysfunction. The amplitude of pupillary diameter reduction reflects parasympathetic function, while the latency to reach maximum dilation measures sympathetic activity. Pupillometry uses infrared dynamic pupillometers, which can quantify the change in the pupil diameter during the course of a light reflex and divide it into several separately analyzed parameters, including the latency from light stimulus to onset of pupillary dilation, the slope of the parasympathetic (constrictive) phase, pupillary reflex amplitude, and the slope of redilation (sympathetic phase) *(3,13)*. Conjunctival application of drugs can localize to preganglionic or postganglionic lesion as well as help to determine autonomic dysfunction (sympathetic vs parasympathetic) when the lesion is postganglionic. Cocaine, phenylephrine, pilocarpine, and hydroxyamphetamine solutions are frequently used.

Lacrimal secretion may also be impaired in autonomic dysfunction, either directly or indirectly. The main lacrimal gland has parasympathetic innervation and functions primarily during reflex tear secretion. Reflex tears are stimulated by sensory stimuli through afferent impulses transmitted in the first division of the trigeminal nerve (V_1) and the efferent pathway is parasympathetic. In addition, tearing can be a component of coughing, yawning, and vomiting. Lacrimal secretion can be assessed with Schimer's test, and damage from deficient secretions can be visualized using instillation of rose bengal followed by slit-lamp examination. Decreased reflex tear production is seen in any process that affects parasympathetic muscarinic function, such as Lambert-Eaton myasthenic syndrome, panautonomic neuropathies, multiple system atrophy, Rilay-Day syndrome, and Guillain-Barré syndrome *(13)*.

Renal and Urinary Function

Activation of the parasympathetic fibers to the bladder produces contraction of the detrusor muscle. Activation of the sympathetic fibers produces relaxation of the detrusor and contraction of the trigone with contraction of internal sphincter. Thus voiding is a complex process coordinated in the pons, which requires detrussor contraction (parasympathetic excitation and sympathetic inhibition) and sphincter relaxation (sympathetic inhibition). The use of medications with anticholinergic effects may unmask urinary bladder dysfunction in autonomic failure. Nocturnal polyuria is a common finding in autonomic disorders and can lead to reduction in extracellular fluid volume. The urological evaluation of patients with autonomic bladder dysfunction in the NSU starts with measurement of the urinary post-void residual volume. In the absence of bladder outlet obstruction, increased residual volumes indicate either bladder motor denervation or loss of sphincter relaxation usually associated with a lower motor neuron process such as diabetic autonomic neuropathy. This may result in chronic urinary tract infections. Once NSU patients are more stable, urodynamic measurements (cystometry) are valuable in investigating the function of the bladder musculature and sphincter mechanisms.

Chemical Measurements

Various neurotransmitters and hormones can be measured in response to stimuli such as head-up tilt that results in sympathoneural activation and normally increases levels of NE in plasma. Standing and lying catecholamines and their metabolites, renin, aldosterone, and vasopressin are tested. Supine plasma NE blood concentrations depend on the release from unstimulated sympathetic postganglionic noradrenergic terminals. On the other hand, the standing NE values reflect activation of these terminals mediated by CNS command. In control subjects, supine plasma NE levels almost double after assuming an upright position, reflecting increase in sympathetic nerve required to counteract the effects of blood pooling in the lower extremities induced by gravity. Patients with PAF usually have low supine plasma NE levels, whereas patients with multiple system atrophy (MSA) and AF have normal or slightly elevated NE levels. However, in CNS disorders the plasma NE levels do not increase in response to standing whereas the inverse is present in the PNS disorders since the remaining peripheral nerves have intact central connections. These findings can help to distinguish between peripheral and central forms of dysautonomia. Measurements of plasma aldosterone and renin activity is useful in Addison's disease and adrenocortical failure, with basal plasma renin levels being markedly elevated, and low or absent plasma aldosterone concentration *(1,2,7)*.

SPECIFIC CONDITIONS ASSOCIATED WITH AUTONOMIC DYSFUNCTION

Cerebrovascular Diseases

It is well known from animal and clinical studies that cerebrovascular diseases can disturb cardiovascular and autonomic function (Table 2). Cardiac arrhythmias and myocardial injury are common complications of cerebrovascular syndromes mediated in large part by ANS and add significantly to their morbidity and mortality. Cerebral ischemia, in particular, is associated with arterial hypertension, bradycardia, and respiratory depression *(14)*. The ischemic response is usually not the result of stimulation of the receptors outside the brain (i.e., baroreceptors), but is rather contained and integrated within the CNS (cortex, hypothalamus, medulla). This is related to the cardiovascular responses observed with increased intracranial pressure (ICP), where the Cushing's triad (hypertension, bradycardia, and altered respirations) is also the result of direct brain stimulation (*see also* Chapter 5). This response is regarded as one of the forms of neurogenic hypertension. It has been suggested that this changes result from distortion of the medulla oblongata and that an elevated arterial BP serves as a compensatory mechanism to increase cerebral blood flow (CBF) and maintain CPP. Signs of elevated ICP may occur as early as 12–24 h after stroke onset, with initial signs of hiccups, vomiting, increased drowsiness, and altered pupillary reflexes.

Horner's syndrome is also a well-recognized manifestation of sympathetic division injury in specific cerebrovascular lesion locations *(15)*. Other aspects of AF have been given less attention but disorders of sweating (hyper- or hypohidrosis), temperature regulation (hyper and hypothermia), genitourinary problems (voiding and sexual dysfunction), and mood disorders (depression, anxiety) are fairly common after stroke *(16–22)*. SAH is a typical example of an acute CNS lesion associated with massive increase in sympathetic tone *(4,23)* (*see also* Chapter 20).

Autonomic changes in many stroke patients can be anticipated based on the location of the lesion *(1,24–27)* (*see also* Chapter 8). Both experimental and clinical studies indicate that certain parts of the cerebral hemisphere, such as insular cortex, amygdala, and lateral hypothalamus have great influence on the ANS control. Evidence also exists for cortical asymmetry in the regulation of cardiovascular function, as many experimental and clinical stroke studies demonstrate that sympathetic activation is lateralized after brain infarction with right-sided dominance for sympathetic effect. It is believed that most cardiovascular dysrrhythmias are associated with "sympathetic surge" as reflected by increased plasma catecholamines concentrations. Increased incidence of supraventricular

Table 2
The Most Common ANS Manifestations in Cerebrovascular Disorders

Autonomic signs/symptoms	Pathophysiological mechanism	Structure involved
Cardiovascular		
Arrhythmias, hypertension, myocardial injury	Increased sympathetic tone ("sympathetic surge")	Frontal cortex, insula
Sudden cardiac death		Right hemisphere strokes associated with greater ("malignant") ECG changes
Sweating		
Hyper-, hypohidriosis	Descending vasomotor pathways involving autonomic skin vasomotor reflexes	No specific location, usually not present in occipital lesions
Thermoregulation		
Hyper-, hypothermia		Hypothalamus
Pupillary abnormalities		
Miosis, mydriasis,	Central: hypothalamus, brainstem	Brainstem
Horner's syndrome (miosis, ptosis, anhidriosis)	Peripheral: middle cranial fossa lesions, carotid artery in the neck, cervical sympathetic chain, anterior C8-T1-T3	PICA and vertebral artery strokes (Wallenberg's syndrome)
Genitourinary		
Voiding problems	Removal of cortical inhibition on PMC	ACA strokes involving anterior cingulate and paracentral regions of frontal lobes—most common
Sexual dysfunction	Pathways involved in sexual arousal	Hypothalamus, limbic system, R > L
Mood disorders		
Depression, anxiety	Disruption of reciprocal pathways linking midline limbic structures with subcortical nuclei	Limbic system—cingulate gyrus, hippocampus, amygdala cortex, subcortical and paralimbic structures, brainstem R > L

PMC, pontine micturition center; PICA, posterior inferior cerebellar artery; ECG, electrocardiogram; R, right cerebral hemisphere; L, left cerebral hemisphere.

tachycardias in right-sided strokes raises also the speculation that decrease in cardiac parasympathetic activity may be partially responsible for probable reciprocal rise in sympathetic tone. Right hemispheric strokes, especially those involving the region of the insula are associated with less favorable outcome attributed to high incidence of life threatening cardiac arrhythmias, myocardial damage (contraction band necrosis), and increased susceptibility to sudden cardiac death. In patients with acute stroke, the incidence of sudden death as a result of arrhythmic causes has been reported to exceed 6% (28). The insular cortex is frequently involved in stroke because of thromboembolic middle cerebral artery occlusion, which is a frequent cause of ischemic stroke, and the importance of insula on sympathovagal balance has been well documented. Therefore patients with insular strokes, especially within the right hemisphere, may require more intensive cardiovascular monitoring in the NSU setting with prophylactic treatment to prevent sudden death (16,29,26).

Seizures

Seizures are often accompanied by autonomic changes. These changes can be present as the predominant seizure manifestation, or more often, as an accompaniment to other seizure signs and symptoms (30). Autonomic symptoms have been described in subclinical, simple partial, complex partial, and primary or secondarily generalized seizures, with the majority of symptoms referable to cardiovascular and gastrointestinal manifestation. These autonomic phenomena probably occur through the spread of an ictal discharge from cerebral cortex to highly interconnected hypothalamus and limbic system (31). Abdominal symptoms are one of the most common early symptoms of partial seizures. Descriptions range from vague unusual or unpleasant feelings to well-defined pain, nausea and vomiting, belching, hunger, or fear. The next most common ictal autonomic symptomatology includes cardiovascular and thoracic symptoms. Chest pain and palpitations are most commonly reported, with sinus tachycardia being the most frequently reported sign of electrographic seizure. Complex arrhythmias occur less frequently, but an excessive mortality among patients with epilepsy has been attributed to cardiovascular factors. Premature atrial or ventricular arrhythmias, conduction blocks, changes in ST segment, and T-wave abnormalities have been demonstrated (5,30,31). Seizure-induced disruption of cardiovascular function is particularly significant since it may be related to the phenomenon of sudden, unexpected, and unexplained death that occurs in some epileptic patients (28,32). It is believed that SNS activity, rather then PSNS discharge, may cause a fatal cardiac response. Neurogenic pulmonary edema has been proposed as alternative mechanism for sudden death in epileptics. It is likely that this process begins with centrally mediated excessive adrenergic surge and is followed by other cardiovascular phenomena. Hyperventilation or prolonged apnea can also be the contributing factors (5,32). Vasomotor symptoms, including blanching, flushing, erythema, or cyanosis are also frequently reported autonomic abnormalities associated with seizures. Hypersecretion, with increased bronchial secretions, perspiration, and lacrimation are often a part of generalized tonic-clonic seizures (GTC) (27). Also, pupillary symptoms (miosis, mydriasis, hippus) may occur during seizures, and especially unilateral ictal pupillary dilation can cause significant diagnostic dilemma. The most commonly recognized urinary symptom occurring with seizures is urinary incontinence (31).

Endocrine disorders, such as pheochromocytoma or carcinoid syndrome, should be considered in the differential diagnosis of autonomic seizures. Pheochromocytoma causes paroxysmal hypertension, sweating, pallor, and headache. Carcinoid syndrome can present with bronchoconstricion, flushing, and diarrhea. A rare syndrome of paroxysmal autonomic dysfunction is termed diencephalic seizures. It is characterized by attacks of sudden hypertension, flushing, and tachycardia. It is unlikely to have true epileptic basis as seizures have never been documented by electroencephalography. Although the exact mechanism of this disorder is still unclear, it is thought to be associated with hypothalamic, thalamic, or brainstem injury and represents a release phenomenon. Most cases in clinical practice are related to severe closed head injury, usually associated with diffuse axonal injury in the subcortical white matter. Treatment can be difficult because this syndrome usually does not respond to typical anticonvulsants. It may respond to bromocriptine, morphine, or chlorpromazine administration *(31,33)*.

Guillain-Barré Syndrome

Guillain-Barré syndrome (GBS) a.k.a acute inflammatory demyelinating polyradiculoneuritis (AIDP) is an acute polyneuropathy characterized by ascending progressive, and relatively symmetric motor weakness that may involve respiratory or bulbar muscles *(34–36)* (*see also* Chapter 27). Dysautonomia is a well-recognized feature in patients with fully developed GBS, occurring in over one half of patients. However, most of them have only minor aspects of autonomic failure including mild orthostatic hypotension, altered sweating, peripheral cyanosis from vasomotor instability, and sinus bradycardia or tachycardia *(37)* (Table 3).

Dysautonomia is more common in patients with severe motor deficits and respiratory failure and life-threatening dysautonomia, an extreme form of autonomic disturbances in GBS, occurs most frequently in the acute evolving phase. It is important to exclude secondary causes of ANS changes including, sepsis, hypoxia, GI bleeding, pulmonary emboli, or disturbances in fluid or electrolyte status before assuming that they are due to the disease process of GBS itself.

ANS involvement may take the form of autonomic overactivity and/or underactivity, sometimes alternating with each other. Common autonomic abnormalities include cardiac dysrhythmias, with sustained sinus tachycardia being probably the most common. Sinus tachycardia is usually harmless and direct treatment may not be necessary unless it causes myocardial ischemia as seen on ECG, or leads to atrial flutter or fibrillation. In contrast, vagally mediated arrhythmias are among the most ominous cardiac complications in GBS. Excessive unregulated vagal activity, likely generated by ectopic activity in a diseased vagus nerve, could lead to episodes of sudden bradycardia, bronchorea, hypotension, and sinus arrest or asystole that may occur with or without an obvious "vagotonic" stimulus. These vagal spells may be noted in response to direct vagotonic procedures like tracheal suctioning, gagging, or Valsalva-like maneuvers. A cardiac pacemaker should be placed prophylactically in patients with demonstrated second or third-degree atrioventricular block or profound bradycardia. Arrhythmias other than sinus tachycardia (possible effect of excessive sympathetic outflow) or vagal spells (sympathetic hypofunction) are much less frequent but are also present. These other arrhythmias and ECG changes include ventricular tachycardia, changes in ST segment, prolonged Q-T intervals, axis deviation, flat or inverted T waves, and various forms of conduction blocks. Other forms of ANS involvement are changes in arterial BP and continuous BP recordings have identified unpredictable swings of hypertension and hypotension. Hypertension may be identified at presentation and later close cardiovascular monitoring can differentiate sustained hypertension (relatively rare, 5–8%) from the paroxysmal form (25–30%). Paroxysmal hypertension is often associated with severe muscle weakness and ventilatory dependence, and can lead to suspicion of pheochromocytoma. Paroxysmal hypertensive episodes may be followed by abrupt hypotension (especially postural hypotension) or "vascular collapse" with sudden death. Some hypotensive episodes are preceded by "vagotonic" procedures, such as tracheal stimulation with intubation, gagging, or suctioning and/or vasoactive agents, as patients with GBS and AF are extremely sensitive to vasoactive drugs. The precise mechanisms of blood pressure disturbances are not known, but it is postulated that alterations in afferent baroreflex activity and disinhibition of central cardiodepressor system, may be the cause of hypertension. At rest, low blood pressure and normal heart rate predominate, but as soon as circulatory effector levels (i.e., norepinephrine) increase, receptor hypersensitivity may provide a dramatic exaggerated response *(35–37)*. If immediate BP reduction is necessary, short-acting titratable agents such as nitroprusside should be used.

Bladder and bowel dysfunction is also common and different ANS problems have been reported. Bladder abnormalities can produce urinary retention (very common) or overflow incontinence due to detrussor muscle hyporeflexia. The most common GI complications reported are constipation, some-

Table 3
The Most Common ANS Manifestation in the Guillain-Barré Syndrome

Autonomic signs/symptoms	Pathophysiological mechanism	Structure involved
Cardiovascular		
Tachycardia, hypertension, arrhythmias (asystole), ECG changes sensitivity to vasoactive drugs	Excessive sympathetic outflow ectopic/unregulated vagal activity	Paroxysmal hypertension (afferent baroreflex abnormality, elevated serum renin and NE), preganglionic sympathetic efferent fibers
Bradycardia, hypotension, orthostatic hypotension	Parasympathetic hyperfunction and/or sympathetic hypofunction "vagal spells"	Paroxysmal hypotension vagus and glossopharyngeal nerves
Vasoactive		
Facial flushing Chest tightening	Parasympathetic overactivity	Sudomotor fibers
Gastrointestinal		
Constipation, ileus, gastroparesis diarrhea, fecal incontinence	Extrinsic autonomic nerve control dysfunction	Enteric division of ANS
Genitourinary		
Urinary retention (most common) overflow incontinence (detrusor hyporeflexia)	Denervation of ANS control of perineal and periurethral muscles	Bladder autonomic nerve supply
Sweating and temperature		
Hyper-, hypohidriosis, anhidriosis	Compromised autonomic skin vasomotor reflexes	Sympathetic cholinergic fibers
Pupillary, ocular and lens accommodation abnormalities		
Miosis, mydriasis, ympathetic chain, cervical and ciliary ganglia, ptosis, blurred vision	Cervical sympathetic chain and	S
	ganglia involvement and/or postganglionic parasympathetic blockage	CN III

GBS, Guillain-Barré syndrome; CNs, cranial nerves; NE, norepinephrine; ECG, electrocardiogram; CN III, 3rd cranial nerve/oculomotor; ANS, autonomic nervous system.

times ileus and gastroparesis, rarely fecal incontinence. Other symptoms include pupillary and lens accommodation abnormalities (i.e., iridoplegia), facial flushing, lacrimal and salivary gland abnormalities, sexual dysfunction, temperature and sweating alterations, and syndrome of inappropriate antidiuretic hormone secretion, leading to hyponatremia. Treatment of these other forms of dysautonomia is rarely indicated and is limited to symptomatic relief in most cases.

Pure pandysautonomia (acute dysautonomic neuropathy) is a rare variant of immune polyradiculoneuropathy characterized by predominant autonomic symptoms (abdominal pain, nausea and vomiting, constipation, diarrhea) and few, if any, somatic motor complaints seen after prodromal viral syndrome. Abdominal distention, ileus, and gastroparesis may develop. Orthostatic changes in BP lead to complaints ranging from lightheadedness to severe orthostatic hypotension with recurrent syncope. Additional early autonomic manifestations include urinary problems, erectile dysfunction, acrocyanosis due to vasomotor instability, and reduced sweating, lacrimation, and salivation. Muscle strength and sensation are usually normal, but deep tendon reflexes are often reduced or absent later in the disease. Specialized ANS test results are uniformly abnormal in these patients.

Management of Dysautonomia in Guillain-Barré Syndrome

Many of the features of autonomic dysfunction in GBS are self-limited and require no intervention. For example, resting tachycardia or transient hypertension does nor require active treatment, except in patients with prior cardiovascular diseases. Management of patients with GBS and severe dysautonomia requires increased vigilance to detect potentially dangerous complications, as autonomic dysfunction competes only with respiratory failure and thromboembolism as a cause for intensive care requirements. For this reason, most patients with GBS require admission to the NSU. Respiratory failure should be anticipated in any patient with GBS progressive limb or craniobulbar weakness (as discussed in Chapter 27). Routine ECG monitoring may disclose severe rhythm disturbances requiring pharmacologic or pacemaker therapy. Patients with significant blood pressure fluctuations and serious dysrhythmias present a challenge to the neurointensivist. The combination of beta-blockers, angiotensin-converting enzyme inhibitors, and pacemaker may provide protection from extremes. Potent sympathomimetic agents generally should be avoided because of the risk of rebound hypertension, but vasopressors may be required for treatment of persistent hypotension. The routine use of Swan-Ganz monitoring may be beneficial, as intravascular volume should be carefully maintained, particularly during positive-pressure ventilation. If plasma exchange is selected as treatment option, physicians need to be acutely aware of possible volume depletion or electrolyte imbalance during procedure. Micturitional dysfunction can be managed with an indwelling urinary catheter or intermittent catheterization. Patients with GI manifestations should be managed with a bowel regimen including stool softeners and laxatives. Narcotics or medications impairing GI motility should be used sparingly. In cases of ileus GI tract rest should be instituted, electrolyte imbalances corrected and total parenteral nutrition entertained. Dysautonomias generally resolve as other features of GBS improve, however, blood pressure lability may persist much longer or constitute a chronic residual sequela of the disease, which, in our experience, may be steroid responsive *(35–37)*.

Botulism

The potent neurotoxin produced from the anaerobic, spore-forming bacterium *Clostridium botulinum* produces a neuroparalytic disease called botulism. This exotoxin blocks presynaptic release of ACh at both, somatic and autonomic synapses. The clostridial toxins are generally regarded as "the most poisonous poisons," and can cause death in humans in doses as small as 0.05–0.1 μg *(38–40)*. Although there are eight strains of bacteria, almost all cases of botulism in humans are caused by one of three serotypes (A, B, or E). The clinical presentation of severe botulism is often stereotypical despite five different clinical categories that are now recognized *(1,38–40)* (*see also* Chapter 28).

Autonomic signs and symptoms can range from mild constipation, dry mouth, nausea and vomiting to profound cholinergic failure with pupillary abnormalities, paralytic ileus, and urinary retention (Table 4). The pupils are paralyzed in half of the patients and impaired accommodation is responsible for blurred vision, an early symptom. Fluctuating BP with postural hypotension and decreased vasomotor tone can also be present. Although constipation is the most frequent GI symptom, nausea, vomiting, and diarrhea may present early in the disease course. Autonomic dysfunction in patients with botulism is further suggested by beat-to-beat heart rate R-R interval variability, depressed or absent sympathetic skin responses, and decreased plasma noradrenaline levels.

The mainstay of treatment for severe botulism is supportive care, with special attention to respiratory status. Adjunctive or experimental forms of therapy include pharmacological treatment with guanidine and 4-aminopyridine (4-AP). Both drugs enhance the release of ACh from nerve terminals and 4-AP is though to block potassium channels and increase calcium influx via voltage-gated presynaptic terminal membrane channels leading to increase of ACh quanta. Both drugs have little effect in reversing respiratory paralysis or autonomic abnormalities but are known to have potentially serious side effects; seizures in case of 4-AP, and bone marrow suppression and nephritis with guanidine. Administration of commercially available botulinum antitoxin is controversial because of the lack of proven efficacy in many cases and the danger of serious side effects, including allergic reactions and anaphylaxis. To be potentially beneficial, antitoxin must be given early in the course of the disease, whereas the botulinum neurotoxin is still in the blood and before it is bound at the nerve terminals. Autonomic dysfunction is treated symptomatically. For instance, just like in GBS, patients with GI manifestations should be managed with a bowel regimen, avoidance of medications that impair peristalsis, correction of electrolyte imbalances, and bowel rest if necessary. Also patients should be kept well hydrated, particularly in those with fluctuating BP.

With the improvement in the intensive care management during the last century, fatality rates have decreased from 50% to close to 10% in recent years. Recovery from botulism is prolonged (weeks or months) but usually complete. The long recovery time is related to time needed for sprouting from nerve terminal at motor end plates. Recovery of autonomic function in most cases takes longer than that of neuromuscular transmission *(38–40)*.

Paraneoplastic Syndromes With Autonomic Dysfunction

Lambert-Eaton myasthenic syndrome, enteric neuropathy, and malignant sensory neuronopathy constitute three well-described paraneoplastic syndromes associated with both somatic and autonomic involvement. We discuss the predominant features of these disorders, concentrating on the ANS involvement.

Lambert-Eaton Myasthenic Syndrome

Lambert-Eaton myasthenic syndrome is associated with generalized muscle weakness but, unlike that of myasthenia gravis, the weakness improves when the muscle is exercised *(41–43)*. The pathogenesis of LEMS involves an immune attack on the presynaptic terminal of the neuromuscular junction. Antionconeural immune response with circulating IgG antibodies to presynaptic voltage-gated calcium channels (VGCC) interferes with calcium-dependent ACh release at both muscarinic and nicotinic sites. This leads to muscle weakness (proximal > bulbar > distal), especially the lower extremities, fatigability, and decrease of deep tendon reflexes. Classically, augmentation of muscle strength during maximal voluntary contraction (muscle facilitation), and post-tetanic potentiation of reflexes can be seen. The diagnosis of LEMS is made based on clinical features, anti-VGCC autoantibody test, and characteristic EMG findings. Serum antibodies can be detected in more than 90% of LEMS patients using standard radioimmunoassay. The electrophysiology of LEMS is essentially diagnostic, showing reduced resting compound muscle action potential (CMAP) amplitudes, decremental response on slow repetitive nerve stimulation, and pathognomonic marked increase of CMAP

Table 4
The Most Common ANS Manifestation in Botulism

Autonomic signs/symptoms	Pathophysiological mechanism	Structure involved
Cardiovascular		
Bradycardia, ECG changes hypotension/hypertension, orthostatic hypotension	Fluctuations in vasomotor tone parasympathetic hyperfunction and/or sympathetic hypofunction	Peripheral ANS, decreased parasympathetic baroreflex buffering ability
Gastrointestinal		
Paralytic ileus, gastroparesis with gastric dilatation dry mouth	Extrinsic autonomic nerve control dysfunction cholinergic failure	Enteric division of ANS
Genitourinary		
Urinary retention (most common) overflow incontinence detrusor hyporeflexia	Denervation of ANS control of perineal and periurethral muscles Cholinergic failure	Bladder autonomic nerve supply
Sweating		
Anhidriosis	Cholinergic failure with compromised autonomic skin vasomotor reflexes	Sympathetic cholinergic fibers
Pupillary, ocular and lens accommodation abnormalities		
Dry eyes, mydriasis ptosis, blurred vision ophthalmoplegia	Cervical sympathetic chain and ganglia involvement Cholinergic failure	Sympathetic chain, cervical and ciliary ganglia, multiple CNs

CNs, cranial nerves; ECG, electrocardiogram; ANS, autonomic nervous system.

amplitude after brief maximal voluntary contraction or rapid repetitive nerve stimulation (postexercise facilitation), an increase in CMAP amplitude that typically is greater than 100% of baseline.

Approximately 70–80% of patients with LEMS have autonomic symptoms and neuropathic elements, such as absent reflexes—features that are not seen in myasthenia gravis. Autonomic symptoms in LEMS were first summarized by Rubenstein et al., and considered to be specific cholinergic dysautonomia *(42)*. Fully developed autonomic failure in LEMS is characterized by dryness of the mouth (the most common autonomic manifestation), blurred vision, urinary retention, impaired sweating, and constipation. Sexual dysfunction can also be seen with erectile impotence and ejaculation dysfunction. Nearly 60–70% of patients with LEMS have underlying tumor, usually small cell carcinoma of the lung. LEMS may also present with respiratory failure requiring admission to the NSU and assisted ventilation. In some cases, prolonged apnea and respiratory failure can be precipitated by muscle relaxants (i.e., curare) used during general anesthesia.

Early detection and treatment of underlying cancer is critical. Eradication of cancer constitutes LEMS management, with addition of symptomatic and supportive management of concomitant ANS symptoms with enhancement of cholinergic function or immunosuppresion. Anticancer treatment sometimes results in improvement in the neurological symptoms of LEMS. Pyridostygmine, although not as effective as in myasthenia gravis, is used for its cholinergic effects. Intravenous or oral steroids with combination of azathioprine can result in symptomatic improvement or remission in some patients, although the clinical response is usually quite slow. For patients with severe symptoms and initial respiratory depression requiring intensive care, plasmapheresis or intravenous immunoglobulin (IVIg) produces clinical and electrophysiological improvement. Rapid symptomatic improvement (within an hour of oral ingestion) can also be achieved with 3,4-diaminopyridine (3,4-DAP).

Malignant Inflammatory Sensory Polyganglionopathy

Malignant inflammatory sensory polyganglionopathy (MISP) is another paraneoplastic neurologic disorder with subacute clinical presentation. Three major clinical presentations of MISP include combinations of ataxia, hyperalgesia with sensory symptoms, and gastrointestinal dysmotility. In addition to sensory ataxia with or without hyperalgesia or GI motility disturbances, MISP patients can also present with variable motor weakness, cerebellar ataxia, brainstem signs, myelopathy, and generalized dysautonomia (orthostatic hypotension, tonic pupils, sudomotor dysfunction, gastrointestinal symptoms). Because MISP may occasionally present as predominantly GI symptoms with intestinal pseudo-obstruction, neurological diagnosis can be substantially delayed. Abdominal complaints include nausea, vomiting, abdominal pain, and severe constipation. Acute intestinal obstruction has been reported, but no apparent causes could be discovered at laparotomy, suggesting motility disorder. Not unexpectedly, the main pathology has been inflamation with marked neuronal loss and Schwann cell proliferation in Auerbach's myenteric plexus *(44)*.

Neuroleptic Malignant Syndrome

Development of potent antipsychotic medications in the 1950s and 1960s revolutionized care of many psychiatric patients, but also introduced to medical community the neuroleptic malignant syndrome (NMS). This syndrome is thought to be an adverse idiosyncratic drug reaction associated with the use of neuroleptic drugs, resulting in sudden release of calcium from sarcoplasmic reticulum *(47)*. It is a life-threatening condition characterized by signs of encephalopathy, as manifested by mental and behavioral changes, skeletal muscle rigidity with increased serum levels of creatine kinase, severe hyperthermia, and profound autonomic instability. Contributing factors include ambient heat, and dehydration, underlying brain damage, and dementia. It typically occurs within the first 3–9 d of therapy but can also occur in a patient taking neuroleptics for a long time, as well as after a single dose of antipsychotic agent. Its incidence is estimated at approx 1% of patients treated with neuroleptics. The NMS-like syndrome has also been reported in the setting of withdrawal of antiparkinsonian medications, especially L-Dopa therapy. Autonomic hyperactivity is an important feature of NMS, and in addition to causing hyperthermia, it can also lead to tachycardia, cardiac dysrhythmias, diaphoresis, and fluctuating blood pressure. The pathophysiology of NMS is not fully understood, but it is believed to be a result of dopaminergic blockage in the basal ganglia and in the hypothalamus. This may result in an increase in heat production through muscle contraction and impairment of heat-dissipation mechanisms. NMS is an emergent neurological condition and early recognition and management is essential for recovery.

The treatment of NMS requires immediate discontinuation of antipsychotic drug(s), dopaminergic pharmacotherapy with oral bromocriptine and/or intravenous administration of dantrolene, and vigorous supportive measures. Admission to NSU may be necessary for close cardiovascular monitoring, surface and core cooling, and meticulous supportive care with aggressive hydration. The patients with NMS must be carefully monitored throughout the course of the disease (2 wk is the average time course of the syndrome) for possible complications, including electrolyte abnormalities, cardiac arrhythmias, sepsis, renal failure (secondary to high serum creatine kinase, muscle damage with high myoglobin load, and hemoglobinuria), aspiration pneumonia and pulmonary embolism. Because acute renal failure is the most common medical complication in NMS, aggressive hydration and close monitoring of fluid balance is crucial for its prevention. Autonomic instability leads to increased insensible losses associated with profound hyperthermia. Antipyretic agents combined with aggressive cooling can be very helpful. The mortality rate in NMS is estimated at 15–20%, with the most significant cause of morbidity and mortality being acute renal failure secondary to rhabdomyolysis, followed by aspiration pneumonia, sudden cardiac death from myocardial damage, or fatal arrhythmias *(1,45–47)*.

Serotonin Syndrome

The serotonin syndrome constitutes a constellation of symptoms including encephalopathy, motor hyperactivity with hyperreflexia, nausea and vomiting, and marked dysautonomia. Neuromuscular symptoms are seen in more than a half of cases and include rigidity, tremor, and myoclonus. Because of many overlapping aspects of the clinical presentation it can sometimes be confused with NMS and other encephalopathic states; therefore, obtaining comprehensive medication history can be crucial in the differential diagnosis (Table 5). The serotonin syndrome is thought to be a toxic effect of potent serotonomimetic agents due to a hyperstimulation of serotonin receptors (5HT-1a) in the brain and spinal cord, and is therefore different in etiology from NMS, an idiosyncratic reaction. Initial cases were reported in patients receiving high-dose tryptophan and monoamine oxidase inhibitor (MAOI) *(48)*. MAOI increase serotonin levels by inhibiting the breakdown of serotonin causing in some cases irreversible enzyme inhibition. More recent literature has also implicated in the etiology of SS newer antidepressant pharmacotherapy agents like the tricyclic antidepressants (TCAs), and selective serotonin reuptake inhibitors (SSRIs).

The autonomic manifestations of SS include tachycardia, tachypnea, elevation in temperature, diaphoresis, flushing, diarrhea, changes in blood pressure, and pupillary abnormalities. The serotonin syndrome is often mild and self-limited, with an uneventful recovery upon withdrawal of the causative agents. In rare cases, however, it can have a fulminant course with severe neuromuscular involvement, decreased level of consciousness, and marked autonomic instability. Acute renal failure, rhabdomyolysis, severe hyperkalemia, cardiac arrhythmias, disseminated intravascular coagulopathy (DIC), and seizures have been reported. Such patients will require careful NSU monitoring of cardiovascular and autonomic parameters, seizure precautions, mild sedation, and proper intravenous hydration. Syndrome-specific treatments have been proposed, including the use of serotonin antagonists (methysergide), propranolol, nitroglycerin, benadryl, and judicious use of benzodiazepines (lorazepam, clonazepam). No definite syndrome-specific recommendations exist at present, and aggressive supportive measures remain the mainstream of treatment.

Table 5
Distinguishing Features of Neuroleptic Malignant Syndrome and Serotonin Syndrome

Feature	Neuroleptic malignant syndrome	Serotonin syndrome
Mechanism and pathophysiology	Idiosyncratic drug reaction (idiopathic, *nor* dose related! sudden release of calcium from sarcoplasmic reticulum Dysregulation of dopaminergic system (central dopamine blockage or depletion)	Toxic effect of serotonin receptors hypersensitivity in the brain and spinal cord Enhancement of serotoninergic neurotransmission
Class of drugs involved	Antipsychotics/neuroleptics (i.e., haloperidol, chlorpromazine, risperidone, olanzepine) Withdrawal of antiparkinsonian medications (i.e., L-dopa, Sinemet)	SSRIs TCAs MAOIs
Clinical features	Triad: Hypertension (autonomic instability) Encephalopathy Skeletal muscles rigidity	Encephalopathy, hyperreflexia/rigidity, tremor, nausea, vomiting, marked autonomic instability
Differential clinical features	Extrapyramidal signs Very high fever Dysphagia Incontinence Sialorrhea	Myoclonus Hyperreflexia Ataxia *Hyperserotoninergic state* (i.e., carcinoid tumor): diarrhea, diaphoresis, vomiting
Most common ANS signs and symptoms	*Severe* hyperthermia, blood pressure instability, tachycardia, diaphoresis	*Mild* hyperthermia, diaphoresis
Laboratory findings	Increased CK, leukocytosis, myoglobinuria	Nonspecific
Average duration	Longer, usually less than 2 wk	Short, less than 72 h
Mortality	12–20%	
Specific treatment	Withdrawal of the offending drugs and aggressive supportive measures (NSU)* Dantrolene sodium Bromocriptine Amantadine	Withdrawal of the offending drugs and aggressive supportive measures (NSU)* Beta-blockers (propranolol) Benzodiazepines (clonazepam) Serotonin antagonists (cyproheptadine, methysergide)[+]

*Both syndromes can be fatal if not acutely and properly treated.
[+]Controversial; no well-design studies yet available.
NMS, neuroleptic malignant syndrome; SS, serotonin syndrome; SSRIs, selective serotonin reuptake inhibitors; TCAs, tricyclic antidepressants; MAOIs, monoamine oxidase inhibitors; CK, creatine kinase; NSU, neurosciences critical care unit.

Wernicke's Encephalopathy

Wernicke's encephalopathy (WE) is an acute or subacute syndrome that occurs in poor nutritional states with inadequate thiamine (vitamin B1) intake (most frequently seen in chronic alcoholics), states of gastrointestinal malabsorption, patients on long-term parenteral nutrition, or increased thiamine metabolic requirements (49,50). WE was first described in 1881 by the German neurologist, Karl Wernicke. He reported three patients (two chronic alcoholics) with signs and symptoms of acute mental confusion, ataxia, and ophthalmoplegia that resulted in their death. Autopsy revealed multiple small hemorrhages in the periventricular gray matter (mainly around third and fourth ventricles and the aqueduct). Wernicke's clinical description of the classic triad of symptoms (confusion, ophthalmoplegia, ataxia) is still the mainstay of clinical diagnosis and recognition. However, most patients will only present with one or two symptoms (50) (Table 6). WE may be precipitated acutely in high-risk thiamine-deficient patients by intravenous glucose administration. Stupor or coma, although rare presentations, will require NSU care.

Autonomic involvement is likely in patients with hypothermia and postural hypotension. The latter is quite a common finding in patients with WE and is often closely associated with alcoholic neuropathy. It probably reflects impairment of sympathetic outflow with involvement of brainstem and hypothalamic ANS pathways, as well as peripheral sympathetic vasomotor control in advanced stages of peripheral alcoholic neuropathy. Early involvement of sympathetic efferent fibers is often confirmed by the sweat tests, and postural hypotension is more likely to occur if the splanchnic outflow is also involved. Hypothermia may be sometimes the initial presenting feature, and occurs mainly in advanced cases (i.e., patients in stupor or coma), commonly with associated hypotension and bradycardia. In chronic alcoholics, neuropathy can also affect cranial nerves with vagus nerve being most commonly affected secondary to length-dependent, dying-back pathophysiology of the majority of peripheral neuropathies. The most distal myelinated segments of the vagus nerve are involved, but shorter and more proximal sympathetic fibers are not affected until later in the illness, when the peripheral neuropathy is already advanced. Clinical manifestations of alcoholic vagal neuropathy (often with the involvement of recurrent laryngeal nerve) include weakness of the tone of voice, hoarseness, and dysphagia. Other manifestations of parasympathetic dysfunction in alcoholics include abnormal pupillary reflexes, impaired esophageal and gastrointestinal motility, and impotence. Autonomic involvement can be confirmed with impaired HR response to VM, to postural changes, to deep breathing, and to atropine. Alcoholics with vagal neuropathy have increased mortality rates (49,50).

Immediate treatment with thiamine is a primary treatment of choice and should be continued daily in the acute phase of the disease. Recommended doses of thiamine include loading dose of 100–500 mg intravenously or intramuscularly, followed by 100 mg/d for 3–5 d. Thiamine is the only treatment known to alter the outcome of this disorder, and the need for administration of thiamine in patients with unexplained stupor or coma should be emphasized. When the global confusional state clears, some patients are left with Korsakoff's psychosis, characterized by poor memory with tendencies to confabulate, decreased learning ability, and general disorientation. Both clinical entities constitute Wernicke-Korsakoff syndrome. WE can be fatal in up to 20% of patients even when appropriate treatment is instituted.

Acute Intermittent Porphyria

Acute hepatic porphyrias constitute a heterogenous group of genetic metabolic disorders caused by enzymatic defects in the heme biosynthetic chain. A partial deficiency of one of the seven enzymes in the pathway causes characteristic clinical and biochemical features. Clinical symptoms alone are not sufficiently specific to distinguish between the various forms, and appropriate biochemical testing is necessary (Watson-Schwartz test, increased urinary excretion of aminolaevulinic acid and porphobilinogen). Acute attacks, which are often provoked by drugs, hormones, alcohol, smoking,

Table 6
The Most Common Clinical and ANS Manifestation in the Wernicke-Korsakoff Syndrome

Autonomic signs/symptoms	Summary of the most common clinical signs and symptoms	
	Pathophysiological mechanism	Structure involved
	W-KS is associated with lesions in CNS (hypothalamus, mammillary bodies, cerebellar vermis) and PNS (dying-back peripheral neuropathy; long, distal vagus fibers are affected first, and shorter, proximal sympathetic fibers get involved later)	
Cardiovascular		
Postural hypotension	"Alcoholic peripheral neuropathy"	Hypothalamus, brainstem, postganglionic sudomotor fibers
Arrhythmias/heart blocks	Malfunctioning sympathetic outflow at central and/or peripheral levels (late)	
ECG changes		
Gastrointestinal		
Impaired esophageal motility, gastroparesis	Extrinsic autonomic nerve control Dysfunction (parasympathetic) "Vagal neuropathy"	Vagus, enteric division of ANS
Genitourinary		
Incontinence	Disordered parasympathetic function	Bladder autonomic nerve supply
Sweating and temperature		
Hypothermia	Hypothalamic lesion	Posterior hypothalamus
Hypohidriosis	Early involvement of sympathetic efferent fibers	Sympathetic efferent fibers
Pupillary and ocular abnormalities		
Abnormal pupillary reflexes blurred vision	Sympathetic/parasympathetic imbalance	Brainstem, CNs, peripheral ocular effector organs

W-KS, Wernicke-Korsakoff syndrome; CNs, cranial nerves; ECG, electrocardiogram; CNS, central nervous system; PNS, peripheral nervous system; ANS, autonomic nervous system.

"Classic triad": confusion, ophtalmoplegia, ataxia (all three seen only in 16% of patients; combination of two seen in 27%, one "classic" manifestation seen in 37 % and no "classic" signs evident in 18 %).

Initial symptoms: confusion—66%, staggering gait—51%, ocular manifestations—40% (nystagmus—85%, bilateral abducens nerve palsy—54%, conjugate gaze palsy—45%), polyneuropathy—36%, exhaustion—20%, alcohol withdrawal manifestations—13%.

pregnancy, or calorie restrictions, are associated with a substantial morbidity and mortality, therefore the need for rapid and accurate diagnosis is essential, particularly because heme arginate can induce a definitive remission if given early into an attack. Any medication that induces the hepatic microsomal cytochrome P450 system can provoke a porphyric attack. Clinically similar acute attacks occur in four distinct types: acute intermittent porphyria (AIP), hereditary corpoporphyria, variegate porphyria, and plumboporphyria *(48)*. The cardinal features of CNS symptoms, peripheral neuropathy, and abdominal involvement characteristic of an acute attack are similar in all of the hepatic porphyrias.

The commonest porphyria type is AIP, an autosomal dominant disease of porphyrin metabolism resulting from the deficient activity of the enzyme hydroxymethylbilane synthase (a.k.a. porphobilinogen deaminase) *(51)* *(see also* Chapter 28). AIP is manifested by recurrent attacks of GI (severe abdominal pain, vomiting), neurologic (polyneuropathy, muscular weakness, hyporeflexia, cranial nerve palsies, convulsions, dysautonomia), and psychiatric symptoms (mental status changes). CNS symptoms include agitation, psychotic features, which may eventually progress to seizures and coma. The neuropathy, which usually follows shortly after acute attack, is typically a predominantly motor neuropathy resembling GBS. The combination of back pain and limb weakness may also suggest GBS, but the porphyrias often cause greater proximal than distal weakness, opposite to typical weakness seen in GBS. Flaccid quadriparesis and respiratory failure may prompt NSU admission and intubation.

ANS dysfunction presents predominantly as a sympathetic overactivity with tachycardia, hypertension, and abdominal colic. Parasympathetic symptoms are prominent. Clinical features of autonomic neuropathy include abdominal pain, nausea and vomiting, constipation/diarrhea, bladder distention, and sweating disorders. The occurrence of postural hypotension and/or labile hypertension suggests that, similarly to GBS, baroreceptor afferents are most likely involved. The pathogenic mechanisms, leading to peripheral neuropathy in porphyria are not completely understood, but heme protein deficiencies and neurotoxic excess of aminolevulinic acid can have detrimental effects on nervous tissue. Interestingly, ANS dysfunction in AIP occurs during the attacks and may reverse immediately afterwards, suggesting that nonstructural alterations in nerve function.

Management of the acute attack usually requires hospitalization *(52,53)*. Symptomatic relief of pain and vomiting with adequate hydration may be required. Drug treatment should be very cautious with only safe medication use (nonporphyrogenic) after reference to a special drug list. Opiates are safe and are the most effective analgesics for pain control during an acute attack, and should be used in sufficient dosages to provide significant pain relief. For maintenance of high-energy intake, oral and/or intravenous (via central line) glucose and heme arginate are the mainstay of treatment. Heme arginate is thought to be preferable to hematin, as it is more stable and has fewer side effects. Assisted ventilation may be necessary in patients with impending respiratory compromise. Sympathetic overactivity causing hypertension and tachycardia can be treated with oral or intravenous propranolol. Reserpine and guanethedine are also considered safe antihypertensive drugs for use in patients with acute porphyric attack. The management of seizures and mental status changes can be difficult secondary to limited number of drugs that can be used safely in these conditions. Some reports recommend the use of gabapentin for seizure control in AIP *(54)*. In some patients, residual neuropathic pain (low back, thighs, shoulders pain) with symptoms of autonomic neuropathy (cool extremities and excessive sweating), is present after the acute attack has settled. The prevention of acute attacks by counseling of affected individuals about the precipitating factors and family screening are the most beneficial measures of disease prevention. Molecular diagnosis allows easier identification of individuals at risk. Heavy metal intoxications with lead, arsenic, and thallium poisoning, may have similar clinical presentation to porphyria with abdominal and neuropathic symptoms, and increase in urinary coproporphiryns.

Primary Autonomic Failure

Full clinical spectrum of primary autonomic failure (PAF) includes, in addition to orthostatic hypotension, disturbances of sweating, bladder and bowel control, and sexual functions *(1)*. Postural hypotension in PAF is often greatest in the morning, because of nocturnal diuresis, after food ingestion secondary to splanchnic vasodilation, and in a hot environment because of cutaneous dilation not compensated for in other regions. In some patients, postural hypotension may be unmasked by exercise because vasodilation in skeletal muscles is not appropriately counteracted by autonomic reflexes. Other, non-neurogenic causes of postural hypotension must be considered in the differential diagnosis. The natural history of PAF reveals that clinical signs progress slowly over several years, and the CNS is generally unaffected. This is in contrast with AF associated with degenerative neurological disorders such as Parkinson's disease (PD), Lewy body disease (LBD), and multiple system atrophy (MSA). It is worth noting that at an early stage an accurate prognosis of AF is often difficult to establish. Disease may look like PAF for many years, with relatively static clinical course, or with time may develop into PD, or MSA. Conversely, the clinical features of AF may be detected later in some patients with CNS disorders.

There is good clinical and pathological evidence that most patients with primary AF (as opposed to secondary AF) have significant loss of intermediolateral cell columns in the thoracolumbar regions, the final common pathway for the sympathetic nervous system. Paravertebral ganglia are also affected. It has been therefore speculated that the pathological process (metabolic, viral, immunological, or other) that leads to this selective cell loss differs in PAF (and probably in AF with PD) from that in AF associated with MSA. Additionally, loss of ganglionic neurons seen often in PAF and preserved in MSA, suggests more distal pathological process in PAF than in MSA. This is in agreement with the common clinical belief that CNS is not affected in PAF. The evaluation and proper diagnosis of the primary cause of autonomic symptoms is therefore needed in order to plan appropriate treatment generally attained through formal testing of the ANS in an autonomic laboratory. Both PAF and central autonomic syndromes are treated mainly symptomatically to maintain the quality of life for as long as possible. Patients with PAF have relatively good prognosis, often with essentially 20-yr life expectancy, despite the disabilities resulting from AF.

Patients with PAF seldom require NSU admission related to dysautonomia only. However, when they are hospitalized for other reasons (i.e., sepsis), management of their vital parameters (BP, HR, temperature, and so on) becomes more difficult. The same general principles of treatment outlined for other forms of AF should be followed.

Spinal Cord Injury

Spinal cord injury (SCI) is covered in more detail in Chapter 23 of this book; therefore, we will concentrate briefly on specific autonomic features that accompany disorders of spinal cord, especially spinal shock (acutely after SCI) and autonomic dysreflexia (delayed SCI complication). Spinal shock is defined as an immediate flaccid paralysis and abolition of reflex activity below the level of the lesion, following SCI (predominantly complete cord transection, but has also been described after incomplete lesions). Tendon reflexes are most commonly affected with the anal reflex being relatively spared in many cases. Return of reflexes is gradual over a 3- to 6-wk period, with development of increased reflex activity (spasticity). Autonomic dysreflexia is a condition of massive paroxysmal reflex sympathetic response to noxious stimuli occurring in patients with high spinal cord injuries, above the major splanchnic sympathetic outflow (T4–T6). It can occur in both complete and incomplete SCI usually after resolution of the spinal shock phase, but "early" dysreflexia has also been described *(55)*. Clinical features depend in large part upon the profound reflex sympathetic cholinergic and adrenergic responses, provoked in most episodes by stimulation from genitourinary and/or alimentary structures. Most common signs and symptoms include paroxysmal hypertension (sometimes two to three times baseline values), cardiac dysrhythmias, tachycardia/bradycardia, pilomotor and sudomotor changes (pallor/flashing, sweating in areas around and above the lesion), paresthesias in the neck and shoulders, headache, chest pain, and visual disturbances. Removal of the noxious stimuli usually results in abrupt decline of the dysautonomic symptoms. SCI patients are at increased risk for other serious neurological complications accompanying autonomic dysreflexia, including stroke (ischemic or hemorrhagic), and seizures *(56)*. Bradycardia in respirator-dependent patients with high spinal cord injury may require a combination of oxygen, atropine, and if necessary, a temporary demand pacemaker.

REFERENCES

1. Mathias CJ. Disorders of autonomic nervous system. In Bradley WC, Daroff RB, Fenichel, GM, Marsden CD, eds. *Neurology in Clinical Practice*, 3rd ed. Boston: Butterworth Heinemann, 2000, pp. 2131–2165.
2. Appenzeller O, Oribe E. *The Autonomic Nervous System: An Introduction to Basic and Clinical Concepts*, 5th ed. New York: Elsevier, 1997.
3. Chemali KR, Chelimsky TC. Autonomic testing. In Katirji B, Kaminski HJ, Preston DC, Ruff RL, Shapiro BE, eds. *Neuromuscular Disorders in Clinical Practice*. Boston: Butterworth Heinemann, 2002, pp. 193–210.
4. Benarroch EE. The central autonomic network. In Low PA, ed. *Clinical Autonomic Disorders. Evaluation and Management*, 2nd ed. Philadelphia: Lippincot-Raven, 1997, pp. 17–22.
5. Wannamaker BB. Autonomic nervous system and epilepsy. *Epilepsia* 1985;26(Suppl):S31–S39.
6. Benarroch EE. Central disorders of autonomic function. In Katirji B, Kaminski HJ, Preston DC, Ruff RL, Shapiro BE, eds. *Neuromuscular Disorders in Clinical Practice*. Boston: Butterworth Heinemann, 2002, pp. 421–428.
7. Polinsky RJ. Neurochemical and pharmacological abnormalities in chronic autonomic failure syndromes. In Low PA, ed. *Clinical Autonomic Disorders. Evaluation and Management*, 2nd ed. Philadelphia: Lippincot-Raven, 1997, pp. 585–595.
8. Harati Y, Machkas H. Spinal cord and peripheral nervous system. In Low PA, ed. *Clinical Autonomic Disorders. Evaluation and Management*, 2nd ed. Philadelphia: Lippincot-Raven, 1997, pp. 25–45.
9. Calaresu FR, Yardley CP. Medullary basal sympathetic tone. *Annu. Rev. Physiol.* 1988;50:511–524.
10. Novak P, Lepicovska V, Dostalek C. Periodic amplitude modulation of EEG. *Neurosci. Lett.* 1992;136:213–215.
11. Novak P. Topography of slow modulation of EEG in normal subjects during rest and head-up tilt. *Clin. Auton. Res.* 1994;4:2000–2002.
12. Smith SA, Smith SE. Pupil function: tests and disorders. In Bannister R, Mathias CJ, eds. *Autonomic Failure. A Textbook of Clinical Disorders of the Autonomic Nervous System*, 4th ed. Cambridge, UK: Oxford University Press, 1999, pp. 245–253.
13. Cross SA. Evaluation of pupillary and lacrimal function. In Low PA, ed. *Clinical Autonomic Disorders. Evaluation and Management*, 2nd ed. Philadelphia: Lippincot-Raven, 1997, pp. 259–268.
14. Korpelainen JT, Sotaniemi KA, Huikuri HV, et al. Abnormal heart rate variability as a manifestation of autonomic dysfunction in hemispheric brain infarction. *Stroke* 1996;27:2059–2063.
15. Bassetti C, Staikov IN. Hemiplegia vegetativa alterna (ipsilateral Horner's syndrome and contralateral hemihyperhydrosis) following proximal posterior cerebral artery occlusion. *Stroke* 1995;26:702–704.
16. Orlandi G, Fanucchi S, Strata G, et al. Transient autonomic nervous system dysfunction during hyperacute stroke. *Acta. Neurol. Scand.* 2000;102:317–321.
17. Smith CD. A hypothalamic stroke producing recurrent hemihyperhydrosis. *Neurology* 2001;56:1394–1396.
18. Korpelainen JT, Sotaniemi KA, Myllyla VV. Hyperhidrosis as a reflection of autonomic failure in patients with acute hemispheral brain infarction. An evaporimetric study. *Stroke* 1992;23:1271–1275.
19. Brittain KR, Peet SM, Castleden CM. Stroke and incontinence. *Stroke* 1998;29:524–528.
20. Marinkovic SP, Badlani G. Voiding and sexual dysfunction after cerebrovascular accidents. *J. Urol.* 2001;359–370.
21. Korpelainen JT, Nieminen P, Myllyla VV. Sexual functioning among stroke patients and their spouses. *Stroke* 1999;30:715–719.
22. MacHale SM, O'Rourke Sj, Wardlaw JM, et al. Depression and its relation to lesion location after stroke. *J. Neurol. Neurosurg. Psychiatry* 1998;64:371–374.
23. Hirashima Y, Takashima S, Matsumura N, et al. Right sylvian fissure subarachnoid hemorrhage has electrocardiographic consequences. *Stroke* 2001;32:2278–2281.
24. Korpelainen JT,Sotaniemi KA, Makikallio A, et al. Dynamic behavior of heart rate in ischemic stroke. *Stroke* 1999;30:1008–1013.
25. Naver HS, Blomstrand C, and Wallin BG. Reduced heart rate variability after right sided-stroke. *Stroke* 1996;27:247–251.
26. Cheung RTF, Hachinski V. The insula and cerebrogenic sudden death. *Arch. Neurol.* 2000;57;1685–1688.

27. Stefan H, Pauli E, Kerling F, et al. Autonomic auras: left hemispheric predominance of epileptic generators of cold shivers and goose bumps? *Epilepsia* 2002;43:41–45.
28. Tokgozoglu SL, Batur MK, Topcuoglu MA, et al. Effects of stroke localization on cardiac autonomic balance and sudden death. *Stroke* 1999;30:1307–1311.
29. Oppenheimer SM, Gelb A, Girvin JP, et al. Cardiovascular effects of human insular cortex stimulation. *Neurology* 1992;42:1727–1732.
30. Baumgartner C, Lurger S, Leutmezer F. Autonomic symptoms during epileptic seizures. *Epileptic Disord.* 2001;3:103–106.
31. Liporace JD, Sperling MR. Simple autonomic seizures. In Engel J Jr, Pedley A, eds. *Epilepsy: A Comprehensive Textbook*, 3rd ed. Philadelphia: Lippincot-Raven, 1997, pp. 549–555.
32. Lathers CM, Schraeder PL, Boggs JG. Sudden unexplained death and autonomic dysfunction. In Engel J Jr, Pedley A, eds. *Epilepsy: A Comprehensive Textbook*. 3rd ed. Philadelphia: Lippincot-Raven, 1997, pp. 1943–1955.
33. Tong C, Konig MW, Roberts PR, et al. Autonomic dysfunction secondary to intracerebral hemorrhage. *Anesth. Analg.* 2000;91:1450–1451.
34. Chalela JA. Pearls and pitfalls in the intensive care management of Guillain-Barré syndrome. *Semin. Neurol.* 2001;21:399–405.
35. Gorson KC, Ropper AH. Guillain-Barré syndrome (acute inflamatory demyelinating polyneuropathy) and related disorders. In Katirji B, Kaminski HJ, Preston DC, Ruff RL, Shapiro BE, eds. *Neuromuscular Disorders in Clinical Practice*. Boston: Butterworth-Heinemann, 2002, pp. 544–566.
36. Ropper AH: Intensive care of acute Guillain-Barré syndrome. *Can. J. Neurol. Sci.* 1994;21:S23–S27.
37. Zochodne DW. Autonomic involvement in Guillain-Barré syndrome: A review. *Muscle Nerve* 1994;17:1145–1155.
38. Shapiro RL, Hatheway C, Swerdlow DL. Botulism in the United States: a clinical and epidemiologic review. *Ann. Intern. Med.* 1998;129:221–228.
39. Cherington M. Clinical spectrum of botulism. *Muscle Nerve* 1998;21:701–710.
40. Cherington M. Botulism. In Katirji B, Kaminski HJ, Preston DC, Ruff RL, Shapiro BE, eds. *Neuromuscular Disorders in Clinical Practice*. Boston: Butterworth-Heinemann, 2002, pp. 942–952.
41. Eaton LM, Lambert EH. Electromyography and electric stimulation of nerves in diseases of motor unit: observations on myasthenic syndrome associated with malignant tumors. *JAMA* 1957;163:1117–1124.
42. Rubenstein AE, Horowitz SH, Bender AN. Cholinergic dysautonomia and Eaton-Lambert syndrome. *Neurology* 1979;29:720–723.
43. Maddison P, Newsom-Davis J. Lambert-Eaton myasthenic syndrome. In Katirji B, Kaminski HJ, Preston DC, Ruff RL, Shapiro BE, eds. *Neuromuscular Disorders in Clinical Practice*. Boston: Butterworth-Heinemann, 2002, pp. 931–941.
44. Smith BE, Windebank AJ. Dorsal root ganglion disorders. In Katirji B, Kaminski HJ, Preston DC, Ruff RL, Shapiro BE, eds. *Neuromuscular Disorders in Clinical Practice*. Boston: Butterworth-Heinemann, 2002, pp. 478–500.
45. Bertram M, Schwarz S, Werner H. Acute and critical care in neurology. *Eur. Neurol.* 1997;38:155–166.
46. Schmidt HB, Werden K, Muller-Werden U. Autonomic dysfunction in the ICU patient. *Curr. Opin. Crit. Care* 2001;7:314–322.
47. Carbone JR. The neuroleptic malignant and serotonin syndromes. *Emerg. Med. Clin.* 2000;18:317–325.
48. LoCurto MJ. The serotonin syndrome. *Emerg. Med. Clin.* 1997;15:665–675.
49. Harper CG, Giles M, Finlay-Jones R. Clinical signs in the Wernicke-Korsakoff complex: a retrospective analysis of 131 cases diagnosed at necropsy. *J. Neurol. Neurosurg. Psych.* 1986;49:341–345.
50. Victor M, Adams RD, Collins GH. The Wernicke-Korsakoff syndrome and related neurologic disorders due to alcoholism and malnutrition. *Contemp. Neurol. Series* Philadelphia: FA Davis 1989; vol. 3.
51. Suarez JI, Cohen ML, Larkin J, et al. Acute intermittent porphyria: clinicopathologic correlation. *Neurology* 1997;48:1678–1883.
52. Thadani H, Deacon A, Peters T. Diagnosis and management of porphyrias. *BMJ* 2000;320;1647–1651.
53. Elder GH, Hift RJ. Treatment of acute porphyria. *Hosp. Med.* 2001;62:422–425.
54. Zadra M, Grandi R, Erli LC, et al. Treatment of seizures in acute intermittent porphyria: safety and efficacy of gabapentin. *Seizure* 1998;7:415–416.
55. Silver JR. Early autonomic dysreflexia. *Spinal Cord* 2000;38:229–233.
56. Colachis SC, Fugate LP. Autonomic dysreflexia associated with transient aphasia. *Spinal Cord* 2002;40:142–144.

11

Management of Medical Complications in the Neurosciences Critical Care Unit

Jose L. Diaz, Marcela Granados, and Jose I. Suarez

INTRODUCTION

Neurosciences critical care units (NSU) were designed for the care of neurologic and neurosurgical patients and, as we will discuss, virtually any medical complication can occur during their hospitalization in this unit. However, neurologic and neurosurgical patients have specific conditions that predispose them to developing certain complex clinical entities, which may not only influence mortality but also functional outcome in this patient population.

The most frequent medical afflictions in neurocritically ill patients include aspiration pneumonia, indwelling catheter infection, gastrointestinal bleeding, serum electrolyte and acid base disturbances, acute renal failure (ARF), venous thromboembolism (pulmonary embolism and deep venous thrombosis) and coagulophaties. This chapter presents an overview of how these medical conditions should be interpreted and managed in the NSU.

ASPIRATION PNEUMONIA

Predisposing Factors

Aspiration pneumonia (AP) is frequently seen in neurocritically ill patients within the first 3 d of admission to the NSU. Neurologic disorders predispose patients to developing disruption of cough and gag reflexes. The risk of aspiration is related to the degree of unconsciousness. It has been demonstrated that respiratory tract infections are frequent in multiple trauma patients especially in those with Glasgow Coma Scale (GCS) score less than 9 (1). This is also seen in patients with other neurological disorders. Approximately 50,000 people per year die because of aspiration pneumonia after stroke (2). The etiology of AP in this patient population is multifactorial. However, a major factor is dysphagia and as many as 40–70% of stroke patients present with this abnormality.

Patients with pure medullary infarction have high occurrence of aspiration when they present with dysphonia, soft palate dysfunction, and facial hypestesia. All these findings on neurological examination correlate with lesions of the middle and the lower medullary segments (3,4). Pneumonia may develop in patients with bilateral basal ganglia strokes due to frequent aspiration during sleep (5). Other neurologic disorders that can predispose to aspiration pneumonia include those presenting with bulbar muscle weakness, such as myasthenia gravis. Less frequently, amyotrophic lateral sclerosis, multiple sclerosis and Parkinson's disease patients may also require admission to NSU because of AP. There are other factors that appear to be associated with AP in NSU patients including feeding

From: *Current Clinical Neurology*
Critical Care Neurology and Neurosurgery
Edited by: J. I. Suarez © Humana Press Inc., Totowa, NJ

techniques, and disturbances of gastric motility. Although there still is controversy, the method of administration of nutritional support may impact upon the risk of aspiration. In one study, the incidence of pneumonia in poststroke patients was significantly higher with oral feeding than tube feeding *(6)*. Therefore, in high risk NSU patients prophylactic placement of feeding tubes is recommended to decrease the incidence of AP.

Early percutaneous endoscopic gastrostomy (PEG) tube placement (within 2 wk of disease onset) may be worthwhile in patients at risk for aspiration since many require long-term enteral feeding. Although the use of PEG placement has not been demonstrated to prevent the occurrence of AP in dysphagic stroke patients, it is more effective than nasogastric tube in reaching the patient's nutritional goal *(7)*. It is also important to consider gastrointestinal (GI) dysmotility. This is particularly frequent in patients after traumatic brain injury (TBI) and in those with history of diabetes regardless of underlying intracranial pathology. A high gastric residual volume due to gastroparesis leads to regurgitation and aspiration, thus the importance of inserting postpyloric feeding tubes in these patients.

Videofluoroscopic swallowing study is considered the gold standard in the dysphagia evaluation *(8)*. However, this technique does not always identify subtle abnormalities in pharyngeal and laryngeal anatomy and sensation. Besides, the patient must be transported to the radiology suite. Flexible endoscopic evaluation of swallowing is a useful alternative for evaluation of dysphagia, and can be performed in the NSU. This method can rule out aspiration with 97% accuracy if accompanied by a rigorous physical examination *(9)*. It is important to realize that patients who suffer from acute disorders causing dysphagia, especially after stroke and TBI, tend to improve with time. Nevertheless, early diagnosis of dysphagia linked to aspiration is important for appropriate management.

Diagnosis

The diagnosis of AP is a challenge for the neurointensivist. It is imperative to have a high index of clinical suspicion along with radiographic evidence of pulmonary infiltrates in patients at risk for aspiration because most episodes are not witnessed. Chest radiographs in patients maintained in a recumbent position can show new pulmonary infiltrates in the posterior segments of the upper lobes and the apical segments of the lower lobes. In contrast, those patients who experience AP while their heads are elevated usually experience lower lobes involvement. Pulse oximetry monitoring is useful for detection of aspiration in dysphagic stroke patients who present with abnormal arterial oxygenation. However, careful interpretation is necessary in older patients, particularly those with chronic pulmonary diseases and smokers *(10)*.

The risk of aspiration remains high after extubation in the NSU and it is necessary to remember that alterations of the swallowing reflex may persist for 48 h. Therefore, it is usually recommended that tube feedings be held 6 h before and after extubation. Another situation where diagnosis of AP can be particularly difficult is following tracheotomy. This surgical procedure has been a traditionally indicated management for airway protection in patients with dysphagia after neurologic injury. However, it has been demonstrated that episodes of aspiration can develop in tracheally intubated patients due to swallowing alterations *(11)*. It has been recommended that tracheal secretions be inspected for blue discoloration in patients fed with blue dyed feedings. However, this method fails to detect most episodes of enteral feeding aspiration. Glucose oxidase test strips have also been advocated since it has been shown to be more sensitive *(12)*.

Treatment

Management of NSU patients at risk for aspiration should be aimed at prevention by proper aspiration precautions and positioning along with prophylactic intubation in patients with poor GCS and inability to protect their airways. NSU patients either on mechanical ventilation or on oxygen supplementation must be placed in a semirecumbent position. In mechanically ventilated patients, other strategies to prevent ventilator associated pneumonia such as adequate hand washing between patient contacts, and avoidance of gastric distention are important in order to prevent pulmonary infection *(13)*. Once aspiration is suspected, aggressive therapy with ventilator support, tracheal suctioning and adequate fluid correction should be instituted. A recent study demonstrated that variations in extubating TBI patients affect the incidence of nosocomial pneumonia since most of them could be related to aspiration *(14)*. Patients with delayed extubation (> 3 d) developed more pneumonias than patients extubated within 48 h (38 vs 21%, $p < 0.05$). There was a similar reintubation rate in both early and delayed extubation groups. These data suggest that removing endotracheal tubes as soon as clinically feasible may be important in this patient population to prevent pulmonary infection.

Empiric antibiotic coverage is usually recommended for patients with fever, leukocytosis, and positive blood or sputum culture. However, it is crucial to entertain some clinical features of NSU patients before beginning antibiotic therapy. First, older patients usually do not mount a fever or leukocytosis despite an overwhelming infection. The aged with pneumonia after aspiration present with atypical features, including confusion, lethargy and general deterioration of condition. Second, fever is observed in 25% of patients within 48 h after stroke and the most probable cause of fever associated to infection is pneumonia *(15)*. Third, these patients may also experience other medical complications such as urinary tract infection, sinusitis, intravenous line infection and venous thrombosis. Therefore, it is recommended that a thorough and integral approach be undertaken to investigate each of these conditions.

The choice of antibiotics is based on the need to cover the most common organisms associated with aspiration of oral pharyngeal contents in hospitalized patients, such as *Enterobacteriaceae*, *Pseudomona aeruginosa*, *Staphylococcus aureus*, and anaerobes. There is evidence that pneumonia caused by methicillin-sensitive *S. aureus* (MSSA) may be the most frequent infection in patients with a decreased level of consciousness *(16)*. However, after 7 d of mechanical ventilation *P. aeruginosa* is the most frequently isolated microorganism in ventilator-associated pneumonia. Recommended empirical antibiotic regimen for hospital-acquired AP includes the combination of piperacillin/tazobactam or meropenem with or without vancomycin administered intravenously (Table 1). Alternative regimens include cefepime plus metronidazole or ciprofloxacin plus clindamycin in penicillin or cephalosporin allergic or intolerant patients *(17)*. Antibiotic agents with specific anaerobic activity should be indicated in patients with severe periodontal disease, putrid sputum, necrotizing pneumonia or pulmonary abscess. Sampling of the lower respiratory tract and quantitative sputum culture in an intubated patient may allow for targeted antibiotic therapy.

ELECTROLYTE IMBALANCE

Sodium

Hyponatremia

This condition is the most common electrolyte disorder in acute brain disease and can result from a wide range of mechanisms. However, there are two main disorders associated with hyponatremia in NSU patients (Fig. 1). The first is the syndrome of inappropriate secretion of antidiuretic hormone (SIADH) and the second is the cerebral salt wasting syndrome (CSWS). Both SIADH and CSWS deserve attention because they have different managements.

SIADH causing isovolemic hyponatremia has been traditionally considered the most common form of hyponatremia in NSU patients. Its presentation is associated with the following conditions: subarachnoid hemorrhage (SAH), brain tumors, stroke, intracranial hemorrhage (ICH), inflammatory and demyelinating diseases, acute intermittent porphyria, TBI, spinal cord injury (SCI), postoperative state, pain, severe nausea, acute respiratory failure, use of drugs like carbamazepine, opiate derivatives, serotonin reuptake inhibitors and more recently lamotrigine *(18,19)*.

Because most patients with SIADH appear to meet the general criteria for CSWS, a thorough clinical examination and laboratory evaluation are necessary to distinguish between the two. Atten-

Table 1
**Empirical Antibiotic Therapy for Aspiration Pneumonia
in NSU Patients With Normal Renal Function**

Agent	Dosage
Piperacillin/Tazobactam	3.375 g IV q 6 h
Cefepime +	1–2 g IV q 12 h
clindamycin	600 mg IV q 8 h
or metronidazole	500 mg IV q 8 h
Imipenem	0.5 g IV q 6 h
Meropenem	1 g IV q 8 h
Third-generation cephalosporins + clindamycin	

tion to volume status is very important. Patients with SIADH are considered euvolemic, so that the symptoms of dehydration are not observed whereas patients with CSWS present symptoms and physical findings compatible with negative fluid balance. It is important to follow water input/ output ratio, weight and mucosae and skin condition. In addition, patients with CSWS and invasive hemodynamic monitoring can show pulmonary capillary wedge pressures less than 8 mmHg or central venous pressures less than 6 mmHg. Several laboratory tests are also useful in the evaluation of volume status and salt balance. Elevations in the hematocrit, the blood urea nitrogen/creatinine ratio, and the serum protein suggest dehydration and argue against the presence of SIADH. A urine sodium concentration more than 20 mEql/L suggests SIADH whereas an increased serum potassium concentration suggests CSWS *(20)*.

CSWS is associated with a variety of intracranial disorders including tuberculous meningitis, metastatic adenocarcinoma of the lung, TBI, and transesphenoidal surgery. However, this syndrome has been classically described in patients with SAH *(21)*. Hyponatremia occurs in as many as 30% of patients with SAH and may be associated with cerebral edema. Currently, some authors believe CSWS occurs as frequently or more than SIADH in neurosurgical patients. CSWS is a complex syndrome and has been linked to elevations of serum atrial natriuretic peptide as well as ouabain-like compound and direct hyperactivity of the sympathetic nervous system *(20)*. There have been reports of SIADH and CSWS in the same patient, occurring successively, particularly after SAH.

The cornerstone of the treatment of SIADH is correction of the underlying cause and fluid restriction (approx 800 cc/d). If this fails to improve the abnormal serum sodium, the patient becomes symptomatic or the patient's serum sodium concentration is less than 120 mEq/L, a 3% hypertonic saline solution may be used. This may also be helpful in decreasing brain edema.

The CSWS is treated with fluid replacement and maintenance of a positive salt balance. Intravenous hydration with normal or 3% hypertonic saline solution is indicated. Caution should be exerted here not to correct the sodium faster than 0.5 mEq/L/h. It is important to follow serum sodium levels closely, along with volume status and hemodynamic parameters. Rapid corrections of serum sodium (>1 mEq/L/h) have been associated with central pontine myelinolisis *(22)*.

SAH patients, as discussed in Chapters 20 and 24, merit special attention. Hypervolemic therapy is frequently used to reduce their risk of ischemic complications. However, this approach may cause excessive natriuresis and osmotic diuresis. Inhibition of natriuresis with fludrocortisone can reduce the sodium and water intake required to achieve hypervolemia while preventing hyponatremia at the same time *(23,24)*.

Hypernatremia

This abnormality is less common in the NSU than hyponatremia. The main scenario for hypernatremia in neurosurgical patients is the one associated with diabetes insipidus (DI) *(see* Fig. 1).

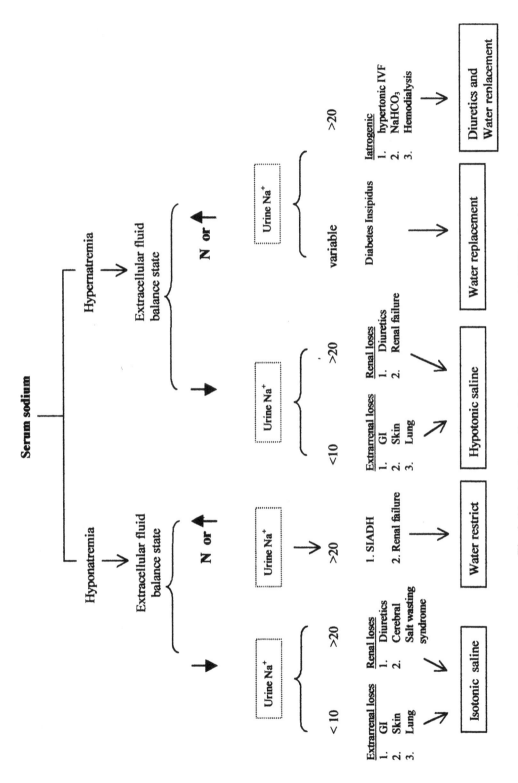

Fig. 1. Algorithm for sodium imbalance management in NSU patients.

The incidence is close to 4% in this patient population and is most commonly found after SAH, severe TBI, postoperative excision of craniopharyngioma or pituitary adenoma and ICH. Prompt recognition of DI is very important because it is associated with an overall mortality of 72.4% and with impending brain death in most patients with SAH and TBI (25).

Timing of DI presentation varies according to different intracranial pathologies. In patients with TBI a temporary DI can appear and resolve as the edema clears. This may occur within 12–24 h and is more marked at 48–72 h. This condition may obey to functional dysfunction without structural damage. In those patients with postoperative DI there are four distinguishing syndromes (26):

1. The most frequent condition is transient postoperative polyuria that begins 1–3 d after surgery and lasts from 1–7 d.
2. A triphasic pattern. Polyuria begins 1–2 d after surgery and lasts 1–7 d followed by a period of normal urinary output. This is followed by recurrence of large polyuria between 24 h to several days later. This latter condition usually persists.
3. Polyuria, which may begin within the first 2–3 d postoperatively followed by a small decrease in the total urinary volume over the next several days.
4. Permanent polyuria, which presents within the first 2 d and persists without changes.

The diagnosis of DI in the NSU may be difficult. As a rule of thumb, whenever the diuresis exceeds the fluid intake an abnormal cause of polyuria should be suspected. When polyuria begins in the immediate postoperative period, it is necessary to establish whether it is secondary to water or solute excretion. Monitoring of urinary specific gravity is a useful tool to help diagnose DI in the NSU. When diuresis is secondary to water excretion, the urinary specific gravity is between 1000 and 1005, the urinary osmolarity is between 50 and 150 mOsm/L, and the serum sodium is normal or increased. The differential diagnosis comprises chronic renal insufficiency, multiple myeloma, the recovery phase of acute tubular necrosis and fluid overload. Special attention should be paid to fluid administration during the intraoperative period, particularly electrolyte free solutions (26).

The treatment of acute DI is expectant until polyuria is apparent. Urinary output is closely monitored along with specific gravity readings. Other variables such as body weight, electrolytes, BUN, and hematocrit are measured every day in this prepolyuria phase. When polyuria appears, the management is determined by the patient's medical condition. Alert patients can be encouraged to regulate their fluid intake by mouth in response to thirst mechanisms. However, it is important to strictly monitor fluid balance. If urinary output exceeds 300 mL/h for 2–3 h or the patient is lethargic, aqueous vasopressin is started, recording weight twice daily to provide a guide of hydration status. The two fundamental aspects to understand in the management of DI patients are that the primary loss in this disease is water and that the process is dynamic. Fluid intake should be almost solely dextrose-water solutions if given IV or tap water if given by mouth. The commonest error in management is to administer saline solutions because they may aggravate the renal loss of water. Older and cardiac patients may not tolerate great fluid replacement. Therefore, in these patients it is preferable to keep fluid intake at lower levels. Vasopressin can be used at any time provided that close monitoring of fluid balance is undertaken to avoid water intoxication. Aqueous vasopressin is the first choice in the early stages of DI for its short duration of action (4–6 h), so that errors in fluid balance can be corrected. Initial doses are usually 5–10 U per dose and preferably intramuscularly, preventing a vasopressor response (26). In awake patients, nasal spray preparations can be used every 6–12 h.

Other causes of hypernatremia in the NSU include increased insensible losses of water in febrile patients, osmotic diuresis related to mannitol administration, diarrhea (either infectious or nutritionally related), and overuse of diuretics in patients who receive this therapy chronically. There are many formulas to calculate water deficit (27). However, the most practical formula is based on the current body water and the desired body water (see Appendix). Replacement of body water deficit should be 50% over 24 h and the rest over the next 24–48 h with close monitoring of serum sodium concentration every 4–6 h.

Potassium

Hypokalemia

Hypokalemia is frequently seen in NSU patients. As many as 20% of stroke patients can present with hypokalemia during hospitalizations even when diuretic therapy is excluded. Lower plasma potassium concentration on admission to the hospital has been associated with an increased risk of death, independent of age, stroke severity, hypertension, or smoking history *(28)*. Significant hypokalemia (3.1 ± 0.4 mEq/L) has also been reported in severe TBI patients (GCS < 7) upon admission to the hospital. This hypokalemia is transient, resolving within the first day and may be secondary to the large catecholamine discharge that accompanies severe head trauma *(29)*.

Patients with hypokalemia often have no symptoms but with serum potassium concentration below 3 mEq/L generalized weakness and lassitude can appear. It is important to understand that symptoms usually correlate with the rapidity of the hypokalemia. Therefore, NSU patients with polyuria secondary to DI or diuretic therapy are at the highest risk of developing symptomatic hypokalemia. Other patients at risk are those treated with β-2 adrenergic agonists or theophyllin, especially the elderly who have a decreased muscle mass and total body potassium *(30)*.

Hypokalemia should be aggressively repleted intravenously in NSU patients. Potassium chloride is the salt most commonly used, at rates between 5 and 10 mEq/h depending on clinical manifestations. Moreover, hypokalemia may be associated with hypophosphatemia. In this case, potassium phosphate is indicated. Although there is no simple formula to replete potassium, typically 40–100 mEq of daily supplemental potassium chloride are needed to maintain serum concentration near or within the normal range. If diuretic therapy is absolutely necessary, a second diuretic drug that inhibits potassium excretion, such as spironolactone or amiloride should be started. Intravenous potassium replacement in patients with cathecolamine infusions or elderly patients warrants close monitoring of serum potassium concentration. Finally hypomagnesemia and hypocalcemia may be the cause of refractory hypokalemia and should also be repleted aggressively *(29)*.

Hyperkalemia

This is another important issue in NSU patients. Supplemental potassium administration may be the most common cause of severe hyperkalemia in NSU patients, since it may especially occur in elderly individuals with underlying renal insufficiency. Other frequent cause is medications including potassium-sparing diuretics, beta-blocking agents, angiotensin-converting enzyme inhibitors (ACEI) and nonsteroidal anti-inflammatory drugs (NSAIDs). On top of that, patients with status epilecticus can present with lactic acidosis and hyperkalemia with or without rhabdomyolisis as a systemic complication of seizures.

Patients with neuromuscular disorders are predisposed to developing hyperkalemia. For instance, severe rhabdomyolysis can be induced in myopathic muscle by the application of succinylcholine during endotracheal intubation resulting in hyperkalemia, myoglobinuria and serum creatine kinase (CK) elevation, sometimes followed by sudden cardiac arrest *(31)*. This can occur in patients with motor deficits after stroke or any other neurologic injury since it has been shown that they upregulate extraunional acetylcholine receptors after 48–72 h, so that massive liberation of potassium and cardiac arrest can be produced *(32)*. Some authors stress the importance of noticing changes in neurologic physical examination before administering this agent. However, this does no ensure that succinylcholine-induced hyperkalemia will not occur.

Management of hyperkalemia depends on the serum potassium concentration and electrocardiographic (EKG) changes. The acute management includes antagonism of potassium effects in the cardiac muscle, increase of transcellular shift of potassium, and enhancement of its clearance (Table 2).

Table 2
Treatment of Hyperkalemia in NSU Patients

Agent	Mechanism	Dosage	Onset of action	Considerations
Calcium gluconate (10%)	Direct antagonism	10–20 mL IV over 2–5 min	Immediate	Monitor continuously with EKG
Sodium bicarbonate (8.4%)	Redistribution	50 mL IV over 1–5 min	Minutes	Alkaline load
Glucose/insulin	Redistribution	50 mL D50W with 10 U regular insulin IV infusion	Minutes	Monitor blood sugar
β-2 Agonists	Redistribution	4 mg albuterol nebul.	30 min	Hypokalemia
Sodium polystyrene sulfonate (Kayexalate)	Increased elimination	15–60 g PO tid or qid	2–12 h	1 mEq K^+ absorbed per g of Kayexalate
Dialysis	Increased elimination	–	2–4 h	–

Magnesium

Hypomagnesemia may be seen in NSU patients. The most important causes in neurocritically ill patients include excessive renal losses of magnesium (i.e., polyuric patients) or internal redistribution (i.e., cathecholamine infusions, stress of severe TBI or extensive neurosurgeries). The clinical manifestation may begin insidiously or suddenly, or more frequently there are no overt symptoms. These symptoms can include neuromuscular hyperactivity with tremors, myoclonic jerks, convulsions, nystagmus, dysphagia, Chvostek's sign, and Trousseau's sign. Psychiatric manifestations range from apathy to delirium and coma. Cardiac arrhythmias including ventricular tachycardia and sudden death are known to occur.

Hypomagenesemia must be suspected in NSU patients with hypokalemia, especially after potassium supplementation, and in patients with unexplained hypocalcemia. The incidence of hypomagnescmia is higher in patients with severe TBI compared to patients with trauma without TBI *(33)*. It is common practice to maintain serum magnesium concentration more than 2.0 mEq/L. Patients should receive 2 g of magnesium sulfate ($MgSO_4$) in 100 mL isotonic saline solution and infuse over 2 h *(see* Appendix). This dose can be repeated every 8 h, after following serum magnesium levels. Although serum magnesium concentration may normalize 24–48 h after initial dosing, it may take several days to replenish the total body magnesium stores.

Calcium

Hypocalcemia

The incidence of hypocalcemia (ionized calcium < 1.16 mmol/L) has been reported in up to 88% of critically ill ICU patients, including neurosurgical patients *(34)*. Hypocalcemia correlates with severity of illness, but not with a specific clinical condition. It is recognized that calcium regulation is disturbed in critical illness because of several factors: impaired parathyroid hormone secretion or action, impaired vitamin D synthesis or action, or calcium chelation/precipitation. Ionized hypocalcemia most commonly presents with cardiovascular or neuromuscular dysfunction. Mild ionized hypocalcemia (concentrations greater than 0.8 mmol/L) is usually asymptomatic and frequently does not require treatment. Although there is no clear evidence, clinical concern regarding intracellular calcium dysregulation during cerebral ischemia poses the question as to whether aggressive calcium supplementation may worsen neurological outcome in NSU patients *(35)*. Besides, calcium replacement may impair the inotropic effect of cardiac medications when administered simultaneously *(35)*. On the other hand, in patients with status epilepticus, it is mandatory to evaluate serum calcium concentrations because of the possibility of hypocalcemic seizures. In fact, there are reports of hypocalcemia as a precipitant factor of nonconvulsive status epilepticus *(36)*.

The most commonly available calcium solutions for intravenous use are 10% calcium chloride and 10% calcium gluconate *(see* Appendix). Calcium chloride has three times more elemental calcium than calcium gluconate. One ampule of 10% calcium chloride contains 272 mg of elemental calcium and one ampule of calcium gluconate 90 mg. A bolus dose of 200 mg of elemental calcium (diluted in 100 mL of isotonic saline solution and given in 10 min) should raise total serum calcium concentration by 1 g/dL. Total and ionized serum calcium concentrations should be observed closely and repleted as necessary.

Hypercalcemia

Hypercalcemia is less common in NSU patients than hypocalcemia. In our experience, primary hyperparathyroidism and malignancies account for 90% of hypercalcemia cases. Other causes include hyperthyroidism, immobilization and Addison disease. The malignances most often associated with hypercalcemia include lung (35%), breast (25%), hematological (myeloma—lymphoma) (14%), head and neck (6%), and renal (3%) *(37)*. Immobilization may be an important cause of hypercalcemia in young NSU patients as a result of decreased bone formation and persistent bone resorption.

Hypercalcemia is common within 4 mo after SCI and in those patients younger than age 16 after motor neurologic deficit. Therefore, this condition should be sought and treated aggressively should these patients be admitted to the NSU.

Clinical presentation of hypercalcemia depends on the serum calcium concentration, the rate of rise, and patient's comorbidities. The highest elevations of calcium are associated with a range of symptoms from drowsiness to stupor and coma. Other symptoms include polyuria constipation, nausea, vomiting, and acute pancreatitis. Evaluation of the Q-T interval on EKG is very important to assess the severity of hypercalcemia. Severe hypercalcemia causes shortened Q-T interval *(38)*.

All NSU patients with altered mental status must be evaluated for hypercalcemia. Ideally, ionized calcium should be determined because it is considered the most accurate test of serum calcium concentration. Simultaneously, serum magnesium and phosphorous concentrations should also be measured in all cases of hypercalcemia.

The main goal of treatment of hypercalcemia is to minimize its deleterious effects on the renal, cardiovascular system, and central nervous systems (CNS). Immediate treatment must be started if the total serum calcium concentration is above 14 mg/dL. It is critical to determine the underlying cause of hypercalcemia, so that patients can be treated appropriately *(39)*.

The first step in the management of hypercalcemia is to increase renal calcium clearance. Calciuresis can be obtained with IV hydration (6 L of NS per 24 h) to achieve urinary outputs of 4–5 L/24 h. This intervention can reduce calcium concentration between 1.6 and 2.4 mg/dL. Patients with congestive heart failure (CHF) must be closely observed during this strategy because of the risk of pulmonary edema. The administration of diuretics further increases renal calciuresis. Furosemide (40–80 mg IV) is the drug of choice in these cases. In those NSU patients with concomitant oliguric acute renal failure (ARF) or severe CHF, dialysis is mandatory.

The second measure is treatment with calcitonin. It reduces resorption of calcium from bone and increases excretion of urinary calcium along with other electrolytes. This strategy is effective for 4–7 d. Calcitonin can be used safely in patients with ARF, and its effects are limited to transient nausea, facial flushing and occasional hypersensitivity at the injection site. Salmon calcitonin leads to serum calcium concentration reduction within a few hours of SQ or IM administration (4 U every 12 h) *(40)*.

Biphosphonates can also be used because of their inhibitory effect on osteoclastic activity. The most frequently used agents, etidronate and pamidronate (60–90 mg IV over 2–4 h), are available for parenteral use. Their benefit is obtained after 2 or 3 d. Doses may be repeated if serum calcium does not decline after this time. There are approaches that combine biphosphonates and calcitonin, achieving the benefits of rapid effect of calcitonin with the more delayed effects of biphosphonates.

More toxic agents include mithramycin and gallium nitrate. These are only administered when all other measures have failed because of their important adverse effects *(41)*. Finally, it has been shown that hypercalcemia from multiple myeloma, lymphoma and granulomatous disorders improves with steroid therapy *(38)*.

Phosphate

Routine detection and treatment of hypophosphatemia in the NSU is common practice, although there is no strong clinical evidence at present to support its routine correction in the absence of clinical symptoms or signs. Undeniably, this condition is very common in NSU patients and deserves especial attention. Severe hypophosphatemia has been associated with tissue hypoxia, leukocyte dysfunction, hemolysis, predisposition to sepsis, and cardiomyopathy. Other manifestations are neurological, such as generalized weakness, encephalopathy, rhabdomyolysis and peripheral neuropathy, which can mimic Guillain-Barré syndrome (GBS). The most common causes of hypophosphatemia include poor oral intake before admission to the NSU, the use of phosphate binding antacids, and transcellular shift of phosphorous from the extracellular to the intracellular compartment as a consequence of hyperglycemic states (parenteral glucose solutions, parenteral nutrition and catecholamines infusions) *(42)*. Severe hypophosphatemia can occur after TBI and may develop more commonly as

Table 3
Recommended Thromboprophylaxis

Patient population	Recommendation
Postoperative	IPC + ES + LDUH (5000 U SQ every 12 h, 24–48 hours after surgery)
Acute ischemic stroke	LDUH, or Danaparoid + IPC + ES
Spinal cord injury	LMWH
Neuromuscular disorders	LDUH, or LMWH + IPC + ES

LDUH, low-dose unfractionated heparin; LMWH, low-molecular-weight heparin.

a sequel to the redistribution of phosphate. This fall in serum phosphate coincides with the induction of respiratory alkalosis secondary to mechanical ventilation. Another clinical scenario relevant to the NSU is hypothermia-induced hypophosphatemia, usually associated with hypomagnesemia. This may be due to increased urinary excretion through hypothermia-induced polyuria.

Due to the potentially dangerous adverse effects associated with hypophosphatemia, intravenous phosphate replacement is recommended in NSU patients with this condition. Commonly used treatment regimens for hypophosphatemia (< 2 mg/dL) include an intravenous dose of 0.9 mg/kg/h, for 4–6 h with monitoring of serum phosphorous concentration every 6 h. Sucralfate should be discontinued if phosphate replacement is continued with oral preparations *(42)*.

To summarize, the neurointensivist must recognize the inter-relationship between the major fluid and electrolyte disturbances and neurologic manifestations affecting all components of the nervous system. Disorders of sodium and osmolality may cause CNS depression with encephalopathy as the major clinical manifestation. Disorders of potassium may lead to peripheral nervous system (PNS) depression with muscle weakness as the major clinical manifestation. Disorders of calcium may be associate with both CNS and PNS compromise. Hypercalcemia and hypermagnesemia cause CNS and PNS depression with encephaplopathy and muscle weakness, respectively. On the other hand, hypocalcemia and hypomagnesemia may induce CNS and PNS irritability with seizures and tetany, respectively *(43)*.

VENOUS THROMBOEMBOLISM

Venous thromboembolism (VT) is a spectrum of diseases that can be classified into two categories: deep venous thrombosis (DVT) and pulmonary embolism (PE). NSU patients are in the highest risk group for VT. Therefore, neurointensivists should always be providing adequate prophylaxis in every subgroup of this patient population. In general, all NSU patients should be treated with at least two of three established VT prophylactic measures unless contraindicated: thigh-high elastic stockings (ES), intermittent pneumatic compression devices (IPC), and low dose unfractionated SQ heparin (LDUH) (Table 3). There are three main groups of neurocritically ill patients with their proper approach to VT that deserve special attention and are therefore presented below: postoperative, acute ischemic stroke, and SCI patients.

Postoperative Patients

Neurosurgical patients are known to be at increased risk of post-operative DVT and PE. Risk factors that appear to increase DVT rates in this subgroup include intracranial surgeries, malignant tumors, long surgeries, and the presence of leg weakness and increased age *(44,45)*. The incidence of lower extremity DVT may be as high as 29% in patients undergoing major cranial or spinal operations, mainly associated with leg weakness and long operations. Similarly, patients with malignant tumors, particularly glioma, may have an incidence of 31% of DVT *(46)*.

Physical methods of prophylaxis have been recommended over heparin because of concerns of intracranial or spinal bleeding. IPC have demonstrated to be effective in these patients, with an average risk reduction of 68% compared with controls (47). The use of ES alone is less effective than ES plus low molecular weight heparins (LMWH). The use of LDUH is supported in neurosurgical patients because of the absence of increased risk of bleeding with these agents, particularly 24–48 h after surgery (48) (see Chapter 24). Therefore, IPC plus or minus ES can be recommended for prophylaxis of DVT in neurosurgical patients. The combination of LDUH and mechanical prophylaxis may also be more effective than either method alone. Other alternatives include LDUH and LMWH alone (49).

Acute Ischemic Stroke

Stroke patients may develop DVT in the paretic or paralyzed limb. Randomized trials of thromboprophylaxis in this patient population have been carried out. LDUH (5000 U subcutaneous twice daily), was associated with a 71% reduction in DVT relative to control patients (50). LMWH trials have demonstrated a reduction in VT events in patients with acute ischemic stroke. However, theses medications are associated with an increased risk of extracranial bleeding and may be case fatality and symptomatic ICH (51). A nonrandomized prospective study of 681 ischemic stroke patients showed that the combination of LDUH, ES, and IPC was associated with fewer symptomatic DVT and PE than LDUH plus ES (52). In the international stroke trial, there was a significant reduction in the incidence of fatal and nonfatal PE with SQ LDUH (53). However, patients with the higher dose regimen (12500 U given subcutaneously every 12 h) had an increased bleeding risk. Danaparoid has also demonstrated efficacy on thromboprophylaxis. In two danaparoid vs placebo trials, the combined relative risk reduction for the danaparoid was 78%, whereas in the two danaparoid vs LDUH trials, there was a 44% reduction (53,54). In summary, LDUH, and danaparoid can be used in stroke patients along with mechanical prophylactic measures for DVT and PE prevention. LMWH cannot be recommended in the routine treatment of these patients.

Acute Spinal Cord Injury

Acute SCI patients have the highest risk of DVT in the NSU. PE continues to be a leading cause of death in this patient population. Prospective studies have shown a 67–100% incidence of documented DVT in this group. Both adjusted heparin and LMWH are more effective prophylactic agents than LDUH (55,56). However, in patients with incomplete motor SCI, initiation of thromboprophylaxis should be delayed for 72 h until there is no suspicion of perispinal hematoma as determined by imaging studies.

Deep Venous Thrombosis

The diagnosis of DVT in NSU patients based solely on anamnesis and physical examination can be difficult mainly due to concurrent neurologic deficits. Also, in patients recovering from acute disease presenting symptoms such as calf pain or tenderness can be missed or misinterpreted as related to other pathologies rather than VT.

NSU patients need appropriate screening tests to rule out DVT. Although venography remains the gold standard for the diagnosis of DVT, duplex ultrasonography is a valuable technique in the NSU. Duplex ultrasonography is essentially helpful for symptomatic patients with proximal DVT with a sensitivity of 88–100% (57). Critically ill patients may need more frequent evaluations for DVT in comparison to noncritically ill ones and false negative results may be encountered in patients with calf DVT.

Upper extremity DVT has recently been recognized as being a more common and less benign disease than previously reported, especially because of the use of indwelling catheters in NSU patients. This condition can be suspected in patients with arm swelling (< 30% of patients). Catheter-related DVT may occur as soon as 1 d after cannulation and is usually asymptomatic (58). The use of femoral lines increases the risk of iliofemoral DVT.

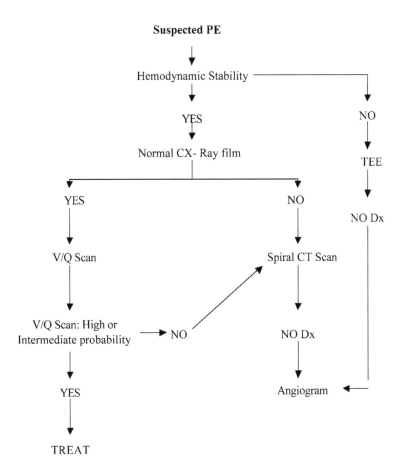

Fig. 2. Algorithm for PE management. CXRay; chest roentgenogram; TEE, transesophageal echocardiography; V/Q, ventilation/perfusion scan; spiral CT scan, spiral chest CT scan; Dx, diagnostic.

Pulmonary Embolism

PE continues to be a frequent cause of morbidity and mortality in neurosurgical patients and represents a real challenge to physicians in the NSU. The clinical diagnosis of PE is notoriously inaccurate and although its incidence may be small, its mortality is not (up to 59.4%) *(59)*. Furthermore, two thirds of all fatal pulmonary emboli cause death within 30 min of the embolic episode, leaving little time for diagnostic work-up and effective treatment.

Diagnostic Tools

There are some diagnostic modalities available for the diagnosis of PE (Fig. 2). Among those the most commonly used in neurocritically ill patients are spiral chest computed tomography (CT) scanning and ventilation/perfusion lung scan (V/Q scan). Spiral chest CT scanning has sensitivity and specificity greater than 95% for clots located in the main lobar and segmental pulmonary arteries. However, it cannot visualize subsegmental emboli (only 6% in PIOPED study) *(60)*. Spiral chest CT offers the additional advantage of assessing lung parenchyma, which is important in the work-up of patients with respiratory deterioration. If the spiral CT is nondiagnostic for PE and there is a high index of suspicion for this entity, pulmonary angiography is indicated because it remains the gold standard for the diagnosis of PE. However, this test is invasive, expensive and requires experienced staff.

Echocardiography may also be a valuable tool with hemodinamically significant PE (less than 50% of patients). PE may cause characteristic echocardiographic changes in patients without prior cardiopulmonary disease and only in this patient population can be adequately interpreted *(57)*. Such echocardiographic changes include dilatation of the right ventricle and the pulmonary outflow tract, and paradoxical motion of the interventricular septum. Transesophageal echocardiography may be more sensitive than transthoracic echocardiography at detecting echocardiographic changes in PE.

The value of the ventilation-perfusion (V/Q) scan is questionable in NSU patients on mechanical ventilation for respiratory failure. This is a frequent occurrence after sudden hypoxemia associated with PE because of the presence of cardiac or pulmonary compromise. These patients usually have underlying abnormal chest radiography, which may make interpretation of V/Q scan imaging very difficult if not impossible.

Chest radiographs may remain unchanged in 15% of PE patients *(57)*. However, the usual radiologic changes of PE that should be sought include atelectasis, pleural-based areas of opacity, and the classic sign of hyperlucency and decreased vascularity caused by local oligoemia. The neurointensivist must have a high index of suspicion for PE in any symptomatic ventilated patient with sudden hypoxemia without evidence of a clear underlying problem to explain it.

Blood D-dimer determination has been proposed as another diagnostic aid in the setting of PE. However the only role of D-dimer testing in the diagnosis of PE is to rule out the entity since its negative predictive value is greater than 95% *(57)*. Arterial blood gases analysis can not be used as definitive support for the diagnosis of PE. Patients without previous cardiopulmonary disease may not present with abnormal arterial-alveolar oxygen gradient even in the setting of angiographic confirmation of PE. This situation is common in both TBI and neurosurgical patients.

Therapeutic Maneuvers

The treatment of DVT and PE is based on both intravenous and oral anticoagulation since the 1960s. However this therapy may be contraindicated in many NSU patients because of the risk of intracranial bleeding. Consequently, inferior vena cava filters (IVCF) are indicated for this patient population. Also patients who are at risk of dying from recurrent PE can obtain benefit from this strategy *(61)*. In most clinical settings, patients who undergo IVCF insertion are also anticoagulated in order to prevent DVT at the insertion site, IVC thrombosis, and the propagation of clot from the filter. Neurosurgical patients can not receive anticoagulation after IVCF placement in the early post-surgical stage. A clear discussion between the neurointensivist and primary neurosurgery and neurology teams should be undertaken to decide upon the most appropriate therapy for each individual patient.

In conclusion, PE is a common condition in NSU patients and needs to be investigated thoroughly and treated promptly. We show in Fig. 2 a summary of the diagnostic workup for NSU patients suspected of having PE.

ACUTE RENAL FAILURE

ARF is another challenging co-morbidity that NSU patients may face. It has been determined that 14.9% and 16.6% of NSU patients develop prerenal and renal insufficiency respectively and that ARF worsens the prognosis carrying a mortality of 71–100% *(62)*. The most common conditions that predispose neurocritically ill patients to deterioration of their renal function after neurosurgical procedures, stroke or diagnostic interventions include concurrent renal disease, older age (> 70 yr), or peripheral vascular disease. However, NSU patients without these factors can also develop renal insufficiency. For instance, ARF has been reported as the cause of postoperative death in 10% of elderly patients with meningioma.

Table 4
Major Causes of Acute Renal Failure in NSU Patients

1. Prerenal failure

    1.1 Hypovolemia
        Hemorrhage
        Dehydration
        Diarrhea
        Diuretics
    1.2 Low cardiac output
        Arrhythmias
        Pulmonary embolism
        Myocardial or valvular disease
        Pulmonary hypertension
    1.3 Renal vasonstrictive states
        Cirrhosis with ascites
        Vasoconstrictive drugs: norepinephrine, amphotericine B, cyclosporine
    1.4 Intrinsic decrease of renal perfusion
        Cyclo-oxygenase (COX) inhibitors
        ACE inhibitors

2. Intrinsic renal failure

    2.1 Acute tubular necrosis (ATN)
        Drugs: contrast agents, aminoglycosides, acetaminophen
        Endogenous toxin: myoglobin
        Ischemia: hemorrhage
    2.2 Obstruction of renal vasculature from atherosclerosis
    2.3 Diseases that affect the glomeruli
        DIC
        Glomerulonephritis
        SLE
    2.4 Interstitial nephritis
        β-lactams
        Captopril
        Sulfonamides, trimetropin
        Rifampin
        COX inhibitors

3. Postrenal failure

        Urolithiasis
        Prostatic hyperplasia
        Neurogenic bladder

ACE, angiotensin-converting enzyme; DIC, disseminated intravascular coagulopathy; SLE, systemic lupus erythematosus.

Patients at high risk for acute ARF in the NSU include those with acute ischemic stroke, severe hypertension, SAH, sepsis, drug use, myasthenia gravis, GBS, and those receiving osmotherapy (Table 4). Stroke patients are frequently hypertensive with or without renal compromise. Cocaine users can present to NSU with several medical complications including ischemic stroke, coronary ischemia, and ischemia-induced renal failure. Patients with myasthenia gravis may have glomerulonephritis associated to this entity at variable intervals after the onset of the disease *(63)*. Patients with severe GBS particularly those with dysautonomia may develop ARF, which is associated with high mortality *(64)*.

Because the serum creatinine concentration in the NSU population may be depressed, caution should be exerted when using it as an estimate of the glomerular filtration rate especially when administering potentially nephrotoxic drugs. For instance, patients with SAH usually have sympathetic overdrive that may impair renal function. Besides, some centers routinely use epsilon-aminocaproic acid for prevention of rebleeding in SAH patient. This drug has been associated with a spectrum of muscle disease that ranges from mild myopathy to life threatening rhabdomyolisis and renal failure *(65)*. Osmotherapy with mannitol for patients with intracranial hypertension leads to ARF. Serum osmolality should be measured frequently after mannitol administration and maintained less than 320 mOsm/L to avoid ARF.

Intravenous immunoglobulins (IVIg) made from pooled human plasma is administered for GBS and chronic inflammatory desmyeliating polyneuropathy. There have been more than 100 reported cases of renal dysfunction following IVIg *(66)*. However, newer preparations and aggressive patients' hydration have reduced this association.

Rhabdomyolysis may lead to increased myoglobin, which may also cause ARF *(67)*. This condition must be suspected in any patient in coma with brown discoloration of the urine, fever, and edema of extremities. Laboratory results with elevated serum CK and serum creatinine out of proportion to BUN and orthotoluidine positive urine support the diagnosis of rhabdomyolisis *(67)*. Patients with TBI may develop increased serum urea levels. This abnormality seems to be associated with a hypercatabolic state due to shock, central dysregulation or both. Serum creatinine levels are only significantly increased in patients with lethal outcomes *(68)*. Patients with intracranial hypertension complicating fulminant hepatic failure have a mortality of 90% in the presence of ARF unless rapid treatment is started for both renal and brain failure. ARF is one of the most important complications of intravascular administration of contrast agents. NSU patients are scheduled frequently for diagnostic procedures such as CT scan and angiograms. Consequently, every effort should be taken to maintain euvolemia and avoid unnecessary imaging evaluations in order to decrease the incidence of ARF. Useful equations and formulas to properly diagnose etiology of ARF are presented in the Appendix section.

Treatment of Acute Renal Failure

The treatment of ARF in neurocritically ill patients is changing. In neurosurgical patients with ARF dialysis entails specific problems, mainly increased intracranial pressure (ICP) and progressive brain edema as a result of rapid lowering of serum osmolality. Another major concern is a tendency to hemorrhagic complication in response to either systemic heparinization or insufficient dialysis *(68)*.

Most patients with ARF are managed with supportive medical care including maintenance of fluid and electrolyte balance, especially in the polyuric phase. Blood pressure support is also important along with avoidance of any potentially nephrotoxic medications. Indications for dialysis include metabolic encephalopathy, severe metabolic acidosis, pulmonary edema, and anuria (Table 5).

There is mounting evidence supporting continuous renal replacement therapy (CRRT) as the method of choice for the treatment of ARF in NSU patients *(69)*. CRRT appears to be superior to intermittent dialysis in NSU patients because of less cerebral edema and hemorrhage. In addition, nutritional goals are achieved more effectively. CRRT has been used in unstable patients with ICH, patients with acute liver failure and cerebral edema and ARF following neurosurgery. The major disadvantage of CRRT is the need for anticoagulation of the extracorporeal circuit. However, epoprostenol appears to confer a reduced risk of hemorrhage without reducing circuit lifespan in these patients compared with the effects of standard and fractionated heparins. Another alternative for anticoagulation during CRRT is administration of low doses of LMWH.

Table 5
Indications for Renal Replacement Therapy in the NSU Patients

1. Metabolic acidosis, pH < 7.2
2. BUN (mg/dL) > 100
3. Creatinine (mg/dL) > 5.6
4. Potassium (mEq/L) > 6.5
5. Oliguria: urinary output less than 500 mL/d
6. Anuria: no urinary output for more than 12 h.
7. Pulmonary edema not responsive to diuretics
8. Uremic encephalopathy
9. Uremic pericarditis
10. Uremic neuropathy

Laboratory data refers to serum values.

ACID-BASE DISORDERS

Acid-base balance in NSU patients merits attention because alterations in the extracellular pH will produce significant responses in the CNS and viceversa. Cerebral pH is regulated by a modulation of the respiratory drive triggered by the early alteration of interstitial fluid pH. This is mostly the result of the high permeability of the blood–brain barrier to CO_2. CSF pH is rapidly corrected in the cases of severe metabolic acidosis and alkalosis, whereas it is not the case during respiratory alkalosis or acidosis where the cerebral pH varies in the same direction as the blood. Therefore, the brain is better protected against metabolic than respiratory acid-base derangements. During systemic metabolic acid base imbalances, cerebral pH is well controlled because the blood brain barrier is slowly and poorly permeable to electrolytes. In contrast, during respiratory acidosis HCO_3^- increases in extracellular fluid, which leads to carbonic anhydrase activation and chloride shift in glial cells *(70)*. In the following few paragraphs we will discuss some of those acid-base alterations common to NSU patients (Table 6). In the Appendix section we present easy calculations to determine adequate compensatory mechanisms during acid-base derangements.

Respiratory Acidosis

Respiratory acidosis is the most common and important acid-base disorder in neurocritically ill patients. Many NSU patients have compromised level of consciousness upon admission. Consequently they develop hypercapnia and respiratory acidosis. Abnormalities in ventilation and gas exchange result in hypoxia, hypercapnia and respiratory acidosis, and these, in turn increase cerebral blood flow (CBF) and may raise ICP. Therefore securing the airway and breathing is of the utmost importance because this is the mainstay of treatment of respiratory acidosis. NSU patients who develop acute respiratory distress syndrome (ARDS) become a real challenge for the neurointensivist. The appropriate therapy for ARDS comprises permissive hypercapnia and adequate PEEP; but both measures can produce intracranial hypertension. The key point to remember is that the rate of change of $PaCO_2$ will lead to sudden alterations of ICP (i.e., hypercarbia will elevate ICP while mild hypocarbia will decrease it). ICP monitoring can help to tailor ventilatory therapy.

All patients with neuromuscular disorders are at risk for both hypoxia and hypercarbia with respiratory acidosis. Sleep apnea is being recognized more frequently as an important cause of respiratory decompensation. There are reports of patients with myotonic dystrophy and sleep apnea requiring management in the NSU. Patients with motoneuron disease may start with acute or progressive respiratory failure without a clear cause or may appear to have similar symptoms as described in obstructive sleep apnea syndrome *(71)*. The treatment of choice is noninvasive mechanical ventilation.

Table 6
Acid-Base Disorders in NSU Patients

Respiratory acidosis
    Low level of consciousness
    ARDS
    Neuromuscular disorders
    Alveolar hypoventilation syndrome (Ondine's curse)
    Sleep apnea
Respiratory alkalosis
    ICH
    Ischemic stroke without extreme compromise of consciousness
    Beginning of ventilatory support
    Meningitis
    TBI
    Pain
    PE
    Early sepsis
Metabolic acidosis
    Status epilepticus
    Hypovolemic shock (TBI associated with multiple trauma)
    Spinal cord injury
    Renal failure
    Ketoacidosis
Metabolic alkalosis
    Vomiting, NG suction
    Diuretics
    Rapid correction of chronic hypercapnia
    Severe hypokalemia

ARDS, adult respiratory distress syndrome; ICH, intracranial hemorrhage; TBI, traumatic brain injury; PE, pulmonary embolism; NG, nasogastric.

Patients with cerebral infarction can develop central alveolar hypoventilation syndrome or Ondine's curse. This is a relatively rare disease characterized by dysfunction of brainstem respiratory centers. This condition should also be entertained in patients who experience apnea during weaning from mechanical ventilation. Cases of chronic inflammatory demyelinating polyradiculopathy may be associated with primary alveolar hypoventilation also.

Respiratory Alkalosis

Respiratory alkalosis is frequent in some NSU patients. Patients with ICH and ischemic stroke may present with respiratory alkalosis in the acute stages of the stroke without extensive compromise of consciousness *(72)*. TBI patients tend to be young and healthy and there is the tendency to hyperventilate them acutely with high tidal volumes which leads to respiratory alkalosis a few hours after initiation of ventilatory support. These patients are at risk of cerebral ischemia (30% of them) because of the CBF-lowering properties of deliberate hypocapnia. It is advised to maintain $PaCO_2$ between 30 and 35 in this patient population to avoid such complication. Patients in mechanical ventilation in whom sudden respiratory alkalosis develops are at risk for severe hypophosphatemia and even seizures. Continuous end-tidal CO_2 monitoring is recommended in mechanically ventilated NSU patients.

Metabolic Acidosis

Metabolic disorders in NSU patients are common in a subgroup of patients. Acid-base abnormalities in patients with status epilepticus frequently include mixed respiratory and metabolic acidosis *(73)*. This state usually resolves spontaneously after general management of status epilepticus. Patients with spinal cord injury, TBI and multiple traumas may present with hypovolemic shock and subsequent metabolic acidosis. SCI patients receive high doses of methylprednisolone and cathecolamines in their management in the NSU. There is evidence for severe hyperglycemia and nonketotic metabolic acidosis in otherwise nondiabetic patients with multiple blunt injuries and associated SCI. The management of acid-base disorder in NSU patients must be directed to correct the primary diagnosis, to avoid extreme measures that compromise CNS function and to discontinue unnecessary medications (*see also* Appendix).

GASTROINTESTINAL BLEEDING

GI bleeding may develop in NSU patients after admission. Neurosurgical patients who undergo surgery for non-traumatic conditions may experience 6.8% endoscopically and surgically proven postoperative GI complications *(74)*. A team approach to GI bleeding made up of the neurointensivist, surgeons, gastroenterologists and interventional radiologists should optimize management and improve patient outcome *(75)*. NSU patients at risk for GI bleeding include TBI patients, patients on mechanical ventilation, those receiving ongoing therapy with ulcerogenic drugs, patients with history of ulcer related bleeding, and individuals in coma *(76,77)*. These subgroups of NSU patients would benefit a great deal from prophylactic therapy with acid suppression therapy. GI bleeding in NSU patients is usually associated with erosive gastritis localized in the gastric fundus and body *(78)*. GI bleeding usually includes a combination of gastric acid production and mucosa hypoperfusion *(79)*.

Initial Evaluation

Initial assessment includes a good medical history and a detailed physical examination. A history of GI bleeding is important because 60% of patients can experience rebleeding from the same initial location *(80)*. Physical examination in older and diabetic patients could demonstrate orthostatic hypotension with minimal blood loss. The abdomen should be evaluated carefully and complemented with a rectal examination.

Laboratory testing should include EKG, coagulation profile, platelet count, BUN, and serum creatinine and liver function tests. Patients with previous renal or hepatic dysfunction can present with GI bleeding unexpectedly. Patients with severe bleeding associated with hypotension, syncope or evidence of hypoperfusion should be studied with serum CK, to rule out myocardial infarction *(81)*.

Initial Management

Nasogastric Aspiration

A nasogastric tube should be placed to evaluate gastric content and confirm bleeding source. However, 50% of patients with duodenal bleeding do not present bloody material *(82)*. Patients with coffee ground aspirate and melanotic stools have a mortality close to 10%, whereas patients with red aspirate and red rectal bleeding have a mortality of 30% *(83)*.

General Measures

All patients should be NPO, and a urinary catheter should be placed in those with hemodynamic instability. Supplemental oxygen is also necessary in patients with severe bleeding in order to guarantee peripheral tissue oxygenation.

Fluid Resuscitation

Two peripheral veins must be canalized with angiocath no. 14–18 in patients with active bleeding, and aggressive hydration should be undertaken. Central venous pressure monitoring help to guide fluid administration and metabolic acidosis improvement should be obtained in the first 24 h to avoid organ dysfunction. Pulmonary artery pressure monitoring is helpful in patients with cardiac failure, renal failure or cirrhosis when an aggressive resuscitation is needed.

Blood Transfusion

Patients with massive and persistent bleeding must be transfused immediately. Also patients with persistent bleeding or hypotension despite fluid infusion must be transfused. However, if initial hemoglobin is within the normal range, it is prudent to hold initial transfusion. The goal in NSU patients is to transfuse early and keep hemoglobin concentrations more than 10 g/dL.

Management of Patients on Warfarin or Aspirin Therapy With Gastrointestinal Bleeding

In those cases where GI bleeding needs to be controlled immediately, fresh frozen plasma should be transfused. Long-term control of coagulopathy can be obtained with low doses of vitamin K (0.5–1.0 mg SC or IV). This schedule guarantees anticoagulation if it should be needed once the acute event is controlled *(84)*. Desmopressin is indicated in those cases with aspirin-related bleeding *(85)*. However, patients without response to desmopresin should receive platelet transfusion.

Acid Suppression Empiric Therapy

H2 blockers are the agents of choice for treatment of lesions that cause GI bleeding (gastritis, duodenitis, peptic ulcer), and should be used as empiric therapy in NSU patients who present GI bleeding *(86,87)*. If patients are endoscopically treated, a high-dose infusion of omeprazole reduces the risk of recurrent bleeding *(88)*.

Endoscopy

Indications

Following initial resuscitation, every patient with significant GI bleeding must be evaluated with esophagogastroduodenoscopy (EGD). However, patients with massive bleeding or active bleeding with unstable vital signs need an emergent evaluation.

Precautions

Patient's respiratory status should be evaluated appropriately before EGD, and patients with respiratory distress or risk for aspiration must be endotracheally intubated. EGD is contraindicated in cases of gastrointestinal perforation, unstable angina, severe and untreated coagulopathy, uncontrolled respiratory decompensation and patients with severe agitation.

Surgery Consultation

This would be indicated in cases of GI bleeding associated with one of the following conditions: suspected gastrointestinal perforation, penetration, obstruction, or malignancy; massive or recurrent bleeding; persistent bleeding despite initial management; bleeding with EGD stigmas of rebleeding; esophageal variceal bleeding, and patients with associated abdominal pain.

COAGULOPATHIES

Coagulopathies can be important complications in NSU patients. Recent knowledge of the relationship between coagulation and inflammation underscores the importance of a thorough knowledge of these topics by the intensivist.

Coagulation

Coagulation factors are involved in a series of enzymatic reactions, of such form that the product of one initiates another, with thrombin being the essential substance. Genetic or acquired deficiencies of these factors will lead to hemorrhagic syndromes, whereas their overexpression will be associated with increased thrombotic risks *(89)*.

It has been established that at least six plasmatic proteins (prothrombin, factor VII, factor IX, factor X, factor V, and factor VIII) and a tissue protein (tissue factor, TF), mediate the procoagulant process. There are other compounds that, although not essential, play a contributory role in the procoagulant response. These include high-molecular-weight kininogen, factor XII prekalikrein, and factor XI. By contrast, four plasmatic proteins (antithrombin III, protein C, protein S and the tissue factor pathway inhibitor) and a vascular tissue protein, trombomodulin (Tm), mediate the anticoagulant process. Other molecules that contribute to the anticoagulant response are heparin-cofactor II, β2-macroglobulin and α-1-antitripsin *(90)*. In addition to these proteins, cell membrane binding sites are essential, because they become activated with vascular tissue injury, inflammatory mediators and platelets.

The coagulation system is highly regulated, with the objective of activating only small amounts of substances, thus avoiding the propagation of the hemostatic plug beyond the site of vascular injury. This regulation is very important because there is sufficient potential amount of coagulation factors in 1 cc of whole blood to coagulate all the sanguineous fibrinogen in 10–15 s.

Once the clot is formed, the vascular repairing process and clot lysis begins. There are three mainly activating substances of the fibrinolitic system: Hageman's factor fragments, urinary plasminogen activator or urokinase (UK) and tissue plasminogen activator (tPA). The main physiologic regulators, tPA and UK, diffuse from endothelial cells and convert the clot-absorbed plasminogen in plasmin.

Stroke

Ischemic Stroke

The most dangerous coagulopathy in ischemic stroke patients is thrombolytic-related ICH. A recent meta-analysis of thrombolysis for acute ischemic stroke trials has been published *(91)*. Data on several pre-specified outcomes including intracranial hemorrhages (ICH) within the first 7–10 d after treatment were sought in each identified randomized, controlled trial. Overall, there was an increase in the risk of symptomatic ICH (OR 3.53, 95% CI 2.79–4.45) after thrombolysis. The available data do not allow much further subgroup analysis, although there is reasonable evidence to indicate that aspirin or heparin administration within 24 h of thrombolytic therapy causes a significant increase in intracranial hemorrhage and death (*see also* Chapter 18).

Hemorrhagic Stroke

Hematologic abnormalities are directly linked to at least 8% of all ICH *(92)*. Coagulopathy-related ICH is most often caused by warfarin therapy, which increases relative ICH risk by sixfold to 11-fold overall, with risk paralleling the degree of anticoagulation. Absolute risk for warfarin-related ICH ranges from 0.3% to 1.7% per year, depending on the reason for anticoagulation *(92)*. Antiplatelet agents affect the risk for ICH to a much lesser extent than anticoagulant medications. Congenital and acquired factor deficiency disorders, thrombocytopenic and thrombocytopathic disorders, and lymphoproliferative disorders all represent other significant, albeit less common, hematologic causes of ICH (*see also* Chapter 19).

Management

Treatment of thrombolysis and others coagulopathies-related ICH includes the immediate administration of cryoprecipitate, fresh frozen plasma, and/or platelets to reverse the coagulopathic state in addition to the other measures of treatment of ICH *(92)* (*see also* Chapter 19).

Trauma

Trauma in all its forms produces tissue injury, and therefore bleeding. Nevertheless, if trauma is severe enough and shock and hypoperfusion states coexist, there is tendency to blood clot formation and a thrombotic state is produced, leading to disseminated intravascular coagulation (DIC).

Critically ill trauma patients can experience significant reductions of antithrombin III concentration *(93)*. Most of these patients can also have ARDS and more thromboembolic than hemorrhagic complications *(93–96)*. TBI produces a series of events that leads to the development of DIC, sometimes producing fatal hemorrhagic complications. Nonsurvivors have been found to have the lowest serum concentration of fibrinogen, antithrombin III, protein C and S, and high levels of D-dimer, along with prolonged PT and PTT *(97)*.

Another contributing factor to coagulopathy in TBI patients is massive transfusion *(98)*. The normal platelet function is virtually absent in the blood bank. Thrombocytopenia correlates with the number of red blood cell units transfused and can be clinically significant in an adult after 15–20 U *(99)*. However, it may be that coagulation abnormalities in multitransfused patients are more related to the magnitude of the trauma and DIC development than to the transfusion itself. This casts doubt over the common practice of routine plasma and platelets administration in the massively transfused patient *(100,101)*.

Approximately 66% of trauma patients arrive to the hospital presenting a core body temperature lower than 36°C. This is important because hypothermia affects the coagulation factors *(102)*. This is frequently underestimated because the coagulation tests are done at 37°C, which means that they may be interpreted as normal in a patient with a body temperature lower than 34°C and with a bleeding diathesis *(103)*. This implies that in such cases, rewarming may be more important than transfusion of plasma and blood substitutes. It is also important to remember that platelet dysfunction is associated with hypothermia, as evidenced by defects in primary hemostasis with temperatures lower than 34°C *(104,105)*.

DIC may occur in trauma patients due to a combination of factors, such as the severity of the trauma itself, shock state and hypoperfusion, massive transfusions, tissue damage, surgery or infection *(106,107)*. Basically, this DIC is caused by the liberation of thromboplastic substances secondary to some stimulus that triggers the coagulation cascade and lastly the fibrinolytic system. When this stimulus is prolonged, the consumption of coagulation factors becomes very important and the activation of the fibrinolysis system produces, in addition to the fibrin and fibrinogen degradation products, an alteration of fibrin polymerization leading to bleeding as the predominant clinical manifestation.

Treatment of coagulopathy related to trauma is based on transfusion of blood and blood components, and although the required number of packed red blood cell units varies depending on tissue perfusion, the prophylactic administration of plasma or platelets has not demonstrated any benefit. In most patients, therapy must be directed to the underlying pathology. Thus, if the platelet count is low, platelets should be transfused (1 U per each 10 kg of weight), if PT and PTT are prolonged, then fresh-frozen plasma should be transfused (10–15 mL/kg of weight), and if fibrinogen is low, then cryoprecipitate should be transfused (1 U per each 10 kg of weight). Clinicians should bear in mind that usually tests results lag behind the clinical event. Finally, there are some uncontrolled studies that have reported on the use of anti-fibrinolytic agents, like epsilon-aminocaproic acid, aprotinin and tranexamic acid, just when there is clear laboratory documentation of exaggerated fibrinolysis with some efficacy *(108,109)*.

INDWELLING CATHETER INFECTION

Intraventricular catheter (IVC), central venous line and urinary catheter placement are common procedures for the management of NSU patients but they carry an infection risk. In a reported case series of 545 NSU patients 113 nosocomial infections were identified in 90 patients *(110)*. This represents a moderate-to-high overall incidence (20.7/100 patients) with 1 bloodstream infections per 100 patient, and 7.3 urinary tract infections per 100 patients.

Central Venous Catheters

Guidelines for preventing infections associated with the insertion and the maintenance of central venous catheters have been developed *(111)*. These guidelines include recommendations as follows:

1. Use a single-lumen catheter unless multiple ports are essential for the management of the patient.
2. If total parenteral nutrition is being administered, use one central venous catheter or lumen exclusively for that purpose.
3. Use a tunneled catheter or an implantable vascular access device for patients in whom long-term (>30 d) vascular access is anticipated.
4. Consider the use of an antimicrobial impregnated central venous catheter for adult patients who require short-term (<10 d) central venous catheterization and who are at high risk for catheter-related bloodstream infection (CR-BSI).
5. Unless medically contraindicated, use the subclavian site in preference to the jugular or femoral sites for nontunneled catheter placement, because of the lower risk for CR-BSI.
6. Consider peripherally inserted central venous catheter (PICCs) as an alternative to subclavian or jugular vein catheterization.
7. Use optimum aseptic technique, including a sterile gown, gloves, and a large sterile drape, for the insertion of central venous catheters (CVC).
8. Clean the skin site with an alcoholic chlorhexidine gluconate solution prior to central venous catheter insertion. Use an alcoholic povidone-iodine solution for patients with a history of chlorhexidine sensitivity. Allow the antiseptic to dry before inserting the catheter.
9. Before accessing the system, disinfect the external surfaces of the catheter hub and connections ports with an aqueous solution of chlorexidine gluconate or povidone- iodine, unless contraindicated by manufacturer´s recommendations.
10. Use either a sterile gauze or transparent dressing to cover the catheter site.
11. Do not routinely replace nontunnelled CVC as a method to prevent catheter-related infection.
12. Use guide wire assisted catheter exchange to replace a malfunctioning catheter, or to exchange an existing catheter if there is no evidence of infection at the catheter site or proven CR-BSI.
13. If catheter-related infection is suspected, but there is no evidence of infection at the catheter site, remove the existing catheter and insert a new catheter over a guide wire; if tests reveal catheter related infection, the newly inserted catheter should be removed and, if is still required, a new catheter inserted at a different site.

Treatment of catheter related infection include removing catheter and antimicrobial therapy administration covering both Gram-positive cocci and Gram-negative bacilli. Vancomycin and a cephalosporin or an aminoglycoside with broad-spectrum penicillin should be added for initial empiric therapy while awaiting the culture results. Appropriate length of therapy for coagulase-negative and coagulase-positive staphylococcal bacteremia should be 10–14 d and minimum of 2 wk, respectively. Catheter-related sepsis due to Gram-negative bacilli such as *P. aeruginosa* and *Stenotrophomona maltophilia* may be difficult to treat. Antimicrobial treatment with aminoglycoside, third generation cephalosporin, or extended-spectrum penicillin is required. In addition combination therapy is appropriate. *Candida* catheter-associated infections should be treated with fluconazole or amphotericin B. Overall clinical results of patients with latter complication are improved if catheters are promptly removed. Length of therapy remains controversial. However, most intensivists treat patients for 2 wk past the time culture results turn negative.

Ventriculostomies

IVC placement has an overall infection rate between 4.1 and 10%. Although a maximum rate of 10.3% by day 6 of catheter insertion has been reported the optimal duration of IVC in order to decrease infection rate remains controversial. Consequently some authors recommend new catheter insertion by d 5 only if it is necessary for monitoring or therapeutics *(112)*. Intraparenchymal fiberoptic catheter use has demonstrated a lower infection rate than IVC (4.4% vs 0.6%) *(113) (see also* Chapters 5, 6, and 24*)*.

Miscellaneous

SCI patients with complete dependence remain at the highest risk for urinary tract infection (UTI). In addition, other patients with bladder dysfunction such as those with multiple sclerosis can develop UTI. Another device used in some NSU patients is the continuous jugular bulb catheter monitoring as described in Chapter 6. It has been demonstrated that the risk of bacteremia related to this catheter is negligible. However, subclinical thrombosis is the major concern.

REFERENCES

1. Rello J, Ausina V, Castella J, Net A, Prats G. Nosocomial respiratory tract infections in multiple trauma patients. Incidence of level of consciousness with implications for therapy. *Chest* 1992;102:525–529.
2. Schmidt E, Smirnov V, Ryabova V. Results of the seven-year prospective study of stroke patients. *Stroke* 1988;19:942–949.
3. Kim H, Chung CS, Lee KH, Robbins J. Aspiration subsequent to a pure medullary infarction: lesion sites, clinical variables, and outcome. *Arch. Neurol.* 2000;57:478–483.
4. Meng Nh, Wang TG, Lien IN. Dysphagia in patients with brainstem stroke: incidence and outcome. *Am. J. Phys. Med. Rehabil.* 2000;79:170–175.
5. Nakagawa T, Sekizawa K, Arai H, et al. High incidence of pneumonia in elderly patients with basal ganglia infarction. *Arch. Intern. Med.* 1997;157:321–324.
6. Nakajoh K, Nakagawa T, Sekizawa K, et al. Relation of pneumonia and protective reflexes in post-stroke patients with oral or tube feeding. *J. Intern. Med.* 2000;247:39–42.
7. Park RH, Allison MC, Lang J, et al. Randomised comparison of percutaneous endoscopic gastrostomy and nasogastric tube feeding in patients with persisting neurological dysphagia. *BMJ* 1992;304:1406–1409.
8. Dray TG, Hillel AD, Miller RM. Dysphagia caused by neurologic deficits. *Otolaryngol. Clin. North Am.* 1998;31:507–524.
9. Kaye G, Zorowitz R, Baredes S. Role of flexible laryngoscopy in evaluating aspiration. *Ann. Otol. Rhinol. Laryngol.* 1997;106:705–709.
10. Collins MJ, Bakheit AM. Does pulse oximetry reliably detect aspiration in dysphagic stroke patients? *Stroke* 1997;28:1773–1775.
11. Nash N. Swallowing problems in the tracheomized patient. *Otolaryngol. Clin. North Am.* 1988;17:701–709.
12. Potts RG, Zaroukian MH, Guerrero PA, Baker CD. Comparison of blue dye visualization and glucose oxidase test strip methods for detecting pulmonary aspiration of enteral feedings in intubated patients. *Chest* 1993;103:117–121.
13. Kollef MA. The prevention of ventilator-associated pneumonia. *N. Engl. J. Med.* 1999;340:627–634.
14. Coplin WM, Pierson DJ, Cooley KD, et al . Implications of extubation delay in brain injured patients meeting standard weaning criteria. *Am. J. Respir. Crit. Care Med.* 2000;161:1530–1536.
15. Grau AJ, Buggle F, Schnitzler P, Spiel M, Lichy C, Hacke W. Fever and infection early after ischemic stroke. *J. Neurol. Sci.* 1999;171:115–120.
16. Boque MC, Bodi M, Rello J. Trauma, head injury, and neurosurgery infections. *Semin. Resp. Infect.* 2000;15:280–286.
17. Gilbert DN, Moellering RC, Sande MA. The Sanford Guide to Antimicrobial Therapy, 31st ed. Hyde Park, VT: Antimicrobial Therapy, 2001.
18. Androgue HJ, Madias NE. Hyponatremia. *N. Engl. J. Med.* 2000;342:1581–1589.
19. Suarez JI, Cohen ML, Larkin J, Kernich CA, Hricik DE, Daroff RB. Acute intermittent porphyria: clinicopathologic correlation. *Neurology* 1997;48:1678–1683.
20. Harrigan MR. Endocrine and metabolic dysfunction syndromes in the critically ill. Cerebral salt wasting syndrome. *Crit. Care Clin.* 2001;17:125–138.
21. Nelson PB, Seif SM, Maroon JC, et al. Hyponatremia in intracranial disease: perhaps not the syndrome of inappropriate secretion of antidiuretic hormone. *Neurosurgery* 1981;55:938–941.
22. Laureno R, Illowsky K. Myelinolysis after correction of hyponatremia. *Ann. Intern. Med.* 1997;126:57–62.
23. Woo MH, Kale-Pradhan PB. Fludrocortisone in the treatment of subarachnoid hemorrhage- induced hyponatremia. *Ann. Pharmacother.* 1997;31:637–639.
24. Mori T, Katayama Y, Kawamata T, Hyrayama T. Improved efficiency of hypervolemic therapy with inhibition of natriuresis by fludrocortisone in patients with aneurysmal subarachnoid hemorrhage. *J. Neurosurg.* 1999;91:947–952.
25. Wong MF, Chin NM, Lew TW. Diabetes insipidus in neurosurgical patients. *Ann. Acad. Med. Singapore* 1998;27:340–343.
26. Shucart WA, Jackson I. Management of diabetes insipidus in neurosurgical patients. *J. Neurosurg.* 1976;44:65–71.
27. Androgue HJ, Madias NE. Hypernatremia. *N. Engl. J. Med.* 2000;342:1493–1499.
28. Gariballa, Robinson TG, Fotherby MD. Hypokalemia and potassium excretion in stroke patients. *J. Am. Geriatr. Soc.* 1997;45:1454–1458.
29. Pomeranz S, Constantini S, Pappaport ZH. Hypokalemia in severe head trauma. *Acta. Neurochir.* 1989;97:62–66.
30. Gennari JF. Hypokalemia. *N. Engl. J. Med.* 1998;339:451–458.

31. Savarese JJ, Caldwell, Lien CA, Miller R. Pharmacology of muscle relaxants and their antagonist. In Miller RD, ed. *Anesthesia*. Philadelphia: Churchill Livingstone, 2000:412–490.
32. Fink EB. Magnesium deficiency. Etiology and clinical spectrum. *Acta. Med. Scand.* 1981;647:125–137.
33. Polderman KH, Bloemers FW, Peederman SM, Girbes AR. Hypomagnesemia and hypophosphatemia at admission in patients with severe head injury. *Crit. Care Med.* 2000;28:2022–2025.
34. Zivin JR, Goolley, Zager RA, Ryan MJ. Hypocalcemia: a pervasive metabolic abnormality in the critically ill. *Am. J. Kidney Dis.* 2001;37:689–698.
35. Zaloga P. Hypocalcemia in critically ill patients. *Crit. Care Med.* 1992;20:251–262.
36. Kline CA, Esekogwu VI, Henderson SO, Newton KI. Non-convulsive status epilecticus in a patient with hypocalcemia. *J. Emerg. Med.* 1998;16:715–718.
37. Mundy GR, Martin TJ. The hypercalcemia of malignancy: pathogenesis and management. *Metabolism* 1982;31:1247–1277.
38. Tohme J, Bilezikian J. Critical illness and calcium metabolism. In Ober K, ed. *Contemporary Endocrinology: Endocrinology of Critical Disease*. Totowa, NJ: Humana Press, 1997:233.
39. Bilezikian J. Management of acute hypercalcemia. *N. Engl. J. Med.* 1992; 326:1196.
40. Baran DT. Disorders of mineral metabolism. In Irwin RS, Cerra FB, Rippe JM, eds. *Intensive Care Medicine*, 4th ed. Philadelphia: Lippincott-Raven, 1999:1283.
41. Hasling C, Charles P, Mosekilde L. Etidronate disodium in the management of malignancy-related hypercalcemia. *Am. J. Med.* 1987;82:51–54.
42. Bugg NC, Jones JA. Hypophosphatemia. Pathophysiology, effects and management on the intensive care unit. *Anaesthesia* 1998;53:895–902.
43. Riggs JE. Neurologic manifestations of fluid and electrolyte disturbances. *Neurol. Clin.* 1989;7:509–523.
44. Agnelli G. Prevention of VTE after neurosurgery. *Thromb. Haemost.* 1999;82:925–930.
45. Valladares JB, Hankinson J. Incidence of lower extremity deep vein thrombosis in neurosurgical patients. *Neurosurgery* 1980;6:138–141.
46. Ruff RL, Posner JB. Incidence and treatment of peripheral venous thrombosis in patients with glioma. *Ann. Neurol.* 1983;13:334–336.
47. Turpie AG, Hirsh J, Gent M. Prevention of deep venous thrombosis in potential neurosurgical patients: a randomized trial comparing graduated compresion stockings alone or graduated compresion stockings plus intermittent pneumatic compression with control. *Arch. Intern. Med.* 1989;149:679–681.
48. Macdonald RL, Amidei C, Lin G, et al. Safety of perioperative subcutaneous heparin for prophylaxis of VTE in patients undergoing craniotomy. *Neurosurgery* 1999;45:245–252.
49. Geerts W H, Heit JA, Clagett GP, et al. Prevention of venous thromboembolism. *Chest* 2001 119:1325–1755.
50. Mc Carthy ST, Turner JJ, Robertson D, et al. Low-dose heparin as prophylaxis against deep-vein thrombosis after acute ischemic stroke. *Lancet* 1977;2:800–801.
51. Bath PM, Iddenden R, Bath BJ. Low-molecular-weight heparins and heparinoids in acute ischemic stroke: a meta-analysis of randomized controlled trials. *Stroke* 2000;35:1770–1778.
52. Kamran SI, Downey D, Ruff RI. Pneumatic sequential compression reduces the risk of deep venous thrombosis in stroke patients. *Neurology* 1998;50:1683–1688.
53. International stroke trial collaborative group. The international stroke trial (IST): a randomized trial of aspirin, subcutaneous heparin, both or neither among 19 435 patients with acute ischemic stroke. *Lancet* 1997;349:1569–1581.
54. The publications committee for the trial of ORG 10172 in acute ischemic stroke treatment (TOAST) investigators. Low molecular weight heparinoid, ORG 10172 (danaparoid), and outcome after acute ischemic stroke; a randomized controlled trial. *JAMA* 1998;279:1265–1272.
55. Green D, Lee MY, Ito VY, et al. Fixed vs adjusted-dose heparin in the prophylaxis of thromboembolism in spinal cord injury. *JAMA* 1998; 260:1255–1258.
56. Green D, Lee MY, Lim AC, et al. Prevention of thromboembolism after spinal cord injury using low-molecular-weight heparin. *Ann. Intern. Med.* 1990;113:571–574.
57. Tapson VF, Carroll BA, Davidson BL, et al. The diagnostic approach to acute venous thromboembolism. Clinical practice guideline. American Thoracic Society. *Am. J. Respir. Crit. Care Med.* 1999;160:1043–1066.
58. Ellis MH, Manor Y, Witz M. Risk factors and management of patients with upper limb deep vein trombosis. *Chest* 2000;117:43–46.
59. Inci S, Erbengi A, Berker M. Pulmonary embolism in neurosurgical patients. *Surg. Neurol.* 1995;43:123–128.
60. Goodman LR, Curtin JJ, Mewissen MW, et al. Detection of pulmonary embolism in patients with unresolved clinical and scintigraphic diagnosis: helical CT versus angiography. *AJR* 1995;164:1369–1374.
61. Wet CJ, Pearl RG. Postoperative thrombotic complications. *Anesth. Clin. North Am.* 1999;17:895.
62. Hausmann D, Schulte am EJ. The prognostic value of various intensive medicine parameters in long-term intubated neurosurgical patients. *Anesthesie Intensivther. Notfallmed.* 1982;17:139–144.
63. Valli G, Fogazzi GB, Cappellari A, Rivolta E. Glomerulonephritis associated with myasthenia gravis. *Am. J. Kid. Dis.* 1998;31:350–355.

64. Khajehdehi P, Shariat A, Nikseresht A. Acute renal failure due to severe Landry-Guillain-Barre syndrome. *Nephrol. Dialysis Trasplant.* 1998;13:2388–2391.

65. Britt CW Jr, Light RR, Peters BH, Schochet SS Jr. Rhabdomyolysis during treatment with epsilon-aminocaproic acid. *Arch. Neurol.* 1980;37:187–188.

66. Levy JB, Pusey CD. Nephrotoxicity of intravenous immunoglobulin. *QJM* 2000;93:751–755.

67. Briggs TB, Smith RR. Exertional rhabdomyolysis associated with decerebrate posturing. *Neurosurgery* 1986;19:279–299.

68. Davenport A. The management of renal failure in patients at risk of cerebral edema/hypoxia. *New Horiz.* 1995;3:717–724.

69. Caruso DM, Vishteh AG, Greene KA, Matthews MR, Carrion CA. Continous hemodialysis for the management of acute renal failure in the presence of cerebellar hemorrhage. *J. Neurosurg.* 1998;89:649–652.

70. Rabary O, Boussofara M, Grimaud D. Acid-base equilibrium and the brain. *Ann. Fr. Anesth. Reanim.* 1994;13:111–122.

71. Tallon-Barranco A, Ayuso-Peralta L, Jimenez-Jimenez, et al. Respiratory form of onset of motor neuron disease. *Rev. Neurol.* 2000;30:51–53.

72. Huang R. Acid-base imbalance in acute cerebrovascular disease. *Chung-Hua Shen Ching Ching Shen Ko Tsa Chih* 1991;24:351–357,384.

73. Wijdicks EF, Hubmayr RD. Acute acid-base disorders associated with status epilecticus. *Mayo Clin. Proc.* 1994;69:1044–1046.

74. Chan KH, Mann KS, Lai EC, Ngan J, Tuen H, Yue CP. Factors influencing the development of gastrointestinal complications after neurosurgery: results of multivariate analysis. *Neurosurgery* 1989;25:378–382.

75. Lichtenstein DR, Berman MD, Wolfe MM. Approach to the patient with acute upper gastrointestinal hemorrhage. In Taylor MB, Gollan JL, Steer ML eds. Gastrointestinal Emergencies, 2nd ed. Baltimore: Williams & Wilkins, 1997: 99–129.

76. Fadul CE, Lemann W, Thaler HT, Posner JB. Perforation of the gastrointestinal tract in patients receiving steroids for neurological disease. *Neurology* 1988;38:348–352.

77. Inayet N, Amoateng-Adjepong Y, Upadya A, Manthous CA. Risks for developing critical illness with GI hemorrhage. *Chest* 2000;118:473–478.

78. Miller TA, Tornwall MS, Moody FG: Stress erosive gastritis. *Curr. Probl. Surg.* 1991;28:459–509.

79. Miller TA: Mechanisms of stress-related mucosal damage. *Am. J. Med.* 1987;83(suppl 6A):8–14.

80. McGuirk TD, Coyle WJ. Upper gastrointestinal tract bleeding. *Emerg. Med. Clin. North Am.* 1996;14:523–545.

81. Cappell MS. A study of the syndrome of simultaneous acute upper gastrointestinal bleeding and myocardial infarction in 36 patients. *Am. J. Gastroenterol.* 1995;90:1444–1449.

82. Cuellar RE, Gavaler JS, Alexander JA, Brouiellette DE, Chien MC, Yoo KC. Gastrointestinal tract hemorrhage: the value of a nasogastric aspirate. *Arch Intern Med* 1990;150:1381–1384.

83. Kankaria AG, Fleischer DE. The critical care management of nonvariceal upper gastrointestinal bleeding. *Crit. Care Clin.* 1995;11:347–368.

84. Shetty HG, Backhouse G, Bentley DP, Routledge PA. Effective reversal of warfarin-induced excessive anticoagulation with low dose vitamin K1. *Thromb. Haemost.* 1992; 67:13–15.

85. George JN, Shattil SJ: The clinical importance of acquired abnormalities of platelet function. *N. Engl. J. Med.* 1991;324:27–39.

86. Lu WY, Rhoney DH, Boling WB, Johnson JD, Smith TC. A review of stress ulcer prophylaxis in the neurosurgical intensive cares unit. *Neurosurgery* 1997;41:416–425.

87. Tryba M, Cook D. Current guidelines on stress ulcer prophylaxis. *Drugs* 1997;54:581–596.

88. Lau JY, Sung JJ, Lee KK, et al. Effect of intravenous omeprazole on recurrent bleeding after endoscopic treatment of bleeding peptic ulcers. *N. Engl. J. Med.* 2000;343:310–316.

89. Fenton WJ , Ofosu FA, Brezniak DV. Understanding Thrombin and hemostasis. *Hematol. Oncol. Clin. North Am.* 1993;7:1107–1119.

90. Jenny NS, Mann KG. Coagulation cascade: an overview. In Loscalzo J, Schafer AI, eds. *Thrombosis and Hemorrhage.* Baltimore: Williams & Wilkins, 1998:3.

91. Wardlaw JM. Overview of Cochrane thrombolysis meta-analysis. *Neurology* 2001;57(5 Suppl 2):S69–S76.

92. Gebel JM, Broderick JP. Intracerebral hemorrhage. *Neurol. Clin.* 2000;18:419–438.

93. Owings JT, Gosselin R. Acquired antithrombin deficiency following severe traumatic injury: rationale for study of antithrombin supplementation. *Semin. Thromb. Hemost.* 1997;23(suppl 1):17–24.

94. Gando S, Tedo l, Kubota M. Posttrauma coagulation and fibrinolysis. *Crit. Care Med.* 1992;20:594–600.

95. Miller RS, Weatherford DA, Stein D, Crane MM, Stein M. Antithrombin III and trauma patients: factors that determine low levels. *J Trauma* 1994;37:442–445.

96. Gando S, Nakanishi Y, Tedo I. Cytokines and plasminogen activator inhibitor-1 in posttrauma disseminated intravascular coagulation: relationship to multiple organ dysfunction syndrome. *Crit. Care Med.* 1995;20:1835–1842.

97. Kearney TJ, Bento L, Grode M. Coagulopathy and catecholamines in severe head injury. *J. Trauma* 1992;32:608–611.

98. Counts RB, Haisch C, Simon TL, Maxwell NG, Heimbach DM, Carrico CJ. Hemostasis in massively transfused trauma patients. *Ann. Surg.* 1979;190:91–99.

99. Phillips TF, Soulier G, Wilson RF. Outcome of massive transfusion exceeding two blood volumes in trauma and emergency surgery. *J. Trauma* 1987;27:903–910.

100. Martin DJ, Lucas CE, Ledgerwood AM, Hoschner J, McGorrigal MD, Grabow D. Fresh frozen plasma supplement to massive red blood cell transfusion. *Ann. Surg.* 1985;202:505–511.
101. Redd RL 2nd, Ciavarella D, Heimbach DM, et al. Prophylactic platelet administration during massive transfusion. *Ann. Surg.* 1986;203:40–48.
102. Watts DD, Trask A, Soeken K, Perdue P, Dols S, Kaufmann C. Hypothermic coagulopathy in trauma: effect of varying levels of hypothermia on enzyme speed, platelet function, and fibrinolytic activity. *J. Trauma* 1998;44:846–854.
103. Reed RL 2nd, Bracey AW Jr, Hudson JD, Miller TA, Fischer RP. Hypothermia and blood coagulation: dissociation between enzyme activity and clotting factor levels. *Circ. Shock* 1990;32:141–152.
104. Luna GK, Maier RV, Pavlin EG, Anardi D, Copass MK. Incidence and effect of hypothermia in seriously injured patients. *J. Trauma* 1987;27:1014–1018.
105. Patt A, McCroskey B, Moore E. Hypothermia induced coagulopathies in trauma. *Surg. Clin. North Am.* 1988;68:775–785.
106. Dhainaut JF. Introduction to the Margaux conference on critical illness: activation of the coagulation system in critical illnesses. *Crit. Care Med.* 2000;28(9 Suppl):S1–S3.
107. Harrigan C, Lucas CE, Ledgerwood AM, et al. The effect of hemorrhagic shock on the clotting cascade in injured patients. *J. Trauma* 1989;29:1416–1421.
108. Verstraete M. Clinical application of inhibitors of fibrinolysis. *Drugs* 1995;29:236–261.
109. Dunn CJ, Goa KL. Tranexamic acid: a review of its use in surgery and other indications. *Drugs* 1999;57:1005–1032.
110. Dettenkofer M, Ebner W, Hans FJ, et al. Nosocomial infections in a neurosurgery intensive care unit. *Acta. Neurochir.* 1999;141:1303–1308.
111. Pratt RJ, Pellowe C, Loveday HP, et al. The epic project: developing national evidence-based guidelines for preventing healthcare associated infections. Phase I: guidelines for preventing hospital-acquired infections. *J. Hosp. Infect.* 2001;47:S3–S82.
112. Paramore CG, Turner DA. Relative risk of ventriculostomy infection and morbidity. *Acta. Neurochir. (Wien)* 1994;127:79–84.
113. Khan SH, Kureshi IU, Mulgrew T, Ho SY, Onnyiuke HC. Comparison of percutaneous ventriculostomies and intraparenchymal monitor: a retrospective evaluation of 156 patients. *Acta. Neurochir. (Wien)* 1998;71:50–52.

12

Sedation and Analgesia in the Critically Ill Neurology and Neurosurgery Patient

Mitzi K. Hemstreet, Jose I. Suarez, and Marek A. Mirski

INTRODUCTION

Sedation of critically ill patients with neurologic or neurosurgical pathology is often a controversial topic, as one of the primary tenants of care of these patients is the capacity to perform repeated neurologic examinations to assess for a change *(1)*. Routine sedation of all intubated patients, for example, is not recommended, as somnolence may be the first indication of a worsening intracranial process. However, there are a number of situations when sedation and analgesia are necessary for either patient safety or comfort. These include patients with traumatic brain injury (TBI), who are often agitated and at risk of injury to self or the medical staff caring for them. Many TBI patients are also withdrawing from chronic alcohol and drug use, and this must be factored in to the choice and duration of sedation. Patients who must remain intubated for either neurologic or systemic reasons, and are at risk of self-extubation or show significant anxiety or discomfort while mechanically ventilated, may also require gentle sedation and analgesia. Patients with severe intracranial hypertension may require deep sedation and analgesia or even general anesthesia to control intracranial pressure (ICP) (*see also* Chapter 5). Similarly, patients with generalized status epilepticus may require general anesthesia to the point of electrographic burst-suppression to control seizure activity (*see also* Chapter 25).

Before initiation of sedation in neurologically affected critically ill patients, alternative explanations for agitation, confusion, or sympathetic hyperactivity must be excluded. Hypoxemia or hypercarbia related to decreased respiratory drive or poor airway protection must be detected and treated appropriately. Metabolic disarray, including acidosis, hyponatremia, hypoglycemia, hypercalcemia, hyperamylasemia, hyperammonemia, or hepatic or renal insufficiency may contribute to behavioral changes in critically ill patients *(2–6)*. Infection is also a frequent trigger of delirium in hospitalized and critically ill patients *(4)*. Cardiac ischemia, hypotension, and associated cerebral hypoperfusion may also contribute to mental status changes, and must be ruled out as a cause of delirium in critically ill neurologic patients *(7)*. Concomitant administration of other psychoactive medications such as antidepressants *(8–10)*, anticonvulsants *(11–13)*, peptic ulcer prophylactics *(14,15)* and interactions with promotility agents *(16)*, corticosteroids *(9,17,18)*, or even antibiotics *(19–25)* and antiretroviral agents *(26)*, may adversely affect cognition and behavior. Another important factor that needs to be addressed is pain, particularly in TBI and postoperative patients. Adequate sedation and analgesia in these patients is necessary.

The choice of intravenous (IV) sedatives is vast, and includes narcotics, benzodiazepines, barbiturates, neuroleptics, α2-adrenergic agents, and the novel compound, propofol, whereas the choice of

From: *Current Clinical Neurology*
Critical Care Neurology and Neurosurgery
Edited by: J. I. Suarez © Humana Press Inc., Totowa, NJ

analgesics is basically limited to narcotics. Each has advantages and disadvantages in the neurologic patient, and these will be addressed. It is generally recommended that shorter-acting agents be used in the neurosciences critical care unit (NSU) setting to facilitate neurologic examinations *(1,27)*, although in certain situations the longer-acting compounds may be preferable. In this chapter, each sedative or analgesic agent will be compared in relation to its mechanism of action, pharmacokinetics, routes of administration, titratability, adverse reactions, hemodynamic stability, effects on ICP and seizure threshold, and recommended monitoring during drug administration and recovery. Where relevant, the reversibility, drug-drug interactions, and cost-effectiveness will also be discussed. We present a summary of the main characteristics of preferred sedatives and analgesics in NSU patients in Tables 1 and 2.

NARCOTICS (OPIOIDS)

A large number of natural opioids (e.g., morphine sulfate, codeine), semi-synthetic opioids (e.g., fentanyl, hydromorphone, oxycodone), and completely synthetic (e.g., meperidine) opioid-like compounds are available. These compounds act primarily as analgesics, but also serve as sedative-hypnotics at low dosages. Their major disadvantage, particularly in neurologic patients, is their suppression of the hypercarbic respiratory drive. Advantages include easy titratability, provision of patient comfort, and reversibility. This discussion shall be limited to the most readily available agents recommended for analgesia and sedation of NSU patients (fentanyl, remifentanil, and morphine).

Mechanism of Action

All opioids act by binding to opioid receptors in the central and peripheral nervous systems as agonists, partial agonists, or agonist-antagonists *(28)*. These receptor interactions are the basis for the pharmacological effects of opioids (analgesia, decreased level of consciousness, respiratory depression, miosis, gastrointestinal hypomotility, antitussive effects, euphoria or dysphoria, and vasodilatation), and vary by the specific opioid receptor subtypes bound by each drug *(29–35)*. For the purposes of this chapter, discussion shall focus on fentanyl, remifentanil, and morphine, all *mu*-opioid receptor agonists *(28)*.

Pharmacokinetics

Opioids are readily absorbed through mucosal surfaces, from the gastrointestinal tract, or through subcutaneous (SQ), intramuscular (IM), intrathecal (IT), epidural, and IV routes of administration *(28)*. Fentanyl is also easily absorbed via transdermal application. Morphine and other opioids are rapidly distributed to the brain, with the more lipophilic compounds (i.e., fentanyl, remifentanil) having the shortest time of onset. Peak effect following IV administration of morphine is approx 15 min; that for fentanyl is 5 min, and remifentanil is 1–2 min.

After enteral administration, the bioavailability of morphine sulfate is only approx 20–40% due to first-pass hepatic metabolism *(36)*. IM and IV morphine sulfate is rapidly and readily available *(37)*. Morphine is 20–36% protein bound in plasma, and has a volume of distribution of 1–6 L/kg, depending on route of administration *(36)*. However, the majority of systemically administered morphine does not cross the blood–brain barrier (BBB) *(38,39)*.

Morphine is eliminated in the liver by *N*-demethylation, *N*-dealkylation, *O*-dealkylation, conjugation, and hydrolysis *(40,41)*. The majority of clearance is by glucuronidation to the active metabolites, morphine-3-glucuronide (approx 50%) and morphine-6-glucuronide (5–15%), which are renally excreted; the latter is a more potent analgesic than the parent compound *(42)*, and may accumulate in patients with renal insufficiency *(43,44)*. The half life of morphine varies greatly by route of administration, ranging from 1.5–4.5 h for IV, IM, and SQ injection, to 15 h or more for sustained-release oral preparations *(45,46)*.

Time to onset following oral administration of fentanyl is 5–15 min, with a peak response at 20–30 min *(47)*. For IM injection of fentanyl, onset is at 7–8 min, and effects last 1–2 h. Transdermal fentanyl has a much slower onset of action, 12–24 h *(48)*, although rate of absorption increases with higher skin temperature (i.e., febrile patients). Steady state is reached at 36–48 h, and duration of action is up to 72 h after removal of transdermal fentanyl *(49)*. Following IV administration, the onset of action of fentanyl is immediate, although peak effects take several minutes to manifest *(50)*. Duration of action after a single IV dose of fentanyl is 30–60 min, which increases after repeated or prolonged dosing due to accumulation in fat and skeletal muscle.

Fentanyl is extensively plasma protein bound (80–86%) *(51)*, with a total volume of distribution of 3–6 L/kg in adults *(52)*. Fentanyl is metabolized via *N*-dealkylation by the hepatic cytochrome P450 system, producing norfentanyl and other inactive metabolites, which are renally excreted *(53)*. Half-life is approx 200 min following IV injection, and up to 17 h for transdermal administration. As up to 10% of fentanyl is excreted unchanged in the urine, its duration of action may be prolonged following high cumulative doses in patients with renal insufficiency *(54)*. Fentanyl does not appear to be removed from the plasma compartment by hemodialysis *(55)*.

Remifentanil is only given by IV injection or infusion, with a time to peak onset of action of 1–3 min *(56)*. Duration of action is only 3–10 min after a single dose, increased slightly after prolonged infusions. Remifentanil is 92% plasma protein bound, with a volume of distribution of 25–60 L *(57,58)* and a distribution half-life of 1 min. Obese individuals require a reduction in remifentanil dosing, which should be based on ideal rather than actual body weight. Remifentanil is rapidly metabolized by plasma esterases to an inactive carboxylic acid, which is 90% renally excreted *(58)*. Metabolism is independent of the cumulative remifentanil dose, and unaffected by hepatic or renal function.

Routes of Administration

Morphine and fentanyl are available as oral preparations, and as sterile parenteral formulations for SQ, IM, IV, IT, and epidural administration. For sedation and analgesia, the IV route is recommended from rapid onset and easy titratability. Because of its short duration of action, remifentanil is given only as an IV infusion.

Titratability

Due to its rapid onset and short duration of action, which is independent of hepatic and renal clearance, remifentanil is easily titratable. Preliminary use of continuous remifentanil infusion for sedation of both intubated and unintubated patients in an NSU setting have shown promising results, with blunting of hemodynamic instability and intracranial hypertension associated with agitation, coughing, and tracheal suctioning *(59)*. Fentanyl is more readily available than remifentanil in many medical centers, and many physicians are more comfortable with this opioid due to its longer history. Fentanyl may be given by either bolus dosing or continuous IV infusion. However, fentanyl is less easily titrated due to its longer duration of action and accumulation in lipid and muscle stores over time, requiring greater periods of drug interruption to permit frequent neurologic assessment. Morphine is the most difficult of these opioids to titrate, again due to its longer duration of action, dependence on hepatic and renal clearance, and prolonged clearance of active metabolites. For these reasons, infusions of morphine are not recommended for NSU patients, although intermittent administration may facilitate patient comfort and hemodynamic stability.

Adverse Reactions

These include pruritus, excessive somnolence, respiratory depression, chest wall and other muscular rigidity (primarily fentanyl and its congeners), dysphoria or hallucinations (primarily morphine), nausea and vomiting, gastrointestinal dysmotility, hypotension, histamine release causing urticaria

Table 1
Main Characteristics of the Main Sedatives and Analgesics Used in NSU Patients

Drug	Type of medication	Sedation	Analgesia	Mechanism of action	Protein binding	Metabolism	Active metabolite
Fentanyl	Opioid	+	+++	Mu receptor agonist	80–86%	Hepatic	
Remifentanyl	Opioid	+	+++	Mu receptor agonist	92%	Plasma esterases	
Morphine sulfate	Opioid	+	+++	Mu receptor agonist	20–30%	Hepatic	Morphine-3-glucuronide Morphine-6-glucuronide
Diazepam	Benzodiazepine	+++	+	GABA$_a$ receptor agonist	99%	Hepatic	Desmethyldiazepam, oxazepam, hydroxydiazepam
Lorazepam	Benzodiazepine	+++		GABA$_a$ receptor agonist	91–93%	Hepatic	
Midazolam	Benzodiazepine	+++		GABA$_a$ receptor agonist	97%	Hepatic	1-Hydroxymethyl-midazolam
Thiopental	Barbiturate	+++		GABA$_a$ receptor agonist	30–40%	Mostly hepatic. Also kidney, brain	
Pentobarbital	Barbiturate	+++		GABA$_a$ receptor agonist	35–45%	Mostly hepatic	
Phenobarbital	Barbiturate	+++		GABA$_a$ receptor agonist	20–40%	Mostly hepatic and urine (unchanged)	

(continued on next page)

224

Haloperidol	Neuroleptic (butyrophenone)	+++		Blocks dopamine, adrenergic, serotonin, acetylcholine, and histamine receptors	92%	Hepatic
Droperidol	Neuroleptic (butyrophenone)	+++		Blocks dopamine, adrenergic, serotonin, acetylcholine and histamine receptors	92%	Hepatic
Clonidine	α-2 agonist	++	++	α-2 receptor agonist (pre- and post-synaptic	20–40%	Hepatic (50%) and urine (unchanged, 50%)
Dexmedetomidine	α-2 agonist	++	++	α-2 receptor agonist (pre- and post-synaptic	94%	Hepatic
Propofol		+++		Unclear	Not found	Hepatic and extrahepatic

+, mild; ++, moderate; +++, high.

Table 2
Dosages, Main Advantages, and Disadvantages of Most Commonly Used Anaglesics and Sedatives in NSU Patients

Drug	Starting dose	Titration	Half-life	Advantages	ICP effects	Seizure threshold effect	Adverse events
Fentanyl	12.5–50 μg IV q 20–30 min	Infusion 0.01–03 μg/kg/min and titrate q 15–30 min, up to 50–100 μg/h	30–60 min (single IV dose). Repeated is hours	Reversible, rapid onset, short duration	Indirect elevation (hypercarbia)	Myoclonus, no seizures	Respiratory depression, chest wall rigidity, gastric dysmotility, hypotension
Remifentanyl	0.5–1.0 μg/kg IV bolus	Infusion 0.05–0.2 μg/kg/min	3–10 min after single dose	Reversible, rapid onset, short duration	Indirect elevation (hypercarbia)	Myoclonus, no seizures	Respiratory depression, chest wall rigidity, gastric dysmotility, hypotension
Morphine sulfate	5–20 mg IM q 4 h 2–10 mg IV q 4 h	Caution: metabolites may accumulate For post-operative pain (PCAP): 0.2–3.0 mg and 5–20 min lockout intervals	1.5–4.5 h IV, IM, SQ	Reversible	Elevates ICP	Myoclonus, no seizures	Respiratory depression, gastric dysmotility, hypotension, hallucinations
Diazepam	2 mg IV 30–60 min		30–60 h	Reversible	Indirect elevation (hypercarbia)	Treat seizures	Respiratory depression, hypotension, confusion
Lorazepam	0.25–0.5 mg IV q 1–2 h		10–20 h	Reversible	Indirect elevation (hypercarbia)	Treat seizures	Respiratory depression, hypotension, confusion

(continued on next page)

Drug	Dose	Infusion	Half-life	Properties	ICP effect	Indication	Adverse effects
Midazolam	0.5–1 mg IV q 5–30 min	Infusion 0.25–1.0 μg/kg/min	1–2.5 h	Reversible, shorter duration, and titratable	No direct effect on ICP. Indirect elevation (hypercarbia and hypotension)	Treat seizures	Respiratory depression, hypotension, confusion
Thiopental	1–5 mg/kg IV		8–12 h		ICP reduction	Treat seizures	Respiratory depression hypotension gastric dysmotility, bronchospasm, angioedema
Pentobarbital	3–30 mg/kg IV	Infusion 1–2 mg/kg/h to burst-suppression EEG	15–50 h		ICP reduction	Treat seizures	Respiratory depression, hypotension, gastric dysmotility, bronchospasm, angioedema
Phenobarbital	1–3 mg/kg IV or IM (sedation) 15–20 mg/kg IV (status epilepticus)		53–120 h		ICP reduction (large doses)	Treat seizures	Respiratory depression, hypotension, gastric dysmotility, bronchospasm, angioedema
Haloperidol	0.5–5.0 mg IV		12–36 h		Not studied	Unpredictable	Extrapyramidal signs; may lower seizure threshold

(continued on next page)

Table 2 (*Continued*)
Dosages, Main Advantages, and Disadvantages of Most Commonly Used Anaglesics and Sedatives in NSU Patients

Drug	Starting dose	Titration	Half-life	Advantages	ICP Effects	Seizure threshold effect	Adverse events
Droperidol	0.625–2.5 mg IV		4–12 h		No effect	Unpredictable	Extrapyramidal signs; may lower seizure threshold; QT prolongation
Clonidine	0.1 mg PO q 8–24 h Increase 0.1 mg/d q 1–2 d up to 0.6 mg/d		12–16 h	Useful in setting of alcohol or drug withdrawal	No effect	Little data: increases epileptiform activity in known focal seizures?	Dry mouth, bradycardia, hypotension, rebound hypertension
Dexmedeto-midine	1 µg/kg IV over 10 min	Infusion 0.2–0.7 µg/kg/h	2 h	Useful in setting of alcohol or drug withdrawl	No effect	No human studies	Dry mouth, bradycardia, hypotension, adrenal suppression, atrial fibrillation
Propofol	1.0–2.5 mg/kg IV (anesthesia induction) 5 µg/kg/min for 5 min IV (sedation)	Increase infusion by 5–10 µg/kg/min q 5–10 min to maintenance 25–100 up to 100–300 µg/kg/min	4–10 min	Very short duration, easy titratability	Lowers ICP	Conflicting results but most likely treats seizures	Hypotension respiratory depression, metabolic rhabdomyolysis, anaphylaxis, sepsis, pain at venous site

ICP, intracranial pressure; IV, intravenous; IM, intramuscular; SQ, subcutaneous; PCAP, patient-controlled analgesia pump.

and flushing (primarily meperidine and morphine), anaphylaxis (rare), and immune suppression after repeated dosing *(28,60)*.

Hemodynamic Stability

Although morphine may induce hypotension even at low therapeutic doses (partly due to promotion of histamine release) *(60,61)*, fentanyl and remifentanil tend to have little effect on blood pressure at sedative doses. Fentanyl also tends to reduce heart rate, which is favorable in the setting of cardiovascular disease.

Effects on Intracranial Pressure

Caution has been issued regarding administration of morphine to TBI patients due to increases in ICP, although the mechanism is unclear. In general, opioids per se have no effects on ICP or cerebral blood flow (CBF) *(28)*, but any hypercarbia related to respiratory depression by opiates may lead to cerebral vasodilatation and its sequelae.

Effects on Seizure Threshold

Very high doses of both morphine and fentanyl *(62–64)* have been shown to induce seizure-like activity in patients undergoing general anesthesia. As none of these cases had documented electrographic seizure activity, some others have suggested that the reported "seizures" were actually manifestations of narcotic-induced rigidity or myoclonus *(65)*. Indeed, nonepileptic myoclonus has been reported in numerous cases when very high doses of IV or IT morphine were given *(66,67)*. In contrast, the active metabolite of meperidine, normeperidine, is associated with an excitatory syndrome which includes seizures; as normeperidine has an elimination half-life of 15–20 h, which is prolonged in both renal and hepatic insufficiencies, the use of meperidine in NSU patients is not recommended.

Recommended Monitoring During Drug Administration and Recovery

Because of their potential to suppress respiratory drive, it is recommended that all patients receiving narcotic sedation have frequent (preferably continuous) monitoring of pulse oximetry and respiratory rate. Additional frequent hemodynamic assessments including blood pressure and heart rate are prudent from the potential for hypotension, bradycardia, and tachycardia with selective narcotic agonists.

Reversibility

One of the advantages of sedation with opioid narcotics is their rapid reversibility with the prototypic antagonist, naloxone. Although the recommended dosage for reversal of narcotic overdose is generally 0.4 mg or above *(28)*, in NSU patients the starting dosage should be much lower (i.e., 0.04–0.08 mg by IV push) to avoid "overshoot" phenomena such as hypertension, tachycardia, and emergence agitation, which may precipitate or worsen intracerebral hemorrhage, intracranial hypertension, or myocardial ischemia. Dosage may be titrated to the desired level of arousal and reversal of respiratory depression, with effects seen within 1–2 min of each subsequent administration.

Drug–Drug Interactions

Combined use of morphine and neuroleptics may produce greater than expected decreases in blood pressure *(28)*. Additionally, the depressant effects of narcotics on respiration and level of consciousness may be potentiated by concurrent administration of phenothiazine neuroleptics, tricyclic antidepressants, and monoamine oxidase inhibitors *(28)*.

Dosage Recommendations for Specific Agents

Dosage recommendations are for narcotic-naïve patients. As a general guideline, fentanyl and remifentanil are approx 100 times more potent than morphine.

Fentanyl

Although fentanyl may also be given by oral, transdermal, IM, IT, and epidural routes, IV administration is recommended for NSU patients. For mild sedation and analgesia, recommended starting dosage is 12.5–50 μg IV every 30–60 min, or a continuous infusion of 0.01–0.03 μg/kg/min or 25–50 μg/h (with or without initial IV bolus), titrating to effect every 15–30 min. Continuous infusions above 50–100 μg/h are not recommended in narcotic-naïve patients unless they are endotracheally intubated or otherwise have a protected airway, and mechanical ventilation is possible. For deeper sedation, as an adjunct to general anesthesia, or in narcotic-tolerant patients, continuous infusions greater than 100 μg/h may be used.

Remifentanil

For induction of general anesthesia, IV bolus of 0.5–1.0 μg/kg is given followed by titration of continuous infusions of 0.05–0.2 μg/kg/min. No adjustment is needed for renal or hepatic insufficiency, although decreasing the dose by 50% is recommended for patients older than 65 yr of age.

Morphine Sulfate

For analgesic dosing, titration doses of 5–20 mg IM every 4 h or 2–10 mg IV over 4–5 min every 4 h is recommended. SQ morphine is usually given up to 10 mg every 4 h. For oral dosing, give 5–30 mg of the immediate release (IR) formula every 4 h. To convert to extended release (ER) enteral morphine, divide the total daily dose of IM, IV, or IR morphine into 12–24 h dosing. These dosages are for narcotic naïve individuals, and may be increased substantially (with appropriate monitoring) in patients tolerant to opioids. Due to hepatic metabolism and renal clearance, dosages should be reduced in patients with hepatic or renal insufficiency or those at the extremes of age.

BENZODIAZEPINES

As with the opioids, there are a large number of benzodiazepines in therapeutic use due to their diverse pharmacologic properties, durations of action, and routes of administration. These medications are sedatives, not analgesics, with one exception, IV diazepam, as will be mentioned below. This chapter shall limit discussion to the most readily available intravenous agents (diazepam, lorazepam, and midazolam) used for sedation in the NSU setting.

Mechanism of Action

The majority, if not all, of the effects of benzodiazepines are through potentiation of the central nervous system actions of the inhibitory neurotransmitter, γ-aminobutyric acid (GABA). Benzodiazepines experimentally increase the frequency of opening of the GABA chloride channel in response to binding of GABA (68). Subsequent effects include anxiolysis, sedation, muscle relaxation, anterograde amnesia, respiratory depression (especially in children, patients with chronic pulmonary disease, hepatic insufficiency, or when combined with other sedatives), anticonvulsant activity (not all benzodiazepines), and analgesia (only intravenous diazepam) (68). Very high doses of several benzodiazepines will also lead to coronary vasodilatation and neuromuscular blockade through interaction with peripheral sites (68).

Pharmacokinetics

Because of their high lipid:water solubility, IV benzodiazepines are rapidly distributed in the brain, followed by redistribution to muscle and fat. Diazepam is most rapidly redistributed due to its higher lipophilicity, requiring repeated dosing in status epilepticus, often leading to higher cumulative doses and greater respiratory depression (*see also* Chapter 25). Lorazepam and midazolam have slower redistribution out of the brain due to greater water solubility. All benzodiazepines are highly bound to plasma proteins, and all are extensively metabolized by hepatic microsomal enzymes *(68)*.

Routes of Administration

Diazepam, lorazepam, and midazolam are all available in oral, IM, and IV preparations.

Titratability

IV midazolam is the most easily titratable because of its shorter duration of action, and is most appropriate for use as a continuous infusion. Because of their much longer half-lives, it is recommended that lorazepam and diazepam be used only as intermittent dosing in NSU patients.

Adverse Reactions

These include headache, nausea or vomiting, vertigo, confusion, excessive somnolence to obtundation, respiratory depression, hypotension, hypotonia/loss of reflexes, or muscular weakness *(68)*.

Hemodynamic Stability

Low (oral hypnotic) doses of benzodiazepines have little effect on blood pressure, but higher IV (sedative or anesthetic) doses may cause hypotension and increased heart rate *(68)*.

Effects on Intracranial Pressure

Because of its more prevalent use in neuroanesthesia and sedation in the NSU, the effects of midazolam on ICP and CBF have been more carefully studied than those of other benzodiazepines. These studies indicate that midazolam, by itself, has little or no effect on ICP *(69–71)*. However, decreases in mean arterial pressure associated with midazolam administration may impair cerebral perfusion *(70,71)*, and hypercarbia associated with the respiratory-depressant effects of benzodiazepines may actually increase ICP in the TBI patient *(71)*.

Effects on Seizure Threshold

Benzodiazepines are well established as treatment for convulsive status epilepticus *(72–74)*, with lorazepam currently recommended as first line treatment of this life threatening condition (*see also* Chapter 25). This is generally supported by animal studies, which demonstrate that benzodiazepines inhibit some types of experimentally induced seizure activity, but not others *(68)*. Benzodiazepines have also widely been used to prevent or treat alcohol withdrawal seizures *(75)*, although some evidence suggests that tolerance develops rapidly, with subsequent decreased anticonvulsant efficacy.

Recommended Monitoring During Drug Administration and Recovery

As with opioid narcotics, the potential for respiratory depression and hypotension with benzodiazepines necessitates careful monitoring of pulse oximetry and blood pressure in individuals sedated with these agents. This is especially prudent in patients maintained on continuous midazolam infusions, and those who are not mechanically-ventilated.

Reversibility

Benzodiazepines are reversible with the selective antagonist, flumazenil *(68,76)*. Caution must be exerted with flumazenil, however, as this agent may precipitate rapid rises in ICP, systemic hypertension, and lowering of seizure threshold *(76,77)*, particularly in TBI and neurosurgical patients. Additionally, because of its short duration of action, patients may become resedated from longer-acting benzodiazepines after flumazenil has been metabolized *(76)*.

Drug–Drug Interactions

As with nearly all sedative agents, additive or synergistic effects may occur with benzodiazepines and any other medication which may alter level of consciousness, suppress respiratory drive, or decrease systemic blood pressure. As such, these agents should be used with caution in individuals who already have altered mental status, have questionable airway protective mechanisms (if not intubated and mechanically ventilated), or who are hypovolemic, septic, or otherwise hemodynamically-unstable and on multiple other medications. Additionally, psychotic reactions have been reported with the combined use of benzodiazepines and valproic acid *(68)*.

Dosage Recommendations for Specific Agents

Diazepam

For sedation, use doses of 2 mg IV every 30–60 min as needed or 5–10 mg orally up to three to four times a day. Half-life is 30–60 h.

Lorazepam

For sedation, give 0.25–0.5 mg IV every 1–2 h as needed, or 2–4 mg orally up to three times a day. Half-life is 10–20 h.

Midazolam

Administer 0.5–1 mg IV every 5–30 min as needed (0.07 mg/kg IM). Maintenance infusions may be titrated from 0.25–1.0 µg/kg/min. Half-life is 1–2.5 h.

BARBITURATES

All centrally acting agents in this class possess dose-dependent sedative, hypnotic, or anesthetic actions; those recommended for use in neurologic emergencies also have anticonvulsant and cerebroprotective properties. The three most commonly used barbiturates in the NSU setting are phenobarbital, pentobarbital, and sodium thiopental, which will be discussed.

Mechanism of Action

Similar to the benzodiazepines, barbiturates produce their central depressant effect by facilitation of chloride conductance through inhibitory GABA ion channels *(68)*. However, barbiturates and benzodiazepines bind to separate sites on the GABA channel, with barbiturates prolonging channel opening time rather than increasing frequency. Additionally, at higher concentrations, some barbiturates (i.e., pentobarbital) may trigger opening of the inhibitory chloride channel in the absence of GABA *(68)*. Through central enhancement of GABA-ergic transmission, barbiturates produce their sedative-hypnotic, anesthetic, anticonvulsant, and respiratory-depressant effects.

Pharmacokinetics

Thiopental is highly lipid soluble, and is rapidly (within thirty seconds) distributed to the brain following IV administration. Redistribution to other tissues occurs within 30 min *(68)*, with the majority of patients awakening from a single IV dose of thiopental within 10 min *(78)*. Although thiopental is classified as an ultra-short acting barbiturate, repeated or prolonged administration may lead to deposition in fat stores, and an effective half-life of 24 h or more *(78,79)*. Low doses of thiopental are eliminated by linear pharmacokinetics, but larger doses or prolonged administration follow a nonlinear pattern. Thiopental is biotransformed in liver, kidney, brain, and other tissues, and excreted renally as inactive metabolites *(68,78,79)*.

Pentobarbital is classified as a short acting barbiturate, and is a major metabolite of thiopental. This barbiturate has historically been used as a continuous infusion in patients with refractory cerebral hypertension *(80)*. Pentobarbital has similar pharmacokinetics behavior as thiopental.

Phenobarbital is classified as a long acting barbiturate, and being less lipophilic than the other members of this class it may require up to 20–30 min for equilibration in the brain *(68)*. Metabolism is primarily hepatic, although a significant amount of phenobarbital is excreted unchanged in urine *(81)*; osmotic diuretics such as mannitol, or alkalinization of the urine *(68)* may enhance this elimination. Cumulative dosing of phenobarbital in patients with renal insufficiency may lead to higher than desired serum levels.

Barbiturates are highly bound to plasma proteins, and as such may potentiate the effects of other highly-bound substances. Weak acids such as aspirin or warfarin *(68)* may displace protein binding of barbiturates.

Routes of Administration

Phenobarbital and pentobarbital are available in oral, IM, and IV formulations. Thiopental is administered IV at a concentration of 25 mg/mL *(78)*, although both thiopental and pentobarbital are also available for rectal dosing *(68)*.

Titratability

Because of their long half-lives, barbiturates are not easily-titratable, and therefore not recommended for routine sedation of NSU patients. Their predominant uses in this patient population have been for reduction of refractory intracranial hypertension, and control of convulsive status epilepticus *(see also* Chapters 5 and 25). Thiopental, given as a single IV bolus dose, is widely used as an induction agent for intubation or general anesthesia.

Adverse Reactions

Potential adverse reactions to barbiturates include bronchospasm, angioedema, cough, hiccough, laryngospasm, loss of protective airway reflexes at higher doses, respiratory depression, hypotension (may be severe), loss of reflexive cardiovascular compensation for hypovolemia and positive pressure ventilation, decreased cardiac contractility (partially reversible by β-adrenergic agonists and cardiac glycosides), decreased CBF, gastrointestinal hypomotility, oliguria or anuria (due to both decreased renal blood flow and direct effects on renal tubular transport), and loss of thermoregulatory control *(68,78)*.

With initial dosing, barbiturates inhibit hepatic cytochrome P-450 activity, followed by enzyme induction with repeated or cumulative dosing (altering metabolism of many other drugs and endogenous steroids). Very high doses of barbiturates (as used to induce electroencephalographic [EEG] burst-suppression) will lead to loss of the neurologic examination, making clinical assessment all but impossible. Due to enhanced porphyrin synthesis, barbiturates are absolutely contraindicated in individuals with porphyria variegata or acute intermittent porphyria *(68,78)* *(see also* Chapter 28).

Hemodynamic Stability

In low doses, barbiturates have little effect on blood pressure and heart rate. At the higher supra-anesthetic doses used in NSU emergencies (to induce EEG burst-suppression), IV barbiturates may lead to severe hypotension requiring vasopressors or inotropic support. Placement of a pulmonary artery catheter is often required to manage hemodynamic support in this situation.

Effects on Intracranial Pressure

Thiopental has beneficial effects on ICP by decreasing both CBF and cerebral metabolic rate (CMRO$_2$) *(78)* *(see also* Chapters 3–5). Cerebral metabolic oxygen demand is reduced by 25–30% within seconds of a single intravenous dosage of 3–5 mg/kg, with maximal reduction in CMRO$_2$ (approx 55%) following bolus doses of 10–20 mg/kg *(78)*. Pentobarbital infusions have historically been used to reduce refractory intracerebral hypertension, although the hemodynamic and other adverse consequences may be life-threatening in themselves.

Effects on Seizure Threshold

Low doses of barbiturates may produce a paradoxical excitation by EEG, but higher doses (as used in the NSU setting) lead to suppression of cortical neuronal firing, progressing to burst suppression and electrocerebral silence at very high doses *(68)*. Pentobarbital infusions have thus been used to treat status epilepticus *(see also* Chapter 25).

Recommended Monitoring During Drug Administration and Recovery

Because of their marked suppression of respiratory function, monitoring of continuous pulse oximetry is mandatory with administration of parenteral barbiturates. At higher doses, this class of pharmacologic agents may have profound effects on cardiovascular function, necessitating frequent or invasive monitoring of blood pressure and cardiac output.

Drug–Drug Interactions

Concurrent administration of other central nervous system depressants will potentiate the sedative, respiratory, and hemodynamic consequences of barbiturates. Dosage adjustments should thus be made (i.e., reduction by 10–50%) when bolusing or titrating barbiturates in patients also receiving narcotics, benzodiazepines, or sympatholytic agents *(78)*. Isoniazid, methylphenidate, and monoamine oxidase inhibitors also enhance the depressant effects of barbiturates *(68)*. Through induction of the hepatic microsomal cytochrome P-450 system, barbiturates increase the metabolism and elimination of a large number of compounds. Those relevant to NSU patients include corticosteroids, warfarin, digoxin, metoprolol, phenytoin, tricyclic antidepressants (whose metabolism may also be inhibited), vitamin D (leading to hypocalcemia), and vitamin K (leading to clotting factor II and VIII deficiencies and coagulopathy).

Dosage Recommendations for Specific Agents

Thiopental

When given as a single IV bolus of 1–5 mg/kg, thiopental acutely reduces ICP for 5–10 min. Repeated dosing may lead to cumulative adverse effects on cardiovascular function, which may be deleterious to cerebral perfusion. IV induction dosage is 3–5 mg/kg, although lower dosages must be used in individuals with reduced cardiac output, hypotension, hypovolemia, and the elderly from relative differences in volume of distribution and fractional cerebral perfusion *(78)*. Half-life for plasma clearance of thiopental is 8–12 h, but is effectively much shorter after a single dose (minutes) due to redistribution from the brain *(68)*.

Pentobarbital

For refractory intracranial hypertension, pentobarbital is given as an initial IV loading dose of 3–30 mg/kg, followed by a maintenance infusion of 1–2 mg/kg/h. Half-life is 15–50 h, and infusion rates must be adjusted based on plasma drug levels.

Phenobarbital

For sedation, 1–3 mg/kg IV or IM, with repeated dosing titrated to effect is usually recommended. For convulsive status epilepticus, administer an IV loading dose of 15–20 mg/kg over 10–15 min, with subsequent dosing based on plasma drug levels. Half-life is 53–120 h.

NEUROLEPTICS/ANTIPSYCHOTICS

Again a large number of medications are available in this general category, and their use in NSU patients is somewhat controversial due to their theoretical lowering of seizure threshold. However, in patients with significant pulmonary disease, dementia, or with agitation or delirium significant enough to risk self injury or aggression towards medical personnel, the lack of respiratory depression and antipsychotic features of the neuroleptics make them attractive sedatives for some patients. Discussion shall be limited to the two agents used most commonly in the NSU and anesthesia realms, the butyrophenones, haloperidol and droperidol.

Mechanism of Action

Neuroleptics produce both therapeutic and adverse effects by blocking cerebral and peripheral (but not spinal) dopamine, adrenergic, serotonin, acetylcholine, and histamine receptors, with variable selectivity depending on the agent *(82)*. These effects include sedation (tolerance develops with repeated dosing), anxiolysis, restlessness, suppression of emotional and aggressive outbursts, reduction of delusions, hallucinations, and disorganized thoughts (over repeated dosing), antiemetic properties, hypotension (varies by agent), and extrapyramidal side effects. Haloperidol and droperidol have limited anticholinergic properties compared with other neuroleptics, reducing the occurrence of blurred vision, urinary retention, and gastrointestinal hypomotility *(82)*.

Pharmacokinetics

Haloperidol is highly lipophilic, plasma-protein bound, and readily crosses the placenta to enter the fetal circulation *(82)*. Sedative effects may be seen within minutes of IV administration. Although plasma half life varies from 12–36 h (depending on hepatic microsomal and conjugation activities), the effective half life may be much longer (1 wk or more) due to accumulation in brain and other tissues with a high blood supply. The very young and very old have a reduced capacity to metabolize haloperidol and related agents.

When administered IV, droperidol has a rapid onset of action (1–3 min), although peak effects may not be noted for 30 min. Duration of action varies from 2–12 h, and elimination appears to follow linear kinetics even at high doses *(83)*. Systemic elimination mirrors hepatic blood flow, and thus metabolism is presumably similar to that of haloperidol.

Routes of Administration

Haloperidol is available for oral, IM, and IV administration. Droperidol is given IM or IV.

Titratability

Because of their onset within minutes of IV administration, both haloperidol and droperidol are readily titratable with initial bolus dosing. However, as metabolism and elimination may be highly variable, repeated dosing should be done with caution due to potential systemic accumulation.

Adverse Reactions

Extrapyramidal side effects (parkinsonism, acute and tardive dystonias, tardive dyskinesia, akathisia, and perioral tremor) are less common with butyrophenones than with phenothiazine antipsychotics, but may still occur with both haloperidol and droperidol. Other potential side effects including increased prolactin secretion, orthostatic hypotension (rare with haloperidol and droperidol), neuroleptic malignant syndrome *(see also* Chapter 10), and jaundice (rare with butyrophenones) have all been reported for neuroleptics in general *(82)*. Recent warnings have also been issued regarding the potential for QT prolongation and torsades de pointes with even low doses of droperidol, greatly limiting the use of this agent for its perioperative sedation and antiemetic properties *(84)*. As such, droperidol is absolutely contraindicated in patients with pre-existing QT prolongation, and should be used with extreme caution in those at risk for cardiac dysrhythmias.

Hemodynamic Stability

Although chlorpromazine and other typical phenothiazine antipsychotics have been associated with hypotension, negative inotropy, and nonspecific ST and T-wave changes (including QT prolongation), significant hemodynamic side effects are rare with haloperidol and droperidol (82). However, both droperidol and haloperidol may cause systemic hypotension via peripheral vasodilatation when given IV.

Effects on Intracranial Pressure

In a limited clinical study in neurosurgical patients, droperidol had little effect on ICP, although cerebral perfusion pressure was decreased by moderate systemic hypotension (85). The effects of haloperidol on ICP have not been studied.

Effects on Seizure Threshold

In general, neuroleptics induce slowing and synchronization (with associated increased voltage) of the EEG (82). However, effects on the seizure threshold are highly variable, depending on the agent. Haloperidol and related butyrophenones (including droperidol) have unpredictable effects on seizure threshold, and although most studies suggest a low risk (86), these drugs should be used with caution in patients with known seizure disorders.

Recommended Monitoring During Drug Administration and Recovery

Prior to treatment with droperidol, a 12-lead electrocardiogram (EKG) should be performed to evaluate for pre-existent QT prolongation that would preclude use of this medication. Continuous EKG monitoring must be performed for several hours following administration of droperidol, and appropriate treatments for hypotension, QT prolongation, and ventricular dysrhythmias must be readily available. Because of potential hypotension from IV haloperidol or droperidol, frequent blood pressure measurement should also be performed with use of these medications.

Drug–Drug Interactions

Because of their sedative and potential autonomic effects, haloperidol and droperidol may enhance the effects of other sedative agents (including anticonvulsants). Additionally, any medications that induce the hepatic microsomal enzyme system may increase the rate at which neuroleptics are metabolized. Selective serotonin reuptake inhibitors (SSRIs) compete with neuroleptics for hepatic oxidative enzymes, and may therefore increase circulating levels of haloperidol and droperidol (82). As with all medications, nonspecific adverse effects including anaphylaxis, laryngospasm, and bronchospasm have been reported.

Because of the risk of ventricular dysrhythmias, droperidol should not be concurrently administered with any medications that may prolong the QT interval (84). These include, but are not limited to, antihistamines, several antibiotics, class I or III antiarrhythmics (including phenytoin), calcium channel blockers, and many antidepressants. Hypomagnesemia and hypokalemia should be avoided or treated.

Dosage Recommendations for Specific Agents

Haloperidol

For sedation, initial IV doses of 0.5–5.0 mg may be used. Dosage should be low in the elderly and in those with hemodynamic instability or high risk of seizures. Half-life is 12–36 h (but active metabolites may remain for a much longer period).

Droperidol

For sedation in the setting of agitation, a starting dosage of 0.625 mg to a maximum of 2.5 mg IV is recommended. Additional dosages should not exceed 0.625–1.25 mg every 2–4 h.

ALPHA-2 AGONISTS

Clonidine has long been used as an adjunct to general *(87)*, neuraxial *(88)*, and regional anesthesia *(89)* due to its sedative and analgesic properties, but its cardiovascular depressant effects limit its utility when combined with most other agents *(78)*. The recent approval of dexmedetomidine in the Unites States for the postoperative and intensive care unit settings has shown promise as an alternative to traditional sedatives, as it reduces the discomfort of mechanical ventilation while permitting rapid patient arousability for neurologic examination *(90)*. Neither clonidine nor dexmedetomidine alone are capable of inducing general anesthesia, but both agents markedly enhance the efficacy of inhalational anesthetics as well as opioids, decreasing the requirements for these other substances *(78,91,92)*.

Mechanism of Action

Both clonidine and dexmedetomidine are selective α-2 adrenergic receptor agonists, although dexmedetomidine is 8 times more specific than the older compound *(93)*. The sedative and analgesic properties of these compounds result from both presynaptic inhibition of descending noradrenergic activation of spinal neurons, as well as activation of post-synaptic α-2 adrenergic receptors coupled to potassium-channel activating G-proteins *(93–95)*. The summation of these effects is a decrease in sympathetic outflow from the locus coeruleus, a decrease in tonic activity in spinal motoneurons and spinothalamic pain pathways, and subsequent decreases in heart rate and blood pressure. At recommended doses respiratory drive is not compromised, and although patients receiving alpha-two agonists appear sedated, they are easily-arousable to perform neurologic examinations.

Pharmacokinetics

As with the other lipophilic sedatives described previously, clonidine is rapidly distributed to the brain and spinal cord following administration *(96)*. Decreases in blood pressure and heart rate may be noted within 30–60 min following oral dosing, although peak effects are not seen for 2–4 h. Half life varies between 12–16 h in healthy individuals, but may be prolonged to 41 h in patients with impaired renal function. Only approx 5% of plasma clonidine is removed by hemodialysis. Approximately 50% of plasma clonidine is cleared by hepatic metabolism, with the remainder of the drug eliminated unchanged in urine. Clonidine is moderately bound to serum proteins (20–40%), and may compete with other substances for these binding sites.

Dexmedetomidine is only given as an IV infusion, and is thus immediately available. Also highly lipophilic, it is rapidly distributed to the brain with an equilibrium half life of 6-9 min. Elimination half life is 2 h in healthy volunteers, but due to extensive metabolism by the liver this may increase to 7.5 h in individuals with hepatic insufficiency. At recommended doses, elimination follows linear kinetics. Excretion of dexmedetomidine is primarily through the kidney as inactive methyl and glucorinide conjugates. Although in vitro studies suggest inhibition of the cytochrome P-450 microsomal system by dexmedetomidine, this does not appear to have clinically significant effects on the metabolism of other substances utilizing this metabolic pathway. Dexmedetomidine is approx 94% protein bound, and thus may compete with other substances for albumin binding *(93,97)*.

Routes of Administration

Clonidine is available in oral and transdermal formulations in the United States (and in IV form throughout Europe), and dexmedetomidine is given IV.

Titratability

Because it is only available in oral and transdermal preparations in the United States, clonidine is not as easily titratable as the IV sedatives. Individual effects of oral doses are relatively rapid, but undesirable effects on heart rate and blood pressure may not be apparent for several days after initiation of drug therapy. As the time of onset for transdermal clonidine is 24–72 h, this system is not useful as a sedative agent. However, transdermal clonidine may be useful in the setting of alcohol or drug withdrawal in NSU patients, or as an adjunct for reduction of sympathetic hyperactivity in severe TBI patients. Due to its IV route of administration and short half-life, dexmedetomidine is easily titrated.

Adverse Reactions

The most common undesirable effects of clonidine include dry mouth, bradycardia, hypotension, lightheadedness, and anxiety. Acute withdrawal of chronic clonidine administration may lead to rebound hypertension, and possible subsequent stroke or cerebral hemorrhage; dosage should thus be tapered off after prolonged use *(78)*.

Like clonidine, dexmedetomidine has been reported to cause hypotension and bradycardia; treatment is supportive, with decrease or discontinuation of the infusion, IV fluids, and rarely pressors or vagolytics. Paradoxical transient hypertension may be observed if a loading dose of dexmedetomidine is given, and thus infusions are often begun without a bolus. Although dexmedetomidine is not approved for use greater than 24 h, limited experience with longer infusions suggests potential withdrawal sympathetic hyperactivity similar to that seen with clonidine. Also with prolonged use, dexmedetomidine may lead to suppression of adrenocorticoid release. Other reported adverse reactions with dexmedetomidine include nausea, vomiting, fever, dry mouth, anxiety, and atrial fibrillation, although the incidence of these side effects did not differ significantly from placebo. Rare elevation of hepatic enzymes has also been reported.

Hemodynamic Stability

As expected from their inhibition of noradrenergic outflow, both clonidine and dexmedetomidine have been associated with bradycardia and hypotension. Treatment is supportive.

Effects on Intracranial Pressure

In individuals without intracranial pathology, clonidine pretreatment has been shown to significantly decrease lumbar cerebral spinal fluid pressure during lumbar puncture *(98)*. However, in both TBI patients in an NSU, and neurosurgical patients undergoing craniotomy for tumor resection, clonidine had no significant effects on ICP but did impair cerebral perfusion pressure via a reduction in systemic arterial pressure *(99,100)*.

During dexmedetomidine infusion, one study demonstrated no changes in lumbar cerebral spinal fluid pressure in post-transsphenoidal hypophysectomy patients with a lumbar drain *(101)*. However, as with clonidine, significant decreases in cerebral perfusion pressure due to a drop in mean arterial pressure were noted. More extensive studies have not been published.

Effects on Seizure Threshold

Little has been published on the specific effects of clonidine on seizure threshold. However, EEG analysis of healthy volunteers receiving IV clonidine reveals decreased alpha and increased delta activity, consistent with the sedating effects of this medication *(102,103)*. In another study, combining clonidine with methohexital in patients with known focal seizure disorders further increased the number of epileptiform discharges as measured by magnetoencephalography *(104)*.

No human studies have been published regarding the effects of dexmedetomidine on seizure threshold. Animal studies have shown conflicting results. In a rat model of experimental generalized seizures, dexmedetomidine infusion decreased the threshold for epileptiform activity *(105)*. Similar results were found in cats undergoing enflurane anesthesia *(106)*. However, dexmedetomidine increased the threshold for cocaine induced seizures in rats in another study *(107)*.

Recommended Monitoring During Drug Administration and Recovery

Frequent monitoring of blood pressure and heart rate is recommended with initiation of clonidine or dexmedetomidine therapy.

Reversibility

α-2 Agonists are reversible with the selective antagonist, atipamezole *(78,108)*.

Drug–Drug Interactions

Due to their sedating properties, both clonidine and dexmedetomidine may exacerbate the effects of other centrally acting depressants. Additionally, hypotension and bradycardia may be worsened by concomitant administration of antihypertensive and antidysrhythmic medications. Conversely, tricyclic antidepressants combined with clonidine may produce a paradoxical increase in blood pressure. As with all of the aforementioned sedatives, caution must be exercised when combining alpha-2 agonists with multiple medications, particularly in hypovolemic or otherwise hemodynamically unstable patients.

Dosage Recommendations for Specific Agents

Clonidine

Initial oral dosing may be started at 0.1 mg PO every 8–24 h, increasing by 0.1 mg/d every 1–2 d to a maximum of 0.6 mg/d. Transdermal clonidine is started with the 0.1 mg patch, applied to hairless skin and changed every 7 d; dosage may be incrementally increased to the 0.2- and 0.3-mg patches each week.

Dexmedetomidine

Use of dexmedetomidine infusions for more than 24 h has not been approved by the US Food and Drug Administration. A loading infusion may be given as 1 µg/kg over 10 min, although this is not mandatory. For sedation in the NSU, maintenance infusions are titrated from 0.2–0.7 µg/kg/hr. Dosage adjustment may be necessary in individuals with hepatic or renal insufficiency.

PROPOFOL

Propofol has been extensively used both as a sedative agent in critically ill patients as well as a general anesthetic. Although similar to barbiturates in many aspects, this novel compound has many advantages over the older class of drugs, including inherent antiemetic properties and more rapid recovery, especially with repeated or prolonged dosing *(78)*. However, recent reports of fatal metabolic acidosis and myocardial failure following long-term administration of propofol (especially in children) have led to disfavor and a return to alternative methods of sedation *(109,110)*.

Mechanism of Action

A GABA-ergic mechanism of action has been suggested for propofol based on both in vivo *(111)* and in vitro *(112)* binding studies, with evidence that propofol may directly bind to GABA receptors and activate inhibitory chloride channels in the absence of GABA. Other studies suggest a nonspecific but structurally dependent effect on neuronal plasma membrane fluidity *(113)*. The specific mechanism(s) of action of propofol thus remain unclear.

Pharmacokinetics

Similar to thiopental in its lipophilicity, propofol is rapidly distributed to the brain following IV administration, with an equally rapid recovery following redistribution to other less perfused tissues *(78)*. Repeated or continuous dosing of propofol is cleared far more rapidly than thiopental, allowing greater titratability and recovery for intermittent neurologic examination. Propofol is metabolized both in the liver and extrahepatically, and its less-active metabolites are renally excreted *(78)*. Propofol is also highly plasma protein bound, with free circulating levels increased in hypoalbuminic states.

Routes of Administration

Propofol is administered IV at a premixed concentration of 10 mg/mL; it may be dosed by single boluses or as a continuous infusion. Because of its insolubility in water, propofol is suspended as an emulsion in a mixture of soybean oil, glycerol, and egg phospholipids, leaving it susceptible to bacterial contamination. For this reason, propofol must be handled in an aseptic manner, and unused solutions discarded within 6 h after a sterile seal is broken.

Titratability and Dosage Recommendations

Anesthetic intravenous induction dosages range from 1.0–2.5 mg/kg *(78)*, and for short durations of sedation (i.e., bedside or outpatient procedures), repeat administration of 10–50% of the induction dose may be repeated every 5–10 min as needed. For longer procedures, or as continuous sedation, an infusion of 25–100 µg/kg/min (with or without induction dose) is generally effective. For deeper sedation (up to general anesthesia and burst-suppression EEG), infusions of 100–300 µg/kg/min are easily titratable in increments of 5–25 µg/kg/min every 5–10 min.

Adverse Reactions

Pain on injection, which is common and due to the carrier solution, may be lessened by administration through central or larger veins, or pretreatment of peripheral injection sites with intravenous lidocaine (0.5–1.0 mg/kg). Hypotension (which may be severe at high doses), dose-dependent respiratory depression, and rare anaphylactoid reactions are also possible with propofol *(78)*. Additionally, due to the carrier solution, administration of propofol is contraindicated in individuals who have had a severe allergic reaction to eggs or soy products.

Although the side-effect profile for propofol is far more favorable than that for barbiturates, a syndrome of metabolic acidosis, hyperkalemia, rhabdomyolysis, and hypoxia has been described in children *(110)* and more recently in adults *(114)* receiving prolonged infusions of propofol. The etiology of this syndrome is unclear, and in the majority of reported cases the affected individuals were critically ill and on multiple other medications that may have initiated the metabolic disarray. Nonetheless, careful monitoring for electrolyte abnormalities in patients on prolonged propofol infusions is highly recommended.

Hemodynamic Stability

Propofol may cause hypotension due to both vasodilation and a negative inotropic effect *(78)*, and impairs the cardio-accelerator response to decreased blood pressure. This hypotension may be especially pronounced in patients with reduced cardiac output, hypovolemia, on other depressant medications, or the elderly.

Effects on Intracranial Pressure

Like thiopental, propofol decreases $CMRO_2$ and CBF, and is thus a useful adjunct to decrease ICP *(78)*. During craniotomy for tumor resection, propofol infusion had a more favorable profile for both reductions in ICP and preservation of cerebral perfusion pressure compared with volatile anesthetics *(115)*. When used as a sedative for severe TBI patients, propofol has also been demonstrated to have better control of ICP and a more favorable outcome than sedation with morphine *(116)*.

Effects on Seizure Threshold

Due to its general anesthetic properties propofol is generally considered to suppress seizure activity, but conflicting animal studies suggest this may not be absolute. In recent years propofol has also been used with increasing frequency for treatment of refractory status epilepticus *(73,74,117–122)* (*see also* Chapter 25). Other investigators suggest a proconvulsant activity for this anesthetic agent *(123,124)*. Indeed, an animal model of generalized seizures supports both possibilities, with propofol having contrasting effects on seizures produced by antagonists of inhibitory amino acid neurotransmitters compared with excitatory amino acid agonists *(125)*.

Recommended Monitoring During Drug Administration and Recovery

During bolus or continuous infusions of propofol, frequent or continuous monitoring of pulse-oximetry, respiratory rate and depth of respiration, and blood pressure is recommended. For high-dose propofol (i.e., burst suppression EEG), invasive monitoring of blood pressure and cardiac output may be necessary. Physicians administering propofol should be proficient at handling airway problems should they arise.

Drug–Drug Interactions

As with nearly all of the preceding sedatives, propofol may potentiate the sedative and cardiovascular effects of alcohol, opioids, benzodiazepines, barbiturates, other general anesthetics, antihypertensives, and antiarrhythmics. Propofol does not appear to alter the metabolism, elimination, or plasma protein binding of other drugs. Because of the scattered reports of rhabdomyolisis, metabolic acidosis, and myocardial failure following prolonged infusions of propofol, this agent should be used with caution when combined with other medications with similar potential. In addition, the high lipid content of propofol should be kept in mind when administered concurrently with parenteral nutrition containing lipids, as hypertriglyceridemia may occur.

SUMMARY

This chapter provides a brief description of the large number of sedatives commonly used in the NSU setting. It is by no means comprehensive, and further information on specific agents may be found in package inserts and general literature. In critically ill neurology and neurosurgery patients, the necessity for frequent neurologic examination is paramount, and use of shorter-acting agents is preferable. Ultimately the choice of particular sedative or analgesic must be carefully individualized for patient needs, cardiovascular and respiratory status, presence of intracranial hypertension, underlying cerebral pathology, and comorbidities.

REFERENCES

1. Mirski MA, Muffelman B, Ulatowski JA, Hanley DF. Sedation for the critically ill neurologic patient. *Crit. Care Med.* 1995;23:2038–2053.
2. Gehi MM, Rosenthal RH, Fizette NB, Crowe LR, Webb WL Jr. Psychiatric manifestations of hyponatremia. *Psychosomatics* 1981;22:739–743.
3. Atchison JW, Wachendorf J, Haddock D, Mysiw WJ, Gribble M, Corrigan JD. Hyponatremia-associated cognitive impairment in traumatic brain injury. *Brain Inj.* 1993;7:347–352.
4. Aldemir M, Ozen S, Kara IH, Sir A, Bac B. Predisposing factors for delirium in the surgical intensive care unit. *Crit. Care* 2001;5:265–270.
5. Hawkes ND, Thomas GA, Jurewicz A, Williams OM, Hillier CE, McQueen IM, Shortland G. Non-hepatic hyperammonaemia: an important, potentially reversible cause of encephalopathy. *Postgrad. Med. J.* 2001;77:717–722.
6. Rao KV, Norenberg MD. Cerebral energy metabolism in hepatic encephalopathy and hyperammonemia. *Metab. Brain Dis.* 2001;16:67–78.
7. Winawer N. Postoperative delirium. *Med. Clin. North Am.* 2001;85:1229–1239.
8. O'Connel GJ, Campbell PB, Anath JV. Amitriptyline: initial intolerance and subsequent psychosis. *Can. Med. Assoc. J.* 1972;106:115.
9. Malinow KL, Dorsch C. Tricyclic precipitation of steroid psychosis. *Psychiatry Med.* 1984;2:351–354.
10. Preda A, MacLean RW, Mazure CM, Bowers MB Jr. Antidepressant-associated mania and psychosis resulting in psychiatric admissions. *J. Clin. Psychiatry* 2001;62:30–33.

11. Matsuura M. Epileptic psychoses and anticonvulsant drug treatment. *J. Neurol. Neurosurg. Psychiatry* 1999;67:231–233.
12. Besag FM. Behavioural effects of the new anticonvulsants. *Drug Saf.* 2001;24:513–536.
13. Kossoff EH, Bergey GK, Freeman JM, Vining EP. Levetiracetam psychosis in children with epilepsy. *Epilepsia* 2001;42:1611–1613.
14. Sanders LD, Whitehead C, Gildersleve CD, Rosen M, Robinson JO. Interaction of H2-receptor antagonists and benzo-diazepine sedation. A double-blind placebo-controlled investigation of the effects of cimetidine and ranitidine on re-covery after intravenous midazolam. *Anaesthesia* 1993;48:286–292.
15 Kim KY, McCartney JR, Kaye W, Boland RJ, Niaura R. The effect of cimetidine and ranitidine on cognitive function in postoperative cardiac surgery patients. *Int. J. Psychiatry Med.* 1996;26:295–307.
16. Schroeder JA, Wolfe WM, Thomas MH, et al. The effect of intravenous ranitidine and metoclopramide on behavior, cognitive function, and affect. *Anesth. Analg.* 1994;78:359–364.
17. Hall RC, Popkin MK, Stickney SK, Gardner ER. Presentation of the steroid psychoses. *J. Nerv. Ment. Dis.* 1979;167:229–236.
18. Patten SB, Neutel CI. Corticosteroid-induced adverse psychiatric effects: incidence, diagnosis and management. *Drug Saf.* 2000;22:111–122.
19. Jacobson S. Psychotic reaction to penicillin. *Am. J. Psychiatry* 1968;124:999.
20. Saker BM, Musk AW, Haywood EF, Hurst PE. Reversible toxic psychosis after cephalexin. *Med. J. Aust.* 1973;1:497–498.
21. Cohen IJ, Weitz R. Psychiatric complications with erythromycin. *Drug Intell. Clin. Pharm.* 1981;15:388.
22. Vincken W. Psychotic reaction to cefuroxime. *Lancet* 1984;1(8383):965.
23. Sternbach H, State R. Antibiotics: neuropsychiatric effects and psychotropic interactions. *Harv. Rev. Psychiatry* 1997;5:214–226.
24. Gomez-Gil E, Garcia F, Pintor L, Martinez JA, Mensa J, de Pablo J. Clarithromycin-induced acute psychosis in peptic ulcer disease. *Eur. J. Clin. Microbiol. Dis.* 1999;18:70–71.
25. Prime K, French P. Neuropsychiatric reaction induced by clarithromycin in a patient on highly active antiretroviral therapy (HAART). *Sex. Transm. Infect.* 2001;77:297–298.
26. Katz MH. Effect of HIV treatment on cognition, behavior, and emotion. *Psychiatry Clin. North Am.* 1994;17:227–230.
27. Buczko GB. Sedation in critically ill patients: a review. *Med. Health RI* 2001;84:321–323.
28. Gutstein HB, Akil H. Opioid analgesics. In Hardman, JG, Limbird, LE, eds. *Goodman and Gilman's The Pharmaco-logical Basis of Therapeutics*, 10th ed. New York: McGraw-Hill, 2001:569–619.
29. Paterson SJ, Robson LE, Kosterlitz HW. Classification of opioid receptors. *Br. Med. Bull.* 1983;39:31–36.
30. Satoh M, Kubota A, Iwama T, et al. Comparison of analgesic potencies of mu, delta and kappa agonists locally applied to various CNS regions relevant to analgesia in rats. *Life Sci.* 1983;33:689–692.
31. Altura BT, Altura BM, Quirion R. Identification of benzomorphan-kappa opiate receptors in cerebral arteries which subserve relaxation. *Br. J. Pharmacol.* 1984;82:459–466.
32. Porreca F, Mosberg HI, Hurst R, Hruby VJ, Burks TF. Roles of mu, delta and kappa opioid receptors in spinal and supraspinal mediation of gastrointestinal transit effects and hot-plate analgesia in the mouse. *J. Pharmacol. Exp. Ther.* 1984;230:341–348.
33. Pfeiffer A, Brantl V, Herz A, Emrich HM. Psychotomimesis mediated by kappa opiate receptors. *Science* 1986;233:774–776.
34. Mansour A, Khatchaturian H, Lewis ME, Akil H, Watson SJ. Anatomy of CNS opioid receptors. *Trends Neurosci.* 1988;11:308–314.
35. Casy AF. Opioid receptors and their ligands: recent developments. *Adv. Drug Res.* 1989;18:177–289.
36. Glare PA, Walsh TD. Clinical pharmacokinetics of morphine. *Ther. Drug Monit.* 1991;13:1–23.
37. Morrison LM, Payne M, Drummond GB. Comparison of speed of onset of analgesic effect of diamorphine and mor-phine. *Br. J. Anaesth.* 1991;66:656–659.
38. Nordberg G, Borg L, Hedner T, Mellstrand T. CSF and plasma pharmacokinetics of intramuscular morphine. *Eur. J. Clin. Pharmacol.* 1985;27:677–681.
39. Goucke CR, Hackett LP, Ilett KF. Concentrations of morphine, morphine-6-glucuronide, and morphine-3-glucuronide in serum and cerebrospinal fluid following morphine administration to patients with morphine-resistant pain. *Pain* 1994;56:145–149.
40. Brunk SF, Delle M. Morphine metabolism in man. *Clin. Pharmacol. Ther.* 1974;16:51–57.
41. Boerner U, Abbott S, Roe RL. The metabolism of morphine and heroin in man. *Drug. Metab. Rev.* 1975;4:39–73.
42. Pasternak GW, Bodnar RJ, Clark JA, Inturrisi CE. Morphine 6-glucuronide, a potent mu agonist. *Life Sci.* 1987;41:2845–2849.
43. Ball M, McQuay HJ, Moore RA, Allen MC, Fisher A, Sear J. Renal failure and the use of morphine in intensive care. *Lancet* 1985;1(8432):784–786.
44. Portenoy RK, Foley KM, Stulman J, et al. Plasma morphine and morphine-6-glucuronide during chronic morphine therapy for cancer pain: plasma profiles, steady-state concentrations and the consequences of renal failure. *Pain* 1991;47:13–19.

45. Osborne R, Joel S, Trew D, Slevin M. Morphine and metabolite behavior after different routes of administration: demonstration of the importance of the active metabolite morphine-6-glucuronide. *Clin. Pharmacol. Ther.* 1990;47:12–19.

46. Gourlay GK. Sustained relief of chronic pain. Pharmacokinetics of sustained release morphine. *Clin. Pharmacokinet.* 1998;35:173–190.

47. Streisand JB, Busch MA, Egan TD, Smith BG, Gay M, Pace NL. Dose proportionality and pharmacokinetics of oral transmucosal fentanyl citrate. *Anesthesiology* 1998;88:305–309.

48. Gourlay GK, Kowalski SR, Plummer JL, Cherry DA, Gaukroger P, Cousins MJ. The transdermal administration of fentanyl in the treatment of postoperative pain: pharmacokinetics and pharmacodynamic effects. *Pain* 1989;37:193–202.

49. Plezia PM, Kramer TH, Linford J, Hameroff SR. Transdermal fentanyl: pharmacokinetics and preliminary clinical evaluation. *Pharmacotherapy* 1989;9:2–9.

50. Mather LE. Clinical pharmacokinetics of fentanyl and its newer derivatives. *Clin. Pharmacokinet.* 1983;8:422–446.

51. Bower S: Plasma protein binding of fentanyl. *J. Pharm. Pharmacol.* 1981;33:507–514.

52. Halliburton JR. The pharmacokinetics of fentanyl, sufentanil and alfentanil: a comparative review. *AANA J.* 1988;56:229–232.

53. Goromaru T, Matsuura H, Yoshimura N, et al. Identification and quantitative determination of fentanyl metabolites in patients by gas chromatography-mass spectrometry. *Anesthesiology* 1984;61:73–77.

54. Corall IM, Moore AR, Strunin L. Plasma concentrations of fentanyl in normal surgical patients and those with severe renal and hepatic disease. *Br. J. Anaesth.* 1980;52:101P.

55. Joh I, Sila M, Bastani B. Nondialyzability of fentanyl with high-efficiency and high-flux membranes (letter). *Anesth. Analg.* 1998;86:447.

56. Glass PS, Hardman D, Kamiyama Y, et al. Preliminary pharmacokinetics and pharmacodynamics of an ultra-short-acting opioid: remifentanil (GI87084B). *Anesth. Analg.* 1993;77:1031–1040.

57. Lemmens HJ. Pharmacokinetic-pharmacodynamic relationships for opioids in balanced anesthesia. *Clin. Pharmacokinet.* 1995;29:231–242.

58. Westmoreland CL, Hoke JF, Sebel PS, Hug CC Jr, Muir KT. Pharmacokinetics of remifentanil (GI87084B) and its major metabolite (GI90291) in patients undergoing elective inpatient surgery. *Anesthesiology* 1993;79:893–903.

59. Tipps LB, Coplin WM, Murry KR, Rhoney DH. Safety and feasibility of continuous infusion of remifentanil in the neurosurgical intensive care unit. *Neurosurgery* 2000;46:596–602.

60. Flacke JW, Flacke WE, Bloor BC, Van Etten AP, Kripke BJ. Histamine release by four narcotics: a double-blind study in humans. *Anesth. Analg.* 1987;66:723–730.

61. Rosow CE, Moss J, Philbin DM, Savarese JJ. Histamine release during morphine and fentanyl anesthesia. *Anesthesiology* 1982;56:93–96.

62. Rao TLK, Mummaneni N, El-Etr AA. Convulsions: an unusual response to intravenous fentanyl administration. *Anesth. Analg.* 1982;61:1020–1021.

63. Safwat AM, Daniel D. Grand mal seizure after fentanyl administration. *Anesthesiology* 1983;59:78.

64. Hoien AO. Another case of grand mal seizure after fentanyl administration. *Anesthesiology* 1984;60:387–388.

65. Murkin JM, Moldenhauer CC, Hug CC, et al. Absence of seizures during induction of anesthesia with high-dose fentanyl. *Anesth. Analg.* 1984;63:489–494.

66. De Conno F, Caraceni A, Martini C, et al. Hyperalgesia and myoclonus with intrathecal infusion of high-dose morphine. *Pain* 1991;47:337–339.

67. de Armendi AJ, Fahey M, Ryan JF. Morphine-induced myoclonic movements in a pediatric pain patient. *Anesth. Analg.* 1993;77:191–192.

68. Charney DS, Mihic SJ, Harris RA. Hypnotics and sedatives. In Hardman, JG, Limbird, LE, eds. *Goodman and Gilman's The Pharmacological Basis of Therapeutics*, 10th ed. New York: McGraw-Hill, 2001:399–427.

69. Sanchez-Izquierdo-Riera JA, Caballero-Cubedo RE, Perez-Vela JL, Ambros-Checa A, Cantalapiedra-Santiago JA, Alted-Lopez E. Propofol versus midazolam: safety and efficacy for sedating the severe trauma patient. *Anesth. Analg.* 1998;86:1219–1224.

70. Papazian L, Albanese J, Thirion X, Perrin G, Durbec O, Martin C. Effect of bolus doses of midazolam on intracranial pressure and cerebral perfusion pressure in patients with severe head injury. *Br. J. Anaesth.* 1993;71:267–271.

71. Forster A, Juge O, Morel D. Effects of midazolam on cerebral hemodynamics and cerebral vasomotor responsiveness to carbon dioxide. *J. Cereb. Blood Flow Metab.* 1983;3:246–249.

72. Cock HR, Schapira AH. A comparison of lorazepam and diazepam as initial therapy in convulsive status epilepticus. *QJM* 2002;95:225–231.

73. Claassen J, Hirsch LJ, Emerson RG, Bates JE, Thompson TB, Mayer SA. Continuous EEG monitoring and midazolam infusion for refractory nonconvulsive status epilepticus. *Neurology* 2001;57:1036–1042.

74. Prasad A, Worrall BB, Bertram EH, Bleck TP. Propofol and midazolam in the treatment of refractory status epilepticus. *Epilepsia* 2001;42:380–386.

75. Ahmed S, Chadwick D, Walker RJ. The management of alcohol-related seizures: an overview. *Hosp. Med.* 2000;61:793–796.
76. Hoffman EJ, Warren EW. Flumazenil: a benzodiazepine antagonist. *Clin. Pharm.* 1993;12:641–656.
77. Schulte am Esch J, Kochs E. Midazolam and flumazenil in neuroanaesthesia. *Acta Anaesthesiol. Scand. Suppl.* 1990;92:96–102.
78. Evers AS, Crowder CM. General anesthetics. In Hardman JG, Limbird LE, eds. *Goodman and Gilman's The Pharmacological Basis of Therapeutics*, 10th ed. New York: McGraw-Hill, 2001:337–365.
79. Russo H, Bressolle F. Pharmacodynamics and pharmacokinetics of thiopental. *Clin. Pharmacokinet.* 1998;35:95–134.
80. Wermeling DP, Blouin RA, Porter WH, Rapp RP, Tibbs PA. Pentobarbital pharmacokinetics in patients with severe head injury. *Drug. Intell. Clin. Pharmacol.* 1987;21:459–463.
81. Viswanathan CT, Booker HE, Welling PG. Pharmacokinetics of phenobarbital following single and repeated doses. *J. Clin. Pharmacol.* 1979;19:282–289.
82. Baldessarini RJ, Tarazi FI. Drugs and the treatment of psychiatric disorders: psychosis and mania. In Hardman JG, Limbird LE, eds. *Goodman and Gilman's The Pharmacological Basis of Therapeutics*, 10th ed. New York: McGraw-Hill, 2001:485–520.
83. Lehmann KA, Van Peer A, Ikonomakis M, Gasparini R, Heykants J. Pharmacokinetics of droperidol in surgical patients under different conditions of anaesthesia. *Br. J. Anaesth.* 1988;61:297–301.
84. Lischke V, Behne M, Doelken P, Schledt U, Probst S, Vettermann J. Droperidol causes a dose-dependent prolongation of the QT interval. *Anesth. Analg.* 1994;79:983–986.
85. Misfeldt BB, Jorgensen PB, Spotoff H, Ronde F. The effects of droperidol and fentanyl on intracranial pressure and cerebral perfusion pressure in neurosurgical patients. *Br. J. Anaesth.* 1976;48:963–968.
86. Pisani F, Oteri G, Costa C, Di Raimondo G, Di Perri R. Effects of psychotropic drugs on seizure threshold. *Drug Saf.* 2002;25:91–110.
87. Higuchi H, Adachi Y, Dahan A, et al. The interaction between propofol and clonidine for loss of consciousness. *Anesth. Analg.* 2002;94:886–891.
88. Dobrydnjov I, Axelsson K, Samarutel J, Holmstrom B. Postoperative pain relief following intrathecal bupivacaine combined with intrathecal or oral clonidine. *Acta Anaesthesiol. Scand.* 2002;46:806–814.
89. Iskandar H, Guillaume E, Dixmerias F, et al. The enhancement of sensory blockade by clonidine selectively added to mepivacaine after midhumeral block. *Anesth. Analg.* 2001;93:771–775.
90. Venn RM, Grounds RM. Comparison between dexmedetomidine and propofol for sedation in the intensive care unit: patient and clinician perceptions. *Br. J. Anaesth.* 2001;87:684–690.
91. Khan ZP, Munday IT, Jones RM, Thornton C, Mant TG, Amin D. Effects of dexmedetomidine on isoflurane requirements in healthy volunteers. 1: Pharmacodynamic and pharmacokinetic interactions. *Br. J. Anaesth.* 1999;83:372–380.
92. Venn RM, Bradshaw CJ, Spencer R, et al. Preliminary UK experience of dexmedetomidine, a novel agent for postoperative sedation in the intensive care unit. *Anaesthesia* 1999;54:1136–1142.
93. Bhana N, Goa KL, McClellan KJ. Dexmedetomidine. *Drugs* 2000;59:263–268.
94. Palmeri A, Sapienza S, Giuffrida R, et al. Modulatory action of noradrenergic system on spinal motoneurons in humans. *Neuroreport* 1999;10:1225–1229.
95. Tulen JH, van de Wetering BJ, Kruijk MP, et al. Cardiovascular, neuroendocrine, and sedative responses to four graded doses of clonidine in a placebo-controlled study. *Biol. Psychiatry.* 1992;32:485–500.
96. Fujimura A, Ebihara A, Shiga T, et al. Pharmacokinetics and pharmacodynamics of a new transdermal clonidine, M-5041T, in healthy subjects. *J. Clin. Pharmacol.* 1993;33:1192–200.
97. Talke P, Richardson CA, Scheinin M, Fisher DM. Postoperative pharmacokinetics and sympatholytic effects of dexmedetomidine. *Anesth. Analg.* 1997;85:1136–1142.
98. Maruyama K, Takeda S, Hongo T, Kobayashi N, Ogawa R. The effect of oral clonidine premedication on lumbar cerebrospinal fluid pressure in humans. *J. Nippon Med. Sch.* 2000;67:429–433.
99. ter Minassian A, Beydon L, Decq P, Bonnet F. Changes in cerebral hemodynamics after a single dose of clonidine in severely head-injured patients. *Anesth. Analg.* 1997;84:127–132.
100. Favre JB, Gardaz JP, Ravussin P. Effect of clonidine on ICP and on the hemodynamic responses to nociceptive stimuli in patients with brain tumors. *J. Neurosurg. Anesthesiol.* 1995;7:159–167.
101. Talke P, Tong C, Lee HW, Caldwell J, Eisenach JC, Richardson CA. Effect of dexmedetomidine on lumbar cerebrospinal fluid pressure in humans. *Anesth. Analg.* 1997;85:358–364.
102. Bischoff P, Scharein E, Schmidt GN, von Knobelsdorff G, Bromm B, Esch JS. Topography of clonidine-induced electroencephalographic changes evaluated by principal component analysis. *Anesthesiology* 2000;92:1545–1552.
103. Yamadera H, Ferber G, Matejcek M, Pokorny R. Electroencephalographic and psychometric assessment of the CNS effects of single doses of guanfacine hydrochloride (Estulic) and clonidine (Catapres). *Neuropsychobiology* 1985;14:97–107.
104. Kirchberger K, Schmitt H, Hummel C, et al. Clonidine- and methohexital-induced epileptiform discharges detected by magnetoencephalography (MEG) in patients with localization-related epilepsies. *Epilepsia* 1998;39:1104–1112.
105. Mirski MA, Rossell LA, McPherson RW, Traystman RJ. Dexmedetomidine decreases seizure threshold in a rat model of experimental generalized epilepsy. *Anesthesiology* 1994;81:1422–1428.

106. Miyazaki Y, Adachi T, Kurata J, Utsumi J, Shichino T, Segawa H. Dexmedetomidine reduces seizure threshold during enflurane anaesthesia in cats. *Br. J. Anaesth.* 1999;82:935–937.

107. Whittington RA, Virag L, Vulliemoz Y, Cooper TB, Morishima HO. Dexmedetomidine increases the cocaine seizure threshold in rats. *Anesthesiology* 2002;97:693–700.

108. Karhuvaara S, Kallio A, Salonen M, Tuominen J, Scheinin M. Rapid reversal of alpha 2-adrenoceptor agonist effects by atipamezole in human volunteers. *Br. J. Clin. Pharmacol.* 1991;31:160–165.

109. Kang TM. Propofol infusion syndrome in critically ill patients. *Ann. Pharmacother.* 2002;36:1453–1456.

110. Hanna JP, Ramundo ML. Rhabdomyolysis and hypoxia associated with prolonged propofol infusion in children. *Neurology* 1998;50:301–303.

111. Alkire MT, Haier RJ. Correlating *in vivo* anaesthetic effects with ex vivo receptor density data supports a GABAergic mechanism of action for propofol, but not for isoflurane. *Br. J. Anaesthesia* 2001;86:618–626.

112. Mohammadi B, Haeseler G, Leuwer M, Dengler R, Krampfl K, Bufler J. Structural requirements of phenol derivatives for direct activation of chloride currents via GABAA receptors. *Eur. J. Pharmacol.* 2001;421:85–91.

113. Tsuchiya H. Structure-specific membrane-fluidizing effect of propofol. *Clin. Exp. Pharmacol. Physiol.* 2001;28:292–299.

114. Perrier ND, Baerga-Varela Y, Murray MJ. Death related to propofol use in an adult patient. *Crit. Care Med.* 2000;28:3071–3074.

115. Petersen KD, Landsfeldt U, Cold GE, et al. ICP is lower during propofol anaesthesia compared to isoflurane and sevoflurane. *Acta. Neurochir. Suppl.* 2002;81:89–91.

116. Kelly DF, Goodale DB, Williams J, et al. Propofol in the treatment of moderate and severe head injury: a randomized, prospective double-blinded pilot trial. *J. Neurosurg.* 1999;90:1042–1052.

117. Carley S, Crawford I. Propofol for resistant status epilepticus. *Emerg. Med. J.* 2002;19:143–144.

118. Begemann M, Rowan AJ, Tuhrim S. Treatment of refractory complex-partial status epilepticus with propofol: case report. *Epilepsia* 2000;41:105–109.

119. Stecker MM, Kramer TH, Raps EC, O'Meeghan R, Dulaney E, Skaar DJ. Treatment of refractory status epilepticus with propofol: clinical and pharmacokinetic findings. *Epilepsia* 1998;39:18–26.

120. Brown LA, Levin GM. Role of propofol in refractory status epilepticus. *Ann. Pharmacother.* 1998;32:1053–1059.

121. Pitt-Miller PL, Elcock BJ, Maharaj M. The management of status epilepticus with a continuous propofol infusion. *Anesth. Analg.* 1994;78:1193–1194.

122. Mackenzie SJ, Kapadia F, Grant IS. Propofol infusion for control of status epilepticus. *Anaesthesia* 1990;45:1043–1045.

123. Makela JP, Iivanainen M, Pieninkeroinen IP, Waltimo O, Lahdensuu M. Seizures associated with propofol anesthesia. *Epilepsia* 1993;34:832–835.

124. Borgeat A. Propofol: pro- or anticonvulsant? *Eur. J. Anaesthesiol. Suppl.* 1997;15:17–20.

125. Bansinath M, Shukla VK, Turndorf H. Propofol modulates the effects of chemoconvulsants acting at GABAergic, glycinergic, and glutamate receptor subtypes. *Anesthesiology* 1995;83:809–815.

13

Blood Pressure Management in the Neurocritical Care Patient

Wendy C. Ziai and Marek A. Mirski

INTRODUCTION

The brain and cerebral circulation are highly vulnerable to the effects of untreated hypertension, which is an important risk factor for cerebral infarction, intracerebral hemorrhage (ICH), and to a lesser extent subarachnoid hemorrhage (SAH) *(1–4)*. The deleterious effects of acutely elevated blood pressure in the presence of these and other cerebral insults, however, must be balanced against the physiologic regulation of cerebral perfusion pressure (CPP) and risks of reduced cerebral blood flow (CBF). This review will focus on the causes of acute hypertension in a variety of brain injury paradigms, the effects of hypertension on the cerebral vasculature, and the management of acutely elevated blood pressure in neurologic disease. Guidelines for acute blood pressure control are often controversial, vague or nonexistent. It is therefore important to review the relevant pathophysiology in order to make rationale decisions under a variety of clinical conditions in the neurosciences critical care unit (NSU).

CEREBROVASCULAR PHYSIOLOGY

CBF is controlled by the following relationship between CPP and cerebrovascular resistance (CVR):

$$CBF = CPP/CVR$$

CPP is the difference between the mean arterial pressure (MAP) and the backpressure produced by the intracranial contents (venous blood, cerebrospinal fluid, and brain tissue), that is, the intracranial pressure (ICP):

$$CPP = MAP - ICP$$

Under normal conditions, ICP is negligible, and arterial blood pressure determines CPP. CBF is maintained at approx 50 mL/100 g of brain tissue per minute and disturbances of CPP, either through changes in systemic pressure or ICP have little effect on CBF because of the presence of autoregulation. This concept refers to the ability of the intracerebral resistance vessels to change diameter in response to blood pressure changes, and to maintain constancy of cerebral blood flow (CBF) over a wide range of CPP (Fig. 1) *(see also* Chapters 3 and 4 for further details). This physiologic regulatory mechanism was first described in the 1930s by Fog, who observed vasomotor responses in the pial vessels of cats in response to systemic blood pressure manipulations, which appeared to be independent of neurogenic stimuli *(5,6)*. Later, Lassen established the concept with human studies of CBF measurement in the setting of controlled hypotension *(7)*. Cerebral autoregulation has been demon-

From: *Current Clinical Neurology*
Critical Care Neurology and Neurosurgery
Edited by: J. I. Suarez © Humana Press Inc., Totowa, NJ

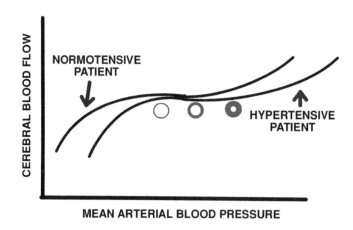

Fig. 1. Cerebral blood flow autoregulation.

strated experimentally to have lower and upper limits, which in the normotensive individual have been estimated at MAP levels of 60 and 150 mmHg, respectively *(8–10)*. As MAP decreases below the lower limit (approx 25% reduction), vasodilatation occurs, but eventually CPP becomes insufficient causing CBF and cerebral blood volume to decrease with resultant cerebral ischemia *(9)*. Additional vasodilation may be induced in the resistance vessels with hypercapnia or certain pharmacologic agents, and oxygen extraction can be increased from the blood to help maintain the cerebral metabolic rate of oxygen consumption ($CMRO_2$). With increasing MAP, vasoconstriction occurs in response to increasing CBF and CBV. As the upper limit of the autoregulatory curve is exceeded, however, increasing intraluminal pressure forcefully dilates segments of arterioles causing damage to the blood–brain barrier with resultant cerebral edema and clinically, hypertensive encephalopathy *(11–13)*.

In chronic hypertension, both the lower and upper end of the autoregulation curve are shifted to the right, toward higher pressure *(9,14–16)*. Anatomically, the smaller resistance blood vessels undergo degenerative changes consisting of thickening and fibrosis of the media (in muscular arteries) and intima, and patchy degeneration of smooth muscle cells producing luminal narrowing and increased vascular resistance *(17)*. Although the resting CBF is the same in normotensive and hypertensive individuals, these structural changes limit the capacity of the resistance vessels for maximal vasodilatation and impair tolerance of lower blood pressures, while improving tolerance to hypertension through vasoconstriction of these same vessels. Long-term antihypertensive treatment can reverse these adaptive changes and shift the autoregulation curve back to its normal range, although only limited reversibility occurs in elderly hypertensive patients *(18,19)*.

The mechanism of autoregulation involves vasoconstriction as MAP increases and vasodilation as MAP decreases involving cerebral arterioles and small arteries; these vasomotor responses are believed to be mediated by myogenic and metabolic mechanisms *(17)*. The myogenic hypothesis by which vessels change caliber in response to changes in the transmural pressure gradient, is supported by observations of a purely myogenic response in vitro and would be consistent with the rapidity of the response on the order of seconds *(20)*. The metabolic hypothesis suggests that changing periarteriolar concentrations of metabolites such as adenosine may mediate autoregulatory vasodilatation; the vasoconstriction response, however, is not well explained by metabolic mechanisms *(21)*.

SPECIFIC CLINICAL ENTITIES

The following acute brain insults are all commonly associated with elevated blood pressure. Although hypertension is frequently associated with the acute neurologic insult and physiologic response to ICP elevation, clinical evaluation of hypertension should consider other possible etiologies requiring unique treatment, including pain (headache), anxiety, withdrawal of medications, and certain illicit drugs.

Hypertension in Acute Brain Insult

In the acute setting, uncontrolled systemic hypertension resulting from neurologic injury is a common occurrence. After a surge in ICP, such as following SAH or other intracranial hemorrhage, ICP may temporarily surpass MAP, so that CPP falls to zero with resultant loss of consciousness. The elevated systemic blood pressure after such events is presumably an autoregulatory phenomenon, and may represent a component of the Cushing response along with bradycardia and irregular respiratory effort if ICP continues to be elevated. Rapid treatment of such hypertension is thought to be detrimental because decreased CPP may worsen brain injury by aggravating ischemia *(22–24)*. Systemic hypertension has been shown to be protective in several brain injury paradigms including mass lesions, infarction, and traumatic brain injury (TBI) *(24–27)*. The rationale for lowering blood pressure in these same conditions is to decrease the risk of new or ongoing hemorrhage, depending on the mechanism of injury. The optimal blood pressure may therefore depend on several factors, including presence of chronic hypertension, suspected intracranial hypertension, age, etiology of hemorrhage, or other injury, and time since onset *(22)*. Blood pressure management is discussed for each type of common brain injury.

Hypertensive Encephalopathy

Hypertensive encephalopathy occurs when a sudden sustained rise in blood pressure exceeds the upper limit of CBF autoregulation (autoregulation breakthrough) resulting in clinical signs of generalized brain dysfunction (headache, decreased mental status, visual disturbance, seizures) and raised ICP (papilledema). This acute organic brain syndrome is associated with hypertensive cerebrovascular endothelial dysfunction, blood-brain barrier disruption and increased permeability resulting in cerebral edema and microhemorrhage formation *(28)*. The characteristic posterior leukoencephalopathy seen on magnetic resonance imaging in the parieto-occipital white matter predominantly is primarily from vasogenic rather than cytotoxic edema *(29)*. Inadequately treated hypertensive encephalopathy can progress to ICH, coma, and death. Thus, unlike other types of neurologic injury, the use of antihypertensive therapy in this condition is not controversial. Because there is some variability in the blood pressure level at which autoregulation is overwhelmed (as low as 160/100 in previously normotensive patients), treatment should be individualized based on the blood pressure level and presence of end-organ damage. The recommended objective is to lower MAP by no more than 20–25% over the first 1–2 h or to decrease diastolic blood pressure to 100–110 mmHg over the same period *(30)*. More aggressive antihypertensive therapy may worsen end-organ damage, and result in worsening neurologic status and even stroke. Recommended agents for rapid reduction of MAP in this setting are sodium nitroprusside, intravenous labetolol, intravenous calcium channel antagonists (nicardipine), and hydralazine in certain patients *(30–32)*. Fenoldopam mesylate has also been approved for management of hypertensive emergencies and appears to be equally effective to sodium nitroprusside *(33,34)*. Other general principles to be applied in hypertensive crisis are: adequate fluid replacement which may lower blood pressure and improve renal function in patients with evidence of hypovolemia; avoidance of diuretics unless left ventricular failure and pulmonary edema are complicating factors, because of the possibility of pressure induced natriuresis and hypo-volemia *(35)*; and cautious use of angiotensin-converting enzyme inhibitors (ACEI) which can cause precipitous falls in blood pressure in hypovolemic patients and those with renal artery stenosis *(28,36)*.

Intracerebral Hemorrhage

ICH has as its most important risk factors, advancing age and hypertension *(3)*. The pathophysiol-ogy of ICH involves most commonly hypertension-induced changes in the small arteries and arteri-oles with formation of microaneurysms at juncture points of major feeding and small penetrating arteries *(37,38)*. Systemic hypertension is common after ICH, often lasting for several days *(39,40)*. High blood pressure on admission and during the first 24 h has been associated with increased mor-tality in some series, but not in others *(41–43)*. The major concern in favor of aggressively treating hypertension is that elevated blood pressure may result in early rebleeding, which occurs in 38% of patients within the first 24 h after presentation *(44)*. The converse issue is whether reducing arterial pressure will reduce CBF with resulting cerebral ischemia *(2,22)* (*see also* Chapter 19).

Although there are many causes of ICH such as cerebral amyloid angiopathy, vascular malforma-tions, aneurysms, anticoagulant use and coagulation disorders, tumors, hemorrhagic transformation of infarcts, and drug abuse, the prevalence of chronic hypertension in this population implies that most patients will have a shifted autoregulatory curve at onset *(17)* (*see* Chapters 3 and 19). Other reasons for abnormal autoregulation are increased ICP causing reduced CPP, and impaired autoregu-lation due to tissue damage *(2,45)*. A hemodynamic study of eight patients with hypertensive ICH who underwent pharmacologic reduction of blood pressure and measurement of CBF by Argon inha-lation in the acute phase suggested presence of autoregulatory responses, but over a limited range *(46)*. The lower limit of autoregulation corresponded to approx 80% of the "post-ictal" blood pres-sure in most patients, suggesting a safety factor of 20% blood pressure reduction before CBF would begin to decrease. Both animal and human studies have reported CBF values close to the threshold of ischemia in the perihematoma region where autoregulation is impaired *(47,48)*. Other studies have found no difference in CBF with blood pressure lowering, one in a dog model of ICH, and the other a human study *(45,49)*. In the latter, CBF was measured with PET and ^{15}O-water in 14 patients with acute ICH. Labetolol or Nicardipine was used to lower MAP by 17% from 143 to 119 mmHg. Auto-regulation of both global CBF and periclot CBF was found to be intact with no significant change in the range of arterial blood pressure reduction studied *(45)*. The clinical impact of such blood pressure lowering has yet to be defined.

The rationale for treating blood pressure is to prevent hematoma growth, increases in ICP and possibly edema formation. The risk of ongoing hemorrhage in the setting of uncontrolled hyperten-sion is difficult to attribute to blood pressure alone. One retrospective and one prospective observa-tional study have not found baseline blood pressure to be associated with hematoma enlargement although early use of antihypertensive agents may have helped prevent this finding *(44,50)*. One retrospective analysis of 186 patients with spontaneous ICH did report systolic blood pressure more than 200 mmHg as an independent factor predisposing to ICH growth in the acute phase *(51)*. Broderick reported that five of six patients with a greater than 40% increase in ICH volume and neurologic deterioration had SBP more than 195 mmHg during the first 6 h of admission *(52)*. Another study found that MAP maintained below 125 mmHg was associated with better outcome *(53)*. The only randomized study looking at blood pressure management reported better outcomes with blood pressure control although the lack of CT data in this early study compromises its validity *(54)*. Tak-ing the combined risks of inadequate CPP with aggressive control of elevated blood pressure, and rebleeding, which may be related to very high systolic blood pressure, the American Heart Associa-tion guidelines recommend maintaining MAP greater than 130 mmHg in patients with a history of hypertension, and CPP more than 70 mmHg in patients with an ICP monitor *(22,55)*. Postoperative blood pressure should be kept below MAP of 110 mmHg. Finally, SBP less than 90 mmHg should be treated with vasopressor agents.

Subarachnoid Hemorrhage

Spontaneous SAH typically results from a ruptured intracranial aneurysm or arteriovenous malformation (*see also* Chapter 20). At the time of rupture, acute arterial hypertension occurs reflecting a compensatory response to the extreme, but usually transient elevation of ICP. If ICP remains elevated, such as may occur with development of hydrocephalus, systemic blood pressure may remain high as a manifestation of the Cushing reflex. Often, however, hypertension is present without overt signs of increased ICP reflecting either a hyperadrenergic state secondary to excess release of catecholamines, and/or response to headache and neck pain. The management of hypertension in patients with SAH may therefore involve therapies other than antihypertensive agents. Early hydrocephalus is managed with placement of an intraventricular catheter. Pain is best treated with a short-acting reversible agent, such as fentanyl or propofol for intubated patients, which have minimal effects on ICP and CBF. Later in the course of SAH, the effects of vasospasm on blood pressure should be taken into consideration as permissive and induced hypertension is often the goal of therapy.

Acute Subarachnoid Hemorrhage (Preclipping/Prevasospasm)

Similar to ICH, dependence of brain perfusion on arterial blood pressure may be more critical because the range between the upper and lower limits of autoregulation narrows *(46)*. If autoregulation is compromised in certain areas, aggressive reduction of MAP may cause ischemia. The risk of not treating blood pressure surges prior to aneurysm clipping is thought to be an increase in the rate of rebleeding. In the Cooperative Aneurysm Study conducted between 1963 and 1970, two of the treatment arms affecting 1005 patients with ruptured aneurysms were pharmacologic lowering of BP and bed rest alone *(56)*. Antihypertensive therapy did not reduce the mortality rate or rate of rebleeding in the intention to treat analysis, but did decrease rebleeding in the treatment analysis. This study was performed in the pre–computed tomography (CT) era and was therefore likely inaccurate for the diagnosis of rebleeding. A subsequent study in the 1980s compared hypertensive treated patients with SAH (to maintain diastolic blood pressure [DBP] < 100 mmHg) to normotensive controls, and reported a lower rate of rebleeding (15% vs 33%; $p = 0.012$), but higher rate of cerebral infarction in the treated patients (43% vs 22%; $p = 0.03$), although the average blood pressures were still higher than in the controls *(57)*. This would suggest an autoregulatory blood pressure response, which should have been left untreated. There was no difference in outcomes between patient groups. In the International Cooperative Study on the Timing of Aneurysm Surgery (1980–1983), the admission blood pressure was an independent predictor of death and disability in the multivariate analysis *(4)*. Higher blood pressure was also associated with altered level of consciousness and older age, both independent predictors of poor outcome. The presence of hypertension therefore most likely reflects the severity of the subarachnoid hemorrhage *(4)*. Recent recommendations for management of blood pressure in the SAH population are to avoid antihypertensive therapy with the exception of "extreme" blood pressure elevation or evidence of end-organ damage such as clinical signs of encephalopathy, retinopathy, cardiac failure, or laboratory findings of proteinuria, elevated creatinine, oliguria, and chest radiography findings of left ventricular failure *(58)*. A more conservative guideline is to treat SBP more than 150 mmHg or above 10% of the premorbid level if the latter is known *(59)*. If ICP is elevated, CPP must be maintained above 70 mmHg, which in some patients may require blood pressure augmentation.

Late Subarachnoid Hemorrhage (Postclipping/Vasospasm)

Once the aneurysm has been secured by clipping or coiling, blood pressure management is directed to optimizing CBF in the setting of vasospasm. Hypervolemia, hypertension, and hemodilution are the cornerstones of triple H therapy based on largely uncontrolled nonrandomized studies *(4,60)*. In one series of 58 patients with progressive neurologic deterioration from angiographically confirmed cerebral vasospasm, induced arterial hypertension reversed neurologic deficits in 47 patients transiently, with permanent improvement in 43 cases *(60)*. The risks of producing a hypervolemic hypertensive state include pulmonary edema, myocardial infarction, aneurysmal rebleeding, cerebral edema, and hemorrhagic transformation of infarcted brain regions *(60,61)*. In the setting of an unsecured aneurysm, the risk of rerupture must be carefully weighed against the risk of cerebral ischemia secondary to vasospasm. In one series, 3/16 patients with unclipped ruptured aneurysms rebled, all with arterial pressures more than 160 mmHg *(60)*. Although it cannot be proven that hypertension was the cause of rebleeding, the potential stress of increased arterial pressure in this setting suggests that blood pressure should be carefully controlled unless neurologic deficits from vasospasm are a certainty.

Ischemic Stroke

Transient hypertension is observed frequently following acute ischemic stroke and may be the result of a combination of factors including anxiety, pain, neuroendocrine factors, alcohol use, stroke location, or a compensatory response to brain hypoxia or increased ICP *(40,62–64) (see also* Chapter 18). It is therefore important to manage stress responses, pain, nausea and vomiting, bladder distention and other sources of anxiety in the immediate care setting. Acutely elevated blood pressure is associated with increased early mortality after stroke although whether this represents a cause or an effect of stroke severity is presently unknown *(1,2,65)*. Early blood pressure elevations often decline spontaneously during the first minutes to hours of monitoring and may not require pharmacologic treatment *(66)*. In other cases, however, this acute hypertension may indicate inadequate perfusion of reversibly damaged ischemic brain regions *(8,67,68)*. Because cerebral autoregulation is impaired in ischemic brain regions, CBF is pressure dependent and further reduction may irreversibly injure the ischemic penumbra and increase stroke volume. A few animal and small patient studies have even provided preliminary data that raising blood pressure with intravenous vasopressors may be effective in improving neurologic function in acute/subacute stroke, especially in patients with large diffusion-perfusion mismatch on magnetic resonance imaging (MRI) *(27,69)*. The goal of such therapy is to raise the MAP by 10–15% using an agent such as phenylephrine and to watch for clinical improvement over a 24- to 48-h period. Patients who improve neurological function may benefit from long-term blood pressure augmentation with agents, such as florinef or midodrine *(70)*. The risk of inducing hypertension include aggravating cerebral edema and hemorrhagic transformation of the infarct as reported in a rabbit embolic stroke model *(71)*. The decision to use antihypertensive therapy in acute stroke therefore must be individualized. Patient groups in which acute treatment of elevated blood pressure should be considered include patients undergoing thrombolysis, patients with severe hypertension, hemorrhagic transformation of the infarct, or patients with conditions such as acute myocardial infarction, aortic dissection, hypertensive encephalopathy, or severe left ventricular failure *(72)*. In the National Institutes of Neurological Disorders and Stroke (NINDS) tissue plasminogen activator (t-PA) trial for ischemic stroke, hemorrhagic transformation was more likely in patients with blood pressure greater than 190 mmHg systolic and 100 mmHg diastolic, although these associations were not statistically significant *(73)*. In these situations, early use of parenteral agents may be warranted *(72)*. Otherwise, oral agents are usually effective. In general, high blood pressure should not be treated unless MAP above 130 mmHg or systolic blood pressure is more than 220 mmHg *(2,74)*. For patients receiving thrombolysis with t-PA, the NINDS t-PA Stroke Study Group Guidelines recommend maintaining blood pressure less than 185/110 mmHg before thrombolysis and less than 180/105 during and after administration of recombinant t-PA (rt-PA) *(75)*. Intravenous labetolol is the agent of choice. In patients who have hemorrhagic transformation of the infarct or other comorbid conditions such as myocardial ischemia, blood pressure must be controlled more judiciously. The rate of blood pressure control is also important as rapid decreases in systemic pressure can worsen neurologic condition and responses to antihypertensives may be exaggerated in these patients *(63,74,76) (see also* Chapter 18).

Traumatic Brain Injury

Systolic blood pressure elevations more than 160 mmHg have been reported in 25% of patients with severe TBI, often associated with tachycardia and tachypnea *(77,78)*. A hyperadrenergic state with elevated norepinephrine levels correlating with low Glasgow Coma Scale (GCS) score, and elevated blood pressure and heart rate has been described with potential implications for management of CBF, CBF, and ICP *(77,79,80)*. Whether this response is adaptive or maladaptive is not fully understood, although sustained hypertension can increase cardiac work and there is evidence of myocardial damage in the form of subendocardial hemorrhages in 50% of autopsied patients with severe TBI *(77)*. Experimentally, elevation of MAP by norepinephrine infusion following TBI in baboons has been shown to increase CBF and ICP *(81)*. To prevent myocardial damage, and mitigate against pressure dependent increases in CBF and ICP, it has been recommended to maintain SBP less than 160 mmHg in TBI patients *(82)*. Beta-blockers are a good choice, especially for patients in a hyperadrenergic state *(83)*. When ICP is elevated, a CPP goal of more than 60 mmHg is associated with improved patient outcome *(84)*. Increasing CPP to improve CBF, however, may not hold for higher levels of CPP as blood brain barrier breakdown will likely result in worsening cerebral edema *(83,84)*. Fluid restriction should not be used as a means of controlling blood pressure as this may result in rapid dehydration, a fall in cardiac output and decreased oxygen delivery, without a fall in blood pressure *(85)* (*see also* Chapter 22).

Carotid Endarterectomy

Hemodynamic instability after carotid endarterectomy is common, and may include hypertension, hypotension, or bradycardia *(86–88)*. Surgical removal of a hemodynamically significant stenosis from the extracranial carotid artery may cause dysfunction of adventitial baroreceptors resulting in hypertension, although metabolic factors such as renin and vasospressin may also be causes *(89–91)*. The risks of postoperative hypertension include stroke, ICH (hyperperfusion syndrome) and encephalopathy *(92)*. A recent hemispheric ipsilateral infarct may be at risk for hemorrhagic transformation because increased blood flow through the operated vessel may cause focal breakthrough of autoregulation impaired by the stroke *(93)*.

Although hemodynamic fluctuations are usually transient, they have been associated with surgical morbidity and mortality *(92)*. In this retrospective study of 291 patients undergoing carotid endarterectomy, the incidence of postoperative hypertension (systolic blood pressure more than 220 mmHg) was 9%, and was significantly associated with stroke or death ($p = 0.04$), in addition to an association with cardiac complications ($p = 0.07$). Independent risk factors for postoperative hypertension included angiographic intracranial stenosis above 50%, cardiac arrhythmia, preoperative systolic blood pressure more than 160 mmHg, neurological instability, and renal insufficiency. It could not be determined whether hypertension was a cause or secondary effect of cerebral ischemia, and therefore it is unknown whether treatment would influence complication rates. It would certainly seem appropriate to treat significant blood pressure elevations in this patient population (i.e., systolic blood pressure more than 160 mmHg) following evaluation for a new intracranial event. Because these patients may have increased sensitivity to beta adrenergic blockers postoperatively, significant bradycardia can be avoided by using alternative agents such as enalaprilat, or hydralazine (*see also* Chapter 24).

Guillain-Barré Syndrome

Autonomic dysfunction in Guillain-Barré syndrome (GBS) can cause fluctuations in hemodynamic parameters, including hypertension, hypotension, cardiac arrhythmias, and even cardiovascular collapse and death *(94)* (*see also* Chapters 10 and 27 for more details). Significant autonomic dysfunction is usually associated with severe motor weakness and respiratory failure *(95–99)*. In one series, 65% of patients had evidence of autonomic dysfunction, most commonly sinus tachycardia, hypertension, or labile blood pressure *(94)*. These disturbances are often transient. The hypertension is believed to be caused by increased sympathetic outflow *(100,101)*. These patients require continuous hemodynamic monitoring. The use of vasoactive agents should be done cautiously owing to the unpredictable occurrence of hypotension, which can occur after administration of antihypertensive agents through the mechanism of denervation hypersensitivity *(102)*. Hypertension often requires no treatment, as it is usually self-limited. If cardiac or end-organ damage is suspected, or for MAP more than 120 mmHg, blood pressure should be treated; sodium nitroprusside has been recommended, although other agents can be used *(103)*.

CHOICE OF ANTIHYPERTENSIVE AGENTS IN THE NEUROINTENSIVE CARE UNIT

The choice of antihypertensive agent is important because some agents have both systemic and cerebrovascular properties potentially affecting cerebral autoregulation and ICP. Blood pressure agents can be subdivided into two groups: those with purely extracerebral effects which do not cross the blood brain barrier, and those which exert direct pharmacologic action on cerebral blood vessels through a variety of mechanisms *(104)*. Acute management of hypertension uses six major classes of blood pressure medication: direct vasodilators (smooth muscle relaxants), ganglionic blockers, α- and β-adrenergic receptor antagonists, calcium channel antagonists, ACEI, and occasionally barbiturates *(105)* (Table 1).

Vasodilators that can cross the blood-brain barrier and act as cerebral vasodilators include sodium nitroprusside, calcium channel antagonists, hydralazine, nitroglycerin, adenosine and diazoxide. With the exception of diazoxide, all of these agents have the potential to increase CBF, impair autoregulation, and may increase ICP.

Diazoxide

This benzothiadiazine derivative related to thiazide diuretics produces vasodilatation by activating adenosine triphosphate sensitive potassium channels with resultant smooth muscle cell hyperpolarization, muscle and arteriolar relaxation *(105)*. The typical bolus dose of 5 mg/kg intravenously causes an abrupt fall in blood pressure of approx 50% and a 30% reduction in CBF in hypertensive rats as MAP falls below the lower limit of autoregulation *(18,104)*. A similar effect on CBF has been reported in man and we therefore do not recommend this drug in neurologic emergencies *(106)*. It has been used in situations where titratable agents could not be used and has a rapid onset of 1–5 min with a duration of 1–12 h *(107)*. Other side effects include myocardial ischemia, severe hyperglycemia, and salt and water retention *(105)*.

Hydralazine

This phthalazine derivative is a direct acting smooth muscle relaxant that acts by inhibiting vascular smooth muscle calcium transport, and also by generating nitric oxide *(105,108,109)*. Nitric oxide activates the guanylate cyclase–cyclic guanosine monophosphate (c-GMP) signaling pathway in vascular smooth muscle to cause vasodilation. Although hypertensive rats maintain normal CBF well below the lower limit of autoregulation, there is a tendency for CBF to rise with high doses and in man a rise in CBF along with increased ICP occurs in the presence of severe TBI and disturbed autoregulation *(110–112)*. Reflex stimulation of the sympathetic nervous system is reported to occur in TBI patients along with increased ICP *(83)*. The most important side effects with acute therapy are reflex tachycardia, myocardial stimulation (increased stroke volume and cardiac output) with possible angina, and sodium and water retention. Combining hydralazine with beta blockers has been suggested to blunt the sympathetic effect. The dose for acute increases in blood pressure is 2.5–10 mg intravenously with repeated doses every 20–30 min. Metabolism occurs predominantly by acetylation; rapid acetylators will therefore have lower plasma concentrations and may require more frequent dosing *(113)*.

Table 1
Antihypertensive Agents for Acute Blood Pressure Control

Drug	Mechanism of action	Onset of action	Duration of action	Dosage	Drug-specific adverse effects
Diazoxide	Activates ATP-sensitive potassium channels	1–5 min	1–12 h	IV Bolus: 50–100 mg q 10 min; continuous infusion: 15–30 mg/min	Severe hyperglycemia, salt and water retention
Hydralazine	Nitric oxide interferes with calcium mobilization in smooth muscle	15–30 min	3–4 h	2.5–10 mg IV bolus (up to 40 mg)	Drug-induced lupus syndrome, serum-sickness-like illness
Sodium nitroprusside	Nitric oxide	Immediate	2–3 min	0.25–10 μg/kg/min IV	Cyanide toxicity
Labetolol	α1, β1, β2 receptor antagonist	5–10 min	2–12 h	10–80 mg IV q 10 min up to 300 mg/d IV infusion: 0.5–2 mg/min	Congestive heart failure, bronchospasm, hypoglycemia, bradycardia
Esmolol	Selective β1 antagonist	Immediate	< 15 min	0.25–0.5 mg/kg IV bolus, then μg/kg/min	Bradycardia, congestive heart failure
Nicardipine	Calcium channel antagonist	1–5 min	3–6 h	5 mg/h IV, 2.5 mg/h q 15 min, up to 15 mg/h	Hypotension, tachycardia
Enalaprilat	Angiotensin-converting enzyme inhibitor	5–15 min	6 h	0.625–1.25 mg IV over 15 min	Renal dysfunction
Clonidine	α2 receptor agonist	3–5 h	8–12 h	0.1 mg po q 12 h; up to 2.4 mg/d	Sedation, bradycardia, rebound hypertension
Phentolamine	α1, α2 receptor antagonist	2 min	10–15 min	5–20 mg IV	Tachycardia, arrhythmias
Thiopental	Activation of GABA receptor	2 min	5–10 min	30–60 mg IV	Myocardial depression
Fenoldopam	DA-1, α2 receptor agonist	15 min	10–20 min	0.01–1.6 μg/kg/min IV; nobolus	Tachycardia, bradycardia; hypokalemia
Trimethaphan	Ganglionic blockade	Immediate	5–10 min	1–5 mg/min IV	Cycloplegia, mydriasis, urinary retention, bronchospasm
Adenosine	Adenosine receptor agonist	< 1 min	1–2 min	Up to 220 mg/kg/min	None
Nitroglycerin	Nitric oxide	1–2 min	3–5 min	5–100 μg/kg/min	Methemoglobin production

Adapted from Tietjen et al. *Crit. Care Med.* 1996 (ref. *105*). *See also* refs. *106–164.*

Sodium Nitroprusside

Nitroprusside is a direct acting nonselective peripheral vasodilator that causes relaxation of arterial and venous vascular smooth muscle *(114)*. The mechanism of action involves the reaction between the nitrate and sulfhydryl groups within red blood cells and the vessel wall, producing cyanide and nitric oxide *(15)*. Nitric oxide activates the enzyme guanylate cyclase that increases concentrations of cyclic guanosine monophosphate (c-GMP), leading to vasodilation in veins and arteries, including the cerebral resistance and capacitance vessels *(116)*. The latter effect may increase CBF and CBV resulting in increased ICP, which, added to the intended decrease in MAP, may compromise CPP in patients with reduced intracranial compliance. Increases in ICP are greatest for < 30% decreases in MAP *(117)*. Nitroprusside also inhibits physiologic vasoconstriction to hypocapnia *(116)*, which may exacerbate intracranial hypertension. Inducing hypocarbia and hyperoxia while administering nitroprusside over a 5-min period can, however, prevent the increase in ICP that occurs with rapid infusion *(117)*. Although detrimental effects on patient outcomes have not been reported in a clinical study of nitroprusside, any deterioration of neurologic status while using this antihypertensive agent warrants switching agents, and/or evaluation of ICP.

Nitroprusside dosing is based on the total acceptable dose rather than the effect on blood pressure. Continuous infusion is required due to the drug's transient effects. The usual infusion rate is 0.5–2 µg/kg/min with a maximum acceptable dose of up to 8 µg/kg/min for 1–3 h *(114)*. The dose of nitroprusside can be lowered by using a beta blocker simultaneously that will also blunts baroreceptor reflex responses. Side effects of nitroprusside include tachycardia, increased myocardial contractility, coronary steal, decreased PaO_2, and impaired platelet aggregation at infusion rates greater than 3 µg/kg/min *(114)*.

Cyanide and thiocyanate toxicity are concerns when the infusion rate exceeds the rate of hepatic conjugation of the cyanide moiety (approx 2 µg/kg/min). Cyanide toxicity should be considered in a patient who becomes resistant to the antihypertensive effects of the drug despite adequate infusion rates. Metabolic acidosis and increased mixed venous PO_2 are indicators. Therefore arterial pH should be monitored at higher infusion rates. The treatment of cyanide toxicity consists of immediate discontinuation of nitroprusside and administration of sodium thiosulfate 150 mg/kg intravenously, which acts as a sulfur donor to convert cyanide to thiocyanate. Thiocyanate, another metabolite of nitroprusside is cleared slowly by the kidney and may accumulate with prolonged infusions or renal failure *(114)*. Plasma thiocyanate levels more than 10 mg/dL may result in muscle weakness and confusion, and with longer exposure, hypothyroidism may occur.

Beta Blockers

Beta-adrenergic receptor antagonists are classified as either nonselective (such as propanolol), or selective on β1 receptors (metoprolol, atenolol, esmolol) or β2 receptors *(118)*. Beta adrenergic blockade removes the effects of catecholamines and sympathomimetics on heart and smooth muscle of airways and blood vessels. Beta blockers such as labetolol, a selective α1 antagonist and nonselective β1 and β2 antagonist, decrease systemic vascular resistance through α1 blockade in addition to beta-blocking the reflex tachycardia induced by vasodilation *(118)*. Labetolol, commonly used for moderately increased blood pressure, does not adversely affect CBF, although large doses often must be used to be effective (up to a maximum 300 mg/d). A dosing regimen of 10–20 mg intravenously every 15–20 min with doubling of each subsequent dose is recommended. In a study of patients with ICH and hypertension treated with propanolol (20–40 mg every 6 h), arterial blood pressure was successfully controlled without increasing ICP *(119)*. Esmolol, a rapid onset short-acting selective β1 receptor antagonist also has minimal known effects on cerebral hemodynamics. The short half-life of this agent (9 min) permits rapid titration (50–200 µg/kg/min following 500 µg/kg bolus dose over 1 min), although the blood pressure-lowering effect is less potent than its effect on heart rate. Metoprolol, another frequently used selective β1 antagonist also has more potent effects on heart rate that blood pressure. It should be noted that the bradycardia associated with the Cushing response (hypertension, bradycardia, irregular respirations) related to increased ICP is exacerbated by beta blockers *(120)* and may be an indication to discontinue attempts at lowering systemic blood pressure. Other side effects include decreased cardiac output (negative inotropic effect) and myocardial contractility potentially leading to cardiac failure, heart block, enhanced pressor effects of epinephrine, peripheral vasoconstriction (β2 blockade), bronchospasm, hypoglycemia, and increased plasma potassium.

Calcium Channel Blockers

Calcium entry blockers (CEB) or calcium antagonists inhibit voltage-dependent calcium channels (mostly L-type) preventing transport of calcium into vascular smooth muscle cells. Pharmacologic effects include vasodilatation, decreased heart rate, decreased myocardial contractility, and decreased cardiac impulse conduction through the atrioventricular node, all contributing to decreased blood pressure *(121)*. CEB do cause cerebral vasodilation with potential increased ICP in patients with TBI *(122–125)*. CEB, such as nicardipine, are however, frequently used to treat hypertensive crisis. Their main advantage over peripheral vasodilators, such as nitroprusside, is the capacity for long-term use and possibly easier control of antihypertension effects compared to nitroprusside *(126)*. The initial dose of nicardipine is 5 mg/h, up to a maximum of 15 mg/h and should be titrated by 1–2.5 mg/h every 15 min *(127)*. The onset of action is 1–5 min and duration of action is 3–6 h. The longer duration of action impairs titratability and as with other rapid acting vasodilators, continuous blood pressure monitoring must be in place along with frequent neurologic examinations, especially if cerebral edema or a space-occupying lesion is present. Sublingual administration of CEB such as nifedipine should be avoided due to rapid absorption which can precipitously drop blood pressure *(72)*.

Side effects of the CEBs include hypotension, headache, nausea and vomiting, and if toxicity occurs, myocardial depression, congestive heart failure, bradycardia, atrioventricular block, and cardiac arrest *(105)*.

Angiotensin-Converting Enzyme Inhibitors

Competitive inhibition of angiotensin I converting enzyme prevents the conversion of angiotensin I to the potent vasoconstrictor angiotensin II, reducing total peripheral resistance, reducing the local vascular effects of angiotensin II, reducing aldosterone concentration and therefore sodium retention, and increasing concentrations of the vasodilator bradykinin *(105)*. Angiotensin-converting enzyme inhibitors (ACEIs) are particularly useful for management of chronic hypertension and congestive heart failure, although the short-acting captopril and intravenous form of enalapril are useful in the acute setting. The major benefits of the ACEI are their minimal effects on heart rate, cardiac output, and pulmonary artery occlusion pressure. Moreover, they are also safe in terms of lacking adverse effects on CBF. Enalapril is a prodrug which is converted by a hepatic esterase to enalaprilat, which then inhibits peptidyl peptidase (hydrolyzes angiotensin I to angiotensin II) *(105)*. The intravenous dose of enalaprilat is 0.625–1.25 mg over 5 min with onset of action in 5–15 min and duration 6 h. A small reduction in heart rate may occur. Captopril is only available orally. A starting dose of 12.5 mg has onset of action in 15 to 30 min with duration 6–10 h, limiting its usefulness for abrupt increases in blood pressure. The cerebral effects of the ACEI include an apparent shift in the autoregulatory curve such that the flat portion is shortened by shifts in both upper and lower limits *(128–131)*. In addition, captopril appears to decrease vascular tone in large cerebral vessels while small resistance vessels constrict *(132)*. In patients with congestive heart failure, CBF is preserved after a single dose, but is increased with chronic treatment *(130,131)*. Effects on ICP have only been studied in patients with normal pressure hydrocephalus who undergo no change in ICP or CBF *(133)*.

Important side effects of ACEI include a skin rash, rarely angioedema, hyperkalemia, proteinuria, cough, and rarely neutropenia *(113)*.

Clonidine

This centrally acting α2 adrenergic agonist specifically acts on inhibitory neurons in the medullary vasomotor center causing a decrease in sympathetic outflow to the periphery, and resultant vasorelaxation in both resistance and capacitance vessels *(113)*. Heart rate and cardiac output are decreased in addition to blood pressure. This class of antihypertensive has been shown to induce cerebral vasoconstriction, reduce baseline CBF and reduce ICP in experimental animals, although cerebral oxygen consumption was unchanged *(134,135)*. Clinical studies have demonstrated conflicting results; oral clonidine for severe hypertension (diastolic blood pressure > 115 mmHg) was associated with increased CBF in patients with low pretreatment CBF, while patients with initially high CBF experienced decreases in CBF *(136)*. In another study comparing intravenous clonidine with oral nifedipine using ^{133}Xe to measure CBF, clonidine decreased CBF to 28% of baseline values *(137,138)*. Finally, a study of a single dose of clonidine in 12 severe TBI patients induced a decrease in MAP and CPP, and in three patients, an increase in ICP, which may have been caused by compensatory autoregulatory vasodilatation in response to the hypotensive effect of the drug.

There are several reasons limiting the usefulness of clonidine for acute management of blood pressure. The intravenous formulation is not available in the United States and the half-life of oral clonidine is 8–12 h. Sedation is an important side effect making this antihypertensive a relatively poor choice, and finally, sudden withdrawal causes rebound hypertension from 8 to 36 h after the last dose. Clonidine, however, may be useful for patients with TBI who experience transient surges of systolic blood pressure, usually the result of alcohol or drug withdrawal, or secondary to the cerebral insult itself which may have damaged the hypothalamus causing sympathetic hyperactivity. The hypertension is often associated with tachycardia, diaphoresis and anxiety, which all respond to this antihypertensive. The starting dose of oral clonidine is 0.1 mg every 8 h, and can be increased up to 0.4 mg every 8 h. Other side effects of clonidine include xerostomia, bradycardia, and reduced anesthetic requirements *(139)*.

Phentolamine

Although less commonly used, this imidazole derivative has equipotent α1 and α2 receptor antagonist properties and produces direct relaxation of vascular smooth muscle making it a useful agent for acute management of hypertension *(105)*. The α1 antagonist effect is five to ten times as potent as that of labetolol. There is no known effect on CBF or ICP in the range of autoregulation, although CBF may be reduced if CPP is significantly decreased *(105)*. The dose for treatment of hypertensive emergencies is 30–70 µg/kg intravenously with onset of action in about 2 min and duration of action for 10–15 min *(105)*. The major drawback for the above indication is the relatively long duration of effect especially in conditions with rapidly fluctuating CPP. Side effects of phentolamine include tachycardia, cardiac arrhythmias, and angina from reflex cardiac stimulation and unopposed beta effects of norepinephrine.

Barbiturates

Barbiturates, although most commonly used as anticonvulsants or for induction of general anesthesia, have a unique role in the management of systemic hypertension especially when intracranial hypertension and space-occupying lesions are also present. Barbiturates act via allosteric activation of the γ-aminobutyric acid receptor causing increased duration of opening of the chloride channel which mediates an inhibitory effect on synaptic activity accounting for the antiepileptogenic effect and probably the depression of cerebral metabolism *(140)*. The effect on cerebral metabolism causes a decrease in CBF and ICP. Because cerebral oxygen metabolism is reduced, the risk for secondary ischemic brain injury is reduced *(141,142)*. Autoregulation is not affected, although animal experiments have demonstrated attenuation of the cerebral vasodilatory responses to hypoxia and hypercapnia *(143)*. The effect on arterial blood pressure is mediated by peripheral venodilation and pooling of blood secondary to the decreased sympathetic nervous system outflow from the central nervous system *(144)*.

Both pentobarbital and thiopental can be used for controlling MAP and ICP when simultaneous management is required and the patient's airway is protected. As a result of significant respiratory depression caused by both agents, endotracheal intubation and mechanical ventilation are generally required especially if longer term administration of these agents is likely. Thiopental, a thiobarbiturate, has rapid onset of action (maximal brain uptake takes 30 s followed by a decrease over the next 5 min as redistribution occurs to inactive tissue sites accounting for the short duration of action). Although a single intravenous dose will not likely affect awakening time, repeated doses of these lipid soluble barbiturates will produce a cumulative drug effect due to the storage capacity of fat *(113)*. A reasonable dose for acute blood pressure control for thiopental is 30–60 mg intravenously; the usual induction dose for general anesthesia is 3–5 mg/kg, which may be required if ICP control is the goal. The long acting oxybarbiturate pentobarbital (elimination half-life: 24 h) should generally not be considered for emergency treatment of hypertension unless management of refractory ICP elevation or status epilepticus is the goal of therapy. Additional monitoring of ICP or continuous electroencephalography for titration of dose is indicated for such patients. Hypotension may be an unwanted effect in these situations, requiring volume infusions or vasopressor support. The dose of pentobarbital depends on the desired effect. For ICP control, a loading dose of 10–40 mg/kg, followed by an infusion of 1–2 mg/kg/h achieves burst suppression on the electroencephalogram.

Adverse effects of the barbiturates, in addition to hypotension and respiratory depression, include compensatory tachycardia, direct myocardial depression, impaired gastrointestinal motility, venous thrombosis, and rarely allergic reactions.

Fenoldopam

Fenoldopam is a rapid-acting potent systemic vasodilator. This benzapine derivative of the catecholamine dopamine (DA) has high affinity for DA-1 receptors and moderate affinity for α2 receptors. In experimental animal preparations, fenoldopam mediates vasodilatation of mesenteric, renal, cerebral and coronary vascular smooth muscle *(145)*. Although it does not cross the blood brain barrier, fenoldopam may have effects on the cerebral circulation via α2 adrenergic receptors found on large and small cerebral vessels *(134,146,147)*. Infusion of this antihypertensive in rabbits with experimental heart failure increased CBF, but had no effect on control animals *(148)*. In a study of fenoldopam infusion in normotensive healthy humans, reduction of systemic blood pressure by 16% was associated with decreased cortical, caudate, and thalamic CBF measured by positron emission tomography *(149)*. This finding was explained by cerebral α2 adrenergic receptor-induced vasoconstriction in these areas, which reflects the known distribution of this receptor type in the cerebral vasculature *(134,146,147,150,151)*. Caution has therefore been advised when considering fenoldopam in patients in which CBF and ICP control are priorities.

Fenoldopam is indicated for rapid short-term management of hypertensive emergencies *(33,152–154)*. It has been recommended as an alternative to nitroprusside in the management of perioperative and intraoperative hypertension. It has not been studied in the setting of hypertensive encephalopathy. Advantages include short half-life (approx 10 min), ability to maintain or improve renal function (renal blood flow and creatinine clearance) during blood pressure lowering, absence of toxic metabolites, and good safety profile with minimal drug interactions *(155)*. Pharmacokinetics are not altered in the presence of renal or hepatic insufficiency *(33)*. In clinical trials, doses from 0.01 to 1.6 µg/kg/min have been studied with effect at a given infusion rate attained in 15 min. A bolus dose should not be used. Fenoldopam causes a dose-related tachycardia, which may be followed by bradycardia (Bezold-Jarisch reflex) *(33)*. Adverse effects include hypokalemia possibly secondary to a pressure natriuresis, headache, flushing, and nausea.

Ganglionic Blockers

Trimethaphan camsylate is an intravenous peripheral vasodilator which produces direct relaxation of capacitance vessels, as well as blockade of sympathetic and parasympathetic autonomic ganglia *(114)*. Both decreased systemic vascular resistance and decreased cardiac output contribute to decreasing blood pressure. Central nervous system effects are unlikely due to the quaternary ammonium structure which limits passage across the blood-brain barrier *(114)*. Studies have reported little or no effect on CBF or ICP although induction of hypotension may cause a transient increase in ICP especially if administered rapidly an in setting of reduced intracranial compliance *(156)*. Trimethaphan is most often used as a continuous intravenous infusion due to its rapid onset and short duration of action. The usual dose is 1–5 mg/min. Duration of effect is 5–10 min. Metabolism includes hydrolysis by plasma cholinesterases *(114)*. Tachyphyllaxis is common and may limit its use *(105)*. Combination treatment of hypertension with nitroprusside (10 : 1 mixture of trimethaphan to nitroprusside) has been suggested to decrease dose requirements of the latter and dose related side effects of both agents, especially cyanide concentrations *(157)*.

Adverse effects of ganglionic blockade include mydriasis, which may complicate neurologic examination, ileus, urinary retention, decreased myocardial contractility, decreased thermoregulatory sweating, and histamine-induced bronchospasm *(105)*.

Adenosine

Adenosine is an endogenous nucleotide with vasodilator actions which maintain the balance between oxygen delivery and demand in the heart and other organs *(114)*. Adenosine can be used to induce controlled hypotension, which has the advantage, notably in the operating room, of rapid onset, stable maintenance and prompt reversal on discontinuation without rebound hypertension *(158)*. Reports of increases in ICP in TBI patients suggest caution in this population *(107)*. Experimental studies, however, reducing MAP to 30 mmHg produced no compromise of cerebral cortical blood flow and oxygen tension *(159)*. The half-life of adenosine in plasma is brief (0.6–1.5 s). Blood pressure control requires intravenous infusion rates of more than 200 μg/kg/min; this level of infusion does not affect cardiac conduction *(160)*.

Side effects of adenosine in awake patients include facial flushing, nausea, headache, chest tightness, and dizziness/lightheadedness *(158,161,162)*. These side effects are caused by hypotension or cerebral vasodilation. Higher doses may cause sinus bradycardia, transient atrioventricular block/asystole, coronary artery steal and bronchospasm *(114)*.

Nitroglycerin

Nitroglycerin is generally avoided in patients with acute brain injury. There are potential uses, however, for controlled hypotension during neurosurgery, and experimentally, nitroglycerin has been investigated for cerebral vasospasm. The mechanism of action of the organic nitrates is via nitric oxide which acts mainly on venous capacitance vessels to produce peripheral pooling of blood, reduced heart size, and decreased cardiac ventricular wall tension. Nitroglycerin is also a cerebral vasodilator and therefore may increase ICP in patients with reduced intracranial compliance. The most likely cause is increased capacitance although dilatation of large intracranial arteries may also be a factor *(163,164)*. A variable effect on CBF has been reported. Animal studies demonstrate preservation of CBF when ICP is normal because CPP is reduced below the limits of autoregulation. If ICP is increased, however, CBF decreases, even within the autoregulatory range and the CBF vasodilatory response to hypercapnia is impaired *(116)*. These changes in ICP are greater with bolus administration than with continuous infusion *(164)*. Continuous infusion is also recommended because of the short elimination half-life of this drug (1–5 min). Metabolism in the liver by nitrate reductase yields glycerol dinitrite and nitrite which are excreted in the urine *(114)*. The nitrite metabolite can oxidize the ferrous ion in hemoglobin to the ferric state producing methemoglobin.

Significant methemoglobinemia is rare with doses less than 5 mg/kg *(105)*. Toxicity is treated with intravenous methylene blue (1–2 mg/kg), which promotes conversion of methemoglobin to hemoglobin.

REFERENCES

1. Britton M, Carlsson A. Very high blood pressure in acute stroke. *J. Intern. Med.* 1990;228:611–615.
2. Powers WJ. Acute hypertension after stroke: the scientific basis for treatment decisions. *Neurology* 1993;43:461–467.
3. Broderick J. Intracerebral hemorrhage. In Gorelick PB AM, ed. *Handbook of Neuroepidemiology*. New York: Marcel Dekker, 1994:141–167.
4. Kassell NF, Torner JC, Haley EC Jr, Jane JA, Adams HP, Kongable GL. The international cooperative study on the timing of aneurysm surgery. Part 1: Overall management results. *J. Neurosurg.* 1990;73:18–36.
5. Fog M. Cerebral circulation. The reaction of the pial arteries to a fall in blood pressure. *Arch. Neurol. Psychiatry* 1937;37:351–364.
6. Fog M. Cerebral circulation II: reaction of pial arteries to increase in blood pressure. *Arch. Neurol. Psychiatry* 1939;41:260–268.
7. Lassen N. Cerebral blood flow and oxygen consumption in man. *Physiol. Rev.* 1959;39:183–238.
8. Strandgaard S, Olesen J, Skinhoj E, Lassen NA. Autoregulation of brain circulation in severe arterial hypertension. *BMJ* 1973;1:507–510.
9. Strandgaard S. Autoregulation of cerebral blood flow in hypertensive patients. The modifying influence of prolonged antihypertensive treatment on the tolerance to acute, drug-induced hypotension. *Circulation* 1976;53:720–727.
10. McHenry LC Jr, West JW, Cooper ES, Goldberg HI, Jaffe ME. Cerebral autoregulation in man. *Stroke* 1974;5:695–706.
11. Westergaard E, van Deurs B, Brondsted HE. Increased vesicular transfer of horseradish peroxidase across cerebral endothelium, evoked by acute hypertension. *Acta. Neuropathol. (Berl)* 1977;37:141–152.
12. Sokrab TE, Johansson BB, Kalimo H, Olsson Y. A transient hypertensive opening of the blood-brain barrier can lead to brain damage. Extravasation of serum proteins and cellular changes in rats subjected to aortic compression. *Acta. Neuropathol.* 1988;75:557–565.
13. Johansson B. Hypertension and the blood brain barrier. In E N, ed. *Implications of the Blood-Brain Barrier and its Manipulation*, Vol. 2. New York: Plenum Press, 1988:557–565.
14. Jones JV, Fitch W, MacKenzie ET, Strandgaard S, Harper AM. Lower limit of cerebral blood flow autoregulation in experimental renovascular hypertension in the baboon. *Circ. Res.* 1976;39:555–557.
15. Barry DI, Strandgaard S, Graham DI, et al. Cerebral blood flow in rats with renal and spontaneous hypertension: resetting of the lower limit of autoregulation. *J. Cereb. Blood Flow Metab.* 1982;2:347–353.
16. Strandgaard S, Jones JV, MacKenzie ET, Harper AM. Upper limit of cerebral blood flow autoregulation in experimental renovascular hypertension in the baboon. *Circ. Res.* 1975;37:164–167.
17. Paulson OB, Waldemar G, Schmidt JF, Strandgaard S. Cerebral circulation under normal and pathologic conditions. *Am. J. Cardiol.* 1989;63:2C–5C.
18. Strandgaard S, Paulson OB. Cerebral autoregulation. *Stroke* 1984;15:413–416.
19. Vorstrup S, Barry DI, Jarden JO, et al. Chronic antihypertensive treatment in the rat reverses hypertension-induced changes in cerebral blood flow autoregulation. *Stroke* 1984;15:312–318.
20. Osol G, Halpern W. Myogenic properties of cerebral blood vessels from normotensive and hypertensive rats. *Am. J. Physiol.* 1985;249:H914–H921.
21. Phillis JW, Walter GA, O'Regan MH, Stair RE. Increases in cerebral cortical perfusate adenosine and inosine concentrations during hypoxia and ischemia. *J. Cereb. Blood Flow Metab.* 1987;7:679–686.
22. Broderick JP, Adams HP, Jr., Barsan W, et al. Guidelines for the management of spontaneous intracerebral hemorrhage: A statement for healthcare professionals from a special writing group of the Stroke Council, American Heart Association. *Stroke* 1999;30:905–915.
23. Lisk DR, Grotta JC, Lamki LM, et al. Should hypertension be treated after acute stroke? A randomized controlled trial using single photon emission computed tomography. *Arch. Neurol.* 1993;50:855–862.
24. Rosner MJ, Daughton S. Cerebral perfusion pressure management in head injury. *J. Trauma* 1990;30:933–940.
25. Schrader H, Zwetnow NN, Morkrid L. Regional cerebral blood flow and CSF pressures during Cushing response induced by a supratentorial expanding mass. *Acta. Neurol. Scand.* 1985;71:453–463.
26. Schrader H, Lofgren J, Zwetnow NN. Influence of blood pressure on tolerance to an intracranial expanding mass. *Acta. Neurol. Scand.* 1985;71:114–126.
27. Drummond JC, Oh YS, Cole DJ, Shapiro HM. Phenylephrine-induced hypertension reduces ischemia following middle cerebral artery occlusion in rats. *Stroke* 1989;20:1538–1544.
28. Vaughan CJ, Delanty N. Hypertensive emergencies. *Lancet* 2000;356:411–417.
29. Schwartz RB, Mulkern RV, Gudbjartsson H, Jolesz F. Diffusion-weighted MR imaging in hypertensive encephalopathy: clues to pathogenesis. *AJNR* 1998;19:859–862.
30. Calhoun DA, Oparil S. Treatment of hypertensive crisis. *N. Engl. J. Med.* 1990;323:1177–1183.

31. Hirschl MM, Binder M, Bur A, et al. Clinical evaluation of different doses of intravenous enalaprilat in patients with hypertensive crises. *Arch. Intern. Med.* 1995;155:2217–2223.

32. Wilson DJ, Wallin JD, Vlachakis ND, et al. Intravenous labetalol in the treatment of severe hypertension and hypertensive emergencies. *Am. J. Med.* 1983;75:95–102.

33. Oparil S, Aronson S, Deeb GM, et al. Fenoldopam: a new parenteral antihypertensive: consensus roundtable on the management of perioperative hypertension and hypertensive crises. *Am. J. Hypertens.* 1999;12:653–664.

34. Pilmer BL, Green JA, Panacek EA, et al. Fenoldopam mesylate versus sodium nitroprusside in the acute management of severe systemic hypertension. *J. Clin. Pharmacol.* 1993;33:549–553.

35. Orth H, Ritz E. Sodium depletion in accelerated hypertension [letter]. *N. Engl. J. Med.* 1975;292:1133.

36. Houston MC. Pathophysiology, clinical aspects, and treatment of hypertensive crises. *Prog. Cardiovasc. Dis.* 1989;32:99–148.

37. Cole F, PO Y. Pseudo-aneurysms in relationship to massive cerebral hemorrhage. *J. Neurol. Neurosurg. Psychiatry* 1967;30:61–66.

38. Fisher CM. Pathological observations in hypertensive cerebral hemorrhage. *J. Neuropathol. Exp. Neurol.* 1971;30:536–550.

39. Britton M, Carlsson A, de Faire U. Blood pressure course in patients with acute stroke and matched controls. *Stroke* 1986;17:861–864.

40. Wallace JD, Levy LL. Blood pressure after stroke. *JAMA* 1981;246:2177–2180.

41. Fogelholm R, Avikainen S, Murros K. Prognostic value and determinants of first-day mean arterial pressure in spontaneous supratentorial intracerebral hemorrhage. *Stroke* 1997;28:1396–400.

42. Terayama Y, Tanahashi N, Fukuuchi Y, Gotoh F. Prognostic value of admission blood pressure in patients with intracerebral hemorrhage. Keio cooperative stroke study. *Stroke* 1997;28:1185–1188.

43. Qureshi AI, Safdar K, Weil J, et al. Predictors of early deterioration and mortality in black Americans with spontaneous intracerebral hemorrhage. *Stroke* 1995;26:1764–1767.

44. Brott T, Broderick J, Kothari R, et al. Early hemorrhage growth in patients with intracerebral hemorrhage. *Stroke* 1997;28:1–5.

45. Powers W, Adams RE, KD Y. Acute pharmacological hypotension after intracerebral hemorrhage does not change cerebral blood flow. In: The American Heart Association Conference. Nashville TN; 1999.

46. Kaneko T, Sawanda T. Lower limit of blood pressure in treatment of acute hypertensive intracranial hemorrhage. *J. Cereb. Blood Flow Metab.* 1983;3:S51–S52.

47. Mayer SA, Lignelli A, Fink ME, et al. Perilesional blood flow and edema formation in acute intracerebral hemorrhage: a SPECT study. *Stroke* 1998;29:1791–1798.

48. Sills C, Villar-Cordova C, W P. Demonstration of hypoperfusion surrounding intracerebral hematomas in humans. *J. Stroke Cerebrovasc. Dis.* 1996;6:17–24.

49. Qureshi AI, Wilson DA, Hanley DF, Traystman RJ. Pharmacologic reduction of mean arterial pressure does not adversely affect regional cerebral blood flow and intracranial pressure in experimental intracerebral hemorrhage. *Crit. Care Med.* 1999;27:965–971.

50. Fujii Y, Takeuchi S, Sasaki O, Minakawa T, Tanaka R. Multivariate analysis of predictors of hematoma enlargement in spontaneous intracerebral hemorrhage. *Stroke* 1998;29:1160–1166.

51. Kazui S, Minematsu K, Yamamoto H, Sawada T, Yamaguchi T. Predisposing factors to enlargement of spontaneous intracerebral hematoma. *Stroke* 1997;28:2370–2375.

52. Broderick JP, Brott TG, Tomsick T, Barsan W, Spilker J. Ultra-early evaluation of intracerebral hemorrhage. *J. Neurosurg.* 1990;72:195–199.

53. Dandapani BK, Suzuki S, Kelley RE, Reyes-Iglesias Y, Duncan RC. Relation between blood pressure and outcome in intracerebral hemorrhage. *Stroke* 1995;26:21–24.

54. McKissock W, Richardson A. Primary intracerebral hemorrhage: a controlled trial of surgical and conservative treatment in 180 unselected cases. *Lancet* 1961;2:222–226.

55. Diringer MN. Intracerebral hemorrhage: pathophysiology and management. *Crit. Care Med.* 1993;21:1591–1603.

56. Torner JC, Kassell NF, Wallace RB, Adams HP, Jr. Preoperative prognostic factors for rebleeding and survival in aneurysm patients receiving antifibrinolytic therapy: report of the Cooperative Aneurysm Study. *Neurosurgery* 1981;9:506–513.

57. Wijdicks EF, Vermeulen M, Murray GD, Hijdra A, van Gijn J. The effects of treating hypertension following aneurysmal subarachnoid hemorrhage. *Clin. Neurol. Neurosurg.* 1990;92:111–117.

58. van Gijn J, Rinkel GJ. Subarachnoid haemorrhage: diagnosis, causes and management. *Brain* 2001;124:249–278.

59. Bernardini G, Mayer SA, RA S. Subarachnoid hemorrhage. In Miller DH RE, ed. *Critical Care Neurology.* Boston: Butterworth-Heinemann; 1999:233.

60. Kassell NF, Peerless SJ, Durward QJ, Beck DW, Drake CG, Adams HP. Treatment of ischemic deficits from vasospasm with intravascular volume expansion and induced arterial hypertension. *Neurosurgery* 1982;11:337–343.

61. Amin-Hanjani S, Schwartz RB, Sathi S, Stieg PE. Hypertensive encephalopathy as a complication of hyperdynamic therapy for vasospasm: report of two cases. *Neurosurgery* 1999;44:1113–1116.

62. Chamorro A, Vila N, Ascaso C, Elices E, Schonewille W, Blanc R. Blood pressure and functional recovery in acute ischemic stroke. *Stroke* 1998;29:1850–1853.
63. Carlberg B, Asplund K, Hagg E. Factors influencing admission blood pressure levels in patients with acute stroke. *Stroke* 1991;22:527–530.
64. Jansen PA, Schulte BP, Poels EF, Gribnau FW. Course of blood pressure after cerebral infarction and transient ischemic attack. *Clin. Neurol. Neurosurg.* 1987;89:243–246.
65. Torner J, Nibbelink DW, LF B. Statistical comparison of end results of a randomized treatment study. In Nibbelink DW, ed. *Aneurysmal Subarachnoid Hemorrhage.* Baltimore: Urban & Schwarzenberg, 1981:249–275.
66. Broderick J, Brott T, Barsan W, et al. Blood pressure during the first minutes of focal cerebral ischemia. *Ann. Emerg. Med.* 1993;22:1438–1443.
67. Hayashi S, Nehls DG, Kieck CF, Vielma J, DeGirolami U, Crowell RM. Beneficial effects of induced hypertension on experimental stroke in awake monkeys. *J. Neurosurg.* 1984;60:151–157.
68. Jorgensen HS, Nakayama H, Raaschou HO, Olsen TS. Effect of blood pressure and diabetes on stroke in progression. *Lancet* 1994;344:156–159.
69. Rordorf G, Cramer SC, Efind JT, Schwamm LH, Buonanno F, Koroshetz WJ. Pharmacological elevation of blood pressure in acute stroke. Clinical effects and safety. *Stroke* 1997;28:2133–2138.
70. Hillis AE, Kane A, Tuffiash E, et al. Reperfusion of specific brain regions by raising blood pressure restores selective language functions in subacute stroke. *Brain Lang.* 2001;79:495–510.
71. Fagan SC, Bowes MP, Lyden PD, Zivin JA. Acute hypertension promotes hemorrhagic transformation in a rabbit embolic stroke model: effect of labetalol. *Exp. Neurol.* 1998;150:153–158.
72. Adams HP, Jr., Brott TG, Crowell RM, et al. Guidelines for the management of patients with acute ischemic stroke. A statement for healthcare professionals from a special writing group of the Stroke Council, American Heart Association. *Stroke* 1994;25:1901–1914.
73. The NINDS t-PA Stroke Study Group. Intracerebral hemorrhage after intravenous t-PA therapy for ischemic stroke. *Stroke* 1997;28:2109–2118.
74. Emergency Cardiac Care Committee and Subcommittees, American Heart Association. Part IV. Guidelines for cardiopulmonary resuscitation and emergency cardiac care. Special resuscitation situations. *JAMA* 1992;268:2242–2250.
75. Adams H, Brott TG, AJ F. Guidelines for thrombolytic therapy for acute stroke: a supplement to the guidelines for the management of patients with acute ischemic stroke. A statement for healthcare professionals from a Special Writing Group of the Stroke Council, American Heart Association. *Circulation* 1996;94:1167–1174.
76. Britton M, de Faire U, Helmers C. Hazards of therapy for excessive hypertension in acute stroke. *Acta. Med. Scand.* 1980;207:253–257.
77. Clifton GL, Robertson CS, Kyper K, Taylor AA, Dhekne RD, Grossman RG. Cardiovascular response to severe head injury. *J. Neurosurg.* 1983;59:447–454.
78. Jennett GT. *Management of Head Injuries.* Philadelphia: FA Davis, 1981.
79. Clifton GL, Ziegler MG, Grossman RG. Circulating catecholamines and sympathetic activity after head injury. *Neurosurgery* 1981;8:10–14.
80. Hortnagl H, Hammerle AF, Hackl JM, Brucke T, Rumpl E. The activity of the sympathetic nervous system following severe head injury. *Intensive Care Med.* 1980;6:169–167.
81. Langfitt T, Weinstein JD, Kassell NF. Cerebral vasomotor paralysis produced by intracranial hypertension. *Neurology* 1965;15:622–641.
82. Marshall LF, Smith RW, Shapiro HM. The outcome with aggressive treatment in severe head injuries. Part I: the significance of intracranial pressure monitoring. *J. Neurosurg.* 1979;50:20–25.
83. Robertson CS, Clifton GL, Taylor AA, Grossman RG. Treatment of hypertension associated with head injury. *J. Neurosurg.* 1983;59:455–460.
84. Clifton GL, Miller ER, Choi SC, Levin HS. Fluid thresholds and outcome from severe brain injury. *Crit. Care Med.* 2002;30:739–745.
85. Davis DH, Sundt TM Jr. Relationship of cerebral blood flow to cardiac output, mean arterial pressure, blood volume, and alpha and beta blockade in cats. *J. Neurosurg.* 1980;52:745–754.
86. Bove EL, Fry WJ, Gross WS, Stanley JC. Hypotension and hypertension as consequences of baroreceptor dysfunction following carotid endarterectomy. *Surgery* 1979;85:633–637.
87. Davies MJ, Cronin KD. Post carotid endarterectomy hypertension. *Anaesth. Intensive Care* 1980;8:190–194.
88. Skudlarick JL, Mooring SL. Systolic hypertension and complications of carotid endarterectomy. *South Med. J.* 1982;75:1563–1565, 1567.
89. Holton P, Wood JB. The effects of bilateral removal of the carotid bodies and denervation of the carotid sinuses in two human subjects. *J. Physiol.* 1965;181:365–378.
90. Lilly MP, Brunner MJ, Wehberg KE, Rudolphi DM, Queral LA. Jugular venous vasopressin increases during carotid endarterectomy after cerebral reperfusion. *J. Vasc. Surg.* 1992;16:1–9.
91. Smith BL. Hypertension following carotid endarterectomy: the role of cerebral renin production. *J. Vasc. Surg.* 1984;1:623–627.

92. Wong JH, Findlay JM, Suarez-Almazor ME. Hemodynamic instability after carotid endarterectomy: risk factors and associations with operative complications. *Neurosurgery* 1997;41:35–41.

93. Piepgras DG, Morgan MK, Sundt TM, Jr., Yanagihara T, Mussman LM. Intracerebral hemorrhage after carotid endarterectomy. *J. Neurosurg.* 1988;68:532–536.

94. Truax B. Autonomic disturbances in Guillain-Barre syndrome. *Semin. Neurol.* 1984;4:462.

95. Ng KK, Howard RS, Wiles CM, et al. Management and outcome of severe Guillain-Barre syndrome. *Q. J. Med.* 1995;88:253.

96. Ropper A, Wijdicks EFM, BT T. *Guillain-Barre Syndrome.* Philadelphia: FA Davis, 1991.

97. Singh NK, Jaiswal AK, Misra S, Srivastava PK. Assessment of autonomic dysfunction in Guillain-Barre syndrome and its prognostic implications. *Acta. Neurol. Scand.* 1987;75:101–105.

98. Susman E, K M. Guillain-Barre syndrome. *Med. J. Aust.* 1940;1:158.

99. Thomashefsky AJ, Horwitz SJ, Feingold MH. Acute autonomic neuropathy. *Neurology* 1972;22:251–215.

100. McQuillan JJ, Bullock RE. Extreme labile blood pressure in Guillain-Barre syndrome. *Lancet* 1988;2:172–173.

101. Mitchell PL, Meilman E. The mechanism of hypertension in the Guillain-Barre syndrome. *Am. J. Med.* 1967;42:986–995.

102. Lichtenfeld P. Autonomic dysfunction in the Guillain-Barre syndrome. *Am. J. Med.* 1971;50:772–780.

103. Fulgham JR, Wijdicks EF. Guillain-Barre syndrome. *Crit. Care Clin.* 1997;13:1–15.

104. Barry DI. Cerebrovascular aspects of antihypertensive treatment. *Am. J. Cardiol.* 1989;63:14C–18C.

105. Tietjen CS, Hurn PD, Ulatowski JA, Kirsch JR. Treatment modalities for hypertensive patients with intracranial pathology: options and risks. *Crit. Care Med.* 1996;24:311–322.

106. Goldberg HI, Codario RA, Banka RS, Reivich M. Patterns of cerebral dysautoregulation in severe hypertension to blood pressure reduction with diazoxide. *Acta Neurol. Scand.* 1977;56:64–65.

107. Clarke KW, Brear SG, Hanley SP. Rise in intracranial pressure with intravenous adenosine. *Lancet* 1992;339:188–189.

108. Spokas EG, Folco G, Quilley J, Chander P, McGiff JC. Endothelial mechanism in the vascular action of hydralazine. *Hypertension* 1983;5:I107–I111.

109. Kruszyna H, Kruszyna R, Smith RP, Wilcox DE. Red blood cells generate nitric oxide from directly acting, nitrogenous vasodilators. *Toxicol. Appl. Pharmacol.* 1987;91:429–438.

110. Barry DI, Strandgaard S, Graham DI, Svendsen UG, Braendstrup O, Paulson OB. Cerebral blood flow during dihydralazine-induced hypotension in hypertensive rats. *Stroke* 1984;15:102–108.

111. Overgaard J, Skinhoj E. A paradoxical cerebral hemodynamic effect of hydralazine. *Stroke* 1975;6:402–410.

112. Skinhoj E, Overgaard J. Effect of dihydralazine on intracranial pressure in patients with severe brain damage. *Acta Med. Scand. Suppl.* 1983;678:83–87.

113. Stoelting R. Antihypertensive drugs. In *Handbook of Pharmacology and Physiology in Anesthetic Practice.* Philadelphia: Lippincott-Raven, 1995:248–256.

114. Stoelting R. Peripheral vasodilators. In *Handbook of Pharmacology and Physiology in Anesthetic Practice.* Philadelphia: Lippincott-Raven, 1995:2257–2268.

115. Tinker JH, Michenfelder JD. Sodium nitroprusside: pharmacology, toxicology and therapeutics. *Anesthesiology* 1976;45:340–354.

116. Hartmann A, Buttinger C, Rommel T, Czernicki Z, Trtinjiak F. Alteration of intracranial pressure, cerebral blood flow, autoregulation and carbon dioxide-reactivity by hypotensive agents in baboons with intracranial hypertension. *Neurochirurgia (Stuttg)* 1989;32:37–43.

117. Marsh ML, Aidinis SJ, Naughton KV, Marshall LF, Shapiro HM. The technique of nitroprusside administration modifies the intracranial pressure response. *Anesthesiology* 1979;51:538–541.

118. Stoelting R. Alpha- and beta-adrenergic receptor antagonists. In *Handbook of Pharmacology and Physiology in Anesthetic Practice.* Philadelphia: Lippincott-Raven, 1995:238–247.

119. Feibel JH, Baldwin CA, Joynt RJ. Catecholamine-associated refractory hypertension following acute intracranial hemorrhage: control with propranolol. *Ann. Neurol.* 1981;9:340–343.

120. van Wylen DG, D'Alecy LG. Regional blood flow distribution during the Cushing response: alterations with adrenergic blockade. *Am. J. Physiol.* 1985;248:H98–H108.

121. Reves JG, Kissin I, Lell WA, Tosone S. Calcium entry blockers: uses and implications for anesthesiologists. *Anesthesiology* 1982;57:504–518.

122. Griffin JP, Cottrell JE, Hartung J, Shwiry B. Intracranial pressure during nifedipine-induced hypotension. *Anesth. Analg.* 1983;62:1078–1080.

123. Bedford RF, Dacey R, Winn HR, Lynch C, 3rd. Adverse impact of a calcium entry-blocker (verapamil) on intracranial pressure in patients with brain tumors. *J. Neurosurg.* 1983;59:800–802.

124. Mazzoni P, Giffin JP, Cottrell JE, Hartung J, Capuano C, Epstein JM. Intracranial pressure during diltiazem-induced hypotension in anesthetized dogs. *Anesth. Analg.* 1985;64:1001–1004.

125. Tateishi A, Sano T, Takeshita H, Suzuki T, Tokuno H. Effects of nifedipine on intracranial pressure in neurosurgical patients with arterial hypertension. *J. Neurosurg.* 1988;69:213–215.

126. Halpern NA, Goldberg M, Neely C, et al. Postoperative hypertension: a multicenter, prospective, randomized comparison between intravenous nicardipine and sodium nitroprusside. *Crit. Care Med.* 1992;20:1637–1643.

127. Wallin JD. Intravenous nicardipine hydrochloride: treatment of patients with severe hypertension. *Am. Heart J.* 1990;119:434–437.
128. Barry DI, Paulson OB, Jarden JO, Juhler M, Graham DI, Strandgaard S. Effects of captopril on cerebral blood flow in normotensive and hypertensive rats. *Am. J. Med.* 1984;76:79–85.
129. Kobayashi S, Yamaguchi S, Okada K, Suyama N, Bokura K, Murao M. The effect of enalapril maleate on cerebral blood flow in chronic cerebral infarction. *Angiology* 1992;43:378–88.
130. Paulson OB, Jarden JO, Godtfredsen J, Vorstrup S. Cerebral blood flow in patients with congestive heart failure treated with captopril. *Am. J. Med.* 1984;76:91–95.
131. Rajagopalan B, Raine AE, Cooper R, Ledingham JG. Changes in cerebral blood flow in patients with severe congestive cardiac failure before and after captopril treatment. *Am. J. Med.* 1984;76:86–90.
132. Paulson OB, Waldemar G, Andersen AR, et al. Role of angiotensin in autoregulation of cerebral blood flow. *Circulation* 1988;77:I55–I58.
133. Schmidt J, Andersen AR, Paulson OB, Gjerris F. Angiotensin converting enzyme inhibition, CBF autoregulation, and ICP in patients with normal-pressure hydrocephalus. *Acta Neurochir.* 1990;106:9–12.
134. Fale A, Kirsch JR, McPherson RW. Alpha 2-adrenergic agonist effects on normocapnic and hypercapnic cerebral blood flow in the dog are anesthetic dependent. *Anesth. Analg.* 1994;79:892–898.
135. McPherson RW, Koehler RC, Traystman RJ. Hypoxia, alpha 2-adrenergic, and nitric oxide-dependent interactions on canine cerebral blood flow. *Am. J. Physiol.* 1994;266:H476–H482.
136. Greene CS, Gretler DD, Cervenka K, McCoy CE, Brown FD, Murphy MB. Cerebral blood flow during the acute therapy of severe hypertension with oral clonidine. *Am. J. Emerg. Med.* 1990;8:293–296.
137. Bertel O, Conen D, Radu EW, Muller J, Lang C, Dubach UC. Nifedipine in hypertensive emergencies. *BMJ* 1983;286:19–21.
138. Bertel O, Marx BE, Conen D. Effects of antihypertensive treatment on cerebral perfusion. *Am. J. Med.* 1987;82:29–36.
139. Davies DS, Wing AM, Reid JL, Neill DM, Tippett P, Dollery CT. Pharmacokinetics and concentration-effect relationships of intervenous and oral clonidine. *Clin. Pharmacol. Ther.* 1977;21:593–601.
140. Olsen RW. GABA-benzodiazepine-barbiturate receptor interactions. *J. Neurochem.* 1981;37:1–13.
141. Pierce E, Lambertsen JG. Cerebral circulation and metabolism during thiopental anesthesia and hyperventilation in man. *J. Clin. Invest.* 1962;41:1664–1671.
142. Wechsler R, Dripps RD, SS K. Blood flow and oxygen consumption of the human brain during anesthesia produced by thiopental. *Anesthesiology* 1951;12:308–314.
143. Donegan JH, Traystman RJ, Koehler RC, Jones MD Jr, Rogers MC. Cerebrovascular hypoxic and autoregulatory responses during reduced brain metabolism. *Am. J. Physiol.* 1985;249:H421–H429.
144. Eckstein J, Hamilton WK. The effect of thiopental on peripheral venous tone. *Anesthesiology* 1961;22:525–528.
145. Cavero I, Thirty C, Pratz J, Lawson K. Cardiovascular characterization of DA-1 and DA-2 dopamine receptor agonists in anesthetized rats. *Clin. Exp. Hypertens.* 1987;9:931–952.
146. Raichle ME, Hartman BK, Eichling JO, Sharpe LG. Central noradrenergic regulation of cerebral blood flow and vascular permeability. *Proc. Natl. Acad. Sci. USA* 1975;72:3726–3730.
147. Toda N. Alpha adrenergic receptor subtypes in human, monkey and dog cerebral arteries. *J. Pharmacol. Exp. Ther.* 1983;226:861–868.
148. Jover BF, McGrath BP. Beneficial effects of fenoldopam on systemic and regional hemodynamics in rabbits with congestive heart failure. *J. Cardiovasc. Pharmacol.* 1988;11:483–488.
149. Prielipp RC, Wall MH, Groban L, et al. Reduced regional and global cerebral blood flow during fenoldopam- induced hypotension in volunteers. *Anesth. Analg.* 2001;93:45–52.
150. McPherson RW, Koehler RC, Kirsch JR, Traystman RJ. Intraventricular dexmedetomidine decreases cerebral blood flow during normoxia and hypoxia in dogs. *Anesth. Analg.* 1997;84:139–147.
151. Zornow MH, Fleischer JE, Scheller MS, Nakakimura K, Drummond JC. Dexmedetomidine, an alpha 2-adrenergic agonist, decreases cerebral blood flow in the isoflurane-anesthetized dog. *Anesth. Analg.* 1990;70:624–630.
152. Post JBt, Frishman WH. Fenoldopam: a new dopamine agonist for the treatment of hypertensive urgencies and emergencies. *J. Clin. Pharmacol.* 1998;38:2–13.
153. Fenoldopam—a new drug for parenteral treatment of severe hypertension. *Med. Lett. Drugs Ther.* 1998;40:57–58.
154. Panacek EA, Bednarczyk EM, Dunbar LM, Foulke GE, Holcslaw TL. Randomized, prospective trial of fenoldopam vs sodium nitroprusside in the treatment of acute severe hypertension. Fenoldopam Study Group. *Acad. Emerg. Med.* 1995;2:959–965.
155. Mathur V, Ellis D, Fellmann J. Therapeutics for hypertensive urgencies and emergencies: Fenoldopam: a novel systemic and renal vasodilator. *CVR&R* 1998:43.
156. Ishikawa T, Funatsu N, Okamoto K, Takeshita H, McDowall DG. Cerebral and systemic effects of hypotension induced by trimetaphan or nitroprusside in dogs. *Acta Anaesthesiol. Scand.* 1982;26:643–648.
157. Fahmy N. Nitroprusside versus nitroprusside-trimethaphan mixture. *Br. J. Anaesth.* 1983;55:381–389.
158. Sollevi A, Ostergren J, Fagrell B, Hjemdahl P. Theophylline antagonizes cardiovascular responses to dipyridamole in man without affecting increases in plasma adenosine. *Acta. Physiol. Scand.* 1984;121:165–171.

159. Eintrei C, Carlsson C. Effects of hypotension induced by adenosine on brain surface oxygen pressure and cortical cerebral blood flow in the pig. *Acta Physiol. Scand.* 1986;126:463–469.

160. Owall A, Gordon E, Lagerkranser M, Lindquist C, Rudehill A, Sollevi A. Clinical experience with adenosine for controlled hypotension during cerebral aneurysm surgery. *Anesth. Analg.* 1987;66:229–234.

161. Sollevi A, Ostergren J, Hjemdahl P, Fredholm BB, Fagrell B. The effect of dipyridamole on plasma adenosine levels and skin micro-circulation in man. *Adv. Exp. Med. Biol.* 1984;165:547.

162. Sollevi A, Lagerkranser M, Andreen M, Irestedt L. Relationship between arterial and venous adenosine levels and vasodilatation during ATP- and adenosine-infusion in dogs. *Acta Physiol. Scand.* 1984;120:171–176.

163. Morris PJ, Todd M, Philbin D. Changes in canine intracranial pressure in response to infusions of sodium nitroprusside and trinitroglycerin. *Br. J. Anaesth.* 1982;54:991–995.

164. Rogers MC, Hamburger C, Owen K, Epstein MH. Intracranial pressure in the cat during nitroglycerin-induced hypotension. *Anesthesiology* 1979;51:227–229.

14

Nutrition and Diet Therapy in the Neurosciences Critical Care Unit

Nancy A. Newman

INTRODUCTION

Nutritional status reflects the extent to which the individual's physiologic needs are met. There needs to be a balance between nutrient intake and nutrient requirements. Nutrition is a significant issue in the source and control of several major clinical outcomes resulting in death or disabilities. Malnutrition is a common accompaniment to the stress of illness among hospitalized patients which contributes to mortality and morbidity. When recognized it is reversible, although it is often not identified. The incidence of untreated malnutrition in hospitalized patients was described more than 25 years ago. Since then, others have reported the occurrence of malnutrition in this patient population with varying degree depending on the circumstances and computations used (1–6).

Nutrient intake is affected by various factors, including cultural, economic, emotional, religious preferences, eating mannerisms and attitudes, disease conditions, appetite, ability to eat, and ability to absorb adequate nutrients. Ideally, nutrient intake will be balanced with nutrient requirements. These needs are affected by factors including stresses, infectious diseases, trauma, fever, expected growth and development, pregnancy, various degrees of strain and activities (1,3,6).

When sufficient nutrients are taken to support physiologic needs along with those needed for increased metabolic requirements then the ideal nutritional state is attained. Adequate growth and development, good health, activities of daily living, and protection from illness or disease are also achieved with this optimal nutritional state.

SCREENING

Patients admitted to a hospital today are generally more acutely ill than in previous years. Evaluating nutrition status by means of screening should be performed routinely on all hospitalized individuals to identify patients who would most benefit from nutrition intervention or assessment. The type of evaluation will differ depending on a basic assessment for the healthy and a more in-depth evaluation for those acutely, critically or chronically ill (6,7).

The screening can be completed by a dietitian, technician, nurse, physician, or qualified health care individual. The significant other can assist in providing needed information for the screening process (8,9). Frequently, in the neurosciences critical care unit (NSU), it is the nurse who completes an initial screening process to identify the individuals who may be at nutritional risk. The individual identified is referred to Nutrition Services for further evaluation and assessment. The screening questions are simple, quick, and complete. The data obtained relies on information that is gathered on a routine basis. The most common nutrition screening questions used in the NSU are listed in Table 1 (8,10).

From: *Current Clinical Neurology*
Critical Care Neurology and Neurosurgery
Edited by: J. I. Suarez © Humana Press Inc., Totowa, NJ

Table 1
Nutrition Screenings

	Yes	No
Are any of these factors placing Pt at nutritional risk—multiple food allergies, dysphagia, cystic fibrosis with wt loss, or FTT		
Pt is pregnant or lactating		
Pt > 80 yr old and admitted for surgical procedure		
Pt has pressure ulcer (s)		
Pt new to therapeutic diet needs and/or requests education (i.e., newly diagnosed diabetes mellitus, renal failure)		
Pt receiving tube feeding/TPN		
Pt has been NPO or on clear liquids > 5 d		
Pt has had unintentional WT loss > 10 lbs in the past month		
Does the patient meet criteria for a nutrition consult		

TPN, Total parenteral nutrition; NPO, nothing by mouth; FTT, failure to thrive; wt, weight; Pt, patient.

NUTRITION ASSESSMENT

After the patient has been identified through the screening process, a comprehensive evaluation is performed. This evaluation is a nutrition assessment. Nutrition assessment is defined by the American Dietetic Association (Council on Practice, 1994) as a comprehensive approach completed by a registered dietitian for defining nutrition status using medical, social, nutritional and medication histories, physical examination, anthropometric measures, and laboratory data. Nutrition assessment involves an accurate evaluation of the degree of malnutrition and should rely on the expertise of a dietitian trained to use the techniques of the anthropometrics, biochemical and global assessment information *(4,11–14)*.

In the hospital many types of malnutrition may occur. A patient may display protein malnutrition (kwashiorkor), protein-calorie malnutrition (marasmus) or a combination of the above (kwashiorkor-marasmus) (Table 2) *(3,5)*. For guideline standards of clinical nutrition care used to evaluate patients, refer to the Appendix section in this book. This information is used as a basis in evaluating the adult medical and/or surgical individual in the general hospital setting and adapted to the intensive care areas including the NSU.

Nitrogen Balance

Nitrogen balance is used as an index of protein status. It determines the amount of nitrogen required to maintain nitrogen equilibrium by assessing urinary nitrogen losses. It determines the severity of protein catabolism and adequacy of an individual nutritional regimen. A positive nitrogen balance indicates nitrogen retention resulting from growth, pregnancy, athletic training and recovery from illness. Negative nitrogen balance indicates nitrogen loss, which may be a result of inadequate quantity or quality of protein intake, inadequate kilocalorie intake, or accelerated protein catabolism. A zero nitrogen balance indicates nitrogen equilibrium. The goal of nutrition therapy is a positive balance of 4 g of nitrogen per day.

Nitrogen balance is the difference between nitrogen intake and output and is computed for clinical purposes as follows.

Table 2
Types of Malnutrition

Type of malnutrition	General appearance	Nutrient deficiency	Occurrence	Visceral protein	Somatic protein	Adipose tissue	Respiratory quotient	Blood chemistry albumin g/L (g/dL)	Prealbumin g/L (g/dL)	Total protein g/L (g/dL)	Glucose monal/L (mg/dL)	Insulin	Immuno-compromised
Kwashiorkor	Corporal edema	Protein	Rapid	↓	OK	OK	0.8–0.85	<28 (<2.8)	<0.1 (<10)	<55 (<5.5)	>7.8 (>140)	High	↓
Marasmus	Cachectic	Protein and calories	Chronic	OK	↓	↓	0.6–0.7	≥35 (≥3.5)	≥0.157 (≥15.7)	≥66 (≥6.6)	4.4–6.7 (80–120)	Normal	↓
Kwashiorkor-Marasmus		Protein and calories	Superimpose on protein/calories	↓	↓	↓							↓

$$\frac{\text{Nitrogen}}{\text{balance}} = \left(\frac{\text{protein intake in 24 h}}{6.25}\right) - \left(\frac{\text{urinary urea} + 2 \text{ g} + 0.02 \text{ g per kg body weight}}{\text{nitrogen in 24 h}}\right)$$

In the formula, nitrogen intake is calculated by dividing protein intake for a 24-h period (enteral and parenteral) by the factor 6.25, which represents the percent of nitrogen in protein. Because approximately 90% of the daily nitrogen output is excreted as urea, nitrogen output is estimated from urinary urea nitrogen for the same 24-h period. To this number a constant urinary nonurea nitrogen loss of 2 g is added. Fecal and integumental losses of skin, hair, and nails are represented by adding 0.02 g of nitrogen per kg of body weight or total of approx 4 g is added. Nitrogen balance calculated by this method is subject to errors in data collection. Calculations underestimate nitrogen excretion for patients with burns, diarrhea, vomiting, fistula drainage, hemorrhage, upper gastrointestinal losses, and other nitrogen losses. All considerably negate the nitrogen balance. Nitrogen balance needs accurate collections. Nitrogen balance is invalid in patients with renal disease.

Nitrogen balance is a valuable means to evaluate whether anabolism has been achieved with nutrition therapy. It is most useful for patients with whom nutrition assessment has been difficult. It should be measured after a feeding regimen has been established and in conjunction with other means of evaluation to assess the adequacy of the nutrition support. Although a positive balance of 2–4 g of nitrogen per day is desirable for the anabolic state, a more manageable goal for the critically ill patient is to have minimal nitrogen loss. Once the stress state is resolved, a positive nitrogen equilibrium may be realized *(6,15–17)*.

Vitamins/Minerals

Adequate intake of vitamins and minerals is necessary. The recommended dietary allowances (RDA) and dietary reference intake (DRI) provide the guidelines. An individual may need supplementation depending on nutritional status on admission, diagnosis, medical history, course of therapy, nutrient delivery during hospitalization, and nutrient intake.

Subjective Global Assessment

In contrast to the anthropometic and biochemical appraisals used for nutritional assessment, there is a screening measure referred to as the Subjective Global Assessment of the nutrition state. It uses a viewing or observation approach that requires good clinical judgment as the information is assembled by interviews. Those originating this technique have developed observation guidelines for health professionals *(18)*.

The Subjective Global Assessment summary includes evaluation of:

1. History
   a. Weight change
   b. Dietary intake change—as it relates to the normal
   c. Any gastrointestinal changes persisting more than 2 wk (including nausea, diarrhea, vomiting, constipation, none)
   d. Any functional changes and for what time
2. Physical examination (e.g., loss of adipose tissue and edema).
3. A Subjective Global Assessment Rating based on overall observation and interview status of well-nourished, moderately malnourished, severely malnourished, or suspected of such a state *(1,6,13,18)*.

Physical Evaluation of Nutritional Status

Physical signs of nutrient deficiencies are often mild, nonspecific, and indistinguishable from non-nutritional problems. The greater the number of signs present which are common to a particular nutrient deficiency, the more likely a true deficiency exists. Findings should be confirmed with anthropometric measurements, dietary history and/or biochemical tests. Physical signs of nutritional deficiencies are listed in Table 3 by area of examination *(1,6,11)*.

Definitions of Protein Status and Adipose Tissue Status

Once the nutrition assessment is completed (*see* Appendix), a nutrition care plan can be produced and activated. Thereafter, it will be fine-tuned according to the patient's needs as outlined below *(14,19–21)*.

Visceral Proteins

Visceral proteins are made up of circulating serum proteins and proteins found in organs. Proteins used to assess nutritional status include albumin, transferrin, prealbumin, and retinol binding protein. Measurements of visceral protein status are used as an index of protein energy malnutrition. Non-nutritive factors can influence the concentration of these proteins including stress, sepsis, hydration status, pregnancy, medications, and reduced protein synthesis due to disease state.

Albumin

Albumin is a useful indicator of protein synthesis. It can determine the severity of malnutrition indicated by degree of depletion of secretory proteins:

Normal	3.5–5.0 g/dL
Mild depletion	2.8–3.4 g/dL
Moderate depletion	2.1–2.7 g/dL
Severe depletion	< 2.1 g/dL

Transferrin

Transferrin is a slightly more sensitive indicator of visceral protein status because of its shorter half life. Serum concentrations can also be used to guide nutritional assessment:

Normal	200–400 mg/dL
Mild depletion:	150–200 mg/dL
Moderate depletion	100–150 mg/dL
Severe depletion	< 100 mg/dL

Prealbumin

Prealbumin is a much more sensitive indicator of protein status with a serum half-life of only 2–3 d. Its synthesis is highly sensitive to the stress of injury and acute infection, and it is one of the first metabolic variables to register increased demands for protein synthesis during stress. Serum prealbumin monitoring can help follow adequacy of nutrition recovery:

Normal	7–22 mg/dL	Age birth to 11 yr
	12–30 mg/dL	Age 12–20 yr
	19–38 mg/dL	Age 21–64 yr
	11–29 mg/dL	Age > 65 yr
Degree of depletion		
Mild depletion	10–15 mg/dL	
Moderate depletion	5–10 mg/dL	
Severe depletion	< 5 mg/dL	

Somatic Proteins

Somatic proteins are skeletal muscle proteins, which can be assessed using different markers such as creatinine-height index (CHI), tricep skin fold (TSF), mid-arm muscle circumference (MAMC), and weight loss. The latter, over time, is useful to assess somatic protein status. Weight loss can be classified as mild, moderate, or severe. Mild percentage of weight loss is (less than) 1% weight decrease in 1 wk; 2% in 1 mo; 5% in 3 mo and 7.5% in 6 mo. Moderate percentage of weight loss is

Table 3
Physical Signs of Nutrient Deficiency

Area and normal appearance	Signs associated with malnutrition	Possible nutrient deficiency or disorder
Face Uniform skin color no swelling overall healthy appearance	Nasolabial seborrhea	Riboflavin Kwashiorkor
Glands Normal size	Thyroid enlarged Parotid enlarged	Iodine Protein (starvation and bulimia)
Gums Healthy pink-red do not bleed not swollen	Red-purple color, spongy; bleeds easily	Vitamin C
Hair Shiny, firm, not easily plucked	Lackluster, thin, easily plucked in clumps, bands of pigmentation	Protein (Kwashiorkor) protein-Kcalories (Marasmus)—less commonly
Lips Smooth not chapped or swollen	Angular stomatitis/cheilosis White or pink lesions at corners of mouth; cheilosis	Riboflavin, niacin, iron, pyridoxine Riboflavin, niacin
Muscular, skeletal systems	Muscle wasting	Protein, kilocalories
Nails Firm, pink, smooth	Brittle, lack luster, longitutional ridges, growth bands Koilonychias	Protein, kilocalories Iron
Nervous system Psychological stability; normal reflexes	Burning and tingling of hands and feet (paresthesia); motor weakness, psychomatic changes, mental confusion, sensory loss, loss of positional sense, loss of vibration, loss of ankle and knee jerks, dementia	Kwashiorkor, thiamine, niacin, vitamin B_{12}

(continued on next page)

272

Body area / Finding	Associated nutrient
Skin	
Smooth, even color	
Xerosis	Vitamin A, essential fatty acids
Follicular hyperkeratosis	Vitamin A, essential fatty acids
Easily bruised skin	Vitamin C
	Vitamin K
Pellagrous dermatosis of skin exposed to sunlight	Niacin, tryptophan
Poor wound healing, pressure ulcers	Protein, vitamin C, zinc
Delayed wound healing, acneform rash, skin lesions, hair loss	Zinc
Nasolabial seborrhea	Riboflavin
Hyperpigmentation of hands and face	Riboflavin, niacin, pyridoxine
Red, swollen skin lesions	Niacin
Orange cast	Excess carotene
Subcutaneous	
Tissue	
Bilateral pitting edema beginning with ankles and feet	Thiamine, protein
Teeth	
Bright no cavities no pain	Fluorine
Caries	Excess sucrose
Mottled enamel (white or brown spots)	Excess fluorine during tooth development
Caries (cavities) missing teeth	Excessive sugar intake
Tongue	
Deep red in appearance; not swollen or smooth	Water
Swollen	Niacin, riboflavin, pyridoxine, B_{12}, folate, iron, tryptophan
Glossitis	Riboflavin
Magenta filiform papillary atrophy	Piacin, riboflavin, vitamin B_{12}, folate, iron
Fungiform papillary	Protein, kilocalories
Hypertrophy	Zinc
Taste impairment	

1–2% in 1 wk; 5% in 1 mo; 7.5% in 3 mo, and 10% in 6 mo. Severe percentage of weight loss is (greater than) 3% in 1 wk; 6% in 1 mo; 8% in 3 mo; and 11% in 6 mo.

Adipose Tissue

Adipose tissue is connective tissue that contains masses of fat cells. Weight as a percentage of ideal body weight (IBW), is a classification for degree of nutritional depletion as follows:

Normal	90–100% IBW
Mild depletion	80–90% IBW
Moderate depletion	70–80% IBW
Severe depletion	<70% IBW
Overweight	>120% = overweight
	>150% = obese
	>200% = morbidly obese

Indirect Calorimetry

Indirect calorimetry is used for individuals who have medical conditions, which make established equations difficult to use to estimate energy needs. Carbon dioxide is produced in proportion to metabolic rate, which is used to compute the resting energy expenditure (REE). The metabolic cart measures oxygen intake and carbon dioxide formation for this computation. Both spontaneous breathing and ventilator-dependent patients can be evaluated using indirect calorimetry in a minimal amount of time. This method measures REE, which comprises basal energy expenditure (BEE), and the metabolic demands of the awakened state, stress, diseased state, thermal dynamic action of food and/or trauma. To allow for physical activity, the REE is multiplied by a 1.0–1.3 activity factor to calculate total energy expenditure (TEE).

Oxidation of each nutrient group develops at a known respiratory quotient (RQ) level. The RQ is the ratio of carbon dioxide expired to the amount of oxygen inspired or $RQ = VCO_2/O_2$. The respiratory quotient can be ascertained from indirect calorimetry to assess nutrient use and applied to modify the patient's nutrition support. The RQ is based on the assumption that all energy comes from the oxidation of carbohydrate, protein and fat. The amount of oxygen absorbed and the carbon dioxide generated are representative and unchanging for each fuel source. The RQ for fat is 0.70; carbohydrate (glucose) oxidation is 0.95–1.00; protein oxidation is 0.80–0.82; a mixed diet oxidation is 0.85; ketosis is less than 0.60. A mixed diet with a respiratory quotient (RQ) of 0.85 is an optimal goal. RQ greater than 1.0 can result when carbohydrate (glucose) intake or total caloric intake is excessive. Usually, in this situation total calories should be decreased. If the RQ is equal to 1.0, it is recommended to decrease carbohydrate and increase lipids (fat). If the RQ is less than 0.82, total energy may need to be increased.

Certain factors during indirect calorimetry measurements need to be considered to make it a reliable evaluation: (1) the patient should be awake, at rest, and in a supine position; (2) patients who are eating should have measurements evaluated 2 h after a meal; (3) nutrition support should not be interrupted during the measurement; (4) individuals having strenuous activity such as physical therapy or dressing changes need measurements obtained at least 1 h following such an activity; (5) measurements should be obtained when vital signs and ventilator settings are stable; (6) indirect calorimetry has a propensity to be inaccurate when the oxygen setting on the ventilator is greater than 50%; (7) indirect calorimetry is not of value with incomplete collection of expired air or if only parts of inspired oxygen are obtained *(19,22–24)*.

Type of Nutrition Support

Various neurologic disabilities can affect the autonomic nervous system, hypothalmus, pituitary and brainstem. These disorders can affect appetite, basal energy expense, digestion and normal stability. Nutritional disorders include cachexia, reduced energy demands as with para or quadriplegia and increased metabolism as with traumatic brain injury (TBI). All these factors can impact on the desired method of nutrition support.

Enteral Feedings

For oral feedings, consider the patient's present diagnosis, medical history and need for modification of consistency of foods based on chewing and swallowing abilities. Nutrition support may need to be considered as a short-term or long-term treatment to avoid inadequate nutrition with the neurologic impaired individual. The gastrointestinal tract (GI) is the preferred route of nutritional support with total parenteral nutrition used if the GI tract is nonfunctional. Use of the enteral route decreases the occurrence of bacterial translocation, improves gut mucosa integrity and enzymatic activity, and improves overall nutrition status when compared to parenteral nutrition. In Fig. 1, we present an algorithm to help with decision-making regarding type of nutrition support to be initiated (4,6,25–29). Many patients cared for in the NSU receive feeding via a tube. For tube feedings, a variety of formulas may be offered (*see* Appendix for a comparison of formulas). It is also crucial that before considering a type of tube feeding, a review of indications, clinical settings when enteral support may be helpful, and contraindications to enteral nutrition is warranted as presented below (28,30–32).

INDICATIONS FOR ENTERAL NUTRITION SUPPORT

- Functional GI tract when the nutrient intake is insufficient (<80%) in meeting needs
- Protein-calorie malnutrition (PCM) with inadequate oral intake for previous 72 h and not expected to progress within the foreseeable future
- Severe dysphagia
- Low output enterocutaneous fistula (<500 mL enteric effluent per day)
- Malnourished patient with acquired immunodeficiency syndrome

CLINICAL SETTINGS WHEN ENTERAL NUTRITION SUPPORT MAY BE HELPFUL

- Postoperative major surgery
- Organ transplantation with anticipated NPO status > 4 d
- Mechanical ventilation
- Short-bowel syndrome with a minimum of 100 cm small bowel and 150 cm ileal length
- Mild pancreatitis
- Esophageal obstruction
- Radiation therapy
- Neoplasms
- Psychiatric diseases resulting in poor oral intake
- Cardiac cachexia
- Multisystem organ failure
- Hepatic failure

CONTRAINDICATIONS TO ENTERAL NUTRITION SUPPORT

- Complete mechanical bowel obstruction
- Insufficient absorptive capacity of bowel
- Ileus or severe intestinal hypomotility
- High output enterocutaneous fistula (> 500 mL enteric effluent)
- Severe acute pancreatitis
- Intolerance to enteral feedings as demonstrated by high residuals, abdominal distension, or ileus

- Severe GI hemorrhage
- Intractable vomiting
- Severe enterocolitis
- Patient prognosis does not warrant aggressive nutritional support
- Where nutrition support is not desired by the patient or legal guardian and is in accordance with individual institution policy and specific state law

BASIC PRINCIPLES TO CONSIDER WHEN PROVIDING MEDICATIONS
TO PATIENTS RECEIVING ENTERAL SUPPORT

- If the patient is able to take medications orally, this is the preferred route
- Liquid medications are the preferred dosage form
- Avoid crushing medications, unless otherwise approved by manufacturer
- Flush the feeding tube with 30 mL water before and after administration of medication
- When several medications are to be administered concurrently, all medications should be delivered separately, and the tube flushed with at least 5 mL water after each dose
- Do not add medications directly to the feeding formula
- Hold tube feedings when giving medications—**this is especially important for phenytoin**.
- Drugs and enteral feeding: one important point to remember is that propofol, a very commonly used sedative in the NSU, is a 1.1 Kcal/mL lipid formulation (10% lipid). Therefore, nutritional requirements need to be adjusted accordingly. Always consult the pharmacist for any questions concerning compatibility of drugs and enteral feeding.

Occasionally a patient may have a problem tolerating the enteral feedings. In Table 4, we present recommendations to help assist you in resolving the patient's problem (30–33).

SELECTION OF ENTERAL FEEDING PRODUCTS

Appropriate selection of an enteral feeding product is important (*see* Appendix). The enteral products are generally classified as follows.

Intact Protein/Lactose Free: These should be used for patients with normal GI function subjected to minimal metabolic stress or injury. They are suitable for minor medical or surgical illnesses and may include fiber-containing formulas.

Intact Protein/Lactose Free/High Caloric Density: These should be used for patients with normal GI function, but who require fluid or volume restriction and who are subjected to minimal metabolic stress or injury. They are suitable for minor medical or surgical illnesses. They are also suitable for patients with normal GI function, but who are subjected to moderate to severe metabolic stress or medical or surgical wound healing needs.

Peptide ("Semielemental" Diet): These should be used for patients with moderate to severely altered GI function and minimal to moderate metabolic stress or injury including low output enterocutaneous fistula, AIDS, malabsorption syndrome, irritable bowel syndrome (IBD), short-gut and mild pancreatitis.

Free Amino Acid (Elemental Diet): These are indicated for patients with moderate to severely altered GI function, and in conditions of moderate to severe metabolic stress.

Intact Protein/Lactose Free/High Caloric Density/Low Electrolyte: These are usually indicated for dialysis patients to provide high-calorie, high-protein feedings in fluid restricted situation with appropriate electrolyte administration.

Intact Protein/Lactose Free/High Fat/Low Carbohydrate/Calorie Dense: These are indicated for patients with significant respiratory and pulmonary conditions with increased CO_2 retention or production.

Total Parenteral Nutrition

Although a significant percentage of patients receive a tube feeding for short or long time, total parenteral nutrition (TPN) may be provided for individuals who are not candidates for enteral feedings (Fig. 1). We present below the most frequent indications, complications, and administration guidelines for TPN/lipids.

Table 4
Managing Enteral Feeding Complications

Mechanical complications	Treatment
High gastric residuals (>150 mL)	a) Hold tube feedings for 1 h and recheck residuals b) R/O mechanical intestinal obstruction or ileus c) Use continuous feedings d) Position the tube distal to the ligament of Treitz e) Consider prokinetic medication (e.g., metoclopramide)
Acute otitis media	a) Use small bore (>10 F) feeding tube b) Consider gastrostomy or jejunostomy feedings
Acute sinusitis	a) Use other nostril for tube placement b) Consider gastrostomy or jejunostomy feedings
Feeding tube obstruction	a) Flush tube with water bolus (~20–30 mL) before and after administration of each medication and after TF is interrupted b) Flush tube with 20–30 mL water every 4 h for continuous feeding or before and after intermittent/bolus feedings c) Use liquid elixirs when possible. Consult pharmacy regarding crushed or diluted medications due to potential alerted drug effects d) Never reinsert stylet to unclog feeding tubes
GI complications/complaints Nausea and vomiting (May be due to gastroparesis, postoperative state, postvagotomy syndrome, medications, nutrient malabsorption, intolerance, or mechanical problems)	a) Administer formula at room temperature b) Administer formula via continuous infusion at a low rate and slowly increase c) Consider a hydrolyzed formula
Abdominal distention, bloating, cramping and gas (Maybe because of rapid bolus or intermittent infusion of cold formula, rapid infusion via syringe, or nutrient malabsorption)	a) Consider prokinetic medication b) Initiate tube feedings at a low rate (20 mL/h) and increase slowly c) Consider postpyloric method of feeding
Constipation (May be from dehydration, inadequate fiber intake, inadequate physical activity, or medications)	a) Assess fluid status and supplement if needed b) Use fiber-containing formulas c) Increase ambulation, if allowed d) Review medications
Diarrhea (related to feedings)	a) Use fiber-containing formula and isotonic formula b) For bolus feedings, reduce rate to < 30 mL/min c) Advance tube feeding rate slowly, by 10–25 mL every 8–24 h d) Consider lower fat formulas if malabsorption is present e) Administer formula at room temperature
Other complications Aspiration pneumonia	a) Verify tube placement radiographically b) Use small bore tube (10 Fr) to reduce aspiration risk from compromise of the lower esophageal sphincter c) Feed with HOB elevated (at least 30 degrees) and keep patient upright for at least 1–2 h after bolus feedings d) Whenever possible use postpyloric feedings

R/O, rule out; GI, gastrointestinal; HOB, head of bed.

INDICATIONS FOR TOTAL PARENTERAL NUTRITION

These include patients who are unable to tolerate enteral feedings. Other indications are patients in whom no oral feedings (NPO) are expected for 5 or more d; severe malabsorption with malnutrition; GI obstruction or ileus for 5 or more d; moderate or severe acute pancreatitis with pain; severely catabolic patients with or without malnutrition when the gastrointestinal tract is not useable (or anticipated to be unusable) within 5–7 d. There are other clinical settings where TPN may also be helpful including: moderate to severe stress such as trauma or major surgery when enteral intake is not expected to be resumed within 7–10 d, enterocutaneous fistula, inflammatory bowel disease, and hyperemesis gravidarum when nausea and vomiting persist less than 7–10 d. A minority of patients will require peripheral parenteral nutrition (PPN) especially those who need short-term (< 7 d) parenteral nutrition and those situations where central access for nutrition support is not available.

TPN ADMINISTRATION

TPN may be given continuously over 24 h (appropriate for most hospitalized patients) or on a cycled schedule *(30–32)*. We present below some recommendations regarding handling of TPN in NSU patients.

Initiating TPN: The following guidelines can be followed when instituting TPN.

- Continuous—dextrose concentrations greater than 10% should be infused at one half the final rate for 12 h, then increased to final rate
- Cycled—TPN should be infused over 12–18 h overnight. When starting, begin at 50 mL per hour for 30 min, increase to 110 mL/h (or final rate if < 100 mL/h) for 30 min, then increase to the final rate (if greater)
- Fat emulsions should be infused on the same schedule as the dextrose solution, but do not need to be tapered

Stopping TPN: Once the decision has been made to discontinue TPN, the following recommendations are useful to avoid complications.

- Reverse the taper schedule
- Monitor for hypoglycemia
- If TPN needs to be stopped immediately, provide 10% dextrose solution and then taper gradually.

Monitoring: Throughout the time of TPN administration there are several parameters that need to be followed very carefully as follows.

- Initially: Chem 23, prealbumin, complete blood cell (CBC) count
- Daily: weight, intake and output
- Twice weekly: Chem 10
- Weekly: Chem 16, CBC count prealbumin

FAT EMULSION

Additional calories and essential fatty acids can be provided with 10% lipids—1.1 Kcal/mL or 20% lipids—2.0 Kcal/mL. The choice of 10% vs 20% fat emulsion depends on the patient's total fluid needs. Ten percent fat emulsion will require roughly twice as much fluid volume as 20% fat emulsion for the same number of calories *(30–32)*.

COMPLICATIONS OF TOTAL PARENTERAL NUTRITION

The major complications of TPN generally relate to catheter infections or electrolyte/metabolic disturbances (Tables 5 and 6). However, other clinically important adverse effects of TPN that need to be considered are deficiency states and liver function abnormalities *(30,32)*. Patients on long-term total parenteral nutrition are at risk for deficiencies of vitamins, minerals, and fatty acids. TPN orders should include lipids and be supplemented with vitamins and minerals. Abnormalities of the liver occur frequently in patients on TPN. The cause is unclear and probably multifactorial. TPN-associated liver abnormalities can be minimized by not over feeding especially with glucose and by cycling

Algorithm Used to Determine Type of Nutrition Support

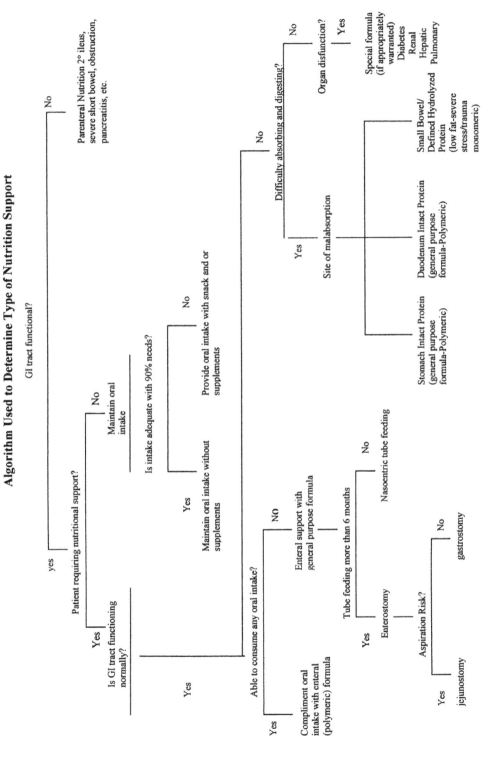

Fig. 1. Algorithm to help with decision making regarding type of nutrition support to be initiated.

Table 5
Catheter Sepsis Associated With Total Parenteral Nutrition

Incidence	3–5% of single lumen catheters	
	15% of triple lumen catheters	
Diagnosis	Sudden unexplained hyperglycemia	
	Fever > 38°C for several hours	
	WBC > 10,000	
	Positive blood culture results	
	Catheter site induration, erythema, or purulence	
Treatment	If blood culture result negative and no signs of sepsis:	If blood culture result positive and/or patient unstable:
	1. Culture per catheter and peripherally	
	2. Change catheter over a wire; culture tip	1. Antibiotics
	3. Monitor patient	2. Consider pulling catheter
		3. Culture again per catheter, catheter tip, and peripherally

Table 6
Metabolic Complications Associated With Total Parenteral Nutrition and Recommendations to Remedy Them

Hyperglycemia (< 160 mg/dL)	Add regular insulin to the TPN in 10-unit increments until glucose < 160 mg/dL; maximum allowable insulin dose per liter of TPN is 40 U (Note: 1 U of regular insulin results in an approx 10 mg/dL decrease in serum glucose)
Hypoglycemia (< 70 mg/dL)	Often occurs when TPN is discontinued suddenly; begin $D_{10}NS$ at previous TPN infusion rate and taper off over 4 h
Hypernatremia (> 145 mEq/L)	Determine the etioliogy of hypernatremia: If from dehydration, add "free water" to the TPN and provide only maintenance sodium (90–40 mEq/L) per TPN If from increased sodium intake, delete sodium from TPN (and all other IV fluids) until serum sodium is < 145 mEq/L
Hyponatremia (< 130 mEq/L)	Determine the etiology of hyponatremia If from dilution, fluid restrict and provide only maintenance sodium (90–140 mEq/L) per TPN If from inadequate intake then add to TPN formula
Hyperkalemia (> 5.2 mEq/L)	Discontinue current TPN and begin $D_{10}NS$ at previous TPN infusion rate; then delete potassium from all IV fluids and reorder TPN without potassium until serum potassium < 5 mEq/L
Hypokalemia (< 3 mEq/L)	TPN solution should not be used for the primary treatment of hypokalemia
Hyperphosphatemia	Discontinue current phosphate containing TPN; reorder TPN without phosphate until serum phosphate < 4.5 mg/dL
Hypophosphatemia (< 2.5 mg/dL)	Increase phosphate concentration in TPN to maximum of 20 mM/L
Hypermagnesemia (> 2 mg/dL)	Discontinue current magnesium containing TPN; reorder TPN without magnesium until serum magnesium < 2 mg/dL
Hypomagnesemia (< 1 mg/dL)	Increase the magnesium content in TPN to a maximum of 12 mEq/L
Hyperchloremic metabolic acidosis (CO_2 < 25 mM/L and Cell > 110 mEq/L)	Minimize NaCl and maximize Na^+ acetate in TPN

TPN. Daily ursodeoxycholic acid (600–900 mg/d) may decrease cholestatic liver function test abnormalities in patients on long-term TPN *(32–36)*.

Refeeding Syndrome

In moderate to severely malnourished patients, refeeding enterally or parenterally may result in stimulated changes in serum phosphate, magnesium and potassium concentrations. Low serum concentrations of these electrolytes may indicate a refeeding phenomenon. This may occur with excessive or rapid administration of nutrients in a patient who is transitioning from a starvation state to an anabolic state. Possible complications include generalized muscle weakness, tetany, myocardial dysfunction including cardiac dysrhythmia, arrhythmia, seizures, excessive sodium and water retention, pulmonary complications, hemolytic anemia, phagocyte dysfunction and death from cardiac or respiratory failure. For patients at increased risk for refeeding syndrome, it is important to monitor electrolytes (magnesium, phosphorus, potassium) daily and replete as needed to decrease the risk of severe shifts *(6,14,17,26,37)*.

The following recommendations should be followed to avoid refeeding syndrome:

1. Anticipate the problem whenever a "patient at risk" is being fed (weight loss and unexpected to regain it).
2. Initial nutrition goals should not exceed 20–30 Kcal/kg/d or between 800 and 1000 Kcal/d initially. These can be increased to stress requirements of 25–35 Kcal/kg/d and 1.5 g Pro/kg/d over 1–2 wk, as tolerated allowing a minimum of 3 d.
3. Monitor phosphorus, magnesium, and potassium closely, especially during the first week of nutrition support and supplement as needed.
4. Provide supplement of vitamins, especially thiamine.
5. Monitor for fluid overload and congestive heart failure *(6,17)*.

NEUROLOGIC DISORDERS

Special Considerations

Neurologic disorders that fall outside the already provided guideline need consideration and will be discussed below. Early nutrition has been linked to a more rapid neurologic recovery and improved survival in TBI patients. Some clinicians estimate energy requirements based on actual weight. Usually, weight above 125% desirable is adjusted and this adjusted weight is used for calculations. Adjusted weight is defined as the actual weight minus desirable weight. This value is multiplied by 25% and then added to the desirable body weight.

Harris-Benedict Equation in Critical Care

The Harris-Benedict equation is frequently used in critical care to calculate patients' calorie requirements (*see* Appendix). The use of the Harris-Benedict equation without the stress and activity factors is more commonly practiced in critically ill patients in which overfeeding can have significant negative effects.

In the NSU, the Harris-Benedict equation × 1.25–1.3 combined activity and stress factor or 28–30 Kcal/kg/d is frequently used. Variable situations for patients arise and have to be considered. Difficulty weaning, pressure sores, mechanical ventilation, low weight or weight loss, increased weight due to positive fluid status or obesity, depleted protein status, impaired renal function, uncontrolled hyperglycemia need consideration when assessing calorie needs. In the NSU, protein needs are determined depending on the patient's condition with a range of 1.1–2.0 g pro/kg desirable body weight or adjusted weight. Some recommendations are presented in Table 7 *(17,29,34)*.

Sepsis

Patients in whom sepsis develops are frequently nutritionally compromised before the development of significant infection. It is important to provide sufficient nutrition for these individuals if they are going to regain better health. Start with the calculation of calories needed either using The Harris-Benedict equation or estimating that the septic individual needs approx 25–35 Kcal/kg/d. Indirect calorimetry can be useful for caloric determination in complicated individuals. Protein needs

Table 7
Nutrition Support in Critical Illness

Calories	25–30 Kcal/kg or BEE X 1.2–2.0
(adjust to maintain respiratory quotient 0.8–0.9)	
Glucose	4–5 g/kg/d or 60–70% of calories. In NSU
(adjust to maintain respiratory quotient 0.8–0.9)	4 g/kg is preferred to avoid hypoglycemia
Fat	15–40% of calories; averaging 30% calories or 1.0
(adjust to maintain respiratory quotient 0.8–0.9)	g/kg body weight with lipids
Amino acids	1.2–2.0 g/kg/d; in NSU 1.2 g/kg/d is used
(adjust to achieve 2 g positive nitrogen balance)	
Vitamin and trace elements	Recommended dietary allowance
	Dietary reference intake
	Add or omit depending in disease condition
Electrolytes	Maintain normal levels particularly K^+, Mg^{2+}, PO_4^-

Summary of recommendation for energy and substrate in the hypermetabolic patient. Respiratory quotient is given by indirect calorimetry. BEE, basal energy expenditure.

in these patients usually approx 1.2–2.0 g/kg of body weight per day. Hyperglycemia should be avoided by moderating carbohydrate/calories and fat recommendations should be between 15% and 30% of total needs. Some investigators have recommended the administration of so-called immunomodulators such as nucleotides, omega-3 fatty acid, glutamine, and arginine *(6,17,26,29)*.

Traumatic Brain Injury

The metabolic response to severe TBI is quite dramatic. Hypermetabolism may sometimes be as high as 100% above normal and this increase is proportional to the severity of brain injury. Nutrition management involves an assessment of the injured individual's caloric needs. Calculation of calorie needs should reflect the resting energy expenditure, which increases by an average of 40–75% [(1.40–1.75 cal × HB (Harris Benedict)] and remains at this level for 10 d after injury. Calories can be estimated at 35–40 Kcal/kg/d to account for the large increase in metabolic rate. However, in patients with brain death or barbiturate-induced coma, resting energy expenditure may decrease by 24–25% (ranging from 20% to 50%) of the predicted energy expenditure and it should be adjusted accordingly. Protein needs in TBI are estimated to be 1.5–2.0 g/kg/d and could range up to 2.2–2.5 g/kg/d. The calorie to nitrogen ratio in these cases should be approx 100:1. Although the gastrointestinal (GI) tract is the preferred route of nutrient delivery in these patients, it is important to note that alteration in GI function may occur without associated abdominal trauma. Patients with severe TBI can be successfully treated with duodenal or jejunal feedings, as needed *(6,37,38,39)*.

Poly-Trauma

There are multiple methods for assessing energy requirements in poly-trauma patients. Indirect calorimetry remains the "gold standard" with the best accuracy for measuring energy requirements. Taking into consideration all forms and phases of traumatic injury, requirements can generally range from 20 to 35 Kcal/kg/d usual body weight. It is recommended that the ideal or adjusted body weight be used for individuals who are obese to avoid overfeeding. Protein requirements for stressed patients is 20–25% of the total nutrient intake as protein or from 1.5 to 2.0 g/kg/d desirable or adjusted body weight. A higher range needs consideration to promote nitrogen equilibrium or to minimize nitrogen losses *(6,15,29,40,41)*.

Spinal Cord Injury

Patients with spinal cord injury (SCI) have prolonged nitrogen excretion, calcium wasting, major weight loss and a decline in basal metabolic requirements. Initial treatment of these patients is to protect them from further spinal cord damage. This is accomplished by treating spinal cord edema, monitoring fluid and electrolytes, preventing respiratory compromise, and giving general support. Maintenance of nutrition health is an important element in preventing the development of pressure ulcers because poor nutrition has a tendency to lead to infection. SCI patients should receive a fiber-enriched diet of at least 30 g containing whole grain, bran products, leafy greens and raw vegetables and fruits. Estimated daily energy requirements for spinal cord injury individual using actual body weight in the acute phase is recommended. After first month of injury, IBW should be adjusted unless the patient is taking steroids. For the paraplegic patient, IBW is suggested to be 4.5 kg below calculated IBW, and for the quadriplegic, the IBW is suggested to be 9 kg below calculated IBW. Calorie requirements are based on this adjusted body weight. For the paraplegic individual, 28 Kcal/kg is used. The quadriplegic individual requires 23 Kcal/Kg *(6,42,43)*.

Miscellaneous Neurological Diseases

These miscellaneous neurologic disease states include cerebral vascular disease, Parkinson's disease (PD), amyotrophic lateral sclerosis (ALS), multiple sclerosis (MS), dementia, Huntington's disease, and Alzheimer's disease. These patients may suffer from similar problems, such as poor nutrition, dysphagia, loss of mobility, decreased cognitive skills, urinary tract infection and bowel and/or bladder disturbances. Nutritional needs for these individuals range between 22 and 25 Kcal/kg of actual or adjusted body weight and are corrected for ambulation. The protein requirements are approximately 0.8 g/kg. Because of important interactions between diet and medications PD patients require especial attention *(6,39,44–49)*. The PD individual should eat a balanced diet with protein of 0.8 g/kg/d and a 5:1 carbohydrate to protein ratio in all meals. The low-protein diet can enhance the effect of levodopa therapy. Protein in the diet should be redistributed to reduce or eliminate the intake during the daytime *(6,46)*.

Neuromuscular Dysfunction

Neuromuscular dysfunctions include Guillain-Barré syndrome (GBS) and myasthenia gravis (MG). For GBS, energy needs should be assessed by indirect calorimetry or 40–45 nonprotein Kcal/kg. Protein needs range from 2.0 to 2.5 g/kg and can be assessed by 24-h urine urea nitrogen or needs. Chewing and swallowing are often compromised and enteral feedings are needed *(6)*.

CONCLUSION

Nutrition is an important component of overall patient care. Adequate nutrition may improve outcome and possibly shorten length of stay. Many patients are admitted to the NSU in good nutritional status. However, most are at nutritional risk due to their dependence on an alternative means of nutrition because of a neurologic incident. An evaluation by a dietitian and continuous monitoring by the entire medical team regarding adequacy of nutrition support is imperative. The goal of nutrition therapy is to prevent the onset of nutritional depletion or correct it before it reaches significance.

ACKNOWLEDGMENTS

I would like to thank my family for their support especially my daughter Kelli for her assistance, my colleagues in the Nutrition Services Department at University Hospitals of Cleveland especially Kathleen Best RD, LD for her assistance, University Hospitals of Cleveland, The Core Library personnel of University Hospitals of Cleveland and the following pharmaceutical companies: Mead Johnson Nutritionals, Nestle Clinical Nutrition, Novartis Nutrition Corporation, and Ross Products Division of Abbott Laboratories Inc.

REFERENCES

1. Barrocas A, Belchar D. Nutrition assessment practical approaches. *Nutr. Aging Age Dependent Dis.* 1995;11:675–713.
2. Blackburn GL, Ahmad A. Skeleton in the hospital closet—then and now. *Suppl. Nutr.* 1995;11:193–195.
3. Blackburn GL, Bistrian BR, Maine BS Schlamm HT, Smith MF. Nutritional and metabolic assessment of the hospitalized patient. *JPEN* 1977;1:11–22.
4. Butterworth C. The skeleton in the hospital closet. *Nutr. Today* 1974;9:4–8.
5. Cheever KH. Early enteral feeding of patients with multiple trauma. *Crit. Care Nurse* 1999;19:40–51.
6. Mahan K, Escott-Stump S. *Krause's Food, Nutrition and Diet Therapy*, 10th ed. Philadelphia: WB Saunders, 2000.
7. Jones JS, Tidwell B, et al. Nutrition support of the hospitalized patient: a team approach. *J. Miss. State Med. Assoc.* 1995;36:91–99.
8. Hunt DR, Maslovetz A, Rowlands BJ, Brooks B. A simple nutrition screening procedure for hospital patients. *J. Am. Diet. Assoc.* 1985;85:332–335.
9. McMahon K, Brown JK. Nutritional screening and assessment. *Semin. Oncol. Nurs.* 2000;16:106–112.
10. Moore MC. *Nutritional Care: Pocket Guide Series*, 4th ed. St Louis: Mosby, 1997.
11. De Jonghe B, et al. A prospective survey of nutritional support practice in intensive care unit patients: What is prescribed? What is delivered? *Crit. Care Med.* 2001;29:8–12.
12. Corish CA. Symposium on nutrition and surgical practice—preoperative nutritional assessment. *Proc. Nutr. Soc.* 1999;58:821–829.
13. Lipkin EW, Bell S. Assessment of nutritional status—The clinician's perspective. *Clin. Lab. Med.* 1993;13:329–352.
14. The American Dietetic Association. *Handbook of Clinical Dietetics*, 2nd ed. New Haven, CT: Yale University Press, 1992.
15. Clifton GL, Robertson CS, Constant CF. Enteral hyperalimentation in head injury. *J. Neurosurg.* 1985;62:186–193.
16. Konstantinides FN. Nitrogen balance studies in clinical nutrition. *NCP* 1992;7:231–238.
17. Matarese LE, Gottschlich MM. *Contemporary Nutrition Support Practice—A Clinical Guide*. Philadelphia: WB Saunders, 1998.
18. Detsky AS, McLaughlin JR, Baker JP, et al. What is subjective global assessment? *Parent. Ent. Nutr.* 1987;11:8.
19. Trujillo EB, Robinson MK, Jacobs DO. Nutritional assessment in the critically ill. *Crit. Care Nurse* 1999;19:67–78.
20. The American Dietetic Association, CD-HCF/DDP. *Pocket Resource for Nutrition Assessment*. Chicago: American Dietetic Association Practice Group, 1997.
21. Halpern S. *Quick Reference to Clinical Nutrition: A Guide for Physicians*, 2nd ed. Hagerstown, MD: Lippincott Williams & Wilkins, 1987.
22. Gottschlich MM, Matarese LE, Shrouts EP, eds. *Nutrition Support Dietetics-Core Curriculum*, 2nd ed. Gaithersburg, MD: ASPEN (American Society of Parenteral and Enteral Nutrition), 1993.
23. The American Dietetic Association. *Manual of Clinical Dietetics*, 4th ed. Chicago: Library of Congress, 1992.
24. Matarese E. Indirect calorimetry. *JADA* 1997;97:S154–S160.
25. American Society of Parenteral and Enteral Nutrition. Guidelines for the use of parenteral and enteral nutrition in adult and pediatric patients. *JPEN* 1993;17(1 suppl).
26. Skipper A (ed). *Dietitian's Handbook of Enteral and Parenteral Nutrition*, 2nd ed. Gaithersburg, MD: ASPEN (American Society of Parenteral and Enteral Nutrition), 1998.
27. Gottschlich MM, Fuhrman MP, Hammond KA, et al. (eds). *The Science and Practice of Nutrition Support-A Case Based Core Curriculum*. Dubuque, IA: Kendall/Hunt Publishing, 2001.
28. Kocan MJ, Hickisch SM. A comparison of continuous and intermittent enteral nutrition in NICU patients. *J. Neurosci. Nurs.* 1986;18:333–337.
29. Merritt RJ, et al. *The ASPEN Nutrition Support Practice Manual*. Gaithersburg, MD: ASPEN (American Society of Parenteral and Enteral Nutrition), 1998.
30. Nutrition Subcommittee of the Pharmacy and Therapeutics Committee. *Guidelines for Nutrition Support of the Adult Patient*. University Hospitals Health Systems. Cleveland: Mead Johnson Nutritionals, 2001.
31. Suchner U, Senftleben U, et al. Enteral versus parenteral nutrition: Effects on gastrointestinal function and metabolism. *Nutrition* 1996;12:13–22.
32. University Hospitals of Cleveland. Department of Nutrition Services. *Guidelines for Standards of Nutrition Care Manual. Guidelines for Nutritional Screening; Nutritional Plan of Care, Nutrition Assessment.* Chapter 3, University Hospitals of Cleveland, Cleveland, OH, 2001.
33. University Hospitals of Cleveland Department of Nutrition Sources Policy and Procedure Manual. Chapter 8: 1–3, University Hospitals of Cleveland, Cleveland, HO, 2001.
34. Barton RG. Nutrition support in critical illness. *Nutr. Clin. Pract.* 1994;9:127–139.
35. Rombeau JL, Rolandelli RH. *Clinical Nutrition: Enteral and Tube Feeding*, 3rd ed, Philadelphia: WB Saunders, 1997.
36. Rombeau JL, Rolandelli RH. *Clinical Nutrition: Parenteral Nutrition*, 3rd ed, Philadelphia: WB Saunders, 2001.
37. Sunderland PM, Heilbrun MP. Estimating energy expenditure in traumatic brain injury: comparison of indirect calorimetry with predictive formulas. *Neurosurgery* 1992;31:246–253.

38. Pepe JL, Barba CA. The metabolic response to acute traumatic brain injury and implications for nutrition support. *J. Head Trauma Rehabil.* 1999;14:462–474.

39. Rosa AM, Shizgal HM. The Harris Benedict equation reevaluated: resting energy requirements and the body cell mass. *Am. J. Clin. Nutr.* 1984;40:168–182.

40. Norton JA, Ott LG, et al. Intolerance to enteral feeding in the brain-injured patient. *J. Neurosurg.* 1988;68:62–66.

41. Stechmiller J, Treloar DM, Derrico D, Yarandi H, Guin P. Interruption of enteral feedings in head injured patients. *J. Neurosci. Nur.* 1994;26:224–229.

42. Phang PT, Aeberhardt LE. Effect of nutritional support on routine nutrition assessment parameters and body composition in intensive care unit patients. *Can. J. Surg.* 1996;39:212–219.

43. Millinger LA, et al. Daily energy expenditure and basal metabolic rates of patients with spinal cord injury. *Arch. Phys. Med. Rehabil.* 1985;66:420.

44. Gariballa SE, Sinclair AJ. Assessment and treatment of nutritional status in stroke patients. *Post. Grad. Med. J.* 1998;74:395–399.

45. Hayes JC. Current feeding policies for patients with stroke. *Br. J. Nurs.* 1998;7:580–588.

46. Kasarskis EJ, Neville HE. Management of ALS. *Neurology* 1996;47:S118–S120.

47. Lo B, Dornbrand L. Sounding board: guiding the hand that feeds—caring for the demented elderly. *N. Engl. J. Med.* 1984;311:402–404.

48. Waxman MJ, Durfee D, et al. Nutritional aspects and swallowing function of patients with parkinson's disease *Nutr. Clin. Pract.* 1990;5:196–199.

49. Strand EA, Miller RM, Yorkston KM, Hillel AD. Management of oral—pharyngeal dysphagia symptoms in amyotrophic lateral sclerosis. *Dysphagia* 1996;11:129–139.

15

Bioethical Issues in the Neurosciences Critical Care Unit

Jose I. Suarez and Stuart Youngner

INTRODUCTION

Critical care physicians, particularly neurointensivists, are faced with daily complex bioethical issues that often times are very difficult to solve. Despite the amount of time spent dealing with these problems, there is little training in this area in both graduate and postgraduate medical training programs. Therefore, most of what is learned comes from observing senior clinical faculty, making adequate training variable and difficult to assess.

In this chapter, we will try to summarize the key aspects of bioethics pertinent to neurosciences critical care units (NSU) to help practitioners improve their care of patients when tackling these difficult situations. We will start with basic principles of morality and ethical theory as it is currently accepted, followed by discussions on particular issues such as decision making, end-of-life care, and organ procurement among others. This chapter is not intended to present a thorough review of the subject. Readers should refer to other published sources (1–7).

MORALITY

Morality (from Latin *moralis*: relating to morals or principles) is defined by The Collins English Dictionary as the conformity, or degree of conformity, to conventional standards of moral conduct (8). In simpler terms, morality can be related to norms about right and wrong actions that are shared by a group or society (4). Therefore, common morality is a social institution with principles, and rules. There is the other concept of professional morality understood as the general norms for the practice of a particular profession (in this case, medicine) that are accepted by those in that profession who understand their moral responsibilities (1,4). Ethics encompasses a set of moral principles that dictates behavior in a particular group of individuals (2,4). The terms ethics and morality are very close in meaning and many authors use them interchangeably when discussing bioethical issues. In this chapter we will do likewise.

ETHICAL AND MORAL CONCEPTS AND PRINCIPLES

As pointed out by Bernat (2), modern ethical theory stems from the combination of two philosophical thoughts: utilitarianism and deontology. The former determines the morality of an act solely based on its consequences whereas the latter does so based on its intent, and other factors that explain why a person acts. Based on these philosophies, Gert has proposed ten moral rules (1). The first five relate to those that take priority and entail prohibition of causation of major harm: do not kill (including causing permanent loss of consciousness); do not cause pain (including mental); do not disable;

From: *Current Clinical Neurology*
Critical Care Neurology and Neurosurgery
Edited by: J. I. Suarez © Humana Press Inc., Totowa, NJ

do not deprive of freedom; and do not deprive of pleasure. The other five relate to those that when not adhered to may cause harm in some but not all situations: do not deceive; keep your promise; do not cheat; obey the law; and do your duty. A more complex issue is the determination of what constitutes a violation of these moral rules and when they are justified. Such justifications may be acceptable when they are justified for every person under similar circumstances, they favor everyone being allowed to commit such violations under similar circumstances, and when is rational to allow that violation. Gert also proposes some questions to answer these quandaries in such a way that they may be understood by all the moral agents *(1)*:

1. What moral rules are being violated?
2. What are the harms being avoided, prevented, and/or caused?
3. What are the relevant beliefs and desires of the people toward whom the rule is being violated? This is the rational for written informed consent before to medical treatments.
4. Does one have a relationship with the person(s) toward whom the rule is being violated such that one sometimes has a duty to violate moral rules with regard to the person(s) without their consent? This is the basis for parental or guardian consent for medical treatment.
5. Are there any benefits?
6. Is an unjustified or weakly justified violation of a moral rule being prevented?
7. Is an unjustified or weakly justified violation of a moral rule being punished? This relates to law enforcement, not to medicine.
8. Are there any alternative actions that would be preferable?
9. Is the violation being done intentionally or only knowingly?
10. Is it an emergency situation that no person is likely to plan to be in?

Beauchamp and Childress have proposed a different set of moral principles that have become popular and widely accepted *(4)*. These principles are: 1) respect for autonomy; 2) nonmaleficence; 3) beneficence; and 4) justice. Because of their wide recognition and relevance to daily NSU practice, we will discuss them in more detail.

Autonomy, from the Greek *autonomia* (freedom to live by one's own laws), is defined by The Collins English Dictionary as the right or state of self-government *(9)*. Autonomy is related to liberty (independence from controlling influences) and agency (capacity for intentional action) *(4)*. Beauchamp and Childress concentrate on the principle of autonomous choice rather than autonomous person (capacity of self-governance) *(4)*. This is based on the fact that an autonomous person who may sign a written consent without proper understanding is qualified to act independently but fails to do so. Therefore, an autonomous action should be viewed in the context of intentionality, understanding, and without controlling influences that determine it. Also the principle of respect of autonomy should correlate with the right to choose rather than a mandatory duty to choose. Lastly, this fundamental principle must be interpreted along with competency. Individuals who are competent to make decisions are autonomous and their consent is valid.

Nonmaleficence entails a moral obligation not to inflict harm on others (in this case patients) *(4)*. This principle encompasses Gert's five first moral rules as stated previously *(1)*. Based on this principle, another obligation would be not to put others at risk of harm. An example of this is negligence defined as the absence of proper and adequate care, which is due an individual. This departure from professional standards has important implications for specific patient care issues such as withdrawal or withholding of life-sustaining measures as will be discussed below. On the other hand, the principle of beneficence implies a moral obligation to contribute to others' well-being and welfare *(4)*. This leads to the question as to whether autonomy (i.e., patients') should take precedence over beneficence (i.e., professional). Because of the emphasis given to patients' rights to refuse or accept treatments the problem of medical paternalism has become evident as clearly demonstrated by Beauchamp and Childress *(4)*. This has created debate in medical ethics with some authors taking the antipaternalistic position, whereas others justify it when the benefits provided to patients outweighs the loss of autonomy.

The last principle proposed by Beauchamp and Childress is the concept of justice *(4)*. Justice, from the Latin *justitia* (just), is defined by The Collins English Dictionary as the quality or fact of being just *(10)*. The type of justice dealt with in medical ethics is the distributive justice, that is the fair distribution of rights and obligations in society. This has important implications for today's society where issues such as allocation of health care resources, health insurance, and expensive medical technology are becoming more pressing. Although equal access to health care and a right to a minimum decent of health care are the two views currently promoted, the most important points to NSU is allocation and rationing of available resources. This has led to the creation of admission and discharge criteria for admission to the NSU or any other critical care area in the hospital as discussed in Chapter 1. The system proposed by Beauchamp and Childress for rationing scarce medical resources, such as technology offered in NSU, is summarized in Table 1 *(4)*. The constituents of such system that directly apply to NSU have to do with screening potential candidates (admission and discharge criteria) based on whether patients have a reasonable chance of improving or benefiting from treatment (prospect of success) when resources are allocated in an efficient and effective manner to maximize patients' welfare (medical utility). Once patients are admitted then the concepts of queuing and triaging may be considered at some point during patients' stay in the NSU. The former raises the question of whether a patient receiving a scarce treatment has absolute priority over those who arrive later but that may have more urgent need for it or better chances of survival. Triaging decisions, or prioritization, are often based on medical utility. However, these decisions need special consideration since it has been shown that in some cases several factors other than medical utility might lead to an increase in the number of critically ill patients denied admission to a critical area when bed availability is limited *(11)*. Beauchamp and Childress rightly argue that queuing and triaging can be applied only if there are no major disparities in medical utility *(4)*. That is, the system is fair.

PROFESSIONAL BIOETHICS IN THE NEUROSCIENCES CRITICAL CARE UNIT

Decision Making and Advance Directives

Models of Physician–Patient Relationship

In an attempt to describe the "ideal" physician–patient relationship, Emanuel and Emanuel have presented four models based on goals of this interaction, physician's obligations, the role of patient's values, and the concept of patient's autonomy *(12)*. These include the following: the paternalistic model (also called parental or priestly), the informative model (also called the scientific, engineering, or consumer), the interpretive model, and the deliberative model. The paternalistic model ensures that patients receive the best possible care to enhance their health. In this situation, patients have little if at all input and physicians become the predominant figure that discerns what is best for patients. The physicians' obligations would be to act in patients' best interests and to make decisions based on the most accurate information possible. The informative model entails that physicians present patients with all relevant information and they select the treatment they think best. The physician becomes a purveyor of technical expertise and patients have control over final decisions. The interpretive model tries to determine and clarify the patients' values and therefore the best treatment to meet them. In this model physicians act as counselors. The deliberative model implies that the physician–patient interaction is to help patients choose the best treatments available for the particular clinical situation. In this case, physicians become teachers or friends establishing a dialogue with patients on the best course of action to take.

The main argument that can be made when applying these models to the NSU is that many times these patients cannot partake in decision-making because of their impaired level of consciousness *(13)*. Therefore, neurointensivists may opt for the paternalistic model. However, most neurointensivists will most likely use different models with different patients or with the same patient in different settings. For instance, in emergency situations and when there is no surrogate consent

Table 1
System for Rationing Scarce Treatments

Screening potential candidates
    The constituency factor: uses social rather than medical factors
    Progress of science: advancement of knowledge; important during the development
    phase of a new treatment
    Prospect of success: distribution to patients with a reasonable chance of improvement
Selecting recipients
    Medical utility: effective and efficient allocation
    Impersonal mechanisms of chance and queuing: "first come, first served"
    Social utility: persons of critical social importance or social value
    Triage: prioritization

Proposed by Beauchamp and Childress *(4)*.

then the paternatilistic approach may be chosen whereas when deciding on elective treatments a combination of informative and deliberative models may be more appropriate. Regardless of the model used, neurointensivists are under the obligation to transmit objective, comprehensive and accurate information (veracity), to protect patients' privacy and confidentiality, and to act in good faith (fidelity) *(4)*.

Refusal or Acceptance of Life-Sustaining or Life-Saving Treatments

As we have seen above patient preferences are important in the physician–patient relationship and the informed consent is the usual vehicle for their expression *(3)*. Autonomy of patients remains the most important factor driving decision-making in the United States today *(14)*. This has led to the concept of advance directives. This is defined as the establishment of patients' preferences for future medical or surgical care before being rendered mentally incapable after experiencing a serious illness *(15–17)*. This could be stated informally (i.e., discussions with next-of-kin, relatives) or by designating a health care proxy or the Durable Power of Attorney for Health Care in a living will. However, patients admitted to NSU are different from the usual patient that is seen at a doctor's office or in a general medical-surgical ward. The main issue is that most patients who are admitted to the NSU do not choose so because they are considered incompetent to make such decision because of their underlying neurological impairment. In fact, many times the neurointensivist does not relate directly to patients but to their relatives or next-of-kins who become their surrogate decision makers. Another difficult problem is the lack of communication in a critical care setting *(18,19)*. NSU are busy places and neurointensivists may have limited time to meet with families. Also families and caregivers are subjected to stressful situations that present suddenly and unexpectedly. Improvements of communication and rapport with families along with enhanced trust can be gained by setting so-called family conferences where a time is allotted to discussion and updates regarding patients' current clinical condition. These meetings should be held in private rooms and should be attended by as many family members as possible, and the NSU team. Ample time should be allowed for questions. This is the time to discuss treatment options and alternatives, advances directives, and also start introducing concepts of end-of-life decisions. The goals of family conferences in the NSU are summarized in Table 2. The information discussed should be accurate and presented in simple and easy-to-understand language and taking into account patients' and families' attitudes toward the burden of treatment, the possible outcomes, and their likelihood. It has been shown that the number of individuals choosing to undergo certain treatments declines when the likelihood of an adverse outcome increases, particularly when it means functional or cognitive impairment *(21)*.

It is important to point out that family conferences do not begin and end in the specific location set up for it. Rather, NSU nurses and physicians should plan carefully beforehand what to say and how to

Table 2
Main Goals of Family Conferences in the NSU

1. Introduce all members of the NSU team to the family.
2. Discuss goals of conference.
3. Explain dynamics of NSU (i.e., teams involved, visiting hours, equipment available).
4. Summarize for the family patients' clinical condition in plain but accurate language.
5. Discuss specific treatment decisions (i.e., need for dialysis, neurosurgery, mechanical ventilation, end-of-life decisions) based on overall patients' prognosis.
6. Allow ample time for questions from the family.
7. Assess and achieve family's understanding of what was discussed.
8. Give recommendations for treatment.
9. Support the family's decisions.
10. Explain to family need for further meetings and assure them of availability of NSU team for further questioning.
11. Establish a spokesperson or a healthcare proxy (if available).
12. Address patient's and family's cultural and religious needs.
13. Organize NSU team meetings to assess and evaluate quality of conference for performance improvement.

These are responsibilities shared by both nurses and physicians.

say it. As much information as possible should be gathered prior to the meeting regarding natural history and prognosis of disease in question, family's cultural and religious background, and discuss (when available) previous knowledge of the family's attitudes and reactions toward neurologic disease *(19,20)*. After the family conference, NSU team members ought to make themselves available should further questions arise and should reiterate what was discussed to ensure understanding. There should also be careful follow up to address issues such as disagreement among family members, changes in plan of care, and quality of conferences.

End-of-Life Care

Neurointensivists have been trained to improve the health of critically ill neurologic patients. However, their role also includes the care of dying patients, especially when the decision to forgo life-sustaining treatments has been made. As we have seen above patients' autonomy has become center stage of medical care when it comes to treatment decision-making. This also applies to end-of-life decisions since the right of patients to refuse life-prolonging treatments has been widely accepted. Several studies have shown that 75–90% of intensive care unit deaths occur after decisions to forgo treatment *(22–24)*. One study in NSU revealed that 43% of non-brain dead patients that died were terminally extubated *(25)*. Despite this high percentage of withdrawal of intensive care, there have been varying degrees of satisfaction among patients and family members with the medical care received after supportive measures have been withdrawn *(25,26)*. This is important to keep in mind because in NSU, similar to other critical care areas, the decision to forgo life-sustaining treatments is usually made by family members that act as surrogate decision makers on behalf of patients and usually following the best interest standard *(27)*. In many instances these end-of-life decisions are preceded by the issuance of a do-not-resuscitate (DNR) order after a particular intervention has been determined to be highly unlikely to result in a meaningful survival for the patient (futility) *(28,29)*. Because of the importance of care of patients during this terminal phase and in an attempt to streamline management several articles have been published with recommendations *(30–32)*. We will proceed to summarize and emphasize the key features of end-of-life care.

The process of caring for patients once the decision to forgo life-sustaining treatment is being made includes a complex interaction of preparatory steps that involves patients, families and clinical

Table 3
Needs of Participants in End-of-Life Decision Making

Needs of the patient
    1. Receive adequate pain and symptom management
    2. Avoid inappropriate prolongation of dying
    3. Achieve a sense of control
    4. Relieve burden
    5. Strengthen relationships with loved ones
Needs of the family
    1. To be with dying relatives and be helpful to them
    2. To be assured of the comfort of the dying relative
    3. To be informed of the person's condition and of impending death
    4. To ventilate emotions
    5. To be comforted and supported by other family members and health professionals
    6. To find meaning in the death of their loved ones
Needs of the clinical team
    1. To reinforce the message that excellent end-of-life care is an institutional priority
    2. To be multidisciplinary and committed to cooperation and clear communication
    3. To be better educated about end-of-life care
    4. Administrative support
    5. To have opportunity for bereavement and debriefing

teams *(32–38)* (Table 3). Clinical teams must prepare the patients' family for what lies ahead since withdrawal of life-sustaining measures usually represents a new event in their lives. Patients (when able to make autonomous decisions) and their relatives need to be assured that management of pain and suffering would be the priority of healthcare workers and that they will be treated with respect and dignity throughout the dying process. It is also important to respect patient's cultural beliefs since in our multicultural society there are varying views on handling of bodies after death, organ procurement, and autopsy *(34)*. Families should be assured that they will have ample time to spend with their loved ones and appropriate information regarding changes in patient's condition and impending death. Healthcare workers should also make sure that families understand what is being done to the patient and offer assurance regarding their decision to forgo life-sustaining treatment. From the standpoint of the healthcare workers good communication should start before meetings with families to discuss end-of-life decisions. A clear plan of action must be available including discussions regarding adequacy of end-of-life treatment offered to patients.

Once the decision to forgo life-sustaining treatment is made caregivers should concentrate on interventions that will improve symptom relief and ameliorate psychological concerns *(34,39)*. This will include rewriting all medical and nursing orders to guarantee that only comfort-directed treatments are given. In NSU patients these treatments include pain and suffering relief, dyspnea alleviation, suppression of nausea and vomiting, avoidance of skin ulcerations, and treatment of fever and seizures. Continued nutrition may be viewed by some families as important during the dying process. However, most practitioners would agree that loss of hunger is part of the normal response to the dying process and that administering nutrition (via nasogastric tube or central venous lines) to terminally ill patients will not contribute to their comfort *(40–42)*. In NSU most patients undergoing withdrawal of life support are in coma and the most common signs after extubation are agonal or labored breathing and tachypnea *(25)*. It is our practice to aggressively check for pain, discomfort, and abnormal breathing and treat these signs immediately when present. In our NSU we administer an "anticipatory dose" of morphine sulfate (usually 4–8 mg) before withdrawing mechanical ventilation followed by a continuous infusion that is titrated according to nurses' assessment of patient comfort. We also pay close attention to treatment of fever with acetaminophen or external cooling techniques if necessary, and seizure control with adequate anticonvulsants. Withdrawal of other treatments such as hemodialysis, and intraventricular catheters, is usually carried out concomitantly with cessation of mechanical ventilation. Although the adequate method for the latter has not been determined we prefer terminal extubation preceded by adequate sedation as opposed to terminal weaning to avoid prolongation of the dying process *(43–46)*. Some patients will not die immediately or close to the extubation process. The care of these patients should be delivered in private rooms in general floors to allow for families to have sufficient quiet time to spend with their loved one. Whenever possible physicians should contact the palliative care or hospice inpatient team to enhance care of dying patients and their families *(47)*.

After patients die, caregivers have the obligation to immediately inform their families. It is recommended to deliver the news in person, in a private and quite room, and showing compassion and empathy *(48–51)*. The language used should also be simple and easy to understand. For discussions on brain death, organ donation and bereavement programs, see below.

Brain Death

Brain death is defined as the irreversible cessation of all brain and brainstem functions *(52)*. As described in more detail in Chapter 16, this implies that brain-dead patients have experienced a severe coma of known cause, have absent brain stem reflexes, and have sustained apnea *(53)*. Standard clinical criteria of brain death have been determined and are widely accepted *(53)*. However, this has created some controversy since some authors have argued that current definitions of brain death does not include a true loss of all integrative brain functions *(54)*. At the core of this controversy lies the fact that death is a process rather than an event and that there may not be a precise point at which an organism dies *(55)*. Regardless of these issues there is no doubt that brain death criteria were created out of medical utility *(56,57)*. Continued expensive treatment in situations where there is little or no hope of any meaningful recovery can create unnecessary burdens in our society. Also there is the practical issue of organ procurement.

Once a patient meets criteria for brain death families must be notified. Physicians should use clear language and convey the message that brain dead patients are dead *(32)*. We routinely hold at least two family conferences. The first one is carried out after the first examination for brain death declaration. During this meeting we address the issues of absent brain function, need for a repeat examination in approx 6 h, and apnea test. Once brain death is declared, we hold the second meeting for notification of the time of death. Families need to be told that bodily functions are being artificially maintained and that as soon as the devices are turned off they will cease. The most common approach in this instance (especially when organ procurement is not being considered) is to proceed with rapid removal of mechanical ventilation, and oxygenation. It is important to bear in mind that reflexive body movements can be seen either during apnea test or after withdrawal of support and that all healthcare workers and family members should be reminded of this fact so as not to cause alarm.

Organ Procurement

In the NSU, organ procurement is exclusively discussed in situations where patients are declared brain dead. A thorough discussion of organ procurement and transplantation is beyond the scope of this chapter and readers should refer to other sources *(5,6,58,59)*. However, it is important to mention that organ procurement discussions must be decoupled from brain death discussions. We normally explore organ donation possibilities after families have been notified of their loved one's death. A representative of the local transplant resource center usually leads this discussion. The fact that we ask families of all deceased patients for permission to procure organs is in compliance with current federal regulations for institutions caring for Medicare and Medicaid recipients *(60,61)*. Also participation of representatives from the local organ procurement organizations, who are especially trained to carry out this task, increases the chances of families' agreeing to proceed with organ donation *(62)*.

Despite the worldwide community support for organ donation or so-called gift of life, the rate of organ donation is low and there is currently a shortage of suitable organs for transplantation *(63–68)*.

Several factors have been put forth to explain this shortage including hard questions about the ethics of taking organs from the dead and giving them to others, confusion about definition of brain death, inadequacy of current organ procurement system, and family intervention in the organ procurement process *(67–71)*. The solutions proposed to augment organ donation have been directed at solving these issues and include: achieving consensus between health care workers and society as a whole regarding the definition of brain death, establishing alternative sources of organs, mandated choice for organ donation, allocating financial incentives to donors or their families, developing culturally-sensitive programs, and enhancing productivity of existing organ procurement organizations *(67,68,72–77)*.

Futility

When, if ever, may physicians ethically refuse to offer, initiate, or continue life-sustaining interventions? This question, under the rubric of medical futility, has been debated in scores of journal articles, has been addressed by professional societies, and has been the subject of several court cases. The issue remains contested, but several important issues have been clarified in the process. We present some of these points in this review as they are important to neurointensivists while caring for patients in the NSU.

Discussions of Futility Must First Identify Goals

Futility is an ambiguous and, potentially confusing word used out of context. Any claim that a specific intervention is "futile" must identify the goal that the intervention will fail to achieve *(78)*. So, for example, intubating and mechanically ventilating a patient dying of metastatic cancer may be futile if the goal is to cure the patient and send them home but not futile if the goal is to extend the life of the patient for days or weeks.

Discussions of Futility Help Clarify the Goals of Medicine and the Responsibility of Physicians

Physicians are not merely body mechanics. Rather, they are entrusted by society to help and do no harm to the patients they serve. As Schneiderman, one of the strongest proponents of medical futility, has convincingly argued, the goal of medicine is to benefit patients not simply to cause an effect in their bodies *(79)*. From this observation, it follows that physicians are not morally obligated to initiate or continue interventions that are not beneficial to patients, especially if those interventions also cause significant harm.

Futility and Rationing Are Not Synonymous

While eliminating futile treatments would certainly conserve health care resources, futility and rationing are not the same *(80)*. Futility implies that a specific intervention will fail to achieve a specific goal or that the goal itself is not beneficial to the patient. Such a treatment is futile whether or not there is abundance or scarcity of resources. Rationing means that there is *not enough* of a treatment to go around. Therefore, some who could benefit must be denied it. Judgments about futility are, it is argued, objective. Empirical data and clinical experience can demonstrate when a treatment will fail to achieve a goal. Conversely, judgments about who should receive and who should be denied beneficial treatment are questions of distributive justice. In a liberal democracy such questions can only be answered by a democratic political process, not by technical experts.

There Is an Important Distinction Between Positive and Negative Rights

There is an unfortunate confusion between positive and negative rights *(81)*. Until recently, the public discussion of rights at the end of life focused on the right to refuse treatment. The famous court cases from Quinlan to Cruzan were examples where patients or their families refused life-sustaining treatment that physicians or health care institutions insisted on imposing upon them. The right to refuse treatment has been firmly established in the law, professional guidelines, and the written policies of health care institutions. But the right to refuse treatment is a *negative* right. It finds its roots in the common law against battery or in the constitutional rights of privacy. A *positive* right, in contrast, implies that someone else has a duty to do something to or for the patient. While the negative right to refuse treatment is well established, the positive right to demand even clearly beneficial treatment is much less so. Pockets of entitlement to health care have been established—e.g., the right to life-saving treatment in an emergency room, or the right to treatment of end-stage renal disease, but there is certainly no general right to health care in the United States. How can it be argued that patients have a right to demand futile treatment when the right to beneficial treatment has not been established?

The Problem With Defining Futility

Futility is a word with a categorical ring, but closer examination indicates that defining it is not so simple. Schneiderman has noted that futility has both a quantitative and a qualitative sense *(79)*. *Quantitative* futility implies that while a chosen goal may benefit the patient, the chances of a given treatment achieving it are so remote as to be negligible. *Qualitative* futility implies that although the chances of achieving a goal are reasonable, the goal itself is unworthy of medicine because it provides no benefit to the patient. This parsing of futility into two categories is quite helpful for discussing it. The problem is agreeing on what chance is a chance not worth taking on one hand, and with determining what counts as a benefit on the other.

For example, Schneiderman's attempts to define quantitative and qualitative futility are unsatisfactory. He claims that physicians can play the futility trump when the intervention in question failed in their last 100 similar cases. But how often do physicians remember or even have 100 cases like the one at hand? Even if one turns to published case series, the numbers of such series is limited and one can almost always find characteristics of the current case that differ from the series. For example, early claims that elderly persons rarely survive cardiopulmonary resuscitative attempts were generalizations from series of cases where few or no otherwise healthy elderly were included. Moreover, physicians themselves have very different views about what counts as quantitative futility *(82)*.

Schneiderman's examples of qualitative futility are even more problematic. Keeping someone alive in a persistent vegetative state is futile, he argues, because continued life is of no benefit to the patient. While most persons probably agree with the conclusion that life without consciousness would not be beneficial for them, a significant minority (including a minority of physicians) does not. Schneiderman also has argued that permanent dependence on intensive care is a situation where the futility trump could be played. It is hard to imagine a physician telling a conscious patient who will never get off a ventilator that his or her life is not a benefit to them when the patient disagrees.

The problem is that both quantitative and qualitative futility include value judgments that should not be left to physicians alone. With the exception of a retrospective ruling by a jury in Massachusetts in a civil case *(83)*, the courts have rejected physicians' claims to make unilateral futility judgments *(84–86)*. A recent article by Helft and his colleagues entitled, "The Rise and Fall of the Futility Movement," summarizes the problems *(87)*. It points out that the emphasis has shifted to a "process-based approach" in which hospital policies "acknowledge the difficulty of trying to reach a consensus on futility and instead outline steps for conflict resolution." Such policies prohibit unilateral decision making by physicians, emphasizing instead the use of multidisciplinary committees and a step-by-step process for discussion, information sharing, and conflict resolution *(88)*. Helft et al. conclude that:

> The judgment that further treatment would be futile is not a conclusion—a signal that care should cease; instead, it should initiate the difficult task of discussing the situation with the patient. Thus, the most recent attempts to establish a policy in this area have emphasized processes for discussing

futility rather than the means of implementing decisions about futility. Talking to patients and their families should remain the focus of our efforts *(87)*.

We could not agree more with this recommendation.

Dying and Bereavement

The role of the neurointensivist does not end when the patient dies. Rather, it continues until the family's immediate needs are met. Many of these needs include choosing a funeral home, arranging financial matters, and starting the process of grief and bereavement. A multidisciplinary team in the NSU can help families deal with these issues in a very difficult moment in their lives. The mortician's office personnel, social workers, and staff involved in bereavement programs can all be part of this team.

Several factors have been reported as helping families with the bereavement process. One such factor is for families to be able to be present during cardiopulmonary resuscitation *(89,90)*. This has been viewed by some families as a way of helping ease their loved one's dying process *(90)*. Also bereavement can be facilitated by allowing families to spend ample time with their relatives while they are alive and assuring them that everything possible has been done to save the patient's life *(89)*. Some authors recommend offering families the opportunity to view and touch the body after death because this may facilitate grief by confirming the death *(91)*. Lastly, establishing bereavement programs for relatives of NSU patients should include delivering follow-up cards to families with sympathetic comments from nurses and physicians that cared for the patient, facilitating contact with support groups, and even attending funerals whenever possible *(32,92,93)*.

Research in the Neurosciences Critical Care Unit

Experimentation in humans are carried out under the assumption that it will result in improved scientific knowledge to better medical care delivery to society in general even though participating subjects are the mean to obtaining that knowledge. This implies that clinical research has the potential for human exploitation *(94)*. Because of this seven ethical requirements have been formulated to guarantee that human subjects are not just used but rather treated with respect while they help solve important medical questions *(95)* (Table 4). These requirements are universal and must be adapted to NSU patients participating in clinical trials.

Social or Scientific Value

This principle means that a clinical study must evaluate a treatment that might lead to improved health. This implies that scarce resources should be used responsibly and that human exploitation should be avoided *(95)*. This would be supported by Beauchamp and Childress' system of rationing scarce resources *(4)*.

Scientific Validity

All valuable research must be evaluated rigorously to guarantee that it adheres to current accepted scientific principles. This includes methods to obtain information and statistical analysis of the data *(95)*. This would also be supported by Beauchamp and Childress' system of rationing scarce resources *(4)*.

Fair Subject Selection

Patient selection should be fair and not dictated by social, economic, religious, or racial issues. Individuals cannot be excluded from a study unless investigators have a good scientific reason *(95)*. This corresponds to the ethical principle of justice *(4)*.

Favorable Risk–Benefit Ratio

Investigators must minimize risks to participating subjects and enhance potential benefits *(95)*. This is in accordance with the principles of nonmaleficence and beneficence *(4)*.

Table 4
Ethical Requirements for Clinical Research

1. Value (social or scientific)
2. Scientific validity
3. Fair subject selection
4. Favorable risk–benefit ratio
5. Independent review
6. Informed consent
7. Respect for potential and enrolled individuals

Independent Review

Researchers usually have various underlying interests to carry out a particular project including need to complete high-quality research, protect subjects, obtain funding, and advance their careers *(95)*. Because of this, it is important that an independent panel of scientists review the research proposal to avoid potential conflicts of interest. In most institutions the Institutional Review Board (IRB) represents this panel and clinical researcher must present their studies to them prior to enrolling subjects.

Informed Consent

This is a very important principle that is justified by the ethical value of respect for autonomy *(4)*. The main goals of informed consent are to ensure that patients decide whether they want to participate in a study and to guarantee that they only participate when the objectives of such study are consistent with their values and preferences *(95)*. This entails that researchers are morally obliged to provide potential participants with accurate information about the purpose of the study, procedures involved, benefits and risks involved. Ample time should be allowed for these individuals to analyze the information given so that they can make a voluntary and autonomous decision. Most NSU patients pose a challenge for investigators because they cannot make autonomous decisions based on the fact that they are not competent to do so.

In situations where NSU individuals cannot make their decisions (i.e., severe traumatic brain injury, coma, severe stroke) it is important to remember that these patients have their own interests and values and they should be respected *(95)*. In such situations the informed consent entails discussing the study purpose with a proxy decision-maker that uses the substituted judgement of making the decision the subject would if they could *(4)*. However, since the risks associated with research may be largely uncertain proxies have been advised to exercise careful discretion and judgement when deciding for patients.

An even more morally challenging issue is the enrolment of mentally impaired patients in emergency research *(96–102)*. It has been argued that this type of research is vital to society *(101)*. However, obtaining consent is not always practical or possible prior to enrollment from a patient or a legally authorized proxy. It has also being argued that this should not be an absolute barrier to providing emergency intervention since individuals may obtain benefits from participating in a clinical trial whether they receive the test treatment or not *(101)*. In situations of emergency research studies can be conducted under a waiver of informed consent provided that certain criteria are met *(96,97)*. The main criteria are evidence that advance consent procedures are impracticable (i.e., narrow therapeutic window for a treatment) and patients' legally authorized proxy, relatives or friends cannot be located within a reasonable period of time. These rules apply to life-threatening conditions for which there is no alternative method of approved or generally accepted therapy that provides and equal or greater likelihood of benefit or saving the life of patients. These also entail that the researchers consult with the community where the research is being conducted, and establish independent monitoring committees to oversee the study. In our institution the IRB mandates that the investigator and an independent physician must make the determination in writing for the medical record that the study offers potential benefit to patients, the patients' condition is life-threatening, there is inability to communicate with patients, and that there is insufficient time to obtain consent from legal representatives or there is no legal representative. Once this is done, the next of kin must be informed, and has to agree to the study and sign the consent. However, it is clear that this does not constitute informed consent and when able individuals themselves have the right to withdraw consent.

Respect for Potential and Enrolled Individuals

This last requirement involves several features: (1) to permit subjects to withdrawn from the study; (2) to protect subjects' confidentiality; (3) to inform subjects of previously unknown risks of the study; (4) to inform subjects of final results of the study; (5) to maintain the welfare of patients *(95)*. By following these rules, investigators guarantee patients' autonomy and welfare *(4)*.

CONCLUSION

Neurointensivists are faced with important ethical issues in their daily practice in the NSU. The most important issues are end-of-life decisions, brain death, organ procurement, and carrying out ethical research. The basic principles of ethics and good medical practice are similar to those practiced by other physicians. However, specific conditions such as altered mentation make NSU patients particularly challenging. Health care providers working in the NSU should make every effort to become more proficient in bioethics to improve the care of their patients.

REFERENCES

1. Gert B, Culver CM, Clouser KD, eds. *Bioethics. A Return to Fundamentals.* New York: Oxford University Press, 1997.
2. Bernat JL, ed. *Ethical Issues in Neurology.* Boston: Butterworth-Heineman, 2002.
3. Jonsen AR, Siegler M, Winslade WJ, eds. *Clinical Ethics,* 4th ed. New York: McGraw Hill, 1998.
4. Beauchamp TL, Childress JF, eds. *Principles of Biomedical Ethics,* 5th ed. New York: Oxford University Press, 2001.
5. Caplan AL, Coehlo DH, eds. *The Ethics of Organ Transplants: The Current Debate.* Amherst, NY: Prometheus Books, 1998.
6. Youngner SJ, Fox RC, O'Connell LJ. *Organ Transplantation: Meanings and Realities.* Madison, WI: The University of Wisconsin Press, 1996.
7. Youngner SJ, Arnold RM, Schapiro R, eds. *The Definition of Death: Contemporary Controversies.* Baltimore: The Johns Hopkins University Press, 1999.
8. Hanks P, ed. *Collins Dictionary of the English Language,* 2nd ed. London & Glasgow: Collins, 1986:1000.
9. Hanks P, ed. *Collins Dictionary of the English Language,* 2nd ed. London & Glasgow: Collins, 1986:101.
10. Hanks P, ed. *Collins Dictionary of the English Language,* 2nd ed. London & Glasgow: Collins, 1986:829.
11. Marshall MF, Schwenzer KJ, Orsina M, Fletcher JC, Durbin CG Jr. Influence of political power, medical provincialism, and economic incentives on the rationing of surgical intensive care unit beds. *Crit. Care Med.* 1992;20:387–394.
12. Emanuel EJ, Emanuel LL. Four models of the physician-patient relationship. *JAMA* 1992;267:2221–2226.
13. Cook D. Patient autonomy versus parentalism. *Crit. Care Med.* 2001;29:N24–N25.
14. Meier DE, Morrison RS. Autonomy reconsidered. *N. Engl. J. Med.* 2002;346:1087–1089.
15. Prendergast TJ. Advance care planning: pitfalls, progress, promise. *Crit. Care Med.* 2001;29:N34–N39.
16. Annas GJ. Nancy Cruzan and the right to die. *N. Engl. J. Med.* 1990;323:670–673.
17. Annas GJ, Arnold B, Aroskar M, et al. Bioethicists' statement on the US Supreme Court's Cruzan decision. *N. Engl. J. Med.* 1990;323:686.
18. Fins JJ, Solomon MZ. Communication in intensive care settings: The challenge of futility disputes. *Crit. Care Med.* 2001;29:N10–N15.
19. Curtis JR, Patrick DL, Shannon SE, Treece PD, Engelberg RA, Rubenfeld GD. The family conference as a focus to improve communication about end-of-life care in the intensive care unit: ooportunities for improvement. *Crit. Care Med.* 2001;29:N26–N33.
20. Vincent JL. Cultural differences in end-of-life care. *Crit. Care Med.* 2001;29:N52–N55.
21. Fried TR, Bradley EH, Towle VR, Allore H. Understanding the treatment preferences of seriously ill patients. *N. Engl. J. Med.* 2002;346:1061–1066.
22. Pendergast TJ, Luce JM. Increasing incidence of withholding and withdrawal of life support from the critically ill. *Am. J. Respir. Crit. Care Med.* 1997;155:15–20.
23. Prendergast TJ, Claessens MT, Luce JM. A national survey of end-of-life care of critically-ill patients. *Am. J. Respir. Crit. Care Med.* 1998;158:11,163–11,167

24. Faber-Langendoen K. A multi-institutional study of care given to patients dying in hospitals. Ethical and practice implications. *Arch. Intern. Med.* 1996;156:2130–2136.

25. Mayer SA, Kossoff SB. Withdrawal of life support in the neurological intensive care unit. *Neurology* 1999;12:1602–1609.

26. SUPPORT Principal Investigators: a controlled trial to improve care for seriously ill hospitalized patients. The study to understand prognoses and preferences for outcomes and risks of treatments (SUPPORT). The SUPPORT Principal Investigators. *JAMA* 1995;274:1591–1598.

27. Weir RF, Gotlin L. Decisions to abate life-sustaining treatment for nonautonomous patients. Ethical standards and legal liability after Cruzan. *JAMA* 1990;264:1846–1853.

28. Luce JM. Ethical principles in critical care. *JAMA* 1990;263:696–700.

29. American Thoracic Society. Withholding and withdrawing life-sustaining therapy. *Am. Rev. Respir. Dis.* 1991;144:726–731.

30. Faber-Langendoen K, Lanken PN, for the ACP-ASIM End-of-Life Care Consensus Panel. Dying patients in the intensive care unit: forgoing treatment, maintaining care. *Ann. Intern. Med.* 2000;133:886–893.

31. Nyman DJ, Sprung CL. End-of-life decision making in the intensive care unit. *Intensive Care Med.* 2000;26:1414–1420.

32. Truong RD, Cist AF, Brackett SE, et al. Recommendations for end-of-life care in the intensive care unit: The Ethics Committee of the Society of Critical Care Medicine. *Crit. Care Med.* 2001;29:2332–2348.

33. Singer PA, Martin DK, Kelner M. Quality end-of-life care: Patients' perspectives. *JAMA* 1999;281:163–168.

34. Danis M, Federman D, Fins JJ, et al. Incorporating palliative care into critical care education: Principles, challenges, and opportunities. *Crit. Care Med.* 1999;27:2005–2013.

35. Council on Scientific Affairs American Medical Association. Good care of the dying patient. *JAMA* 1996;275:474–478.

36. Hampe SO. Needs of the grieving spouse in a hospital setting. *Nurs. Res.* 1975;24:113–120.

37. Furukawa MM. Meetings the needs of the dying patient's family. *Crit. Care Nurse* 1996;16:51–57.

38. Asch DA. The role of critical care nurses in euthanasia and assisted suicide. *N. Engl. J. Med.* 1996;334:1374–1379.

39. Brody H, Campbell ML, Faber-Langendoen K, et al. Withdrawing intensive life-sustaining treatment—Recommendations for compassionate clinical management. *N. Engl. J. Med.* 1997;336:652–657.

40. McCann RM, Hall WJ, Groth-Juncker A. Comfort care for terminally ill patients: The appropriate use of nutrition and hydration. *JAMA* 1994;272:1263–1266.

41. Printz LA. Terminal dehydration, a compasionate treatment. *Arch. Intern. Med.* 1992;152:697–700.

42. Gillick MR. Rethinking the role of tube feeding in patients with advanced dementia. *N. Engl. J. Med.* 2000;342:206–210.

43. Gilligan T, Raffin TA. Withdrawing life support: Extubation and prolonged terminal weans are inappropriate. *Crit. Care Med.* 1996;24:352–353.

44. Gilligan T, Raffin TA. Rapid withdrawal of support. *Chest* 1995;108:1407–1408.

45. Krishna G, Raffin TA. Terminal weaning from mechanical ventilation. *Crit. Care Med.* 1999;27:9–10.

46. Gianakos D. Terminal weaning. *Chest* 1995;108:1405–1406.

47. Campbell ML, Frank RR. Experience with an end-of-life practice at a university hospital. *Crit. Care Med.* 1997;25:197–202.

48. Campbell ML. Breaking bad news to patients. *JAMA* 1994;271:1052.

49. Krahn GL, Hallum A, Kime C. Are there good ways to give "bad news"? *Pediatrics* 1993;91:578–582.

50. Ptaceck JT, Eberhardt TL. Breaking bad news. *JAMA* 1996;276:496–502.

51. Quill TE, Townsend P. Bad news: delivery, dialogue, and dilemmas. *Arch. Intern. Med.* 1991;151:463–468.

52. Williams MA, Suarez JI. Brain death determination in adults: more than meets the eye. *Crit. Care Med.* 1997;25:1787–1788.

53. Plum F. Clinical standards and technological confirmatory tests in diagnosing brain death. In Youngner SJ, Arnold RM, Schapiro R, eds. *The Definition of Death. Contemporary Controversies.* Baltimore: The Johns Hopkins University Press, 1999: 34–65.

54. Brody BA. How much of the brain must be dead? In Youngner SJ, Arnold RM, Schapiro R, eds. *The Definition of Death. Contemporary Controversies.* Baltimore: The Johns Hopkins University Press, 1999: 72–82.

55. Halevy A, Brody B. Brain death: Reconciling definitions, criteria, and tests. *Ann. Intern. Med.* 1993;119:519–525.

56. Ad Hoc Committee of the Harvard Medical School to Examine the Definition of Brain Death. A definition of irreversible coma. *JAMA* 1968;205:337–340.

57. Youngner SJ. Brain death: A superficial and fragile consensus. *Arch. Neurol.* 1992;49:570–572.

58. O'Connell LJ. The realities of organ transplantation. In Youngner SJ, Fox RC, O'Connell LJ, eds. *Organ Transplantation. Meanings and Realities.* Madison, WI: The University of Wisconsin University Press, 1996:19–31.

59. Caplan AL. Ethical and policy issues in the procurement of cadaver organs for transplantation. In Caplan AL, Coehlo DH, eds. *The Ethics of Organ Transplants. The Current Debate.* Amherst: Prometheus Books, 1998:142–146.

60. Federal Register Final Rule: Hospital Conditions for Participation for Organ Donation (42 CFR Part 482), 2000.

61. Centers for Medicare and Medicaid Services (CMS), HHS. Medicare and Medicaid programs; emergency recertification for coverage for organ procurement organizations (OPOs). Interim final rule with comment period. *Fed. Regist.* 2001;66:67,109–67,111.

62. Gortmaker SL, Beasley CL, Sheehy E, et al. Improving the request process to increase family consent for organ donation. *J. Transpl. Coord.* 1998;8:210–217.

63. Kerridge IH, Saul P, Lowe M, McPhee J, Williams D. Death, dying and donation: organ transplantation and the diagnosis of death. *J. Med. Ethics* 2002;28:89–94.

64. Merle JC. A Kantian argument for a duty to donate one's own organs. A reply to Nicole Gerrand. *J. Appl. Philos.* 2000;17:93–101.

65. Murray TH. Are we morally obligated to make gifts of our bodies? *Health Matrix J. Law Med.* 1991;1:19–29.

66. Pugliese MR, Degli Esposito D, Venturoli N, et al. Hospital attitude survey on organ donation in the Emilia-Romagna region, Italy. *Transpl. Int.* 2001;14:411–419.

67. Spital A. Mandated choice for organ donation: time to give it a try. *Ann. Intern. Med.* 1996;125:66–69.

68. Klassen AC, Klassen DK. Who are the donors in organ donation? The family's perspective in mandated choice. *Ann. Intern. Med.* 1996;125:70–73.

69. Youngner SJ. Some must die. In Youngner SJ, Fox RC, O'Connell LJ, eds. *Organ Transplantation. Meanings and Realities.* Madison, WI: The University of Wisconsin University Press, 1996:32–55.

70. Fiedler LA. Why organ transplant programs do not succeed. In Youngner SJ, Fox RC, O'Connell LJ, eds. *Organ Transplantation. Meanings and Realities.* Madison, WI: The University of Wisconsin University Press, 1996:56–65.

71. Ott BB. Defining and redefining death. In Caplan AL, Coehlo DH, eds. *The Ethics of Organ Transplants. The Current Debate.* Amherst: Prometheus Books, 1998:16–23.

72. Murray TH. Organ vendors, families, and the gift of life. In Youngner SJ, Fox RC, O'Connell LJ, eds. *Organ Transplantation. Meanings and Realities.* Madison, WI: The University of Wisconsin University Press, 1996:101–125.

73. Guy BS, Aldridge A. Marketing organ donation around the globe. *Mark Health Serv.* 2001;21:30–35.

74. Lovasik D. Brain death and organ donation. *Crit. Care Nurs. Clin. North Am.* 2000;12:531–538.

75. Bollinger RR, Heinrichs DR, Seem DL, et al. Organ procurement organization (OPO), best practices. *Clin. Transplant* 2001;15(suppl 6):16–21.

76. Andresen J. Cultural competence and health care: Japanese, Korean, and Indian patients in the United States. *J. Cult. Divers.* 2001;8:109–121.

77. Samaritan Transplant Services, Phoenix, AZ. Development of a culturally sensitive, locality-based program to increase kidney donation. *Adv. Ren. Replace. Ther.* 2002;9:54–56.

78. Youngner SJ. Applying futility: Saying no is not enough. *JAGS* 1994;42:887–889.

79. Schneiderman LJ, Jecker NS, Jonsen AR. Medical futility: its meanings and implications. *Ann. Intern. Med.* 1990;112:949–954.

80. Jecker NS, Schneiderman LJ. Futility and rationing. *Am. J. Med.* 1992;92:189–196.

81. Brett AS, McCullough LB. When patients request specific interventions. *N. Engl. J. Med.* 1986;15:1347–1351.

82. McCrary SV, Swanson JW, Youngner SJ, Perkins JS, Winslade WI. Physicians' quantitative assessments of medical futility. *J. Clin. Ethics* 1994;5:100–105.

83. Gilgun v. Massachusetts General Hospital. Mass. Sup. Ct., April 21, 1995. (No. 92-4820).

84. In re Helga Wanglie, Fourth Judicial District (Dist. Ct., Probate Ct. Div.) PX-91-283. Minnesota, Hennepin County.

85. Angel M. The case of Helga Wanglie: A new kind of "right to die" case. *N. Engl. J. Med.* 1991;325:511–512.

86. Capron AM. Medical futility: Strike two. *Hastings Ctr. Rep.* 1994;September-October:42–43.

87. Helft PR, Siegler M, Lantos J. The rise and fall of the futility movement. *N. Engl. J. Med.* 2000;343:293–296.

88. Halevy A, Brody BA. A multi-institutional collaborative policy on medical futility. *JAMA* 1996;276:571–574.

89. Tsai E. Should family members be present during cardiopulmonary resuscitation? *N. Engl. J. Med.* 2002;346:1019–1021.

90. Doyle CJ, Post H, Burney RE. Family participation during resuscitation: an option. *Ann. Emerg. Med.* 1987;16:673–675.

91. Dubin WR, Sarnoff JR. Sudden unexpected death: intervention with the survivors. *Ann. Emerg. Med.* 1986;15:54–57.

92. Anderson AH, Bateman LH, Ingallinera KL, et al. Our caring continues: A bereavement follow-up program. *Focus Crit. Care* 1991;18:523–526.

93. McClelland ML. Our unit has a bereavement program. *Am. J. Nurs.* 1993;93:62–68.

94. DeCastro LD. Exploitation in the use of subjects for medical experimentation: A re-examination of basic issues. *Bioethics* 1995;9:259–268.

95. Emanuel EJ, Wendler D, Grady C. What makes clinical research ethical? *JAMA* 2000;283:2701–2711.

96. US Food and Drug Administration. Protection of human subjects: informed consent and waiver of informed consent requirements in certain emergency research; final rules. *Fed. Regist.* 1996;61:51,497–51,531

97. Moreno J, Caplan AL, Wolpe PR, and the Members of the Project on Informed Consent, Human Research Ethics Group. Updating protections for human subjects involved in research. *JAMA* 1998;280:1951–1958.

98. Dresser R. Mentally disabled research subjects: The enduring policy issues. *JAMA* 1996;276:67–72.

99. Capron AM. Ethical and human-rights issues in research on mental disorders that may affect decision-making capacity. *N. Engl. J. Med.* 1999;340:1430–1434.

100. American College of Physicians. Cognitively impaired subjects. *Ann. Intern. Med.* 1989;111:843–848.

101. Biros MH, Lewis RJ, Olson CM, Runge JW, Cummins RO, Fost N. Informed consent in emergency research. Consensus statement from the coalition conference of acute resuscitation and critical care researchers. *JAMA* 1995;273:1283–1287.

102. Levine RJ. Research in emergency situations. The role of deferred consent. *JAMA* 1995;273:1300–1302.

16

Coma and Brain Death

Alexandros L. Georgiadis, Romergryko Geocadin, Jose I. Suarez, and Osama O. Zaidat

COMA AND RELATED STATES

Consciousness

Definition

Consciousness represents the summated activity of the cerebral cortex. It is characterized by awareness of self and environment and by the ability to respond to environmental and intrinsic stimuli. Plum and Posner differentiated between two aspects of consciousness: arousal and content (1). Arousal is linked to wakefulness or alertness, whereas the content of consciousness represents the sum of cognitive and affective mental functions. A variety of insults can cause impairment of one or both aspects of consciousness. Among other causes, these include structural brain lesions, metabolic disturbances, hypoxia or hypoperfusion, and traumatic brain injury (Table 1).

The Ascending Arousal System

The ascending arousal system is located in the rostral pons, midbrain, thalamus and hypothalamus. Ascending pathways from monoaminergic cell groups in the brainstem and hypothalamus and cholinergic cell groups of the pedunculopontine, laterodorsal tegmental, and parabrachial nuclei, project to the thalamus and cortex and increase wakefulness and vigilance (2). Impairment of consciousness is caused by damage to those structures or by bilateral hemispheric damage. Even complete transection of the brainstem below the rostral pons almost invariably does not affect consciousness.

States of Decreased Alertness

Overview

The level of alertness is characterized by the intensity of stimulation needed in order to elicit a meaningful response. Thus, the states of decreased alertness form a continuum, which ranges from a normal mental state to unresponsiveness. Coma is defined as a state of unarousable unresponsiveness in which the patient lies with the eyes closed. There is no purposeful response to external or internal stimuli. Stupor is a state in which patients appear to be asleep, but may become alert when vigorously stimulated. As soon as the stimulus ceases, patients lapse back into sleep. Lethargy and obtundation are terms, which are used to describe patients with mild and moderate reduction in alertness, respectively. Both terms are subjective and should therefore be used only with additional clarification.

From: *Current Clinical Neurology*
Critical Care Neurology and Neurosurgery
Edited by: J. I. Suarez © Humana Press Inc., Totowa, NJ

Table 1
Conditions Associated With Decreased Level of Consciousness

Focal neurological signs		
Absent	Possibly present	Present in most cases
Meningitis	Hypoglycemia	Cerebral infarction
Hydrocephalus	Subarachnoid hemorrhage	Intracranial hemorrhage
Hypercarbia	Paraneoplastic syndromes	Epidural hemorrhage
Azotemia	CNS vasculitis	Subdural hemorrhage
Uremia	Seizures and postictal states	Venous sinus thrombosis
Endocrine dysfunction	Heart failure with cerebral	CNS tumors
Hypothermia	hypoperfusion	Encephalitis
Hyperthermia	Hyponatremia	CNS abscess
Intoxication	Hepatic failure	Traumatic brain injury
Systemic infections	Pituitary apoplexy	Diffuse demyelinating
Diabetic ketoacidosis		disorders
		Wernicke's encephalopathy

Vegetative State

The duration of coma is usually limited to 2–4 wk. Depending on the underlying etiology, the outcome will be lethal for some patients, whereas a subset of individuals will regain consciousness with varying degrees of disability. In a third subset of patients, sleep-wake cycles will return, but this wakefulness will be accompanied by an apparent total lack of cognitive function. This state was termed "vegetative state" by Jennett and Plum in 1972 *(3)*. Between 1 and 14% of patients with coma will go into a vegetative state *(4)*. It is obvious that there are serious ethical and legal issues involved in the treatment of those patients. Therefore, a Multi-Society Task Force was established in 1991 with the assignment to provide clear criteria for the diagnosis of the vegetative state *(5)* as well as an algorithm that could aid with determining prognosis *(6)*. The Multi-Society Task Force proposed diagnostic criteria for vegetative state and are summarized in Table 2.

The vegetative state is termed *persistent* when it exceeds 1 mo. In persistent vegetative state there is potential for recovery, especially in cases of traumatic etiology *(5)*. However, 12 mo after traumatic injury and 3 mo after nontraumatic injury, the chance for recovery is exceedingly low and the term *permanent vegetative state* can be applied.

It is thought that the neuropathologic correlate of the vegetative state is diffuse axonal injury in cases of trauma *(7)* and laminar cortical necrosis in cases of nontraumatic injury *(1,5)*. Characteristic of traumatic and nontraumatic cases is the relative sparing of brainstem structures *(1,8)*. In a recent study, Adams et al. proposed that the fundamental structural abnormality underlying the persistent vegetative state, regardless of etiology, is widespread damage to subcortical white matter and the thalami *(8)*.

Minimally Conscious State

This term refers to patients who, albeit severely impaired, do not meet the criteria for being in a vegetative state. According to a recently proposed definition, the minimally responsive state is a condition of severely altered consciousness in which minimal but definite behavioral evidence of self or environmental awareness is demonstrated *(9)*. Cognitively mediated behavior occurs inconsistently but is reproducible. Significant controversy exists regarding the definition and use of this term *(10,11)*.

Akinetic Mutism

Patients with this syndrome are immobile and will usually lie with their eyes closed. Sleep-wake cycles exist. There is little or no vocalization. Motor response to noxious stimuli is absent or mini-

Table 2
Diagnostic Criteria for the Vegetative State as Proposed by the Multi-Society Task Force

Vegetative state:
1. No evidence of awareness of self or environment and inability to interact with others.
2. No evidence of sustained, reproducible, purposeful, or voluntary behavioral responses to visual, auditory, tactile, or noxious stimuli.
3. No evidence of language comprehension or expression.
4. Intermittent wakefulness manifested by the presence of sleep-wake cycles.
5. Sufficiently preserved hypothalamic and brainstem autonomic functions to permit survival with medical and nursing care.
6. Bowel and bladder incontinence.
7. Variably preserved cranial nerve reflexes and spinal reflexes.

Persistent vegetative state:
> 1 mo

Permanent vegetative state:
> 3 mo in nontraumatic insults, >12 mo in traumatic injury

mal. The hallmark of this syndrome is the relative paucity of signs of damage to the descending motor pathways, i.e., the absence of spasticity and rigidity *(12)*. The underlying lesions are quite variable *(1)*. In the early stages of the vegetative state, the two conditions can be indistinguishable.

Locked-In Syndrome

The locked-in syndrome consists of quadriplegia, anarthria, and paresis of horizontal eye movements. Vertical eye movements can be slow and incomplete but are preserved, as is the ability to blink. The patients are awake and fully aware of their surroundings. The most common underlying etiology is destruction of the ventral pons. The locked-in state is usually caused by infarction, but it has been described as a result of pontine hemorrhage, midbrain infarction, central pontine myelinolysis, brainstem mass lesions, multiple sclerosis, encephalitis, and a variety of other pathologies *(13)*. Guillain-Barré syndrome and myasthenia gravis can produce a similar clinical picture. Recovery is rare but has been reported *(13,14)*.

Coma

Initial Approach to the Patient

The evaluation of the patient in coma must begin with the assessment of airway, breathing and circulation as outlined in Chapters 1, 8, and 9. After immediate life-threatening issues have been addressed, a comprehensive general and neurological examination can be performed.

Once vascular access has been obtained, blood samples should be drawn for testing of serum electrolyte concentration including calcium, magnesium, and phosphorus, renal function parameters, liver function tests, including ammonia levels, coagulation profile, and arterial blood gases (ABG). Serum and urine drug screens, serum anticonvulsant concentrations, cardiac enzymes, lactate levels, thyroid and adrenal hormone levels, carboxyhemoglobin levels, and a blood smear can be obtained if deemed appropriate. Potential seizures should be treated immediately. If the cause of coma is not clearly understood, it is recommended to administer 50 mL of a 50% glucose solution intravenously preceded by 100 mg of intravenous thiamine to avoid precipitating Wernicke's encephalopathy in alcoholic or malnourished patients. If opiate overdose is suspected, naloxone should be administered cautiously. Rapid reversal can lead to acute withdrawal syndromes or acute severe pain in chronic pain patients. If there is suspicion of benzodiazepine overdose, flumazenil can be given at a dose of 0.2 mg intravenously. Flumazenil is contraindicated in patients who may have also ingested tricyclic antidepressants because in this case it can precipitate seizures.

A 12-lead electrocardiogram and a chest radiograph are some of the routine tests that should be performed in all patients. Head computed tomography (CT) should be performed as soon as feasible. If magnetic resonance imaging (MRI) is readily available, and depending on the suspected pathology and the patient's state, it might be preferable to head CT. Electroencephalography (EEG) must be performed in all unresponsive patients particularly those with seizures even after clinical activity has ceased in order to rule out subclinical status epilepticus. If the presence of acute ischemic stroke has been established, the appropriateness of use of thrombolytic agents must be assessed. In case infection is suspected antibiotic treatment is initiated immediately and lumbar puncture is performed as soon as possible thereafter. Lumbar puncture can also aid confirm the presence of subarachnoid blood in patients with equivocal head CT scanning findings, or assess intracranial pressure (ICP). It is essential to "tailor" the above tests and measures and the initial preliminary clinical assessment to the individual patient. Conditions that require immediate action must be recognized and treated first. In cases of elevated ICP with associated herniation a very poor or fatal outcome can only be avoided if the appropriate measures are initiated without any delay (*see* Chapter 5 for details in management). Likewise, certain lesions (for example, large cerebellar or epidural hematomas) may constitute a surgical emergency and neurosurgical consultation must be obtained as soon as possible (*see* Chapter 19). Delay in treating a central nervous system (CNS) infection or status epilepticus also worsens outcome significantly (*see* Chapters 25 and 29).

General Examination

The patient's appearance can provide important information (*see also* Chapter 1). The presence of vomitus can be a sign of increased ICP or drug intoxication. Urinary or fecal incontinence are frequently seen after seizures. Core body temperature can be elevated in infections, heat stroke, thyrotoxic crisis, drug toxicity and neurogenic hyperthermia. Hypothermia is most often secondary to exposure to cold. It is important to recognize that hypothermia blunts cortical and brainstem activity. Abnormalities in heart rate and blood pressure can be caused by endocrine, metabolic and cardiac abnormalities. The Kocher-Cushing reflex consists of hypertension, bradycardia and irregular respiration and is associated with elevated ICP and herniation. The presence of neck stiffness can indicate infectious or carcinomatous meningitis, subarachnoid hemorrhage or herniation. Examination of the fundi can reveal subhyaloid hemorrhages (associated with subarachnoid hemorrhage), papilledema (associated with increased ICP) or embolic material in form of Hollenhorst plaques (associated with carotid disease). Important clinical findings and their significance are summarized in Table 3.

The Neurological Examination

To confirm the presence of coma, the absence of any purposeful response must be demonstrated. Further examination should help determine whether the cause of coma lies in a toxic-metabolic insult or in structural damage. In cases of structural damage, the examination can provide clues that help with localization.

EVALUATION OF RESPIRATORY PATTERNS

Observing the patient's pattern of respiration can yield valuable clues for the localization of potential lesions. Breathing patterns observed in patients in coma include Cheyne-Stokes respiration, central neurogenic hyperventilation is sustained, rapid and deep hyperpnea, which results from injury to the midbrain tegmentum, apneusis, cluster breathing, ataxic breathing, and Kussmaul breathing. We have summarized in Table 4 the clinical and pathological features of these breathing patterns.

ASSESSMENT OF THE LEVEL OF CONSCIOUSNESS AND OF MOTOR RESPONSE

Assessment starts with observing the patient for any spontaneous movements. Whereas abnormal movements such as myoclonic jerks and spontaneous posturing may be present, purposeful movements should be absent. The patient is subsequently stimulated verbally and then by gentle shaking. If there is no response, noxious stimuli are applied in the form of supraorbital pressure, temporoman-

Table 3
Common Clinical Conditions Found in Patients in Coma With Their Clinical Findings and Recommended Initial Management

Condition	Possible findings	Recommended testing and/or action
Increased intracranial pressure	Papilledema, sixth cranial nerve palsies, Kocher-Cushing reflex (hypertension, bradycardia, and irregular respirations), presence of vomitus	Imaging study Depending on findings: ventriculostomy placement, intravenous mannitol, hyperventilation
Seizure activity	Eye deviation, pupillary asymmetry, urinary or fecal incontinence, tongue biting	Immediate treatment with antiepileptic drugs, followed by EEG
CNS infection	Meningeal signs, fever, petechial-purpuric rash (meningococcemia), Osler's nodes (subacute bacterial endocarditis), seizures, signs of increased intracranial pressure	Immediate initiation of antibiotics, followed by lumbar puncture
SAH	Meningeal signs, third nerve palsy or other cranial nerve findings, subhyaloid hemorrhages, papilledema or other signs of increased intracranial pressure	Head CT scanning If CT equivocal, then lumbar puncture
Liver failure	Icterus, ascites, gynecomastia, spider nevi, decreased axillary and pubic hair, hepatomegaly, testicular atrophy, fetor hepaticus	Liver function tests including ammonia levels

CNS, central nervous system; EEG, electroencephalography; SAH, subarachnoid hemorrhage.

dibular joint compression, rubbing the sternum, and applying nail bed pressure. Patients with high cervical cord damage or severe peripheral neuropathy may show no response to a sternal rub or nail bed pressure but may grimace to supraorbital pressure. Asymmetric grimacing can be due to damage to the facial nerve or the stimulated sensory pathways. A localizing response to pain, i.e., movement aimed at removing the stimulus, is not consistent with the diagnosis of coma. A more rudimentary withdrawal response can be generated at the spinal level. Asymmetry in withdrawal indicates unilateral damage to the motor or sensory pathways. If there is also a difference in tone or reflexes or a unilateral Babinski sign then the damage can be further localized to the descending corticospinal pathways.

In some patients painful stimulation will elicit a posturing response. Extension of the lower extremities with downward flexion and inward rotation of the feet is common to both decorticate and decerebrate posturing. Decorticate (flexor) posturing is associated with flexion of the arms and indicates damage to the upper midbrain above the level of the red nucleus. Decerebrate (extensor) posturing is associated with extension of the arms and it is caused by damage to the lower midbrain or upper pons. In reality, the localizing value of posturing responses may be limited because there is evidence that they can be caused by hemispheric dysfunction *(1)*. In any case, flexor posturing seems to correlate with more rostral and less severe lesions. Patients' response can fluctuate between decorticate

Table 4
Respiratory Patterns in Coma

Respiratory pattern		Typical underlying injury
Cheyne-Stokes	Waxing of frequency followed by waning and apnea	Metabolic disturbances, large bilateral hemispheric insults, congestive heart failure
Central neurogenic hyperventilation	Rapid and deep hyperpnea	Midbrain tegmentum
Apneusis	2–3 s long end-inspiratory pauses, sometimes alternating with end-expiratory pauses	Midpons, caudal pons
Cluster breathing	Periodic and irregular frequency and amplitude of respirations with irregular pauses between clusters	Lower pontine and rostral medullary lesions
Ataxic breathing	Irregular and uneven respirations with no recognizable pattern (preterminal states)	Reticular formation of the dorso-medial medulla
Kussmaul breathing	Deep, regular inspirations	Metabolic acidosis

and decerebrate and as mentioned previously, posturing can also occur spontaneously. We recommend that practitioners describe the abnormal movements seen rather than just use the terms decorticate and decerebrate.

EXAMINATION OF THE EYES

The pupils are inspected for symmetry, reactivity, size, and shape. The patient's eyes are initially observed in resting position *(15)*. Note is made of any spontaneous movements. Subsequently, reflex ocular movements are examined. A comprehensive review of the mechanisms underlying the control of pupillary reflexes and eye movements is provided in Chapter 30 and will not be dealt with here. Details on caloric stimulation are provided below.

COMPLETING THE ASSESSMENT OF BRAINSTEM FUNCTION

The corneal reflex is tested by touching the cornea with a throat swab, or alternatively by instilling a few drops of sterile water into each eye. Sensory innervation of the cornea is through the first division of the trigeminal nerve (V_1). The normal response is bilateral eye blinking mediated by the seventh nerves. Damage to V_1 causes a decreased or absent response bilaterally, whereas facial nerve damage will abolish the response only in the stimulated eye. Damage to the facial nerve can also cause asymmetry in grimacing to noxious stimulation. The gag reflex is elicited by touching the pillars of the palatal arch with a tongue blade or cotton swab and it allows an assessment of the glossopharyngeal (IX) and vagus (X) nerves. In intubated patients, sensory function of the vagus nerve is assessed by attempting to elicit a cough response with use of a suction catheter ("tracheal reflex").

Further Management

Further management of patients in coma is aimed at addressing the underlying etiologies and providing sufficient support in form of nutrition and physical therapy as outlined in other sections of this book. Patients are monitored and screened as needed in order to avoid complications. Daily bedside transcranial Doppler ultrasound (TCD), continuous ICP monitoring and continuous or intermittent EEG monitoring are used as needed.

Table 5
Outcome from Hypoxic-Ischemic Coma

Time after CPA	No. of brainstem reflex abnormalities[a]	No. of patients/ time interval	Survivors		p value[b]
			N	%	
0–3 h	0	5	4	80	
	1	13	6	46	
	2	7	2	29	= 0.07
	3	3	0	0	
0–6 h	0	10	8	80	
	1	19	7	37	
	2	11	3	27	<0.005
	3	6	0	0	
0–24 h	0	16	13	81	
	1	24	9	38	
	2	14	3	21	<0.0005
	3	9	0	0	
24–48 h	0	29	22	76	
	1	14	3	21	
	2	8	0	0	<0.0005
	3	3	0	0	

[a]Absent pupillary light reflex, absent corneal responses, absence of volitional EOM.

[b]Test of significance compared survival pf patients with reflex abnormalities against those with none; all tests were done by chi square with three degrees of freedom.

Source: Reprinted with permission from ref. *17*.

Patients with a protracted course need to be evaluated for placement of a percutaneous endogastric (PEG) tube and for tracheostomy (*see* Chapters 9 and 11). Complications can be avoided by using drugs for deep venous thrombosis and gastrointestinal tract prophylaxis (*see* Chapter 11). Pressure ulcers are avoided by nursing support and the use of special bedding equipment (*see* Chapter 33).

Outcome from Nontraumatic Coma

The outcome of nontraumatic coma depends mainly on three factors: underlying cause, severity, and duration. Coma induced by toxic or metabolic abnormalities carries the best prognosis with an overall mortality rate of 47%. Hypoxic-ischemic coma has an intermediate prognosis with regard to survival (58% mortality) but is the most likely to result in a persistent vegetative state *(16)*. In Table 5, we present the correlation between presence of brainstem reflexes and prognosis in hypoxic coma *(17)*. Cerebrovascular disease (including ischemic and hemorrhagic syndromes) carries the worst prognosis with a mortality that exceeds 70%. The overall likelihood of good recovery ranges from 5% in patients with subarachnoid hemorrhage or stroke to 25% in patients with toxic-metabolic insults or infectious disease *(16)*.

The severity of coma as assessed by the Glasgow Coma Scale is predictive of outcome as soon as 6 h after onset. All aspects of the scale have an independent predictive value. The overall chance of making a moderate to good recovery falls from 10% on admission to 7% by the third day and to 2% by the 14th day.

Outcome from Traumatic Coma

Posttraumatic coma generally carries a better prognosis in terms of both survival and likelihood of good recovery. In a study of 496 cases of posttraumatic coma of greater than 6-h duration, Pazzaglia et al. found a mortality of 49% *(18)*. Among the survivors, nearly 70% achieved complete social reintegration whereas only 20% remained fully dependent. The following observations were made about prognosis: (1) younger patients were more likely to recover; (2) the more caudal the location of the underlying lesions, the worse the outcome was; and (3) patients with surgical lesions had worse outcomes. Some of the patients included in the study were stuporous and not comatose. Later studies have essentially confirmed these observations. The most important variable for outcome seems to be the age of the patient. As a matter of fact, mortality and severe morbidity seem to increase in a nearly linear fashion with age. It is thought that this is partly because of the fact that serious posttraumatic complications such as subdural hematomas, intracranial hemorrhage, and subarachnoid hemorrhage all become more frequent with age *(19)*. The absence of brainstem reflexes, a low Glasgow Coma Scale score, and the presence of hypoxia or hypotension during the first 24 h after admission are further very important prognostic factors.

BRAIN DEATH

The Evolving Concept of Death

Death had always been associated with the cessation of cardiopulmonary function. With the advent of mechanical ventilation and advanced cardiac support, a new state emerged, in which patients could have sustained cardiopulmonary function in the apparent absence of cerebral function. Although descriptions of such patients can be found in the literature as early as 1956 *(20)*, it was in 1959 that Mollaret and Goulon systematically presented 23 patients with this condition which they coined "coma dépassé," i.e. irreversible coma *(21)*. In this paper, the authors discussed hallmarks of brain death such as the absence of brainstem function, the absence of spontaneous respiration, the cardio-vascular collapse that ensued without the use of pressors and many of the common associated medical complications. Ancient Greeks defined death as the moment when the soul abandons the body. Professor Goulon, faced with the care of those patients appropriately raised the question of "where the patient's soul dwelled" *(20)*. It became apparent that a new definition of death based on neuro-logical criteria was needed.

In the United States, the Uniform Determination of Brain Death Act now acknowledges the principle that death can be diagnosed when neurological criteria for brain death are met *(22)*. Brain death is defined as the irreversible cessation of function of the brain, including the brainstem *(23)*.

Causes and Incidence of Brain Death

The most common causes of brain death in adults are traumatic brain injury and subarachnoid hemorrhage, followed by hypoxic-ischemic brain damage and fulminant hepatic failure. It is estimated that the diagnosis of brain death is made 25–30 times a year in large referral centers *(24)*. In children, the most common cause of brain death is abuse, followed by motor vehicle accidents and asphyxia *(25)*.

Diagnosis of Brain Death: Current Practice

Although United States law acknowledges brain death, it does not define the diagnostic criteria to be applied. Institutions should base their practice on "accepted medical standards." Most institutions follow the recommendations published by the Quality Standards Subcommittee of the American Academy of Neurology in 1995 *(26)*. Those recommendations are outlined below with some minor modifications that reflect common clinical practice. These are guidelines and not standards and they apply to patients older than 18 yr. Guidelines for brain death determination in children will not be further discussed in this text.

Initial Approach to the Patient

The following prerequisites must be met prior to determination of brain death:

1. There must be clinical or neuroimaging evidence of an acute CNS catastrophe that is compatible with the clinical diagnosis of brain death. In most cases, head CT scanning will reveal appropriate findings such as

diffuse edema or mass lesions with severe shift and possibly herniation. However, in some instances, head CT scanning can be incompatible with the clinical examination. In such cases, obtaining a repeat scan is recommended. Lumbar puncture can aid in the diagnosis in case a fulminant infection is suspected. If cerebrospinal fluid studies and repeated neuroimaging fail to reveal any abnormalities, then the diagnosis of brain death should be reconsidered. In patients who are in coma of undetermined origin, a prolonged period of observation and additional confirmatory tests demonstrating absent cerebral flow are recommended *(27)*.

2. Complicating medical conditions that may confound clinical assessment, such as severe electrolyte, acid-base, or endocrine disturbances must be excluded.
3. There must be no evidence of intoxication, drug poisoning or neuromuscular blockade.
4. Core temperature must be 32°C (90°F) or above.
5. Significant hypotension (i.e., systolic blood pressure of <90 mmHg or mean arterial pressure of <60 mmHg) should be absent.

Clinical Examination

The three cardinal findings that must be documented are the presence of coma, the absence of brainstem reflexes, and the presence of apnea. A repeat neurological examination after 6 h is recommended. The apnea testing does not need to be repeated or can be performed after the second clinical examination.

DETERMINATION OF COMA

Using standardized tactile stimuli, the absence of eye opening and cerebral motor response in all extremities must be documented. The accepted stimuli are nail-bed pressure, supraorbital pressure, and temporomandibular joint compression. Sternal pressure is also commonly used. Triple flexion, the babinski sign, preserved deep tendon, abdominal and cremasteric reflexes, as well as responses such as sweating, blushing and tachycardia are consistent with the diagnosis of brain death. Brief, slow movements of the upper limbs, finger flexion and arm lifting can also occur, either spontaneously or after painful stimulation. As long as there is no full decerebrate or decorticate response, these movements can be considered to be generated at the spinal level. Respiratory-like movements, such as shoulder elevation and adduction, back arching, and intercostal expansion, without significant tidal volumes can also be accepted. More complex movements that have been referred to as "Lazarus signs" have also been described in patients who otherwise met all brain death criteria *(20)*. When in doubt, one should obtain confirmatory testing, such as EEG or a blood flow study.

EXAMINATION OF BRAINSTEM REFLEXES

Pupillary reflex to light should be absent (both direct and consensual responses). The pupils should be in midposition (4 mm) to dilated (9 mm). The shape of the pupils can be round, oval, or irregular. Oculocephalic reflex should be absent during testing with head turning and caloric testing. The head should not be turned if spinal instability is known or suspected. Prior to caloric testing, the head should be elevated to an angle of 30 degrees and the tympanic membrane should be visualized with an otoscope to make sure that there is no obstruction of the canal by blood or cerumen. Each ear must then be irrigated with 50–60 mL of ice water. The eyes must be observed for 1–3 min after irrigation and 5 min must be allowed between testing on each side. The corneal reflex is tested with a throat swab or by instilling sterile water into the eyes and should be absent. There should be no jaw reflex. No grimacing should be elicited by applying deep pressure on the nail beds, supraorbital ridge or temporomandibular joint. Stimulation of the posterior pharynx with a tongue blade should produce no response. There should also be no cough response to bronchial suctioning.

DETERMINATION OF APNEA

The technique of apneic diffusion oxygenation is used to confirm the absence of ventilatory drive. Apnea testing should only be performed under the following conditions: (1) core temperature of 36.5°C (97°F) or above; (2) systolic blood pressure of 90 mmHg or above; and (3) positive fluid balance over the previous 6 h. Ten minutes of preoxygenation with FiO_2 of 100% at a low respiratory rate of 10 is recommended. The goal is to achieve a PaO_2 of 200 mmHg or above and to reverse possible hypocapnia. Baseline arterial blood gas (ABG) is then assessed before the test begins. If possible, the $PaCO_2$ should be in the normal range of 35–45 mmHg. The patient is disconnected from the ventilator and a catheter is advanced through the endotracheal tube, delivering oxygen at a rate of 6 L/min. The catheter tip should be at the level of the carina. Oxygen saturation is monitored continuously by means of pulse oxymetry. The chest wall and the abdominal wall are observed for possible motion over the next 8–10 min. At that point, a second ABG sample is obtained and the patient is connected again to the ventilator. Alternatively, the apnea test can be continued until the results of the second ABG are available, and a third specimen can be drawn if the results do not satisfy the criteria for a "positive" test result.

If the apnea test result is "positive," i.e., it supports the diagnosis of brain death, if the second ABG sample shows a $PaCO_2$ of 60 mmHg or above, or if there has been an increase in $PaCO_2$ by at least 20 mmHg. The test is "negative" if any respiratory movements are observed. Testing must be interrupted if: (1) systolic blood pressure drops below 70–90 mmHg; (2) the patient becomes hypoxemic; and (3) significant cardiac arrhythmias occur. If ABG analysis at that time does not show adequate $PaCO_2$ elevation, it is recommended to perform a confirmatory study, such as electoencephalography (EEG) or a cerebral blood flow study.

Pitfalls in the Diagnosis of Brain Death

Confirmatory testing is recommended under the following circumstances that can interfere with the diagnosis of brain death: (1) severe facial trauma; (2) preexisting pupillary abnormalities; (3) toxic levels of any sedative drugs, aminoglycosides, tricyclic antidepressants, anticholinergics, antiepileptic drugs, chemotherapeutic agents, or neuromuscular blocking agents; and (4) sleep apnea or severe pulmonary disease resulting in chronic retention of CO_2.

Confirmatory Testing

Confirmatory tests are optional in adults, unless special circumstances exist, as outlined above. They should always be performed after the clinical assessment has been completed.

CEREBRAL ANGIOGRAPHY

Consistent with the diagnosis of brain death is the finding of absent filling at the level of the carotid bifurcation or the circle of Willis. The external carotid circulation is patent, and filling of the superior longitudinal sinus may be delayed.

ELECTROENCEPHALOGRAPHY

For the purpose of brain death confirmation, electrical activity must be recorded over a minimum of 30 min using a 16- to 18-channeled machine at a sensitivity of 2 μV/mm with a filter setting of 0.1 or 0.3 s and 70 Hz *(28)* *(see also* Chapter 6). In brain death, the electroencephalograph (EEG) shows loss of cerebral electrical activity (electrocerebral silence). It must be noted however, that electrical activity can persist transiently in some cases of clinically confirmed brain death. In a prospective study of 56 patients who fulfilled the clinical criteria for diagnosis of brain death, Grigg et al. reported persistent electrocerebral activity in nearly 20% of cases for as long as 168 h after the clinical diagnosis was made *(29)*.

TRANSCRANIAL DOPPLER

Transcranial Doppler (TCD) is performed at the bedside and has a high sensitivity and specificity *(30)*. As intracranial pressure (ICP) rises, the Doppler waveforms go through distinct changes until intracranial flow is eventually abolished (Fig. 1) *(31)*. Because of the fact that raised ICP is essential in producing these abnormal flow patterns, it has been recently proposed that TCD should not be used for confirming brain death in patients with large craniotomies or ventricular drains *(32)*. We present in Table 6 an algorithm for the use of TCD in brain death determination.

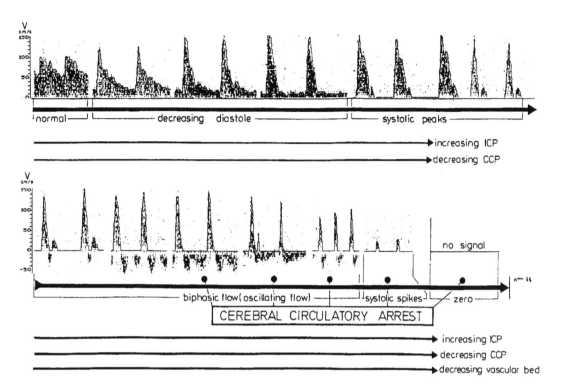

Fig. 1. As intracranial pressure (ICP) rises, it reaches values above the end-diastolic arterial blood pressure (ABP) and therefore starts compromising diastolic flow (middle portion, top figure). When ICP exceeds the diastolic ABP, diastolic flow ceases and only systolic peaks are seen (right end, top figure). Subsequently there is reverberating (oscillating) flow. The biphasic flow velocity spectrum consists of equivalent, opposing inflow and outflow components and the resulting time-averaged mean velocity is zero, i.e., effectively there is already circulatory arrest. In final stages flow consists only of very small brief spikes in early systole followed by no flow at all. The angiographic correlate of oscillating flow and systolic spikes is usually stasis filling (delayed and tapered filling of the intracranial arteries without venous drainage after 26 s). When Doppler signals are absent, angiography usually shows no filling of the intracranial vessels. Reprinted with permission from ref. *31*.

SINGLE PHOTON-EMISSION COMPUTED TOMOGRAPHY

The typical finding is that of absent uptake of isotope in the brain parenchyma ("hollow skull phenomenon").

SOMATOSENSORY-EVOKED POTENTIALS

Consistent with brain death is the bilateral absence of N20-P22 response with median nerve stimulation. The recordings should adhere to the minimal technical criteria for somatosensory evoked potential recording in suspected brain death as adopted by the American Electroencephalographic Society *(28)* (*see* Chapter 6).

Diagnosis of Brain Death Outside the United States

Although brain death is accepted throughout Europe, there is considerable variation in the diagnostic criteria that are used *(33)*. Many countries require the performance of a confirmatory test, and/or involvement of multiple physicians. In some countries repeated testing is mandatory after variable intervals.

Table 6
The Use of Transcranial Doppler for Brain Death Confirmation

Subjects:
Patients who fulfill clinical criteria for diagnosis of brain death and do not have ventricular
drains or large craniotomies that can prevent increases in intracranial pressure.

Examination technique:
Minimal requirement: Bilateral insonation with assessment of at least one artery on each side.
Recommended: Bilateral intra- and extracranial examination, performed twice with a 30-min
interval. Extracranial examination should include the internal and common carotid arteries
and the vertebral arteries.

Intracranial flow patterns consistent with brain death:
Reverberating (oscillating) flow or
Low amplitude (<50 cm/s), brief (<200 ms) spikes in early systole without diastolic flow or
absent intracranial flow in a patient who is known to have a temporal window. It is recommended to further confirm the diagnosis with a study of the extracranial vessels.

Organ Donation

The ethical basis for organ procurement is the concept of beneficence *(34)* (*see* Chapter 15). The
brain-dead person's organs can be used to improve the recipients' health status. This implies that
physicians have the ethical obligation to inform and request from families the possibility of organ
procurement. Also many families are comforted by the fact that amidst a painful and terrible situation
"a gift of life" has been given so that another person can be saved. It is mandatory in the United States
to report brain dead patients to local organ procurement organizations before they are removed from
the ventilator. If the family consents for organ donation cardiovascular and ventilatory support continue until the organs can be obtained. If the family refuses donation, or the patient is found not to be
a suitable candidate donor, then physicians can proceed with extubation. In most cases, organ donation is not performed when the family disagrees even if the patients had completed a Uniform Donor
Card, or had indicated on their drivers' license that they wished to be donors in the event of their
death. However, organ procurement organizations have different consent policies since a uniform
national policy has not yet been established *(34)*. For instance, the new Ohio Donor Registry, authorized by the Ohio Revised Code Sec. 2108.18 (General Assembly 123, Senate Bill 188) went into
effect on July 1, 2002. Such provision states that in Ohio persons who agree to be listed on the
Registry after this date have given legal consent for the anatomical gifts of their organs, tissues or
eyes upon their death. This allows for an anatomical donation to be executed without obtaining additional consent from the deceased's family.

It is generally agreed upon that although the concept of brain death was developed before the
advent of organ transplantation, an increased demand for the latter has promoted the legalization of
the former. A potential conflict of interest between healthcare teams and the deceased person exists
because the donor can be viewed as the only mean to organ donation *(34)*. Adhering to the axiom that
members of the transplantation team cannot be involved in determining brain death and having
empathetic and experienced physicians talk to the family increases the likelihood of obtaining consent for organ donation.

It is important to realize the public still has significant difficulties accepting and comprehending
the concept of brain death. This may be in part because the term is somewhat unfortunate in the sense
that it can be thought of implying a condition other than true death which is by nature irreversible.
This issue will possibly need to be revisited in the future. Conveying to the family that their loved one
is dead (and not brain dead) and that his or her organs can be temporarily preserved by artificial
means for the purpose of donation only might be more appropriate.

REFERENCES

1. Plum F, Posner JB. *The Diagnosis of Stupor and Coma*, 3rd ed. Philadelphia: FA Davis, 1982.
2. Saper CB. Brain stem modulation of sensation, movement and consciousness. In: Kandel ER, Schwartz JH, Jessell TM (eds.). *Principles of Neural Science*, 4th ed. New York: McGraw-Hill, 2000, pp. 889–909.
3. Jennett B, Plum F. Persistent vegetative state after brain damage: A syndrome in search of a name. *Lancet* 1972;1:734–737.
4. Levy DE, Bates D, Caronna JJ, et al. Prognosis in non-traumatic coma. *Ann. Intern. Med.* 1981;94:293–301.
5. The Multi-Society Task Force on PVS. Medical aspects of the persistent vegetative state—First of two parts. *N. Engl. J. Med.* 1994;330:1499–1508.
6. The Multi-Society Task Force on PVS. Medical aspects of the persistent vegetative state–Second of two parts. *N. Engl. J. Med.* 1994;330:1572–1579.
7. Gennarelli TA, Thibault LE, Adams JH, Graham DI, Thompson CJ, Marcincin RP. Diffuse axonal injury and traumatic coma in the primate. *Ann. Neurol.* 1982;12:564–574.
8. Adams JH, Graham DI, Jennett B. The neuropathology of the vegetative state after an acute brain insult. *Brain* 2000;123:1327–1338.
9. Giacino GT, Ashwal S, Childs N, et al. The minimally conscious state. Definition and diagnostic criteria. *Neurology* 2002;58:349–353.
10. Shewmon DA. The minimally conscious state. Definition and diagnostic criteria [letter]. *Neurology* 2002;58:506.
11. Coleman D. The minimally conscious state. Definition and diagnostic criteria [letter]. *Neurology* 2002;58:506.
12. Cartlidge N. States related to or confused with coma. *J. Neurol. Neurosurg. Psychiatry* 2001;71(Suppl 1):i18–i19.
13. Patterson JR, Grabois M. Locked in syndrome: A review of 139 cases. *Stroke* 1986;17:758–764.
14. McCusker EA, Rudick RA, Honch GW, et al. Recovery from the locked in syndrome. *Arch. Neurol.* 1982;39:145–147.
15. Fisher CM. Some neuro-ophthalmological observations. *J. Neurol. Neurosurg. Psychiatry* 1967;30:383–392.
16. Bates D. The prognosis of medical coma. *J. Neurol. Neurosurg. Psychiatry* 2001;71(Suppl 1):i20–i23.
17. Snyder B. Neurologic prognosis after cardiopulmonary arrest: IV. Brainstem reflexes. *Neurology* 1981;31:1092–1097.
18. Pazzaglia P, Frank G, Frank F, Gaist G. Clinical course and prognosis of acute post-traumatic coma. *J. Neurol. Neurosurg. Psychiatry* 1975;38:149–154.
19. Andrews BT. Prognosis in severe head injury. In Cooper PR, Golfinos JG, eds. *Head Injury*, 4th ed. New York: McGraw-Hill, 2000:555–563.
20. Wijdicks EFM. *Brain Death*. Philadelphia: Lippincott Williams & Wilkins, 2001.
21. Mollaret P, Goulon M. Le coma dépassé. *Rev. Neurol.* 1959;101:3–15.
22. Uniform determination of brain death act, 12 Uniform Laws Annotated (U.L.A.) 589 (West 1993 and West Supp. 1997).
23. Guidelines for the determination of death: report of the Medical Consultants on the Diagnosis of Death to the President's Commission for the Study of Ethical Problems in Medicine and Biomedical and Behavioral Research. *JAMA* 1981;246:2184–2186.
24. Wijdicks EFM. The diagnosis of brain death. *N. Engl. J. Med.* 2001;344:1215–1221.
25. Ashwal S, Schneider S. Brain death in children. *Pediatr. Neurol.* 1987;3:5–11.
26. The Quality Standards Subcommittee of the American Academy of Neurology. Practice parameters for determining brain death in adults (Summary statement). *Neurology* 1995;45:1012–1014.
27. Wijdicks EFM. Determining Brain death in adults. *Neurology* 1995;45:1003–1011.
28. American EEG Society. Guidelines in EEG and evoked potentials. *J. Clin. Neurophysiol.* 1994;11:1–143.
29. Grigg MM, Kelly MA, Celesia GG, Ghobrial MW, Ross ER. Electroencephalographic activity after brain death. *Arch. Neurol.* 1987;44:948–954.
30. Petty GW, Mohr JP, Pedley TA, et al. The role of Transcranial Doppler in confirming brain death: Sensitivity, specificity, and suggestions for performance and interpretation. *Neurology* 1990;40:300–303.
31. Hassler W, Steinmetz H, Pirschel J. Transcranial Doppler study of intracranial circulatory arrest. *J. Neurosurg.* 1989;71:195–201.
32. Ducrocq X, Hassler W, Moritake K, et al. Consensus opinion on diagnosis of cerebral circulatory arrest using Doppler-sonography: Task Force Group on Cerebral Death of the Neurosonology Research Group of the World Federation of Neurology. *J. Neurol. Sci.* 1998;159:145–150.
33. Haupt WF, Rudolf J. European brain death codes: a comparison of national guidelines. *J. Neurol.* 1999;246:432–437.
34. Brain death and organ transplantation. In Bernat JL. *Ethical Issues in Neurology*, 2nd ed. Boston: Butterworth-Heinemann, 2002:262–265.

17

Endovascular Therapy and Neurosciences Critical Care

Jawad F. Kirmani, Ricardo A. Hanel, Andrew R. Xavier, Abutaher M. Yahia, and Adnan I. Qureshi

INTRODUCTION

The field of endovascular or neurointerventional therapy for patients harboring various intra and extracranial processes has evolved significantly in the past decade. Currently, most tertiary care facilities offer these therapeutic maneuvers in the United States. Because medical care of this patient population is usually provided in the neurosciences critical care unit (NSU) it seems appropriate to discuss this topic in this book. We will describe current indications as well as pre- and postprocedural management in patients with acute ischemic stroke, arterial stenosis, subarachnoid hemorrhage (SAH), cerebral venous thrombosis (CVT), neoplasms, traumatic arterial lesions, and arteriovenous malformations (AVM).

ACUTE ISCHEMIC STROKE

Stroke is the leading cause of disability and third leading cause of death in the United States. By the year 2050, an estimated 1 million people will suffer from stroke every year because of changes in age and ethnic distribution. Data compiled by the Stroke Prevention Patient Outcomes Research Team indicate that annually there are as many as 550,000 hospitalizations and 150,000 deaths attributable to stroke in the United States *(1)* *(see* Chapter 18).

Intravenous (IV) recombinant plasminogen activator (rt-PA) remains the only approved therapy for the acute ischemic stroke treatment strategy to establish reperfusion. The direct intra-arterial (IA) infusion of thrombolytic therapy may serve as an adjunct or an alternative to IV thrombolysis. This approach has advantages of direct visualization of clot, may allow possible mechanical manipulation of clot for disintegration and a theoretical advantage of delivery of high concentration of drug directly to the clot and thus minimizing possible systematic complications.

Anterior Circulation

Recanalization of acutely occluded arteries in the carotid territory, particularly the middle cerebral artery, by IA delivery of thrombolytic drugs, has advanced dramatically over the last decade. Randomized prospective studies have begun to show potential benefit and positive impact of neuroendovascular intervention. Still, the patient selection, therapeutic window, NSU support, and the management experience of the team seem to determine the course and outcome of IA therapy.

From: *Current Clinical Neurology*
Critical Care Neurology and Neurosurgery
Edited by: J. I. Suarez © Humana Press Inc., Totowa, NJ

Nonrandomized studies for the IA therapy in acute stroke have demonstrated higher recanalization rate than the IV therapy; generally rates of 50–80% recanalization, either partial or complete, have been reported. IA approach allows precise determination of site occlusion, presence of collateral supply, and response to thrombolysis. Recently, the Qureshi grading system has helped correlate clinical outcome to angiographic findings *(2)*. The six grades used in this scheme have also allowed precise angiographic evaluation of perfusion changes (Fig. 1). The rate of ICH in IA therapy has ranged from 2% to 11%. The primary agents used have been rt-PA, urokinase, prourokinase, and reteplase.

The only two randomized controlled trials of IA therapy for acute stroke have been performed with prourokinase *(3)*. The Prolyse in Acute Cerebral Thromboembolism Trial (PROACT) was a phase II trial that enrolled patients that presented within 6 h of symptom onset who had angiographically demonstrable occlusions of the middle cerebral artery. Forty-six patients were randomized in 2:1 fashion to either receive 6 mg of IA prourokinase or placebo. No mechanical disruption was allowed in this trial. Patients had all received a bolus of heparin at 100 U/kg followed by a constant infusion at 1000 U/h for the next 4 h. After the review by external safety monitoring board of 16 treated patients, the guidelines were changed to give initial bolus of 2000 U followed by 500 U/h maintenance dose. Partial or complete recanalization at 120 min was observed in 58% in the treated group and was significantly higher from the placebo group with a recanalization rate of 14%.

Following the initial successful results of the PROACT I, a larger trial PROACT II was undertaken *(4)*. This study was a Phase III multicenter, randomized, double-blinded, placebo controlled trial enrolling 180 patients. The median National Institute of Health Stroke Scale (NIHSS) Score was 17 and the median time to treatment was 5.3 h for both groups. Again, mechanical disruption was not allowed. Patients treated with prourokinase were significantly more likely to have good outcome at 90 d than were placebo-treated patients (40 % vs 25%, $p = 0.043$). The use of thrombolytic agents currently available and research involving the next generation of these agents open a field that shows promise for the improvement of outcomes of patients whose typical prognosis of meaningful recovery without severe disability is poor *(5)*.

Posterior Circulation

Ischemia in the territory of the basilar artery involves the pons, midbrain, cerebellum, thalami, and the occipital lobes. The onset may be abrupt or stuttering over several days. Involvement of reticular formation leads to impairment in level of consciousness. The patients who are in coma for longer than 6 h, who are ventilator-dependent, and who have lost most of their brainstem reflexes are poor candidates for the IA therapy.

The poor prognosis of basilar artery occlusions approaches 80–90% despite use of antiplatelet and anticoagulation *(6,7)*. There is no placebo-controlled equivalent study of posterior circulation stroke *(8)*. In the past few years, a number of uncontrolled series have emerged with promising results especially considering the poor natural history of posterior circulation strokes. It should be noted however that in posterior circulation ischemia, thrombolytics have been successfully given after 6 h of stroke onset and as late as 79 h after the onset *(9)*. The general consensus among the interventionalists, until controlled studies are available, is to treat patients with ischemic stroke in progression, incomplete deficit of brainstem function, basilar artery embolism and acute bilateral vertebral artery occlusion, when presenting within 6 h of symptoms onset.

Nonthrombolytic Interventional Techniques

In a patient with slow or ineffective response to IA thrombolytic agents, or in whom the concern is to minimize the dose of the thrombolytic agent, clot disruption aimed at increasing the surface area has been found to be effective. Balloons either soft, stiffer or wire-directed with cutting edges can be used for fragmenting the clot, depending on its location *(10)*. The balloons have a potential of causing

Grade 0	No occlusion		
Grade 1	MCA occlusion (M3 segment)	ACA occlusion (A2 or distal segments)	1 BA/VA branch occlusion
Grade 2	MCA occlusion (M2 segment)	ACA occlusion (A1 and A2 segments)	≥2 BA/VA branch occlusions
Grade 3	MCA occlusion (M1 segment)		
3A	Lenticulostriate arteries spared and/or leptomeningeal collaterals visualized		
3B	No sparing of lenticulostriate arteries nor leptomeningeal collaterals visualized		
Grade 4	ICA occlusion (collaterals present)	BA occlusion (partial filling direct or via collaterals)	
4A	Collaterals fill MCA	Anterograde filling*	
4B	Collaterals fill ACA	Retrograde filling*	
Grade 5	ICA occlusion (no collaterals)	BA occlusion (complete)	

Fig. 1. Diagrammatic representation of the proposed Qureshi Grading Scheme with grades of increasing severity of arterial occlusion. ACA, anterior cerebral artery; BA, basilar artery; ICA, internal carotid artery; MCA, middle cerebral artery; VA, vertebral artery; *, the predominant pattern of filling. From Qureshi A. *Neurosurgery* 2002;50:1405–1415, with permission.

arterial rupture or dissections; therefore, utmost care should be taken in their use. A microwire may also be used to safely fragment the clot. The procedure has to be gentle to avoid possible perforation or dissection of the target vessel. Passing a microcatheter through the matrix of the clot may help to form channels within the clot increasing the penetration of thrombolytics into it *(5)*. Various snare devices are now available that may be effective in breaking the clot or in some instances even retract the whole clot from the artery. Recently several companies have embarked upon development of rheolytic agents and distal protection devices. Rheolytic agents involve a high-velocity jet of saline to disrupt the clot. The distal protection devices use strategies to deploy and use devices to catch the resultant debris from disruption of the clot down stream from the site of the occlusion and therefore possibly prevent secondary embolic phenomenon.

Discovery of a critical extracranial or intracranial stenosis during the course of acute thrombolytic treatment is not uncommon. These critical stenoses sometimes necessitate acute intervention with angioplasty and even stenting as described later *(11)*. Different antiplatelet agents such as aspirin, clopidogrel and glycoprotein (GP) IIb/IIIa inhibitors are used to prevent rethrombosis of the stent.

Pharmacologic Intervention for Prevention of Thrombosis

Thrombosis can be prevented by inhibiting two major steps, platelet adhesion and aggregation (antiplatelet agents) and tissue factor-induced activation of thrombin and fibrinogen (anticoagulation agents). The intravenous administration of a heparin bolus (70 U/kg) before thrombolysis, to maintain the activated clotting time (ACT) between 250 and 300 s, may be considered. Postthrombolytic use of heparin to prevent reocclusion is recommended for patients with partial recanalization, arterial dissection, or persistent distal emboli not amenable to selective thrombolysis. Intravenous heparin administration should be titrated to maintain activated partial thromboplastin times of 1.5 to 2.3 times the control values *(12)*.

In patients status poststent placement and angioplasty, the high complication rates and the failure to prevent subacute thrombosis by the anticoagulation agents such as heparin, coumadin, and low-molecular-weight heparin, has prompted a search for alternative antithrombotic regimens, with emphasis on antiplatelet agents rather than anticoagulants. This was supported by evidence suggesting that local platelet deposition and activation are the major factors in thrombosis after angioplasty and stent placement. The systematic overview of the Antiplatelet Trialists' Collaboration provides unequivocal evidence that aspirin therapy reduces by one half the odds of arterial or graft occlusion among patients who have undergone a range of vascular operations, including coronary artery or peripheral vessel surgery and angioplasty *(13)*.

Aspirin, unlike the newer antiplatelet agents, does not affect platelet secretion and thus has no effect on local accumulation of platelet-derived mitogenic factors. These mitogenic factors promote cellular proliferation and lead to restenosis and accelerated atherosclerosis after angioplasty. Another limitation of aspirin therapy is that individual responses to it vary unpredictably. Ticlopidine and its recently developed analog clopidogrel are thienopyridine derivatives that inhibit platelet aggregation. The inhibition of platelet aggregation by both agents is concentration dependent. Adequate inhibition with ticlopidine (500 mg daily) or clopidogrel (75 mg daily) requires 2–3 d after the initiation of therapy. Although ticlopidine and clopidogrel have not been compared, recent studies suggest that clopidogrel is more effective than either aspirin or ticlopidine in preventing coronary stent thrombosis caused by high shear stress. New classes of drugs that inhibit GP IIb/IIIa receptors prevent the binding of fibrinogen to these receptors, thereby inhibiting platelet aggregation irrespective of the metabolic pathway responsible for the initiation of platelet aggregation. In Phase II trials with human subjects, abciximab, integrilin, lamifiban, and tirofiban, all of which are administered parenterally, have been demonstrated to be potent inhibitors of platelet aggregation, with acceptable safety profiles. The beneficial reduction in ischemic complications demonstrated in coronary interventions has led to the frequent use of intravenous GP IIb/IIIa as an adjunct to neurointerventional procedures *(13)*. Antiplatelet therapy is now used extensively for prophylaxis of thromboembolic events in the acute and chronic periods after endovascular procedures *(13)*.

General Measures in Neurosciences Critical Care Unit

In addition to the specific therapies and endovascular treatment outlined above the NSU care of acute ischemic stroke patients involve general therapeutic measures (*see also* Chapter 18). After the femoral sheath is removed, and if no closure devices are used, care is taken to properly clamp and hold the leg immobile to avoid the groin hematomas and potential bleeding complications. In cases of either local or systemic bleeding complications, rapid measures are taken including transfusion of fresh frozen plasma to reverse the coagulopathy and blood transfusions to maintain the hematocrit close to or above 30% and hemodynamic stability.

The general aims are to optimize the cerebral perfusion pressure (CPP), oxygenation and metabolism, and to avoid complications *(14)*. Respiratory care includes ensuring patency of airways, enriching inspired air with oxygen, and preventing and treating the pulmonary complications. Deep vein thrombosis prophylaxis is regularly used. When using mechanical ventilation positive end expiratory pressure (PEEP) is usually kept below 10 cm H_2O to minimize the possibility of decreased cerebral venous return and increased intracranial pressure (ICP). Patients with large infarcts need measures to control the increased ICP. Many pharmacological agents, hyperventilation and hypothermia can be employed as temporary measures. Definitive surgical options remain controversial. Management of blood pressure in stroke patients is very critical and CPP should be maintained at greater than 65

Table 1
Exclusion Criteria

NASCET exclusion criteria
Age 80 or greater*
Inability to give informed consent (mentally incompetent)
No angiography of bilateral carotids and intracranial branches available
Intracranial occlusive lesion which is more severe than the carotid lesion
Organ failure of kidney, or lung, or had cancer likely to cause death within 5 yr
Cerebral infarction on either side which deprived patient of all useful function
Symptoms attributable to nonatherosclerotic disease*
Cardiac disease associated with cardioembolic symptoms
Previous ipsilateral carotid endarterectomy*

NASCET temporary exclusion criteria
Uncontrolled hypertension*
Uncontrolled diabetes mellitus*
Myocardial infarction within 6 mo*
Unstable angina pectoris*
Signs of progressive neurologic dysfunction*
Contralateral carotid endarterectomy within 4 mo*
Major surgery within 30 d*

*May be candidates for carotid angioplasty and stent placement.

mmHg. Rapid fluctuations of blood pressures are detrimental. Also aggressive lowering of blood pressure in the initial 48 h of stroke is not recommended *(15–17)*. It is important that patients are maintained normoglycemic, normothermic and disturbances of any serum electrolyte imbalance carefully managed. Initial hydration and subsequent euvolumia is recommended *(18)*.

EXTRACRANIAL AND INTRACRANIAL OCCLUSIVE DISEASE

Extracranial Arterial Stenosis

The results of the North American Symptomatic Carotid Artery Trial (NASCET) have become the standard of safety and efficacy in symptomatic carotid artery intervention *(19)*. The overall perioperative stroke or death rate in NASCET was 6.5% with permanent death or disability of 2% of patients. Lesser complications included postoperative wound complications (9.3%), cranial nerve injury (8.6%), and general medical complications (8.1%) *(19)*. For symptomatic patients with greater than 70% stenosis, carotid endarterectomy yielded an absolute risk reduction for ipsilateral hemispheric stroke *(20)*. In patients with symptomatic carotid stenosis of 50–69%, the absolute risk reduction for ipsilateral stroke was still significant at 6.5%.

These outcomes and safety figures for the various subgroups of the NASCET trial set a high standard that must be equaled or surpassed to become an acceptable standard of care for carotid stenosis. In the absence of a randomized study, carotid angioplasty and stent placement is reserved for the patients who are poor candidates for carotid endarterectomy. Patients were excluded from the NASCET study for any of the reasons depicted in Table 1. The majority of evidence available indicates that carotid angioplasty and stenting offers an apparently reasonable alternative to medical or surgical therapy in patients with symptomatic disease and comorbid factors that increase the risk of endarterectomy *(21,22)*.

Cerebral hyperperfusion is a well recognized but an uncommon complication of both carotid endarterectomy and carotid angioplasty. It is related to transient hyperemia of the ipsilateral circulation after revascularization of the carotid artery. In a small series, risk of hyperemia was directly

**Table 2
Complications Associated With Extracranial
Carotid Angioplasty and Stent Placement**

Intraprocedure
1. Dissection
2. Embolization (distal)
3. Stent thrombosis
4. Bradycardia
5. Hypotension
6. Hyperperfusion brain injury

Postprocedure
1. Distal embolization
2. Stent thrombosis
3. Hyperperfusion related neurologic deficit
4. Postprocedure hypotension
5. Femoral bleeding resistant to compression
6. Femoral arteriovenous fistula
7. Femoral pseudoaneurysm
8. Myocardial infarction
9. Cardiac conduction abnormalities

associated with the degree of stenosis and evidence of extensive small vessel disease in the white matter and/or lacunar infarctions *(13)*.

The significance of microembolic events in the endovascular procedures involving revascularization cannot be understated. It has been shown, with the use of transcranial Doppler ultrasound, that embolic phenomenon occurs frequently and persists with increased frequency compared with baseline for hours or even days after the angioplasty *(23,24)*. Only small portions of these events correlate with easily detectable clinical deficits. Embolic showers to the intracranial circulation are more frequently seen with Doppler monitoring during the angioplasty than during endarterectomy *(25)*. A prospective study of neuropsychological deficits outcome after carotid angioplasty and carotid endarterectomy patients demonstrated that 20–25% of patients had neuropsychological abnormalities at 6 wk after either procedure without any significant differences *(26)*. Different studies have indicated that high grade lesions with greater than 90% stenosis *(27)*, advanced age *(28)*, long or multiple stenosis *(13,28)*, and symptomatic lesions are more highly correlated with clinically significant embolic events. The potential complications associated with extracranial angioplasty and stenting are outlined in Table 2. The case depicted in Fig. 2 illustrates the application of endovascular intervention in carotid endarterectomy restenosis and subsequent revascularization.

Extracranial Vertebral Artery Angioplasty and Stenting

Extracranial atherosclerotic disease of the vertebral artery is common and most often involves the ostium. Surgical options are limited and difficult for patients considered candidates because of their symptoms. Endarterectomy and bypass have been some of the options tried in the past *(31)*. Balloon angioplasty has been an option and has also met with some clinical success in the reported case series. However a high rate of restenosis because of the recoil nature of these lesions particularly when calcified, and propensity to dissect easily if overdilation is attempted is one of the major limiting factors *(30)*. With any operative endovascular attempts of posterior circulation, an immediate postoperative care in the NSU is essential to look for any deficits involving the cerebellum and brainstem.

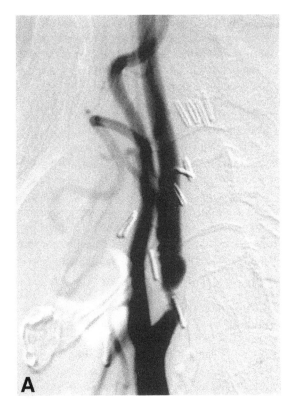 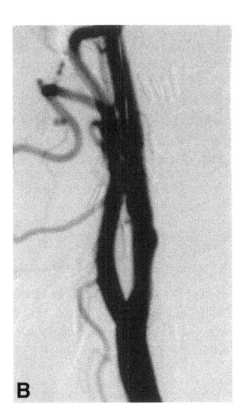

Fig. 2. A 75-yr-old woman who underwent a carotid endarterectomy 5 yr earlier presented with a severe (89%) asymptomatic left carotid restenosis (**A**), which was successfully treated with carotid angioplasty followed by stent placement (**B**).

Dissection of Carotid and Vertebral Artery

Dissection of the cervical carotid artery or vertebral artery can occur spontaneously, following injury, or in association with connective tissue disease affecting the arterial wall. When anticoagulation therapy has failed or is contraindicated options for endovascular occlusion or endovascular reconstruction using stents should be explored.

Intracranial Arterial Lesions

It has been estimated that intracranial atherosclerotic stenotic lesions carry a risk of stroke of 10–56% per year and is strongly correlated with the possibility of death from ischemic heart disease *(31,32)*. A small, retrospective study of warfarin versus aspirin in the treatment of intracranial stenosis indicates a slightly greater efficacy of warfarin in the subset of symptomatic patients *(33)*. In the absence of evidence the endovascular intervention is usually reserved for the symptomatic patients in whom medical therapy failed. The high risk for any intracranial endovascular procedure has to be recognized. Compared with the extracranial arteries, the intracranial arteries are deficient in adventitia and external elastic lamina. This increases the risk of rupture even during minor over sizing of the balloon during angioplasty *(34)*.

If procedural complications are minimized the successful treatment of stenotic disease resistant to medical therapy seems to be effective in different case series reported over the last few years *(12,35,36)*. With a variety of coronary stents now available, the question of whether angioplasty may be safer and more durable if supported by stent deployment arises. Stent placement has been used routinely at some centers for cases of acute vessel occlusion secondary to dissection following angioplasty.

Postprocedure Medication Protocols

Most of the medication protocols have evolved from the cardiac literature involving coronary stenting. The use of clopidogrel or ticlodipine in combination with aspirin 3 d before the procedure and 4–6 wk afterward has become standard of care in most institutions. Abciximab, eptifibatide, and tirofiban have also been used in conjunction with the above medications. Heparinazation during the procedure with ACT higher than 300 s is also used. Lower levels of anticoagulation are used when GPIIb/IIIa inhibitors are used. With the administration of multiple antithrombotic and anticoagulant agents recognition of risks of primary or postembolic hemorrhagic events in the postprocedural period is important. Anecdotally, intravenous glycopyrolate has also been used during carotid stent and angioplasty to reduce reflex bradycardia and hypotension resulting from carotid manipulation.

General Measures in Neurosciences Critical Care Unit

NSU care should focus on careful monitoring of neurological, respiratory, and cardiovascular function. Careful management of groin sheaths to avoid hematomas and compromise of perfusion to the lower extremity is mandatory. These patients are observed in the NSU for at least first 12–24 h. Special emphasis is on the neurological monitoring and any changes in examination should be aggressively investigated and treated. In such situations, head CT scanning should be obtained. Once the possibility of intracranial hemorrhage has been excluded and the patient has persistent neurologic deficits, CPP should be maximized (*see also* Chapters 3, 5, and 19). Sustained perioperative hypertension is preferably treated with continuous intravenous infusions of antihypertensive agents to allow for smooth control (*see also* Chapter 13). Bradyarrhythmias are a distinct possibility in carotid artery manipulations making dopamine the vasopressor of choice due to its strong inotropic and chronotropic actions resulting in an increase in cardiac output and CPP (*see* Chapter 8).

SUBARACHNOID HEMORRHAGE

SAH is a common and often devastating occurrence. Each year, approx 30,000 Americans have nontraumatic aneurysmal SAH *(37)*. Population-based incidence rates for SAH vary from 6 to 16 per 100,000 *(37)*. Despite considerable advances in diagnostic techniques, surgical, endovascular and anesthetic techniques, and perioperative management, the outcome of patients with SAH remains poor, with overall mortality rates of 25% and significant morbidity among approx 50% of survivors (*see also* Chapter 20).

Despite all therapeutic possibilities, a good number of SAH patients develop angiographic or clinical vasospasm, which is responsible for high mortality and morbidity. Early aneurysm surgery followed by hypervolemic, hypertensive therapy has been the treatment of choice to prevent and treat this clinical and radiological entity. Pharmacologic treatment with calcium channel blockers has been shown to improve the final outcome *(38)*. In 1987 the Cooperative Aneurysm Study reported an incidence of angiographic vasospasm of more than 50%, with symptomatic vasospasm in 32% of 1378 SAH patients at 71 centers *(39)*. These values have remained consistent with more contemporary retrospective reviews *(40,41)*.

In a small subset of patients, early vasospasm can be seen immediately following SAH. Usually the vasospasm is delayed and has a typical temporal course, with onset 3–5 d after the hemorrhage, maximal narrowing at 5–14 d, and gradual resolution over 2–4 wk. In about half of cases, vasospasm is manifested by the occurrence of a delayed neurological ischemic deficit, which can lead to stroke, disability and death. In contemporary series, 15–20% of such patients suffer stroke or die from vasospasm despite maximal therapy *(42)*. The delayed ischemic neurological deficit associated with symptomatic vasospasm usually appears shortly after the onset of angiographic vasospasm with the acute or subacute development of focal or generalized symptoms and signs *(43)*. Progression to cerebral infarction occurs in approx 50% of symptomatic cases; recovery without deficit in the remaining individuals may occur despite the persistence of angiographic vasospasm.

Endovascular therapy offers an additional treatment for these patients who continue to have delayed ischemic neurological deficits despite optimal medical management. It is preceded by head CT scanning to ensure that no large hemorrhage, hydrocephalus or recent infarctions are present. Monitoring of intracranial and cadiac hemodynamics is performed closely. Once transferred to the angiography suite heparinization is performed and maintained during the procedure. Presently, the most commonly employed treatments are angioplasty and/or IA administration of papaverine.

Percutaneous Transluminal Angioplasty

With the availability of smaller balloons and more navigable catheters almost all vessels can undergo angioplasty. The mechanism of action of balloon angioplasty is poorly understood. At a cellular level it is thought that fragmentation of collagen fibres and myocytes result in permanent restoration of vessel diameter *(44)*. Because the effects of angioplasty seem to be more sustained this is a preferred treatment. It is however more effective in treating larger proximal segments of the vessels rather than distal ones.

Balloon angioplasty has been associated with complications including aneurysm rupture if incompletely obliterated, vessel rupture or thrombosis, and reperfusion hemorrhage *(45)*. The case depicted in Fig. 3 illustrates application of endovascular intervention in a patient with symptomatic cerebral vasospasm.

Intra-Arterial Papaverine

IA papavarine injection is achieved with small repeated injections with superselective catheter positioning just proximal to the affected area of the vessel *(46)*. Papavarine hydrochlororide is an alkaloid now manufactured synthetically. It acts on the smooth muscle cells through inhibition of cyclic adenosine monophosphate (cAMP) phosphodiesterase activity thereby increasing the levels of cAMP. It may also exert its effect by blocking calcium ion channels.

The results of the endovascular papaverine therapy are derived from case series. Papaverine is usually reserved for the treatment of vessel segments inaccessible to angioplasty and when it is desirable to dilate distal segments of the vessels. The effect of papavarine is usually not sustained and a high rate of recurrence of vasospasm is observed *(47–49)*.

Use of papaverine has been associated with transient rise in ICP and therefore it has been recommended to use ICP monitoring during infusion if indicated. Other reported complications include the possible formation of crystal emboli causing monocular blindness, brainstem dysfunction with respiratory and hemodynamic compromise, and other focal neurologic deficits that are usually transient.

Improvement in NSU monitoring and diagnostic studies has allowed rapid identification of patients who are reaching critical reductions in cerebral blood flow. The effects of endovascular treatment have been limited to documentation of improvement of vessel diameter, improvement of cerebral blood flow, and reversal of neurologic deficits. With further experience and newer devices, the complications related to treatment have decreased. A more rigorous assessment of the effects of the interventional approach would require further trials *(50)*.

CEREBRAL VENOUS SINUS THROMBOSIS

CVT is an infrequent but important disorder that must be recognized and treated promptly. The mortality rate associated with this condition is high, ranging from 5% to 30% *(51)*. CVT includes not only dural sinus thrombosis but also cortical and deep cerebral veins. The real incidence is still unknown but based on autopsy studies it may vary from 0.03% to 9% *(52)* (*see* Chapter 21).

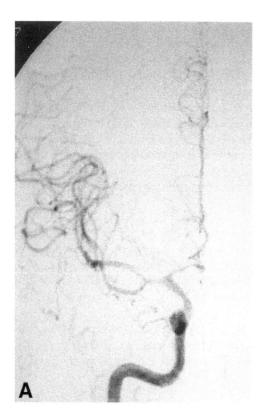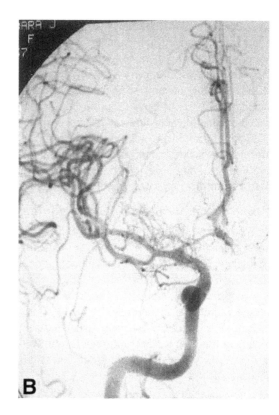

Fig. 3. Severe vasospasm after subarachnoid hemorrhage demonstrated on this right sided antero-posterior view of carotid angiogram (**A**), which was resistant to traditional medical management. The patient underwent angioplasty of the supraclinoidal segment of the right internal carotid artery, and proximal segments of both middle and anterior cerebral arteries with improvement of filling in distal circulation (**B**).

The clinical features of CVT are unspecific, varying from mild headache and focal neurologic signs to catastrophic progressive rise in ICP leading to neurological deterioration and death. The interruption of outflow in the brain circulation leads to augmentation in the pressure of the whole vascular system with venous hypertension, intracranial hypertension and hemorrhagic events.

Several conditions can predispose a person to develop CVT including trauma, neoplasms, and infections. The latter may account for 8.2% of cases (53). Outcome of CVT patients is closely related to initial clinical picture (51,54,55). Patients presenting with headache and papilledema alone have good prognosis whereas those with rapid onset, early reduced Glasgow Coma Scale score, focal neurological signs, seizures, and concomitant infection do not (*see also* Chapter 21). Due to its relative rarity and variable clinical features, the key for the diagnosis is a high level of suspicion (52).

The treatment of choice for CVT remains controversial. The main goal of treatment should be the recanalization of venous drainage system with complete reestablishment of normal brain circulation. The Stroke editorial "Cerebral venous thrombosis: nothing, heparin, or local thrombolysis?" written by Bousser in 1999 shows how weak the evidence is toward each therapeutic option. In most centers, including ours, the treatment of choice is intravenous heparin followed by thrombolysis, if indicated (56). Even though the studies are small, heparin use may be safe even in the presence of intracranial hemorrhage (57–59).

In our institution we reserve the endovascular approach for patients who demonstrate clinical worsening despite adequate intravenous coagulation and treatment of overlying etiology. Those patients presenting with contraindication for systemic anticoagulation may also be treated with thrombolysis. The endovascular route used is the transvenous approach through the femoral vein, navigating the catheter into the venous circulation and final placement in the matrix of the thrombus. The thrombolytics are infused over hours for a better recanalization. The rate of recanalization (partial and total) ranges from 70% to 95% *(60–62)*. There is a low risk of intracranial hemorrhagic complication in published series.

Small series of cases have documented the use of mechanical devices to facilitate the thrombolysis process. Chaloupka et al. described the use of microballoon transluminal angioplasty in a case of superior sagital sinus occlusion reistant to urokinase infusion *(63)*. Malek et al. reported the use of angioplasty and stenting in a case of pansinus thrombosis refractory to anticoagulant therapy, which provided sustained venous outflow *(64)*. A rheolytic thrombectomy catheter, Angiojet (Possis Medical, Minneapolis, MN) has been described as a useful adjuvant in some cases *(65–67)*.

NEOPLASTIC LESIONS

Endovascular treatment of central nervous system (CNS) tumors is targeted at devascularization and superselective delivery of chemotherapy. Endovascular techniques are particularly valuable in preoperative embolization of highly vascular tumors and tumors involving difficult surgical exposures, such as the skull base. Vascular metastatic lesions, such as renal cell carcinoma, are also routinely referred for preoperative embolization. In selected cases of advanced medical illness or inoperative tumors, endovascular therapy may be used alone.

Chemotherapy Infusion

IA delivery of chemotherapeutic agents to treat CNS disorders dates back to the 1940s when direct injection of drugs into the carotid artery was attempted for the treatment of syphilis. Although it is an appealing approach, local IA delivery has not yet contributed to any significant improvement in the survival of patients with CNS tumors *(68)*.

Pedicle Embolization

More appealing than IA chemotherapy is the preoperative vascular pedicle occlusion possible in those tumors with prominent vasculature. However, the majority of brain tumors are intra-axial and not accessible to embolization. According to Choi and Tantivatana this fact is due to peripheral localization of the vessels, which often are not dilated *(69)*. The tumors more commonly embolized are the following *(72)*: (1) intra-axial tumors—hemangioblastoma, gliobastoma multiforme, metastatic tumors; (2) extra-axial tumors—meningioma, hemangiopericytoma, neurogenic tumor, paraganglioma, esthesioneuroblastoma, and malignant bone tumors; and (3) primary bone tumors—aneurysmal bone cyst, hemangioma, chordoma, chondrosarcoma, and osteogenic sarcoma.

Selection of embolic agents is extremely important in the embolization of intracranial tumors, and the neurosurgeon must be involved in this determination. *N*-butryl cyanide (NBCA) and polyvinyl alcohol are widely used. Gelfoam (Upjohn, Kalamazoo, MI) and Avitene are acceptable agents, but the effect is less permanent. Absolute ethanol is a liquid agent that produces an intense angionecrosis and liquefaction of the tumor. However, pericapsular extravasation may occur and the histotoxicity of ethanol raises the level of concern should this occur. Reflux of these agents should be avoided. The choice of embolic material is dependent upon multiple factors. Standard and Hopkins suggest that the optimum period before maximum tumor devascularization and surgical resection of solid tumors is 7–14 d *(70)*. Delays of more than 6–12 wk are associated with vascular recruitment by the tumor *(73)*.

The goal of embolization of neoplastic disorders is to devascularize the tumor capillary bed while preserving the normal arterial circulation. Before the injection of any embolic material, the interventionist should carefully reexamine the anatomy and hemodynamics of the vessel to be embolized, attempting to identify possible dangerous anastomosis, caliber and pattern of tumor vessels, blood

Table 3
Dangerous Anastomoses

Extracranial arteries	Intracranial arteries
Anterior branch of middle meningeal	Ophthalmic (ethmoidal)
Anterior meningeal	Anterior cerebral
Petrosquamosal branch of middle meningeal	Petrous internal carotid (cranial nerve VII)
Occipital	Vertebral
Neuromeningeal branch of ascending pharyngeal	Posterior inferior cerebellar/ anterior inferior cerebellar (cranial nerves IX–XI)

Adapted with permission from Standard S, Hopkins LN. Principles of neuroendovascular intervention. In: Maciunas RJ (ed). *Endovascular Neurological Intervention.* Park Ridge, IL: AANS, 1995, pp. 1–34.

flow characteristics and circulation to adjacent territories (Table 3) *(70)*. Of particular interest are dangerous anastomoses that may exist between vascular territories. However, angiographic visualization must not be relied on exclusively, and provocative testing using lidocaine must be used to demonstrate risk to the cranial nerve and brain blood supply. Additional provocative testing with agents like amobarbital is necessary when potential parenchymal anastomoses are present.

Preoperative assessment of the tumor is of particular importance in planning the embolization and estimating the subsequent risk that may be associated with a certain tumor. In particular, anatomical localization will determine the possible vascular supply that will provide access for embolization. The neuroendovascular physician must be thoroughly familiar with the blood supply to the skull base and meninges as well as the spinal cord to perform adequate angiographic visualization of the tumor. Preoperative assessment must also include a detailed neurological examination of the neurological territory adjacent to the tumor and the vascular territory at risk during the embolization *(71)*. Also preoperative magnetic resonance imaging provides a wealth of information regarding the growth patterns and compartmentalization of the tumor. Relationships to bony landmarks, such as the petrous apex and basal foramina, are critical aspects of any evaluation. The relationship of the tumor to major vascular structures, such as the petrous or cavernous internal carotid artery, will determine whether vessel sacrifice should be contemplated and if balloon test occlusion is necessary.

The tumors that are most commonly embolized, are meningiomas. This benign neoplasia presents, frequently, a huge vascular bed, sometimes leading to catastrophic hemorrhages during surgery. Because radical surgical removal is still the gold standard treatment for these tumors, the endovascular occlusion of nourishing vessels facilitates and abbreviates surgical procedure. Jungreis describes a significant reduction of intraoperative blood loss after endovascular pedicle occlusion *(72)*.

Direct percutaneous puncture with intratumoral injection of embolic agents may be another effective treatment for selected vascular tumors. Casasco et al. have employed direct puncture of vascular intracranial and head and neck tumors with intratumoral injection of NBCA *(73)*. Complete angiographic obliteration of the vascular bed of the tumor volume was achieved with regression of the tumors in 80% of cases.

TRAUMATIC ARTERIAL LESIONS

Traumatic injuries of both intracranial and extracranial parts of cerebral arteries such as dissection and fistula formation are probably underdiagnosed. The coexistence of traumatic brain injuries often obscures this diagnosis *(74)*. When diagnosed early enough, these lesions can be treated both medically and surgically. Medical management with anticoagulants may be hazardous in patients with multiple traumas. According to Fabian et al. in a long-term follow-up review, up to 40% of dissections and almost 100% of pseudoaneurysms do not improve with anticoagulation *(75)*. These abnormalities can become possible source of emboli and flow-related complications. Because most of these lesions occur near or even into the skull base, the surgical approach is difficult. Such arguments support the increasing utilization of endovascular techniques in this clinical setting.

Three types of vascular abnormalities are observed following traumatic injury to the vessels: dissections with variable impact on distal flow, pseudoaneurysms and arteriovenous fistulas. Dissections are observed acutely while pseudoaneurysms and arteriovenous fistulas are frequently observed in the subacute or late phase of an injury. Dissections are the most commonly observed abnormality after blunt arterial lesion. This term implies separation of anatomic structures, in this case, layers of the vessel wall. Dissection can lead to vessel stenosis or occlusion and/or pseudoaneurysm. The most common angiographic appearance of a dissection is a tapering stenosis. In the carotid artery it is seen in up to 0.7% of all patients who had blunt trauma due to motor vehicle collisions *(75,76)*.

With use of endovascular techniques, dissections can be treated using intravascular stents. Often the vessel is frequently occluded, and one or more pseudolumens may be present. The most critical step for endovascular approach is the localization of the true lumen. The use of a soft-tip microwire is usually helpful. Once the wire is across the lesion, the stent is placed along the inner wall of the dissection and trap the flap. This restores the patency of the lumen of the vessel.

Pseudoaneurysms may require endovascular treatment if they are progressively enlarging with local mass effect or are present intracranially where they pose a risk of SAH. Two methods of treatment are available. The first one is the occlusion of the parent vessel in a proximal location, if tolerated. A temporary occlusion is performed prior to the permanent occlusion to confirm the ability of the patient to tolerate the procedure. The second method is placement of intravascular stent to cover the inner segment of the pseudoaneurysm followed by placement of coils between the stent and inner wall of pseudoaneurysm. Some authors have been using covered stent to restore the true lumen of the artery excluding the pseudoaneurysm from circulation *(77,78)*. The use of covered stents is only possible on those vascular segments where perforator vessel occlusion is not a major concern, like in the cervical, petrous and cavernous segments of the internal carotid artery.

Carotid-cavernous sinus fistula (CCF) is an abnormal communication between the internal or external carotid arteries and the cavernous sinus. CCF is the most common intracranial posttraumatic arteriovenous fistula. It consists of a communication between the arterial blood from carotid artery with the venous system represented by the cavernous sinus. Distinction between direct and indirect fistula should be done. The direct fistula comprises of direct shunt from the internal carotid artery to the cavernous sinus. Indirect fistulas are formed from shunts between meningeal branches of internal or external carotid artery to the cavernous sinus. The main objective of the treatment of these lesions is to identify the fistula that connects the carotid artery and cavernous sinus. The fistula is then occluded by ballons, coils or other embolic agents. Parent vessel occlusion is another method that is less commonly used.

ARTERIOVENOUS MALFORMATIONS

CNS AVM occur in approx 0.15% of the American population, and 90% are supratentorial in location *(79)*. Ondra et al. described a 4% hemorrhage/yr rate for cerebral AVM and a combined morbidity and mortality rate of 2.7%/yr *(80)*. Certain angiographic risk factors such as venous stenosis and intranidal aneurysms have been associated with a more malignant course *(81,82)*. AVM can also cause headaches, seizures, and ischemia related to steal.

AVM treatment is often challenging; large and deep-seated AVMs pose special problems and often require mutimodality treatment *(79)*. Embolization has been used to serve the following purposes: (1) adjunct to surgery; (2) reduction of size prior to radiation; (3) palliation; (4) embolization alone for cure. To understand the role of endovascular treatment in AVM management, one should first briefly review the other treatment modalities that are being used to treat them: surgery and radiosurgery.

Table 4
Spetzler Martin Grading Scale

Grade feature	Points
Size	
Small < 3 cm	1
Medium 3–6 cm	2
Large > 6 cm	3
Eloquence of adjacent brain	
Noneloquent	0
Eloquent	1
Pattern of venous drainage	
Superficial	0
Deep	1

Table 5
Incidence of Postoperative Deficit in Relation to the Spetzler
Martin Grading Scale

Grade	Minor deficit (%)	Major deficit (%)
I	0	0
II	5	0
III	12	4
IV	20	7
V	19	12

The efficacy of microvascular AVM resection for preventing hemorrhage and reducing seizures in patients who present with epilepsy has been established *(83–85)*. Although, the feasibility of surgical resection has been significantly advanced it is clear that certain AVM are associated with unacceptable surgical risks. The Spetzler-Martin Scale attempts to quantify this differential risk by analyzing three AVM factors: size, venous drainage and eloquence of the cortex involved *(84)* (Table 4). Larger AVM, deep venous drainage and eloquent cortex have been associated with worse surgical outcomes. There are some biases regarding this classification. The same grade may not apply to all AVM, because large right temporal AVM with deep venous drainage may have lower surgical morbidity than a small AVM near motor cortex. Recent observations have raised questions regarding our traditional view of eloquent cortex because AVMs are congenital lesions. Their presence throughout development may be associated with displacement of function so that an AVM in motor cortex by traditional landmarks may actually not be in physiologically active motor cortex *(86)*. Embolization reduces the operative blood loss associated with AVM resection. This increases safety and ease of operation. For large AVM, embolization can serve the purpose of gradually decreasing flow through the AVM and, hence, decreasing the complications associated with normal perfusion pressure breakthrough *(85,87)* (*see* Chapter 24). Embolized AVM vessels can also serve as a roadmap during surgery. Despite these advantages AVM embolization carries risks. Only AVM that will significantly benefit from embolization before surgery should undergo this treatment. A small AVM in the right frontal lobe with easily accessible arterial feeders may not warrant embolization before surgery.

Radiosurgery has emerged as a relatively safe way to treat small AVM *(88,89)*. This treatment modality is particularly attractive for small deep-seated AVM. AVM with volumes equal to or less than 3 cm^3 have a 78–88% obliteration rate at 3 yr *(90)*. The limitation to this form of treatment is the

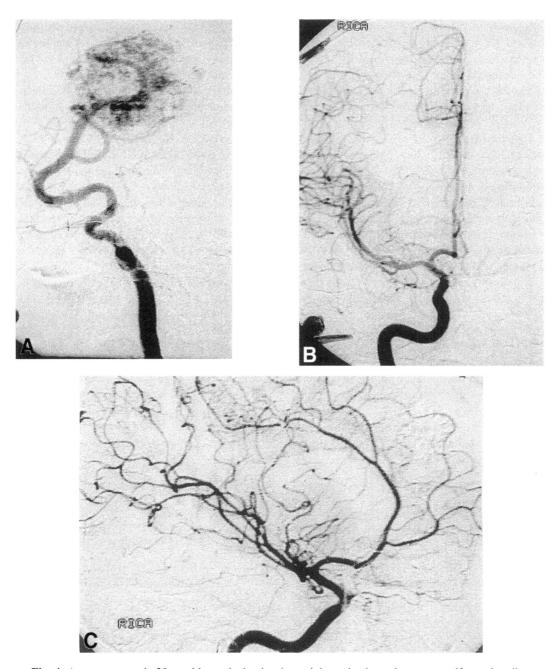

Fig. 4. An asymptomatic 20-yr-old man had a 4 × 4 cm right parietal arteriovenous malformation discovered. It was nourished by pedicles from middle cerebral (**A**), posterior cerebral and external carotid artery. After seven staged pedicle embolizations, he underwent microsurgical resection of the lesion. Follow-up four-vessel angiogram showed no residual lesion. Anteroposterior (**B**) and lateral (**C**) views of right carotid angiogram.

delay of 2–3 yr before complete obliteration during which hemorrhage can occur. Some limited evidence exists to support embolizing large AVMs down to a size, which can be amenable to radiation *(91,92)*. The long-term results of this strategy have not yet been adequately documented.

Endovascular treatment alone is only rarely curative *(92)*. This can be achieved occasionally only in small AVM with one or two feeders. Embolization as a palliative measure can occasionally be justified. Multiple pedicle embolization must be considered to prevent hemorrhages related to dramatic changes in the hemodynamics of the involved hemisphere and the AVM.

The most common embolic agent used for AVM treatment is NBCA. Although there is a steep learning curve involved in its use, many authors have reported on its successful use with low morbidity in recent years. The safety and efficacy of AVM embolization with NBCA has been reported in multiple series *(79,93–95)*. Embolization achieved 50% or greater reduction in AVM size in most patients in these series. Surgeons have reported greater ease of resecting embolized AVM compared with unembolized AVMs *(94)*. In a recent report on the efficacy of combining gamma knife and embolization, complete AVM obliteration was achieved in 46% of patients *(95)*. Complication rates have been reported between 3% and 25% *(96)*. The incidence of postoperative deficit has been correlated with the Spetzler Martin Grading (Table 5). Embolizing the draining vein or the normal branches is the most common complications associated with NBCA *(96)*. The technique of embolizing with NBCA involves subjectively assessing the AVM angioarchitecture which is seen with super selective angiography. Particular attention must be paid to the anatomy of the nidus.

New agents are being developed for the treatment of these lesions. Ethylene vinyl alcohol copolymer dissolved in dimethyl sulfoxide (Onyx-Micro Therapeutics, Irvine, CA), a nonadhesive liquid embolic agent is another agent evaluated in early studies *(96)*. The case depicted in Fig. 4 illustrates application of endovascular intervention in a patient with AVM.

In summary, four indications exist for treatment of AVM: preoperative, before radiation, curative, and palliative. Because embolization carries a risk, an AVM should be embolized only if this will truly result in a benefit to the patient. A small AVM with surgically accessible feeders may be easily embolized but the benefit to the surgeon may be questionable. Close coordination between the interventional specialist, surgeon and radiosurgeon are critical to optimal decision making in AVM treatment. The angiographic and MRI images must be carefully evaluated to understand the hemodynamics and proximity of the AVM to eloquent cortex, the presence of associated aneurysms and the pattern of venous drainage.

REFERENCES

1. Stroke Prevention Patient Outcomes Research Team. *Stroke Prevention: Recommendations*. Research Findings for Clinicians. Fact sheet. Rockville, MD: Agency for Health Care Policy and Research, 2002.
2. Qureshi AI. New grading system for angiographic evaluation of arterial occlusions and recanalization response to intra-arterial thrombolysis in acute ischemic stroke. *Neurosurgery* 2002;50:1405–1414.
3. del Zoppo GJ, Higashida RT, Furlan AJ, Pessin MS, Rowley HA, Gent M. PROACT: a phase II randomized trial of recombinant pro-urokinase by direct arterial delivery in acute middle cerebral artery stroke. PROACT Investigators. Prolyse in Acute Cerebral Thromboembolism. *Stroke* 1998;29:4–11.
4. Furlan A, Higashida R, Wechsler L, et al. Intra-arterial prourokinase for acute ischemic stroke. The PROACT II study: a randomized controlled trial. Prolyse in Acute Cerebral Thromboembolism. *JAMA* 1999;282:2003–2011.
5. Qureshi AI, Ali Z, Suri MF, Kim SH, et al. Intra-arterial third-generation recombinant tissue plasminogen activator (reteplase) for acute ischemic stroke. *Neurosurgery* 2001;49:41–48.
6. Ferbert A, Bruckmann H, Drummen R. Clinical features of proven basilar artery occlusion. *Stroke* 1990;21:1135–1142.
7. Hacke W, Zeumer H, Ferbert A, Bruckmann H, del Zoppo GJ. Intra-arterial thrombolytic therapy improves outcome in patients with acute vertebrobasilar occlusive disease. *Stroke* 1988;19:1216–1222.
8. The National Institute of Neurological Disorders and Stroke rt-PA Stroke Study Group. Tissue plasminogen activator for acute ischemic stroke. *N. Engl. J. Med.* 1995; 333:1581–1587.
9. Cross DT, III, Moran CJ, Akins PT, Angtuaco EE, Derdeyn CP, Diringer MN. Collateral circulation and outcome after basilar artery thrombolysis. *AJNR* 1998;19:1557–1563.
10. Ringer AJ, Qureshi AI, Fessler RD, Guterman LR, Hopkins LN. Angioplasty of intracranial occlusion resistant to thrombolysis in acute ischemic stroke. *Neurosurgery* 2001;48:1282–1288.
11. Qureshi AI, Ringer AJ, Suri MF, Guterman LR, Hopkins LN. Acute interventions for ischemic stroke: present status and future directions. *J. Endovasc. Ther.* 2000;7:423–428.

12. Marks MP, Marcellus M, Norbash AM, Steinberg GK, Tong D, Albers GW. Outcome of angioplasty for atherosclerotic intracranial stenosis. *Stroke* 1999;30:1065–1069.
13. Qureshi AI, Luft AR, Janardhan V, et al. Identification of patients at risk for periprocedural neurological deficits associated with carotid angioplasty and stenting. *Stroke* 2000;31:376–382.
14. Oppenheimer S, Hachinski V. Complications of acute stroke. *Lancet* 1992;339:721–724.
15. Calhoun DA, Oparil S. Treatment of hypertensive crisis. *N. Engl. J. Med.* 1990;323:1177–1183.
16. Dinsdale HB. Hypertensive encephalopathy. *Stroke* 1982;13:717–719.
17. Powers WJ. Acute hypertension after stroke: the scientific basis for treatment decisions. *Neurology* 1993;43:461–467.
18. Pulsinelli WA, Levy DE, Sigsbee B, Scherer P, Plum F. Increased damage after ischemic stroke in patients with hyper-glycemia with or without established diabetes mellitus. *Am. J. Med.* 1983;74:540–544.
19. Paciaroni M, Eliasziw M, Kappelle LJ, Finan JW, Ferguson GG, Barnett HJ. Medical complications associated with carotid endarterectomy. North American Symptomatic Carotid Endarterectomy Trial (NASCET). *Stroke* 1999;30:1759–1763.
20. North American Symptomatic Carotid Endarterectomy Trial Collaborators Beneficial effect of carotid endarterectomy in symptomatic patients with high-grade carotid stenosis. *N. Engl. J. Med.* 1991;325:445–453.
21. Mericle RA, Kim SH, Lanzino G, et al. Carotid artery angioplasty and use of stents in high-risk patients with contralat-eral occlusions. *J. Neurosurg.* 1999;90:1031–1036.
22. Qureshi AI, Suri MF, Ali Z, et al. Carotid angioplasty and stent placement: A prospective analysis of perioperative complications and impact of intravenously administered abciximab. *Neurosurgery* 2002;50:466–473.
23. Markus HS, Clifton A, Buckenham T, Brown MM. Carotid angioplasty. Detection of embolic signals during and after the procedure. *Stroke* 1994;25:2403–2406.
24. McCleary AJ, Nelson M, Dearden NM, Calvey TA, Gough MJ. Cerebral haemodynamics and embolization during carotid angioplasty in high-risk patients. *Br. J. Surg.* 1998;85:771–774.
25. Crawley F, Clifton A, Buckenham T, Loosemore T, Taylor RS, Brown MM. Comparison of hemodynamic cerebral ischemia and microembolic signals detected during carotid endarterectomy and carotid angioplasty. *Stroke* 1997;28:2460–2464.
26. Crawley F, Stygall J, Lunn S, Harrison M, Brown MM, Newman S. Comparison of microembolism detected by transcranial Doppler and neuropsychological sequelae of carotid surgery and percutaneous transluminal angioplasty. *Stroke* 2000;31:1329–1334.
27. Ohki T, Marin ML, Lyon RT, et al. Ex vivo human carotid artery bifurcation stenting: correlation of lesion characteris-tics with embolic potential. *J. Vasc. Surg.* 1998;27:463–471.
28. Mathur A, Roubin GS, Iyer SS, et al. Predictors of stroke complicating carotid artery stenting. *Circulation* 1998;97:1239–1245.
29. Spetzler RF, Hadley MN, Martin NA, Hopkins LN, Carter LP, Budny J. Vertebrobasilar insufficiency. Part 1: Micro-surgical treatment of extracranial vertebrobasilar disease. *J. Neurosurg.* 1987;66:648–661.
30. Vitek JJ. Subclavian artery angioplasty and the origin of the vertebral artery. *Radiology* 1989;170:407–409.
31. Marzewski DJ, Furlan AJ, St Louis P, Little JR, Modic MT, Williams G. Intracranial internal carotid artery stenosis: Longterm prognosis. *Stroke* 1982;13:821–824.
32. Thijs VN, Albers GW. Symptomatic intracranial atherosclerosis: outcome of patients who fail antithrombotic therapy. *Neurology* 2000;55:490–497.
33. Chimowitz MI, Kokkinos J, Strong J, et al. The Warfarin-Aspirin Symptomatic Intracranial Disease Study. *Neurology* 1995;45:1488–1493.
34. Lee RM. Morphology of cerebral arteries. *Pharmacol. Ther.* 1995;66:149–173.
35. Nahser HC, Henkes H, Weber W, Berg-Dammer E, Yousry TA, Kuhne D. Intracranial vertebrobasilar stenosis: angioplasty and follow-up. *AJNR* 2000;21:1293–1301.
36. Levy EI, Horowitz MB, Koebbe CJ, et al. Transluminal stent-assisted angioplasty of the intracranial vertebrobasilar system for medically refractory, posterior circulation ischemia: early results. *Neurosurgery* 2001;48:1215–1221.
37. Detailed Diagnoses and Procedures, National Hospital Discharge Survey, 1990. Hyattsville, Md: US Dept of Health and Human Services; 1992. Series 13, 92–1774. 2002. DHHS publication PHS.
38. Allen GS, Ahn HS, Preziosi TJ, et al. Cerebral arterial spasm—a controlled trial of nimodipine in patients with sub-arachnoid hemorrhage. *N. Engl. J. Med.* 1983;308:619–624.
39. Adams HP Jr, Kassell NF, Torner JC, Haley EC Jr. Predicting cerebral ischemia after aneurysmal subarachnoid hemor-rhage: influences of clinical condition, CT results, and antifibrinolytic therapy. A report of the Cooperative Aneurysm Study. *Neurology* 1987;37:1586–1591.
40. Treggiari-Venzi MM, Suter PM, Romand JA. Review of medical prevention of vasospasm after aneurysmal subarach-noid hemorrhage: A problem of neurointensive care. *Neurosurgery* 2001;48:249–261.
41. Megyesi JF, Vollrath B, Cook DA, Findlay JM. In vivo animal models of cerebral vasospasm: A review. *Neurosurgery* 2000;46:448–460.

42. Haley EC Jr, Kassell NF, Torner JC. The International Cooperative Study on the Timing of Aneurysm Surgery. The North American experience. *Stroke* 1992;23:205–214.

43. Longstreth WT Jr, Nelson LM, Koepsell TD, van Belle G. Clinical course of spontaneous subarachnoid hemorrhage: A population-based study in King County, Washington. *Neurology* 1993;43:712–718.

44. Yamamoto Y, Smith RR, Bernanke DH. Mechanism of action of balloon angioplasty in cerebral vasospasm. *Neurosurgery* 1992;30:1–5.

45. Higashida RT, Halbach VV, Cahan LD, et al. Transluminal angioplasty for treatment of intracranial arterial vasospasm. *J. Neurosurg.* 1989;71:648–653.

46. Milburn JM, Moran CJ, Cross DT III, Diringer MN, Pilgram TK, Dacey RG, Jr. Increase in diameters of vasospastic intracranial arteries by intraarterial papaverine administration. *J. Neurosurg.* 1998;88:38–42.

47. Carhuapoma JR, Qureshi AI, Tamargo RJ, Mathis JM, Hanley DF. Intra-arterial papaverine-induced seizures: case report and review of the literature. *Surg. Neurol.* 2001;56:159–163.

48. Hanel RA, Xavier AR, Mohammad Y, Kirmani JF, Yahia AM, Qureshi AI. Outcome following intracerebral hemorrhage and subarachnoid hemorrhage. *Neurol. Res.* 2002;24:S58–S62.

49. Qureshi AI, Frankel MR. Recognition and management of subarachnoid hemorrhage. *Heart Dis. Stroke* 1994;3:270–274.

50. Qureshi AI, Sung GY, Razumovsky AY, Lane K, Straw RN, Ulatowski JA. Early identification of patients at risk for symptomatic vasospasm after aneurysmal subarachnoid hemorrhage. *Crit. Care Med.* 2000;28:984–990.

51. Benamer HT, Bone I. Cerebral venous thrombosis: anticoagulants or thrombolyic therapy? *J. Neurol. Neurosurg. Psychiatry* 2000;69:427–430.

52. Hsu FP, Kuether T, Nesbit G, Barnwell SL. Dural sinus thrombosis endovascular therapy. *Crit. Care Clin.* 1999;15:743–753.

53. Ameri A, Bousser MG. Cerebral venous thrombosis. *Neurol. Clin.* 1992;10:87–111.

54. Preter M, Tzourio C, Ameri A, Bousser MG. Long-term prognosis in cerebral venous thrombosis. Follow-up of 77 patients. *Stroke* 1996;27:243–246.

55. Smith AG, Cornblath WT, Deveikis JP. Local thrombolytic therapy in deep cerebral venous thrombosis. *Neurology* 1997;48:1613–1619.

56. Bousser MG. Cerebral venous thrombosis: nothing, heparin, or local thrombolysis? *Stroke* 1999;30:481–483.

57. de Bruijn SF, Stam J. Randomized, placebo-controlled trial of anticoagulant treatment with low-molecular-weight heparin for cerebral sinus thrombosis. *Stroke* 1999;30:484–488.

58. Einhaupl KM, Villringer A, Meister W, et al. Heparin treatment in sinus venous thrombosis. *Lancet* 1991;338:597–600.

59. Fink JN, McAuley DL. Safety of anticoagulation for cerebral venous thrombosis associated with intracerebral hematoma. *Neurology* 2001;57:1138–1139.

60. Di Rocco C, Iannelli A, Leone G, Moschini M, Valori VM. Heparin-urokinase treatment in aseptic dural sinus thrombosis. *Arch. Neurol.* 1981;38:431–435.

61. Frey JL, Muro GJ, McDougall CG, Dean BL, Jahnke HK. Cerebral venous thrombosis: combined intrathrombus rtPA and intravenous heparin. *Stroke* 1999;30:489–494.

62. Horowitz M, Purdy P, Unwin H, et al. Treatment of dural sinus thrombosis using selective catheterization and urokinase. *Ann. Neurol.* 1995;38:58–67.

63. Chaloupka JC, Mangla S, Huddle DC. Use of mechanical thrombolysis via microballoon percutaneous transluminal angioplasty for the treatment of acute dural sinus thrombosis: case presentation and technical report. *Neurosurgery* 1999;45:650–656.

64. Malek AM, Higashida RT, Balousek PA, et al. Endovascular recanalization with balloon angioplasty and stenting of an occluded occipital sinus for treatment of intracranial venous hypertension: technical case report. *Neurosurgery* 1999;44:896–901.

65. Baker MD, Opatowsky MJ, Wilson JA, Glazier SS, Morris PP. Rheolytic catheter and thrombolysis of dural venous sinus thrombosis: a case series. *Neurosurgery* 2001;48:487–493.

66. Chow K, Gobin YP, Saver J, Kidwell C, Dong P, Vinuela F. Endovascular treatment of dural sinus thrombosis with rheolytic thrombectomy and intra-arterial thrombolysis. *Stroke* 2000;31:1420–1425.

67. Dowd CF, Malek AM, Phatouros CC, Hemphill JC, III. Application of a rheolytic thrombectomy device in the treatment of dural sinus thrombosis: a new technique. *AJNR* 1999;20:568–570.

68. Hopkins LN, Lanzino G, Guterman LR. Treating complex nervous system vascular disorders through a "needle stick": Origins, evolution, and future of neuroendovascular therapy. *Neurosurgery* 2001;48:463–475.

69. Choi IS, Tantivatana J. Neuroendovascular management of intracranial and spinal tumors. *Neurosurg. Clin. North Am.* 2000;11:167–85.

70. Standard S, Hopkins LN. Principles of neuroendovascular intervention. In: Maciunas RJ, ed. *Endovascular Neurological Intervention.* Park Ridge, IL: AANS, 1995, pp. 1–34.

71. Ahn HS, Kerber CW, Deeb ZL. Extra- to intracranial arterial anastomoses in therapeutic embolization: recognition and role. *AJNR* 1980;1:71–75.

72. Jungreis CA. Skull-base tumors: ethanol embolization of the cavernous carotid artery. *Radiology* 1991;181:741–743.

73. Casasco A, Herbreteau D, Houdart E, et al. Devascularization of craniofacial tumors by percutaneous tumor puncture. *AJNR* 1994;15:1233–1239.

74. Gomez CR, May AK, Terry JB, Tulyapronchote R. Endovascular therapy of traumatic injuries of the extracranial cerebral arteries. *Crit. Care Clin.* 1999;15:789–809.

75. Fabian TC, Patton JH Jr, Croce MA, Minard G, Kudsk KA, Pritchard FE. Blunt carotid injury. Importance of early diagnosis and anticoagulant therapy. *Ann. Surg.* 1996;223:513–522.

76. Duke BJ, Ryu RK, Coldwell DM, Brega KE. Treatment of blunt injury to the carotid artery by using endovascular stents: an early experience. *J. Neurosurg.* 1997;87:825–829.

77. Alexander MJ, Smith TP, Tucci DL. Treatment of an iatrogenic petrous carotid artery pseudoaneurysm with a Symbiot covered stent: technical case report. *Neurosurgery* 2002;50:658–662.

78. Marotta TR, Buller C, Taylor D, Morris C, Zwimpfer T. Autologous vein-covered stent repair of a cervical internal carotid artery pseudoaneurysm: technical case report. *Neurosurgery* 1998;42:408–412.

79. Wallace RC, Flom RA, Khayata MH, et al. The safety and effectiveness of brain arteriovenous malformation embolization using acrylic and particles: the experiences of a single institution. *Neurosurgery* 1995;37:606–615.

80. Ondra SL, Troupp H, George ED, Schwab K. The natural history of symptomatic arteriovenous malformations of the brain: A 24-year follow-up assessment. *J. Neurosurg.* 1990;73:387–391.

81. Thompson RC, Steinberg GK, Levy RP, Marks MP. The management of patients with arteriovenous malformations and associated intracranial aneurysms. *Neurosurgery* 1998;43:202–211.

82. Mansmann U, Meisel J, Brock M, Rodesch G, Alvarez H, Lasjaunias P. Factors associated with intracranial hemorrhage in cases of cerebral arteriovenous malformation. *Neurosurgery* 2000;46:272–279.

83. Sisti MB, Kader A, Stein BM. Microsurgery for 67 intracranial arteriovenous malformations less than 3 cm in diameter. *J. Neurosurg.* 1993;79:653–660.

84. Spetzler RF, Martin NA. A proposed grading system for arteriovenous malformations. *J. Neurosurg.* 1986;65:476–483.

85. Spetzler RF, Zabramski JM. Surgical management of large AVMs. *Acta. Neurochir. Suppl. (Wien.)* 1988;42:93–97.

86. Gandhi RT, Bendok BR, Getch C, Parrish TB, Batjer HH. Correlation of functional MRI with intraoperative cortical mapping in patient with cerebral arteriovenous malformation. *J. Am. Coll. Surg.* 2001;192:793.

87. Batjer HH, Devous MD, Sr., Meyer YJ, Purdy PD, Samson DS. Cerebrovascular hemodynamics in arteriovenous malformation complicated by normal perfusion pressure breakthrough. *Neurosurgery* 1988;22:503–509.

88. Flickinger JC, Pollock BE, Kondziolka D, Lunsford LD. A dose-response analysis of arteriovenous malformation obliteration after radiosurgery. *Int. J. Radiat. Oncol. Biol. Phys.* 1996;36:873–879.

89. Kondziolka D, Lunsford LD, Kanal E, Talagala L. Stereotactic magnetic resonance angiography for targeting in arteriovenous malformation radiosurgery. *Neurosurgery* 1994;35:585–590.

90. Pollock BE. Stereotactic radiosurgery for arteriovenous malformations. *Neurosurg. Clin. North Am.* 1999;10:281–290.

91. Gobin YP, Laurent A, Merienne L, et al. Treatment of brain arteriovenous malformations by embolization and radiosurgery. *J. Neurosurg.* 1996; 85:19–28.

92. Wikholm G, Lundqvist C, Svendsen P. The Goteborg cohort of embolized cerebral arteriovenous malformations: A 6-year follow-up. *Neurosurgery* 2001;49:799–805.

93. Vinuela F, Dion JE, Duckwiler G, et al. Combined endovascular embolization and surgery in the management of cerebral arteriovenous malformations: Experience with 101 cases. *J. Neurosurg.* 1991;75:856–864.

94. Jafar JJ, Davis AJ, Berenstein A, Choi IS, Kupersmith MJ. The effect of embolization with N-butyl cyanoacrylate prior to surgical resection of cerebral arteriovenous malformations. *J. Neurosurg.* 1993;78:60–69.

95. Fournier D, TerBrugge KG, Willinsky R, Lasjaunias P, Montanera W. Endovascular treatment of intracerebral arteriovenous malformations: experience in 49 cases. *J. Neurosurg.* 1991;75:228–233.

96. Jahan R, Murayama Y, Gobin YP, Duckwiler GR, Vinters HV, Vinuela F. Embolization of arteriovenous malformations with Onyx: Clinicopathological experience in 23 patients. *Neurosurgery* 2001;48:984–995.

18

Neurointensive Care of the Acute Ischemic Stroke Patient

Neeraj Badjatia, Thanh N. Nguyen, and Walter J. Koroshetz

INTRODUCTION

The patient with major brain ischemia is at high risk of loss of life or loss of quality of life. In the past two decades, life-threatening stroke has been more frequently treated with an intensive level of care, not only to manage respiratory or cardiac instability but also to optimize the neurological condition. The treatment of acute ischemic stroke is evolving rapidly and intensive care for certain specific stroke subtypes has become standard of care in certain institutions.

Recently, a number of interventions have been demonstrated to improve outcome of the acute stroke patient. Reperfusion therapy is the most prominent new treatment, by either intravenous or intra-arterial means to achieve recanalization of occluded cerebral arteries. Intensive neurologic and cardiopulmonary care in the neurosciences critical care unit (NSU) during the early stages is required to minimize risk after such interventions.

The goals of NSU care of ischemic stroke are fourfold:

1. To reverse brain ischemia before it causes permanent brain injury
2. To prevent secondary or progressive stroke
3. To optimize the patient's medical condition and prevent the common medical sequelae that occur after stroke or after a stroke intervention
4. To optimize functional recovery after the residual permanent injury that has occurred.

The NSU care of stroke is based on attempt to reverse or manage identified pathophysiolgic processes and the field is generally bereft of controlled clinical trials.

EMERGENT EVALUATION

As in many critical care illnesses, but perhaps more so in stroke, the actions taken during the first hours of presentation often dominate the patient's course. NSU care of the stroke patient therefore has greatest success if it is merged with the emergency care. Consensus guidelines should form the basis of standard emergency stroke care. Support of airway, respiration (breathing), and blood pressure (cardiovascular) form the common basis of all emergency care and should not be minimized in the stroke patient (1) (see Chapters 1, 8, and 9). Hypoxia is generally considered detrimental in ischemia and O_2 saturation should be maintained above 90%. In patients with altered mental status, airway protection may require intubation to prevent aspiration. This is especially the case when nausea and emesis accompany the stroke; i.e., along with vertigo in brainstem ischemia, or with increased intracranial pressure (ICP) in patients with intracranial hemorrhage (ICH). The nauseous, drowsy stroke patient lying flat, and often restrained, for brain imaging is at high risk for aspiration. Severe pneumonia or chemical pneumonitis can result (see Chapter 11).

From: *Current Clinical Neurology*
Critical Care Neurology and Neurosurgery
Edited by: J. I. Suarez © Humana Press Inc., Totowa, NJ

Neurologic Examination and History

After assessment of the ABCs, attention should rapidly shift to the potential cause of the patient's neurologic condition. Of importance is the realization that every "acute" neurologic deficit is not caused by stroke. One of the most treacherous pitfalls is to embark on a time consuming "stroke work-up" in a patient with another life-threatening but nonstroke cause of their deficit. Common stroke mimics include migraine, post-ictal state, hypoglycemia, traumatic brain injury, and reversible posterior leukoencephalopathy.

The neurologic history and examination in combination with analysis of the neuroimaging form the core diagnostic component of acute stroke. The initial history and examination is best at identifying a number of conditions associated with high risk and requiring early intervention. The patient with fluctuating vertigo, perioral numbness, diplopia, dysarthria, and quadriparesis likely has impending basilar artery (BA) occlusion and should be considered for immediate anticoagulation. The patient with sudden right-sided hemiplegia, hemisensory loss, aphasia, and eye deviation contralateral to the hemiparesis likely has a large hemispheric ICH or ischemia in distribution of the left middle cerebral artery (MCA). Patients with incomplete syndromes are more difficult to classify accurately and those with bilateral hemispheric lesions, frontal anterior cerebral artery (ACA) stroke or diencephalic stroke can be confused as "encephalopathic." The National Institutes of Health Stroke Scale (NIHSS) is a widely used convention to describe stroke severity (*see* Chapter 34 and Appendix). It was devised to provide consistent, reproducible, assessment of stroke deficits without sophisticated neurologic training.

The neurologic examination is sensitive in identifying patients with the most severe neurologic deficits who warrant evaluation for NSU level of care. However, the examination has limitations in this regard because patients with no or minimal deficit may harbor a life-threatening vascular lesion that is unappreciated because of their good neurologic status. The transient ischemic attack (TIA) is the good example. The patient may have a completely normal neurologic examination when seen despite being found with severe deficits minutes earlier and despite fatal stroke occurring minutes later. Therefore, the addition of brain and neurovascular imaging to the examination and history is essential to assess the degree of damage, the distribution of ischemia, and the vascular lesion.

Neuroimaging

A sophisticated ability to interpret head computed tomography (CT) scanning and magnetic resonance imaging (MRI) images is an inherent feature of acute stroke care. Errors in interpretation can be costly.

There are four primary goals of neuroimaging in the acute stroke patient:

1. Determine if there is ICH.
2. Identify evidence of brain ischemia.
3. Identify the vascular lesion(s), which threaten future brain viability.
4. Determine if the distribution of brain ischemia is more extensive than the distribution of brain injury/infarction.

Imaging studies such as CT, MRI, and ultrasound based techniques are instrumental in helping the neurointensivist to identify the underlying pathophysiology and thereby triage patients appropriately to NSU level of care and set management goals. In addition, infarction occurs as a function of the degree of blood flow reduction and duration of this blood flow reduction (Fig. 1). Modern imaging allows decisions on reperfusion to be made based on how much brain is salvageable. A patient with a small region of infarction, but who has neurologic deficits and perfusion imaging that suggest widespread ischemia, may have a severe stroke syndrome that is still reversible with improved blood flow.

Computed Tomography

Head CT scanning is the most widely accessible and reliable modality in the emergency setting (*see* Chapter 7). The value of CT in assessing brain injury and brain ischemia has rapidly expanded

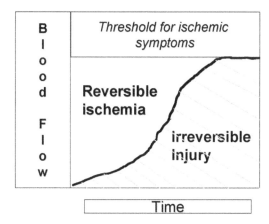

Fig. 1. In a primate stroke model investigators demonstrated that a quantitative irreversible injury occurs in ischemia as a function of both the degree of blood flow reduction and the duration. This simple idea is at the core of the current practice of reversing ischemic injury in the first hours after stroke, before infarction has a chance to complete. (From Jones TH, Morawetz RB, Crowell RM, et al. Threshold of focal cerebral ischemia in awake monkeys. *J. Neurosurg.* 1981;54:773–782).

with the advent of helical devices. In contrast to previous CT studies, recent data indicate that the noncontrast CT scan is rarely normal in patients with major artery stroke. Low-density regions can be found in over 75% of patients with middle cerebral artery distribution stroke scanned within 6 h of onset *(2)*. To recognize these low-density regions it is helpful to set the window and level settings on the CT display to give an almost black/white image, usually approx 30 Hounsfield units each. Low-density lesions on CT due to brain ischemia are always associated with infarction.

One major advance consequent to the introduction of helical scanners is CT angiography (CTA), which can scan fast enough to capture a bolus of dye traveling through the vasculature of interest. The data is acquired by scanning an intravenously delivered bolus of dye as it passes through the aorta, extracranial and then intracranial cerebrovasculature. The study takes approx 5 min to perform and allows for immediate assessment of major vessel occlusion or stenosis by an experienced examiner. Detection of distal intracranial stenoses or occlusions often requires computer processing of the data to provide two-dimensional angiographic images. The technique has been validated against direct angiographic studies with very high specificity. It is used to triage patients to intra-arterial thrombolysis and serves to completely eliminate angiography in patients with open circle of Willis vessels. It is also important in the identification of severe stenosis in the carotid or vertebrobasilar territory, which threaten to cause recurrent infarction. It is also a useful triage tool in patients with only mild-to-moderate deficits to determine whether they harbor a major vascular obstruction that warrants careful monitoring in the NSU.

CT perfusion imaging is the newest advance in the acute evaluation of the stroke patient. Helical scanners are now fast enough to image an intravenous bolus of dye as it travels through the cerebral vascular tree and then out again. The elements of this "bolus tracking technique" allow computation of maps of cerebral blood flow (CBF), volume (CBV) and mean transit time (MTT), similar to those used in MRI perfusion weighted imaging (PWI). The advantage is that the change in signal in the vessel is proportional to the dye concentration in CT but not in MRI. This makes quantitative brain maps of CBF, MTT and CBV possible whereas quantitation has been difficult with MRI. The disadvantage of CT is that the assessment of CBF is limited to a single 2-cm wide slab of tissue for each bolus of contrast. In contrast, echoplanar MRI is fast enough to scan the entire brain every half second to allow computation of qualitative CBF, CBV and MTT in 11 slices covering the entire brain.

A partial resolution and compromise to the single slice limitations of CT can be reached simply by extending the scanning through the entire brain during the bolus of dye used to acquire the CTA. This provides a crude blood volume map called the "whole brain perfusion" map. Regions with blocked vasculature will not fill with dye and appear dark compared to the surrounding brain with normal blood volume. Studies on acute stroke patients have demonstrated that a drop in blood volume in the tissue is highly correlated with the early stage of injury. Lev et al. reported that, in patients in whom an MCA occlusion could be reopened by intra-arterial lysis, the lesion seen on this "whole brain perfusable blood volume" scan constituted the final infarct (2). In those patients in whom lysis was not successful the final stroke size was larger than the "whole brain perfused blood volume" lesion. There is a strong correlation between the lesion seen on this contrast CT scan and on diffusion weighted imaging (DWI). Good patient outcome occurred consistently in patients with MCA occlusion who had a small (<100 cc) whole brain CT perfusion abnormality and in whom thrombolysis was successful. This whole brain CT perfusion abnormality is therefore valuable in assessing early signs of infarct, size of infarct, and in helping to predict best possible outcome with thrombolysis. Noncontrast CT and whole brain CT perfusion give images that are highly predictive of tissue that is already injured. As discussed below, CBF and MTT maps are valuable in assessing regions at risk that are not yet damaged; i.e., low CBF, high MTT, but normal blood volume and normal on noncontrasted CT.

Magnetic Resonance Imaging

MRI has become extremely valuable in the emergency evaluation of the stroke patient due to the advent of DWI and PWI (*see* Chapter 7). Decrease in the diffusibility (lowering of the apparent diffusion coefficient [ADC]) of brain water occurs when ATP levels fall to very low levels and neural cells are no longer able to maintain their ionic gradients. Water flows into cells at this stage of ischemia. This shift in water from the more diffusible extracellular space into the colloidal intracellular space causes the restricted diffusion that is seen as increased signal intensity on DWI and decreased signal intensity on ADC maps. Regions that have progressed to this stage due to ischemia are very difficult but not impossible to salvage. Even in the rare case where early reperfusion leads to normalization of the diffusion abnormality the tissue may still die a late death. As such DWI hyperintensity with reduced ADC due to brain ischemia is a reliable marker of injured tissue. This contrasts to focal status epilepticus where water shifts can occur without cell death and the DWI abnormality may reverse.

Of greatest interest is the finding that when patients present with ischemic stroke in the first hours of symptom onset the DWI is abnormal in over 90% of cases. Although brainstem lacunar strokes can be missed, DWI is especially good in identifying small regions of stroke of only 1 mm or so in diameter. The finding of a unilateral smattering of small dots of DWI hyperintensity in the distribution of the MCA/ACA or MCA/ posterior cerebral artery (PCA) watershed suggests a low-flow syndrome and should trigger a search for the responsible vascular lesion. As such, this finding may motivate NSU care level monitoring of neurological symptoms and blood pressure.

The second important finding is that the DWI abnormal brain tissue may be quite limited as compared to the extent of abnormally functioning ischemic brain. The most dramatic example is the patient with a complete hemispheric syndrome with DWI brightness restricted to the distribution of a few penetrator vessels supplying deep white matter (3). There is a "mismatch" between a more severe pattern of clinical deficit than the DWI abnormality. Serial MRI studies show that the DWI abnormal region in such cases enlarges over hours. Combined PWI shows that this enlargement of the injured brain occurs into brain regions with low CBF and increased MTT. In this instance there is "mismatch" between a smaller DWI lesion indicating injured brain and a larger region with low CBF and increased MTT (Fig. 2). In contrast to the CBF and MTT abnormalities, the CBV is usually close to normal in most of the region with normal DWI. This occurs because slow flow through collateral vessels prolongs the transit time of the blood through the tissue and CBV = CBF × MTT. Stroke

A MRA with left MCA stem occlusion in patient with total left anterior circulation syndrome

B Extensive perfusion abnormality on MTT maps.

C DWI abnormality limited to deep penetrator territory.

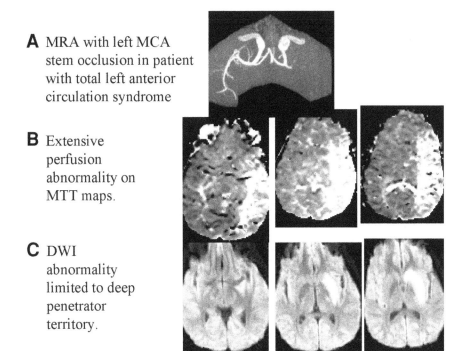

Fig 2. Common pattern of "mismatch" between clinical deficits of aphasia and right hemiparesis in a patient with MCA stem occlusion and infarction limited to the deep MCA penetrator territory with its poor collateral flow. Neurologic deficits correlate much better with the perfusion abnormality as seen on the mean transit time maps using bolus tracking MRI. Such patients are at high risk of progressive infarction on serial DWI and are considered among the best candidates for reperfusion or hypertensive therapy. (**A**) MRA with left MCA stem occlusion in patient with total left anterior circulation syndrome. (**B**) Extensive perfusion abnormality on MTT maps. (**C**) DWI abnormality limited to deep penetrator territory. (From Rordorf G, Koroshetz WJ, Copen W, et al. Regional ischemia and ischemic injury in patients with acute MCA stroke as a defined by early diffusion weighted and perfusion weighted MRI. *Stroke* 29:939–943.)

patients with this mismatch between DWI and MTT or CBF are currently the targets of clinical trials of extending the window of rt-PA past 3 h. Reperfusion improves the perfusion abnormality, eliminates the mismatch and freezes the extent of infarction.

Difficulty occurs due to the lack of specificity of the perfusion abnormality on MRI. Perfusion CT scanning offers more specificity because it is more quantitative. CT research groups have used thresholds of CBV to identify tissue that cannot be salvaged by thrombolysis (*3*) much as discussed above for "whole brain perfused blood volume imaging" (*2*). In addition, perfusion CT imaging allows researchers to set thresholds of CBF to identify tissue which can be salvaged by thrombolysis (*3*). Evidence also suggests that this may be the subgroup that will benefit from hypertensive therapy.

Perfusion Imaging and Positron Emission Tomography

While DWI has been pivotal in the evaluation of brain infarction, its accuracy can be tainted by the artifact of T2 shine through, diffusion anisotropy (*4*), and does not always correlate with irreversible tissue damage. Positron emission tomography (PET) scan is another modality that can reliably demarcate areas of tissue infarct as well as "misery perfusion," which is the area of mismatch of severely hypoperfused brain tissue yet intact oxygen consumption (*5*). Neuronal viability remains preserved for a limited time via a compensated increase in oxygen extraction, and if prompt reperfusion does not occur, neuronal death will ensue. This phenomenon may be seen in up to one third of patients with acute stroke and may persist up to 16 h following onset of symptoms, suggesting an extended therapeutic window *(6)*. However, the use of PET in acute evaluation of ischemic stroke is limited by its cost, need for arterial blood sampling, and inaccessiblity in the emergency setting.

Therapeutic Options

Because of the variability in stroke outcome only a select group of patients is appropriate for NSU level of care. Selection will change as the therapeutic armamentarium is expanded and with the experience of the neurointensivist. Based on the combination of neurologic evaluation and neuroimaging, we selected patients at high risk for deterioration and potentially helped by NSU level of services, as presented in Table 1.

CRITICAL CARE MANAGEMENT ISSUES

Reperfusion Therapy

Intravenous Recombinant Tissue Plasminogen Activator

The NINDS trial demonstrated that treatment with intravenous t-PA within 3 h of stroke onset improved outcome at 3 mo *(7)*. Subsequent analysis of the NINDS trial and further studies have shown that the earlier the treatment is given, the greater likelihood exists for improved outcome. As a result, the slogan "time is brain," has become the driving force for creating acute stroke teams to deliver early and rapid assessment. Adherence to the NINDS inclusion and exclusion criteria is recommended (*see* Table 2). For those meeting the criteria for administration, the dose is 0.9 mg/kg intravenous infusion, with 10% of the dose given as a bolus over the first minute and remaining infusion lasting 1 h. New patient data as well as animal data suggest that transcranial Doppler ultrasound may improve recanalization rates after intravenous t-PA.

Intra-Arterial Lysis of Occlusive Clot

The first promising results of reperfusion therapy were using intra-arterial (IA) urokinase in patients with basilar occlusion. The PROACT II study demonstrated the efficacy of IA prourokinase in treating proximal MCA occlusion within 6 h of onset *(8)*. A statistically significant increase in the chance of returning to independent function was seen; 40% of the treated group as opposed to only 25% in the placebo achieved independence at 3 mo. Recanalization rate was 67% as opposed to the 25–33% recanalization seen in the angiographic studies of intravenous rt-PA. This impressive result in patients with severe stroke, however, did not gain US Food and Drug Administration (FDA) approval. Urokinase became unavailable a number of years ago but has recently been re-released. Its effective dose ranged between 250,000 and 1.25 million units. Many clinicians are using rt-PA for IA delivery. Unfortunately, optimal dosing, duration of infusion and treatment window have not been established.

IA dosing schemes have included giving an infusion of up to 20 mg of rt-PA over 2 h directly into the thrombus *(9,10)*. Our recanalization rates with 20 mg IA rt-PA (47%) were inferior to our previous experience with urokinase (approx 80% recanalization), which led us to try a sequential series of infusions of 4 mg rt-PA into the thrombus followed by balloon angioplasty of the clot. We first successfully attempted balloon angioplasty of clot in patients with top of internal carotid artery (ICA)/MCA/ACA occlusions, so called "T-occlusions," which are clinically disastrous and very resistant to pharmacologic lysis. Further improvement of overall recanalization rates (approx 67%) followed when we pretreated patients with an intravenous infusion of the GPIIb-IIIa platelet antagonist eptifibatide (Integrilin) in addition to heparin (PTT goal, 50–70 s). In post surgical acute stroke patients with ICA, BA, or MCA stem occlusion, angioplasty assisted mechanical lysis is relied on with only small doses, 4–11 mg of rt-PA administered intra-arterially with no GPIIb-IIIa antagonist, and minimal heparin. Note the major reduction in rtPA dose using the intra-arterial route *(4–20)* vs the

Table 1
Diagnostic and Management Issues Surrounding Common Acute Stroke Syndromes

Clinical presentation	Neuroimaging	Potential interventions	Risks
Stroke considered eligible for intravenous rt-PA	Noncontrast CT abnormality less extensive than expected based on extent of neurologic deficits	Intravenous rt-PA Blood pressure control Monitor for thrombolysis-related hemorrhage	Hemorrhage
TIA or minor stroke syndrome	Severe stenosis or occlusion of relevant cerebrovascular vessel Embolic pattern of injury or no injury on DWI DWI abnormality in watershed territory	Antiplatelet and anticoagulant therapy Carotid endarterectomy or vertebral/basilar stent/angioplasty	Recurrent stroke
Total anterior circulation syndrome	Occlusion of major intracranial vessel Only partial MCA territory abnormal on DWI/CT perfusion noncontrasted CT	IA reperfusion therapy Induced hypertension if blood pressure sensitive symptoms	Progressive stroke Postreperfusion hemorrhage
Total anterior circulation syndrome	Total MCA territory abnormal on DWI/CT perfusion/noncontrasted CT	Antiedema therapy Hemicraniectomy	Death from ischemic brain swelling
Ataxia, vertigo nausea	Large PICA stroke on DWI/CT perfusion	Ventriculostomy or cerebellectomy	Progessive vertebrobasilar stroke Cerebellar swelling with hydrocephalus and or brainstem compression
Fluctuating brainstem deficits	Vertebrobasilar stenosis with or without DWI/CT perfusion abnormality in cerebellum and or brainstem or PCA territory	Anticoagulation Stent/angioplasty for clinical worsening Induced hypertension if blood pressure sensitive symptoms	Progressive stroke Reperfusion hemorrhage
Coma and quadriplegia	Basilar occlusion and Substantial but subtotal DWI/CT perfusion abnormality	Intra-arterial thombolysis with or without stent angioplasty	Death or locked-in syndrome
Abulia, decreased upgaze, visual field abnormality	DWI/CT perfusion/non contrasted CT abnormality in thalamus, midbrain or medial occipital/temporal lobe and Top of basilar embolic occlusion	Intra-arterial thrombolysis Anticoagulation if vertebrobasilar stenosis or obstruction to basilar/PCA flow	Basilar occlusion Hemorrhage into infarct
Stroke deficit with neck pain	Blood in wall of carotid or vertebral atery with or without narrowing of lumen on fat-saturated T1 MR sequence Watershed distribution of DWI abnormality Embolic occlusion of major intra-cranial vessel with limited injury on DWI/CT perfusion/noncontrasted CT	Anticoagulation Potential need for stent/angioplasty for low flow symptoms thrombolysis of embolus	Recurrent embolic stroke Progressive low flow stroke Hemorrhage into infarct Subarachnoid hemorrhage from extension of dissection intracranially

DWI, diffusion-weighted MRI; PCA, posterior cerebral artery; PICA, posterior inferior cerebellar artery; MCA, middle cerebral artery; rt-PA, recombinant tissue plasminogen activator; TIA, transient ischemic attack.

Table 2
Inclusion/Exclusion Criteria for the Use of Recombinant
Tissue Plasminogen Activator

Inclusion
Ischemic stroke with clearly defined symptom onset
Measurable deficit on the NIH Stroke Scale
No evidence of intracranial blood on brain CT scan
180 min or less from the time of symptom onset to initiation of IV rt-PA*

Exclusion
Rapidly improving or minor stroke symptoms
Stroke or serious head trauma within 3 mo
Major surgery within 14 d
History of intracranial hemorrhage
Systolic BP > 185 mmHg or diastolic > 110 mmHg at time of treatment initiation
Aggressive BP treatment
(i.e., continuous IV infusion of an antihypertensive to achieve above goal)
Suspected subarachnoid hemorrhage despite a normal CT scan
Gastrointestinal or urinary tract hemorrhage within 21 d
Arterial puncture at a noncompressible site within 7 d
Seizure at the onset of stroke
Use of heparin within 48 h and an elevated PTT–aPTT
PT > 15 s, platelet count < 100,000, glucose < 50 or > 400

rt-PA, recombinant tissue-plasminogen activator; NIH, National Institutes of Health; CT, computed tomography; IV, intravenous; BP, blood pressure; aPTT, activated partial thromboplastin time; PT, prothrombin time.
*Onset time needs to be rigorously defined. Patients are excluded if they awaken with stroke symptoms and are not known to have been "normal" within the previous 3 h.

intravenous route (0.9 mg/kg to 90 mg). We have successfully treated postoperative patients with these low doses without bleeding at the operative site.

The other advantage of the endovascular approach to acute clot lysis is that it allows additional opportunity to acutely reperfuse ischemic brain by angioplasty/stenting of a relevant atherosclerotic stenosis. Passing a thin wire into the ICA and injecting a small amount of rt-PA distally can reopen on occasion even the acutely occluded carotid. The severe ICA or critical vertebral artery (VA) stenosis can be stented open and blood flow returned to the brain within hours of onset of ischemic signs with resolution of neurologic deficits. Of note however, the use of stent/angioplasty is associated with a significant rate of rethrombosis unless antiplatelet agents are used. We administer a GPIIb-IIIa antagonist, eptifibatide, for 24 h followed by clopidogrel and aspirin.

Based on the results of PROACT II, a treatment window of 6 h, i.e., time from symptom onset to initiation of IA infusion, for the carotid circulation appears reasonable. Longer windows may be justified in the presence of a BA occlusion especially in those with fluctuating or progressive symptoms.

Combined Intravenous and Intra-Arterial Lysis of Occluding Clot

Systemic rt-PA and plasminogen in the blood stream can only access the surface at the two ends of an occluding clot. Perhaps for this reason initial angiographic studies showed that the probability of vessel recanalization after intravenous rt-PA decreased the larger the clot and the more proximal the vessel occlusion. If intravenous rt-PA is not effective in patients with MCA, ICA, or BA occlusion then we, and others, routinely attempt IA lysis of clot within the next 3 h. After intravenous rtPA administration special care is needed to make a clean femoral artery puncture. However, in these patients already treated with intravenous rt-PA we find that only mechanical manipulation of the clot with a thin wire or disruption of the clot using an angioplasty balloon can lead to recanalization with minimal injury from distal embolization. Injection into the clot of small additional amounts of rt-PA, 4–11 mg is sometimes needed. Under current investigation is the efficacy of a lower dose of intravenous rt-PA (0.6 mg/kg) as a "bridge" to treatment with IA rt-PA *(11)*.

Acute Revascularization

Given the high risk of ICH, carotid endarterectomy for symptomatic patients is usually considered only several weeks after ischemic stroke. However, in some rare instances of acute ICA occlusion where either perfusion imaging or clinical examination with induced hypertension demonstrates a significant ischemic territory at risk for infarction, emergent revascularization to remove carotid clot may be a very risky yet potentially life-saving procedure *(12–14)*. There have also been case reports of successful emergent revascularization via angioplasty and endovascular stenting. The field will be further advanced by the development of endovascular devices, which remove clot from intracranial vessels obviating the need for thrombolytic drugs. A number of such devices are currently in human studies (*see* Chapter 17). On rare occasions a patient with ICA occlusion (usually due to dissection) with congenitally absent anterior and posterior communicating arteries will develop a progressive low flow stroke syndrome that goes on to complete hemispheric infarction despite maximal hypertensive/hemodilution/hyperosmolar therapy. External carotid to MCA bypass surgery may be the only option remaining to reverse this process.

Cerebral Venous Sinus Thrombosis

Despite the presence of ICH, the usual treatment for cerebral venous sinus thrombosis (CVT) is heparinization to therapeutic levels *(15)*. In neurologically deteriorating patients with CVT catheter-directed thrombolysis in the cerebral venous sinuses along with catheter manipulation for direct clot disruption has been described to be effective in resolving CVT and improving neurological outcome *(16)*. Studies have shown that ICH does not worsen with either therapy in CVT. Readers are referred to Chapter 21 for a detailed discussion on CVT.

Postthrombolysis Care

In the NINDS study, a protocol for postthrombolytic care was established and now has become the standard of care in the first 24 h after intravenous rt-PA (*see* Table 3). The biologic half-life of rt-PA at the site of the thrombus where it binds to fibrin is approx 45 min. As a result, the hemorrhagic complications from rt-PA are more likely to occur in the first few hours and much less likely after 12–24 h. An important factor that correlated with ICH in the PROACT II and the NINDS rt-PA study was elevated serum glucose concentrations. Therefore, the treatment of hyperglycemia is warranted in this setting although whether this reduces the incidence of ICH is not known.

The most common signs of ICH include decreased level of consciousness, headache, vomiting, increased blood pressure, and worsening of focal neurologic deficit. The development of these symptoms should prompt immediate CT imaging and determination of the fibrinogen level, PT/aPTT, platelet count and hematocrit. Reversal of thrombolysis with infusion of cryoprecipitate, fresh frozen plasma should be considered if CT imaging demonstrates a significant ICH and blood work reveals a fibrinogen level less than 100 mg/dL. Neurosurgical consultation should also be obtained, although there are no established guidelines for intervention. Life-threatening systemic bleeding is managed with hemodynamic stabilization, reversal of the thrombolytic process and transfusion of packed red blood cells. The risk of clinically significant ICH in the NINDS trial was 6.4%.

Important additional complications of rt-PA use are anaphylaxis and angioedema *(17)*. These reactions occur rarely and have been estimated to occur in less than 0.02% of patients who receive rt-PA for the treatment of acute myocardial infarction. In the setting of acute ischemic stroke their incidence has been reported to be 1.5–1.9% *(18)*. Patients taking angiotensin converting enzyme (ACE) inhibitors may be particularly susceptible. A protocol for managing a patient with angioedema

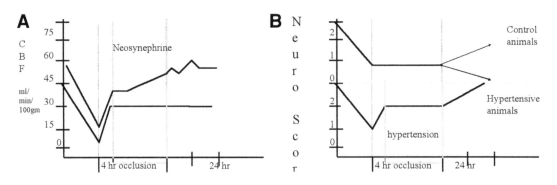

Fig 3. Investigators demonstrate that induced hypertension with Neo-Synephrine can improve cerebral blood flow in primates with MCA occclusion and avert the "no reflow" phenomenon, lack of increase of tissue flow when the MCA is reopened (**A**). This effect of induced hypertension leads to clinical recovery in this animal stroke model. Beneficial effects of induced hypertension on experimental stroke in awake monkeys. (**B**). These experiments from the same group as in Fig. 1 form the basis of induced hypertension in patients with major vascular occlusion by improving collateral flow to the ischemic but not yet damaged cortex as illustrated in Fig. 2. From ref. *25.*

Table 3
Patient Management After Recombinant Tissue Plasminogen Activator Administration

No anticoagulants or antiplatelet agents for 24 h.

Blood pressure monitoring for the first 24 h: every 15 min for 2 h after starting infusion, every 30 min for 6 h, then every hour from the eighth hour until 24 h after rt-PA started.

Aggressive blood pressure management to maintain BP < 185/110 mmHg using following protocol.

If for two readings 5–10 min apart, the systolic blood pressure is between 180–230 mmHg or the diastolic pressure is in the range of 105–120 mmHg: Give labetalol 10 mg intravenously over 1 to 2 min. The dose may be repeated and/or doubled every 10–20 min up to 150 mg. Monitor blood pressure every 15 min during treatment. Observe for hypotension.

If the systolic blood pressure is greater than 230 mmHg or the diastolic pressure is in the range 121–140: Give labetalol 10 mg intravenously over 1 to 2 min. The dose may be repeated and/or doubled every 10 min up to 150 mg. If satisfactory response is not obtained, use nitroprusside. Monitor blood pressure every 10 min during treatment. Observe for hypotension.

If the diastolic blood pressure is greater than 140 mmHg: Infuse sodium nitroprusside (0.5–10 μg/kg/min). Monitor blood pressure every 15 min during treatment. Observe for hypotension.

rt-PA, tissue-plasminogen activator; BP, blood pressure.

has been reported and involves the discontinuation of rt-PA infusion and administration of Benadryl and epinephrine with careful attention to the airway.

After IA lysis the patient is taken directly to neuroimaging. CT scan regularly shows dye staining of infarcted tissue. It is impossible to determine whether ICH has also occurred except with serial CT scans. Angiographic dye usually dissipates to some significant extent over 24 h, but blood does not.

Susceptibility sequence on MRI is a more reliable means of determining whether there has been hemorrhage. Our preference is to discontinue anticoagulants and GPIIb-IIIa antagonists after IA lysis unless a stent has been deployed. Blood pressure limits in the normal range are enforced after lysis to decrease hemorrhage risk and ischemic edema. In the PROACT II study the symptomatic hemorrhage rate was 10% in the treated compared to 2% in the placebo group.

Retroperitoneal hematoma is not an uncommon cause of dropping hematocrit or fever in the patient who undergoes IA lysis/stenting having been treated during the procedure with heparin, GPIIb-IIIa antagonist, and rt-PA. Ischemic edema must also be carefully looked for as it can occur sooner in patients who have been reperfused. In patients in whom a severe ICA stenosis or occlusion has been repaired a hyperperfusion syndrome can appear characterized clinically by hemispheric deficits, headache, and seizure. Fatal ICH can follow unless great care is taken to decrease blood pressure and normalize coagulation system. Imaging in the hyperperfusion syndrome is characterized by markedly elevated blood flow velocity on transcranial Doppler ultrasound, increased CBF, decreased MTT, T2 and ADC hyperintensity on MRI, and increased vascular staining on CT perfusion.

Hemodynamic Management

Blood pressure management in the acute setting remains controversial but requires careful attention (*see* Chapter 13). In ischemic stroke the general consensus is not to treat hypertension unless systolic blood pressure exceeds 210 mmHg or a MAP that exceeds 120 mmHg (*1*). Aggressive treatment of blood pressure in ischemic stroke patients has been associated with worsening symptoms, particularly in patients with longstanding hypertension who exhibit limited autoregulation with the curve shifted to the right (*19,20*). If the decision is made to lower blood pressure it should be done carefully. Short-acting intravenous agents such as labetolol, nitroprusside, enalapril, fenoldopam, or nicardipine are preferred because they can be titrated to achieve a blood pressure goal with less chance of sustained hypotension. Moreover, there is increasing evidence that even inducing hypertension may improve symptoms in some patients by augmenting cerebral perfusion to ischemic tissue (*21*).

On occasion ischemic stroke patients have ischemic deficits that worsen with spontaneous downturns in blood pressure. In these patients, maintaining blood pressure above a threshold associated with neurologic worsening may require fluid bolus or intravenous infusion of pressor agents. We have been impressed with the ability of induced hypertension to quickly reverse neurologic deficits in some patients. Dependency on raised blood pressure to sustain neurologic improvement is usually short lived but can occur over days (*21*). Others have noted that vasopressor responsive patients have DWI/PWI mismatch on MRI and that induced hypertension improves perfusion (*22*).

Instead of awaiting spontaneous fluctuations in deficits with fluctuating blood pressure, we have utilized a trial of intravenous neosynephrine to identify patients in whom neurologic deficits improve with raised blood pressure (*23*). If they also worsen as pressors are removed and then improve again when blood pressure is raised, the patient is considered blood pressure dependent. In the emergency setting or on the hospital floor, we infuse a dilute solution of neosynephrine through a large bore intravenous catheter. The patient is under continuous observation with frequent blood pressure checks over a 20-min period. Patients in whom neurological deficits consistently fluctuate around a threshold blood pressure are transferred to the NSU, vasopressors are infused centrally in a more concentrated solution and strict blood pressure limits followed using IA blood pressure monitoring. Central venous pressure is monitored and used to ensure euvolemia.

Once a patient is committed to induced hypertension it is important to regularly shut off the vasopressors under observation to ascertain that the patient still has pressure sensitive deficits and then to titrate the pressors to the lowest required blood pressure. Once the embolus is lysed or collateral flow paths improve, hypertension has no advantages but can be associated with cardiac decompensation or hemorrhage into stroke. We speculate that the latter is not an issue while the vascular obstruction results in low pressure in the distal ischemic tissue. This becomes an issue when there is recanalization and the injured tissue is then exposed to the elevated pressure. Induced hypertension to increase blood flow is standard therapy in treating ischemia in patients with vasospasm after subarachnoid hemorrhage *(24)*. It has been shown effective in increasing CBF and improving functional recovery in an primate stroke model *(25)* (Fig. 3). Its use requires careful attention to cardiac care. The electrocardiogram needs to be monitored for ischemic changes and chest roentgenogram and exam for signs of congestive heart failure.

Hemodilution helps to improve cerebral flow *(26)*, yet numerous trials with hypervolemic and isovolemic dilution have failed to show significant benefit in humans *(27–29)*. A hematocrit of at least 30% would be targeted, or hemoglobin 10 g/dL, which is the threshold above which arterial oxygen transport can be sustained without risk of cerebral ischemia *(30)*. Continuous infusions of mannitol (1–2 g/h) may also improve blood rheology, but its routine use for ischemic stroke patients is not supported by randomized trials. Other rheologic drugs have been studied, including low molecular weight dextran *(31)*, hydroxyethyl starch *(28)*, and glycerol *(32)* but with limited success and potential for worsening cerebral edema.

Ischemic Cerebral Edema

The development of significant cerebral edema occurs in up to 10–15% of ischemic stroke patients, with the period of maximal swelling occurring on poststroke d 2–5 (*see* Chapter 5 for a detailed discussion on cerebral edema and its treatment). This is most commonly seen in ICA, MCA stem and cerebellar strokes, where the mortality of malignant cerebral edema approaches 80% *(33,34)*. The pathophysiology underlying the development of cerebral edema after ischemic stroke is not well understood; however, the clinical syndromes that result have been well described. Although there are no established guidelines for management of cerebral edema in the acute stroke setting, current practice is to measure serum osmolarity and treat hypo-osmolar states, maintain normal glucose, control hypertension and aggressively treat fever. The goal of such treatment is to prevent the secondary infarctions that result from compression of vascular structures.

Medical Treatment

In the setting of acute deterioration from brain swelling, the first lines of therapy are diuresis with 1 g/kg intravenous bolus of mannitol and hyperventilation to reduce $PaCO_2$ to 30 mmHg. Mannitol reduces ICP by extracting water from the edematous tissue. The effects are usually immediate, but not sustained by one bolus alone. Therefore, it is usually administered on an every 4–6 h schedule with parameters to hold for blood osmolarity greater than 320. It is important to note, however, that the effectiveness is reduced with continued dosing. Moreover, the systemic effect of mannitol may lead to a significant dehydrated state resulting in a decrement in cerebral perfusion pressure and worsening of infarct size.

Other agents that have been reported to produce similar effects to mannitol have included glycerol, hypertonic saline (3% NaCl, 10% NaCl, 23% NaCl) *(35–37)*, and albumin *(38)*. Each of these agents requires multiple dosing and is also limited in its use by transient effectiveness. The use of barbituates, such as pentobarbital, is effective in reducing the metabolic rate, CBV and hence the ICP, but is reserved for only those instances of increase ICP that is refractory to all other medical therapies. It is initially dosed as an intravenous bolus of 3–7 mg/kg with continued boluses based on desired ICP, or initiated as a continuous infusion at 1–5 mg/kg/h. Although it reduces mortality, the use of pentobarbital is not known to improve functional outcome and is associated with potentially significant side effects including the inability to follow a neurological examination, decreased peripheral vascular tone, myocardial depression, illeus, decreased ability to track signs of infection (fever), and obstruction of lower airway passages from mucous plugging.

Hyperventilation to a $PaCO_2$ of 30 mmHg is the quickest acting therapy by which to reduce ICP. This occurs by reducing cerebrospinal fluid (CSF) pH, which results in cerebral vasoconstriction and reduction of CBF. However, this effect is also only transient, and prolonged vasoconstriction in the cerebrovascular bed may lead to exacerbation of ischemia *(39,40)*.

Hypothermia has been directly linked to lowered ICP prompting aggressive treatment of fever. Induced hypothermia with surface and invasive cooling techniques are currently under investigation for the treatment of malignant brain edema *(41)*. Current limitations of this technique include rebound swelling in the rewarming stage, infection (pneumonia being the most common), impaired myocardial contractility, and coagulopathy.

Decompressive Surgery in Internal Carotid Artery Territory Stroke

In patients with massive anterior circulation infarction an early discussion with family members (and occasionally patients) about hemicraniectomy as potential life-saving therapy should be considered. In prospective clinical studies, this technique has been shown to reduce mortality; however, timing of intervention may affect the potential for good functional outcome. In an open, prospective series of 63 patients, early hemicraniectomy (<24 h from symptom onset) significantly reduced length of stay in critical care compared to late surgery, and improved mortality (16% early vs 34.4% late) with a trend toward improved neurological outcome *(42)*. However, another series showed that in elderly patients with space-occupying infarction and without other comorbidities, hemicraniectomy improved survival but not functional outcome *(43)*. When considered, patients are monitored closely and at the earliest signs and symptoms of neurologic deterioration associated with worsening mass effect and effacement of the perimesencephalic cistern, hemicraniectomy with opening of the dura and duraplasty is performed. Successful surgery requires a very wide bone flap and duraplasty, otherwise compression of the swollen brain will occur at the sides of an inadequate craniectomy. The bone is stored in the patient's abdominal fat pad or frozen. The bone flap is usually replaced several weeks to months after removal. During the interim period, the patient wears a protective head gear to prevent injury.

Decompressive Surgery in Cerebellar Stroke

The patient with large inferior cerebellar infarction may be at risk for swelling with brainstem compression, hydrocephalus, and death *(44)*. Similar to large anterior circulation strokes, deterioration in the level of consciousness in large cerebellar strokes usually occurs in the first 2–4 d following onset of symptoms, peaking on day 3 *(45)*. Close monitoring for clinical signs and symptoms of brainstem compression or hydrocephalus is crucial. Clinical findings in acute hydrocephalus include drowsiness, emesis, loss of upgaze, pinpoint pupils, and long tract signs. Some of the hallmarks of brainstem compression include progressive cranial nerve deficits, deteriorating level of arousal, gaze paresis, extensor plantar reflexes, and decerebrate posturing. Serial CT scans are a necessary part of the assessment for hydrocephalus, cerebellar edema, or hemorrhagic transformation. In general, the posterior inferior cerebellar artery (PICA) infarcts have a far greater predilection for swelling as compared to the superior cerebellar artery (SCA) territory infarcts. The edema that develops is not responsive to osmotherapy or steroids, and surgical approaches are considered the effective treatments. Acute hydrocephalus can be reversed rapidly with placement of an external ventriculostomy drain; however, this does not prevent brainstem compression *(46)*. Most advocate decompression for massive cerebellar infarction causing progressive brain stem signs, hydrocephalus or impairment of consciousness. Even comatose patients had a 38% chance of a good recovery with decompressive surgery in one study *(46)*.

After cerebellectomy, patients cannot be safely anticoagulated for days, which may be problematic in some patients. Anticoagulation with intravenous heparin may be indicated in patients with cerebellar infarction who are at risk for fatal BA from severe vertebrobasilar atherosclerotic disease, or vertebral dissection. Patients presenting with fluctuating or progressive brainstem deficits often have severe atheromatous or embolic stenosis of the BA or a VA and are at risk of death from progression of thrombus leading to complete brainstem infarction *(47)*.

Poststroke Seizures

Seizures may occur in 6–9% of acute stroke patients *(48)*. The prompt treatment of seizures is especially important in the setting of large infarctions in order to prevent significant secondary neuronal injury (*see* Chapter 25). The treatment of active seizures is usually a 2 mg intravenous bolus of lorazepam. Further dosing may result in significant respiratory depression and reduced level of consciousness, and therefore should be used cautiously. Most commonly, maintenance therapy with phenytoin is initiated. Given the potentially serious adverse effects of ongoing seizure activity, phenytoin is given as a bolus of 15–20 mg/kg and subsequently dosed to maintain a drug level of 10–20 mg/dL. Therapy may be discontinued after 1 mo if no seizure activity occurs during treatment.

Anticoagulation

The role of fractionated and unfractionated heparin in the management of ischemic stroke has generated much debate. Recent studies and guidelines have not supported its use throughout the hospitalization period for patients with ischemic stroke *(49,50)*. We consider exceptions are those with nonmassive embolic stroke(s) distal to high grade atherosclerotic ICA stenosis, vertebrobasilar thrombosis, ICA or VA dissection as well as non-massive cardiogenic embolic strokes due to atrial fibrillation, noninfectious valvular heart disease, mechanical valves, parodoxical embolus with deep vein thrombosis (DVT), luminal clot demonstrated in the cerebrovascular vessels, aorta or heart. Other patients who merit consideration are those with myocardial infarction and/or myocardial thrombus, both of whom carry a high risk of recurrent embolism in the first 2 wk *(51)*. ICH with anticoagulation in the first day of stroke is exceedingly rare. Vigilant monitoring for cerebral hemorrhage and a strict partial thromboplastin time (PTT) target of 50–70 s is required. Anticoagulation becomes more dangerous after the first 48 h, at which point the risk of hemorrhagic conversion may outweigh the benefit of treatment. PTT values more than 150 s are especially dangerous.

In the PROACT study, secondary ICH (petechial and parenchymal) occurred in 13% (7/54) of patients treated with intravenous heparin and neurologic deterioration was seen in only patients in this subgroup (2%, 1/54). Three large prospective trials on low-molecular-weight heparin over the first weeks of stroke had up to approx 6% incidence of ICH resulting from anticoagulation *(52–54)*. If a repeat scan shows evidence of blood, a massive stroke or completed infarction of the territory supplied by the diseased vessel then heparin is stopped. Protamine sulfate can be used to reverse heparin if required urgently, with a target dose of 1 mg protamine sulfate/100 U of heparin. Subcutaneous heparin or low-molecular-weight heparin (LMWH) for deep venous thrombosis (DVT) prophylaxis is essential in stroke care.

Respiratory Issues

Aspiration pneumonia is the most common respiratory complication that occurs after ischemic stroke, occuring in up to 50% of cases. Patients with posterior circulation strokes, multiple lesions, larger territory infarcts, subcortical strokes, abnormal cough, abnormal gag, and dysphonia tend to have a higher frequency of aspiration and/or pneumonia *(55,56)*. Other clinical markers of aspiration include delayed oral transit and incomplete oral clearance *(57)*. Initial antibiotic coverage should include gram positive respiratory flora, gram negative nosocomial bacteria, and anaerobes. Once further culture data is obtained, antibiotic therapy can be tailored appropriately. Because of the immobility from neurologic injury, there is a relatively high incidence of DVT and resultant pulmonary embolism in the ischemic stroke population. Therefore, all acute ischemic stroke patients should have prophylactic therapy with sequential compression devices. There is no contraindication to the use of subcutaneous unfractionated heparin (UF heparin 5000 IU subcutaneously every 12 h) or LMWH (enoxaparin, 1 mg/kg subcutaneously every 12 h) in the setting of acute ischemic stroke and these agents should be used (*see* Chapter 11).

Only a minority of patients with ischemic stroke require mechanical ventilation. Progressive cerebral edema can result in a deterioration of the level of consciousness that necessitates intubation to protect the airway, and evolving ischemia and/or pressure against brainstem structures may also compromise the patient's respiratory pattern and hemodynamics, prompting invasive respiratory support. Although a subgroup of patients requiring intubation for cardiopulmonary compromise or seizures have been reported to have better neurologic recovery and survival, overall, the need for mechanical ventilation in this population has been associated with a high mortality and poorer outcome *(58)*. As a result, the use of invasive respiratory support in all cases of ischemic stroke is controversial and the decision for mechanical ventilation should be made in concert with the patient or appointed medical guardian.

Because the overwhelming indication for mechanical ventilation in acute ischemic stroke is for airway protection, most patients do well with just pressure support ventilation (*see* Chapter 9). The FiO2 should be maintained to keep the oxygen saturation greater than 90%. While high oxygen concentrations can be injurious to both the airway and lung parenchyma *(59)*, experimental data shows that increasing FiO_2 to 100% may salvage ischemic brain tissue, particularly in the cortex *(60)*. Whether patients with ischemic stroke could benefit from hyperoxia therapy is unknown, and is currently under investigation.

Whereas the criteria for successful extubation in medical patients has been well studied, the corollary for patients with ischemic stroke remains ill defined. The two populations are different, as patients with cardiopulmonary compromise usually have a problem with lung function, whereas ischemic stroke patients have a problem with airway protection. Still, many medical considerations are crucial for successful extubation, including euvolemia, correction of all electrolyte abnormalities and treatment of coexistent infections. Verification of respiratory mechanics remains important with attention to minute ventilation, respiratory rate, oxygenation, maximal inspiratory pressure and rapid shallow breathing index (RSBI), as defined by respiratory rate/tidal volume (f/VT). The latter is particularly useful, with a RSBI less than 100 being a sensitive predictor of successful weaning in medical patients *(61*; *see* Chapter 9).

Additional clinical parameters that may be helpful to guide weaning from mechanical ventilation include presence of a gag (or cough) reflex, decreased suctioning frequency, and good respiratory effort. Localization of stroke may also play a significant role in determining the likelihood of successful extubation. A Glascow coma scale score of ≥ 7 and lack of brainstem deficits have been reported as predictors of successful extubation in posterior circulation strokes *(62)*, while no such predictors have been reported in anterior circulation strokes. Decision and timing for tracheostomy is based on individual cases as there are no established criteria in ischemic stroke patients.

Temperature Management

An elevated core body temperature, or fever, defined as temperature more than 38.5°C occurs frequently in the first 48 h after an ischemic event *(63)*. Fever in the setting of ischemic stroke also has been shown to correlate with increased severity of stroke, size, mortality, and poorer prognosis in patients with ischemic stroke *(64)*. Hyperthermia induces a deleterious chain of events, in which it accelerates metabolism and neuronal injury. Whether hyperthermia is a marker of increased severity of stroke, or is a consequence of large strokes, is unclear. Nonetheless, temperature should be aggressively lowered using cooling blankets, acetaminophen and ice. Moreover, mild hypothermia has been shown to improve neurological outcome *(41)*, and reduce elevated ICP, especially in patients with MCA strokes *(65)*. The use of early hypothermia using inferior vena cava cooling devices is currently being evaluated as a neuroprotective strategy.

The presence of fever carries a wide differential, for which an intensive search for its potential causes is important. Infectious or chemical aspiration pneumonia, urinary tract infections, presence of indwelling catheters, line sepsis, or viral infections are common causes *(41)*. Once a source has been isolated, antibiotics should be administered early and relevant catheters should be removed. Less commonly, there are noninfectious causes of fever, including atelectasis, DVT, drug fever, hyperthyroidism, neoplastic processes, and inflammatory disorders, for which appropriate therapy should be initiated.

Nutritional Support

Early nutritional support should be implemented in all critically ill stroke patients via nasogastric tube. This decreases hemorrhagic gastritis, risk of sepsis, and improves the chance of surviving the NSU. In patients at risk or with cerebral edema, concentrated tube feeds (2 cal/mL) should be requested (most formula are 1 cal/mL, with significant free water) (*see* Chapter 14).

Most patients with major bulbar dysfunction due to brainstem and large hemispheric strokes will likely require weeks to months long enteral feeding, and therefore, once the initial critical period has passed early percutaneous gastrostomy (PEG) placement is indicated. Approximately 20–30% of patients have their PEG removed when they reestablish their ability to swallow safely and the median time needed for its insertion is 4 mo *(66,67)*. Complications include aspiration pneumonia, infection at PEG site (3%), and obstruction of the PEG.

As mentioned previously, many experimental studies have emphasized the role of elevated serum glucose in worsening degree of infarction. Elevated serum glucose may also be associated with worsened brain edema and hemorrhage into infarction. Although recent studies have shown the use of continuous insulin infusions to maintain tight blood glucose controls reduces morbidity and mortality in surgical intensive care patients *(68)*, there is no current clinical data for the use of continuous insulin infusion in the setting of acute cerebral infarction. Nonetheless, every attempt should be made to achieve normoglycemia.

CONCLUSION

The patient with a severe stroke due to occlusion of a major cerebral vessel has a poor outlook for functional recovery and often faces a fatal outcome or one bereft of quality of life. Invasive means of reversing the process of infarction may be warranted in such situations if patient or family surrogates give informed consent. Successful outcome from such interventions requires rapid action and a prepared multidisciplinary team and protocols. The complicated management of hemodynamic, ventilatory, coagulation, as well as neurologic issues, calls for experienced, neurointensive physicians and nursing care as well as constant monitoring. Success is far from routine but in the severe stroke patient the natural outcome may be so bleak that major risk is acceptable if intervention offers even a limited chance for acceptable recovery. Close communication with the family is an absolute requirement but makes the practice much more fulfilling. The opportunity to snatch a patient from stroke related death or permanent institutionalization in a nursing home motivates neurointensivists to develop better tools and more accurate clinical decision-making skills.

REFERENCES

1. Adams HP Jr, Brott TG, Crowell RM, et al. Guidelines for the management of patients with acute ischemic stroke. A statement for healthcare professionals from a special writing group of the Stroke Council, American Heart Association. *Circulation* 1994;90:1588–1601.
2. Lev MH, Segal AZ, Farkas J, et al. Utility of perfusion-weighted CT imaging in acute middle cerebral artery stroke treated with intra-arterial thrombolysis: Prediction of final infarct volume and clinical outcome. *Stroke* 2001;32:2021–2028.
3. Hillis AE, Wityk RJ, Barker PB, et al. Subcortical aphasia and neglect in acute stroke: the role of cortical hypoperfusion. *Brain* 2002;125:1094–1104.
4. Baird AE. Warach S. Imaging developing brain infarction. *Curr. Opin. Neurol.* 1999;12:65–71.

5. Baron JC, Rougemont D, Soussaline F, et al. Local interrelationships of cerebral oxygen consumption and glucose utilization in normal subjects and in ischemci stroke patients: a positron tomography study. *J. Cereb. Blood Flow Metab.* 1984;4:140–149.

6. Baron J. Mapping the ischaemic penumbra with PET: implications for acute stroke treatment. *Cerebrovasc. Dis.* 1999;9:193–201.

7. The National Institute of Neurological Disorders and Stroke rt-PA Stroke Study Group. Tissue plasminogen activator for acute ischemic stroke. *N. Engl. J. Med.* 1995;333:1581–1587.

8. Furlan A, Higashida R, Wechsler L, et al. Intra-arterial prourokinase for acute ischemic stroke. The PROACT II study: A randomized controlled trial. Prolyse in acute cerebral thromboembolism. *JAMA* 1999;282:2003–2011.

9. Phan TG, Wijdicks EFM. Intra-arterial thrombolysis for vertebrobasilar circulation ischemia. *Crit. Care Clin.* 1999;15:719–742.

10. Gonner F, Remonda L, Mattle H, et al. Local intra-arterial thrombolysis in acute ischemic stroke. *Stroke* 1998;29:1894–1900.

11. Lewandowski CA, Frankel M, Tomsick TA, et al. Combined intravenous and intra-arterial r-TPA versus intra-arterial therapy of acute ischemic stroke: Emergency Management of Stroke (EMS) Bridging Trial. *Stroke* 1999;30:2598–2605.

12. Kasper GC, Wladis AR, Lohr JM, et al. Carotid thromboendarterectomy for recent total occlusion of the internal carotid artery. *J. Vasc. Surg.* 2001;33:242–249.

13. Pikus HJ, Heros RC. Stroke: indications for emergent surgical intervention. *Clin. Neurosurg.* 1999;45:113–127.

14. Eckstein HH, Schumacher H, Klemm K, et al. Emergency carotid endarterectomy. *Cerebrovasc. Dis.* 1999;9:270–281.

15. Einhaupl KM, Villringer A, Meister W, et al. Heparin treatment in sinus venous throbosis. *Lancet* 1991;338:597–600.

16. Horowitz M, Purdy P, Unwin H, et al. Treatment of dural sinus thrombosis using selective catheterization and urokinase. *Ann. Neurol.* 1995;38:58–67.

17. Hill MD, Barber PA, Takahashi J, Demchuk AM, Feasby TE, Buchan AM. Anaphylactoid reactions and angioedema during alteplase treatment of acute ischemic stroke. *CMAJ* 2000;162:1281–1284.

18. Fayad PB, Albers GW, Frey JL, Raps EC. Orolingual angioedema complicating rt-PA therapy for acute ischemic stroke. *Stroke* 1999;30:242.

19. Fujii K, Sadoshima S, Okada Y, et al. Cerebral blood flow and metabolism in normotensive and hypertensive patients with transient neurologic deficits. *Stroke* 1990;21:283–290.

20. Hankey GJ, Gubbay SS. Focal cerebral ischaemia and infarction due to antihypertensive therapy. *Med. J. Austr.* 1987;146:412–414.

21. Rordorf G, Cramer SC, Efird JT, et al: Pharmacological elevation of blood pressure in acute stroke. Clinical effects and safety. *Stroke* 1997;28:818–821.

22. Hillis AE, Barker PB, Beauchamp NG, Winters BD, Mirski M, Wityk RJ. Restoring blood pressure reperfused Wernicke's area and improved language. *Neurology* 2001;56:670–672.

23. Rordorf G, Koroshetz W, Ezzeddine M, Segal A, Buonanno F. A pilot study of drug induced hypertension for treatment of acute stroke. *Neurology* 2001;56:1210–1212.

24. Muizelaar J, Becker D. Induced hypertension for the treatment of cerebral ischemia after subarachnoid hemorrrrhage: direct effects on cerebral blood flow. *Surg. Neurol.* 1986;25:317–325.

25. Hayashi S, Nehls DG, Kieck CF, Vielma J, DeGirolami U, Crowell RM. Beneficial effects of induced hypertension on experimental stroke in awake monkeys. *J. Neurosurg.* 1984;60:151–157.

26. Vorstrup S, Andersen A, Juhler M, Brun B, Boysen G. Hemodilution increases cerebral blood flow in acute ischemic stroke. *Stroke* 1989;20:884–889.

27. Asplund K, Israelsson K, Schampi I. Haemodilution for acute ischaemic stroke. *Coch. Database Syst. Rev.* 2000;2:CD000103.

28. Aichner FT, Fazekas F, Brainin M, Polz W, Mamoli B, Zeiler K. Hypervolemic hemodilution in acute ischemic stroke: The Multicenter Austrian Hemodilution Stroke Trial (MAHST). *Stroke* 1998;29:743–749.

29. Scandinavian Stroke Study Group. Multicenter trial of hemodilution in acute ischemic stroke. I. Results in the total patient population. *Stroke* 1987;18:691–699.

30. Dexter F, Hindman BJ. Effect of haemoglobin concentration on brain oxygenation in focal stroke: a mathematical modelling study. *Br J Anaesth* 1997;79:346–351.

31. Zhuang J, Shackford SR, Schmoker JD, Pietropaoli JA. Colloid infusion after brain injury: effect on intracranial pressure, cerebral blood flow, and oxygen delivery. *Crit. Care Med.* 1995;23:140–148.

32. a'Rogvi-Hansen B, Boysen G. Glycerol for acute ischaemic stroke. *Coch. Database Syst. Rev.* 2000;2:CD000096.

33. Hacke W, Schwab S, Horn M, Spranger M, De Georgia M, von Kummer R. Malignant middle cerebral artery territory infarction: clinical course and prognostic signs. *Arch. Neurol.* 1996;53:309–315.

34. Ropper AH, Shafran B. Brain edema after stroke: Clinical syndrome and intracranial pressure. *Arch Neurol.* 1984;41:26–29.

35. Qureshi AI, Suarez JI, Bhardwaj A, et al. Use of hypertonic (3%) saline/acetate infusion in the treatment of cerebral edema: Effect on intracranial pressure and lateral displacement of the brain. *Crit. Care Med.* 1998;26:440–446.

36. Schwarz S, Georgiadis D, Aschoff A, Schwab S. Effects of hypertonic (10%) saline in patients with raised intracranial pressure after stroke. *Stroke* 2002;33:136–140.

37. Suarez JI, Qureshi AI, Bhardwaj A, et al. Treatment of refractory intracranial hypertension with 23.4% saline. *Crit. Care Med.* 1998;26:1118–1122.
38. Belayev L, Liu Y, Zhao W, Busto R, Ginsberg MD. Human albumin therapy of acute ischemic stroke: marked neuroprotective efficacy at moderate doses and with a broad therapeutic window. *Stroke* 2001;32:553–560.
39. Schneider GH, Sarrafzadeh AS, Kiening KL, Bardt TF, Unterberg AW, Lanksch WR. Influence of hyperventilation on brain tissue-PO2, PCO2, and pH in patients with intracranial hypertension. *Acta Neurochir. Suppl.* 1998;71:62–65.
40. Muizelaar JP, Marmarou A, Ward JD, et al. Adverse effects of prolonged hyperventilation in patients with severe head injury: A randomized clinical trial. *J. Neurosurg.* 1991;75:731–739.
41. Krieger DW, De Georgia MA, Abou-Chebl A, et al. Cooling for acute ischemic brain damage (cool aid): An open pilot study of induced hypothermia in acute ischemic stroke. *Stroke* 2001;32:1847–1854.
42. Schwab S, Steiner T, Aschoff A, et al. Early hemicraniectomy in patients with complete middle cerebral artery infarction. *Stroke* 1998;29:1888–1893.
43. Koh MS, Goh KY, Tung MY, Chan C. Is decompressive craniectomy for acute cerebral infarction of any benefit? *Surg. Neurol.* 2000;53:225–230.
44. Lehrich JR, Winkler GF, Ojemann RG. Cerebellar infarction with brain stem compression. *Arch Neurol.* 1970;22:490–498.
45. Jauss M, Krieger D, Hornig C, Schramm J, Busse O. Surgical and medical management of patients with massive cerebellar infarctions: results of the German-Austrian Cerebellar Infarction Study. *J. Neurol.* 1999;246:257–264.
46. Hornig CR, Rust DS, Busse O, Jauss M, Laun A. Space-occupying cerebellar infarction. Clinical course and prognosis. *Stroke* 1994;25:372–374.
47. Kubik CS, Adams RD. Occlusion of the basilar artery—a clinical and pathological study. *Brain* 1946;69:73–121.
48. Lesser RP, Lüders DH, Dinner DS, Morris HH. Epileptic seizures due to thrombotic and embolic cerebrovascular disease in older patients. *Epilepsia* 1985;26:622–630.
49. Coull BM, Williams LS, Goldstein LB, et al. Joint Stroke Guideline Development Committee of the American Academy of Neurology. American Stroke Association. Anticoagulants and antiplatelet agents in acute ischemic stroke: report of the Joint Stroke Guideline Development Committee of the American Academy of Neurology and the American Stroke Association (a division of the American Heart Association). *Stroke* 2002;33:1934–1942.
50. Mohr JP, Thompson JL, Lazar RM, et al. Warfarin-Aspirin Recurrent Stroke Study Group. A comparison of warfarin and aspirin for the prevention of recurrent ischemic stroke. *N. Engl. J. Med.* 2001;345:1444–1451.
51. Cerebral Embolism Task Force. Cardiogenic brain embolism. *Arch. Neurol.* 1986;43:71–84.
52. TOAST. The Publications Committee for the Trial of Org 10172 in Acute Stroke Treatment (TOAST) Investigators. Low molecular weight heparinoid, ORG 10172 (Danaparoid), and outcome after acute ischemic stroke: a randomized controlled trial. *JAMA* 1998;279:1265–1272.
53. Berge E, Abdelnoor M, Nakstad PH, Sandset PM. Low molecular-weight heparin versus aspirin in patients with acute ischaemic stroke and atrial fibrillation: a double-blind randomised study. HAEST Study Group. Heparin in Acute Embolic Stroke Trial. *Lancet* 2000;355:1205–1210.
54. Bath PM, Lindenstrom E, Boysen G, et al. Tinzaparin in acute ischaemic stroke (TAIST): a randomised aspirin-controlled trial. *Lancet* 2001;358:702–710.
55. Mann G, Hankey GJ. Initial clinical and demographic predictors of swallowing impairment following acute stroke. *Dysphagia* 2001;16:208–215.
56. Ding R, Logemann JA. Pneumonia in stroke patients: a retrospective study. *Dysphagia* 2000;15:51–57.
57. Mann G, Hankey GJ. Initial clinical and demographic predictors of swallowing impairment following acute stroke. *Dysphagia* 2001;16:208–215.
58. Gujjar AR, Deibert E, Manno EM, Duff S, Diringer MN. Mechanical ventilation for ischemic stroke and intracerebral hemorrhage. Indications, timing, and outcome. *Neurology* 1998;51:447–451.
59. Jenkinson SG. Oxygen toxicity. *New Horizon* 1993;1:504–511.
60. Singhal AB, Dijkhuizen RM, Rosen BR, Lo EH. Normobaric hyperoxia reduces MRI diffusion abnormalities and infarct size in experimental stroke. *Neurology* 2002;58:945–952.
61. Yang KL, Tobin MJ. A prospective study of indexes predicting the outcome of trials of weaning from mechanical ventilation. *N. Engl. J. Med.* 1991;324:1445–1450.
62. Qureshi AI, Suarez JI, Parekh PD, Bhardwaj A. Prediction and timing of tracheostomy in patients with infratentorial lesions requiring mechanical ventilatory support. *Crit. Care Med.* 2000;28:1383–1387.
63. Grau Aj, Buggle F, Schnitzler P, Spiel M, Lichy C, Hacke W. Fever and infection early after ischemic stroke. *J. Neurol. Sci.* 1999;171:115–120.
64. Reith J, Jorgensen HS, Pedersen PM, et al.: Body temperature in acute stroke: relation to stroke severity, infarct size, mortality, and outcome. *Lancet* 1996;347:422–425.
65. Schwab S, Schwarz S, Spranger M et al. Moderate hypothermia in the treatment of patients with severe middle cerebral artery infarction. *Stroke* 1998;29:2461–2466.
66. Nicholson FB, Korman MG, Richardson MA. Percutaneous endoscopic gastrostomy: A review of indications, complications, and outcome. *J. Gastroenterol. Hepatol.* 2000;5:21–25.
67. James A, Kapur K, Hawthorne AB. Long term outcome of percutaneous endoscopic gastrostomy feeding in patients with dysphagic stroke. *Age Ageing* 1998;27:671–676.
68. Van den Berghe G, Wouters P, Weekers F, et al. Intensive insulin therapy in critically ill patients. *N. Engl. J. Med.* 2001;345:1359–1367.

19

Management of Nontraumatic Intracerebral Hemorrhage

Eliahu S. Feen, Aleksandyr W. Lavery, and Jose I. Suarez

INTRODUCTION

Spontaneous or nontraumatic intracerebral hemorrhage (ICH) is one of the more common causes for admission to the neurosciences critical care unit (NSU). We will review the epidemiology, pathophysiology (including etiology), clinical presentation, method of diagnosis, management, and prognosis of ICH in the present era. This topic has been the subject of excellent reviews in the literature in recent years (1,2).

ICH represents perhaps 10–15% of all strokes. However, ICH carries with it the highest mortality rate of the stroke subtypes. The Oxfordshire Community Stroke Project estimated that about 60% of patients with ICH do not survive beyond one year (3). ICH may extend into the ventricular system, although we will not deal directly with isolated intraventricular hemorrhage.

ICH has generally been classified as primary or secondary. Primary ICH, defined as the spontaneous bleeding from small arterioles classically thought to be damaged by chronic hypertension (HTN) or amyloid angiopathy, is estimated to constitute around 80% of all cases (4). Secondary ICH represents bleeding as a result of some underlying vascular pathology or a few other causes. The underlying causes of secondary ICH that are most commonly described are arteriovenous malformation (AVM), intracranial neoplasm, cavernous angioma, venous angioma, cerebral venous thrombosis, coagulopathy (either inherent or drug-induced, such as patients on chronic warfarin therapy), vasculitis, cocaine or alcohol use, and the hemorrhagic conversion of an ischemic stroke. We list in Table 1 certain important details of some of these causes (4–18). Thrombolysis-related ICH has been discussed in Chapter 18 in this book and will not be dealt with in detail in the present chapter.

EPIDEMIOLOGY AND RISK FACTORS

Several studies have been performed to assess the incidence of ICH (19–21). What has come out of these studies is that the incidence is estimated at 10–20 per 100,000 inhabitants, which appears to increase with age and to be more common in men. African Americans and Japanese in Japan have been identified to have a significantly higher incidence of ICH (3,22). It has been theorized that the higher prevalence of HTN, which is a known risk factor for ICH, among these two populations as compared to whites may explain the higher rates of incidence. Interestingly, there are some data regarding the Japanese population that low serum cholesterol may be a relevant risk factor predisposing the population to ICH (23).

The main risk factor for ICH is HTN. This risk is exacerbated in people who are younger than 55 or smoke (24). Long-term control of HTN does appear to reduce the incidence of ICH (25,26). Two prospective studies, the Hypertension Detection and Follow-up Program and the Systolic Hypertension in the Elderly Program (SHEP) have documented a clear reduction in the risk of ICH with

From: *Current Clinical Neurology*
Critical Care Neurology and Neurosurgery
Edited by: J. I. Suarez © Humana Press Inc., Totowa, NJ

Table 1
Characteristics of Selected Less Common Causes of Spontaneous Intercerebral Hemorrhage

Causes	Age group of greatest incidence	Location/arterial distribution	Recurrence rate
Amyloid angiopathy	Sixth to eighth decades of life	Cortex and subcortical white matter of cerebral lobes; small vessels affected, but not those in the basal ganglia and brainstem (5)	21–31% (6–8)
Intracranial aneurysm (9)	Mean for rupture of aneurysm is about 50 yr of age	Depends upon type of aneurysm (e.g., saccular, mycotic, etc.) but usually affecting medium-sized vessels	50% within 6 mo of rupture for unsecured aneurysms and 3% per yr afterward (10)
Arteriovenous malformation	Symptomatic presentation usually prior to 40 yr of age (not just intracranial hemorrhage)	Heterogeneous	2–4% per year in the absence of surgical correction (10,11)
Cavernous angioma	Symptomatic presentation usually prior to 30 yr of age	Mostly supratentorial locations but a minority occur in cerebellum and brainstem (12)	0.5–1% initial (12), and 4.5% recurrence (13)
Venous angioma	Mean age at diagnosis is in the fourth decade of life with a broad range	Mostly lobar with a frontal predominance and a minority in cerebellum and other locations	Recent estimate of rate of first bleed is 0.15% but recurrence rate not clearly delineated (14,15)
Neoplasms	Varies with tumor type (e.g., malignant astrocytomas are more common in older individuals)	Varies with site involved and with type of tumor. Most common neoplasms: primary: anaplastic astrocytoma/glioblastoma muliforme; oligodendrogliomas, pituitary adenomas; metastatic: lung, kidney, choriocarcinoma, melanoma	Overall estimate of bleeding in intracranial neoplasms may be 1–15%
Drugs of abuse (e.g., amphetamine, cocaine, "ecstasy")	Younger age (usually third through fifth decades of life), corresponding to the prevalence of drug use in this population	Amphetamines-cortical lobes Cocaine-supratentorail Arteries affected vary because etiology may be vasculitis with amphetamines and a vasculopathy and/or hypertensive effect with cocaine (16–18)	Unknown

control of blood pressure *(27,28)*. Other risk factors include alcohol and lower cholesterol levels (an association seen at less than 160 mg/dL) *(29–31)*. In elderly individuals, cerebral amyloid angiopathy represents a significant risk factor for lobar ICH. In this condition, associated with the presence of a pathologically increased amount of β-amyloid protein in small- and medium-sized cerebral arteries, there is a significantly increased risk of lobar hemorrhage and the risk of recurrence is estimated to be as high as 10.5%. A genetic association in this condition with the presence of either ε2 or ε4 alleles of the apolipoprotein E gene appears to triple the risk of lobar hemorrhage *(6)*. Carriers of ε2 or ε4 alleles may have a 2-yr rate of recurrence of 28%.

PATHOPHYSIOLOGY
Location

The most common locations for ICH are: the lobes, basal ganglia, thalamus, pons (and to a lesser extent the other parts of the brainstem, the midbrain and the medulla), and cerebellum *(32)* (Fig. 1). These locations correspond to small perforating arteries branch from large cerebral arteries. It is the bifurcation point of the perforating arteries branching off from the larger arteries that seems most vulnerable to damage. Thus, it is also the most likely point at which some kind of rupture or tear, and consequently bleeding, occurs. It has been observed that there is degeneration of the media and smooth muscles of the arterioles at these points *(33)*. In general, ICH located in basal ganglia, thalamus, cerebellum and pons is most likely related to HTN, whereas lobar presentations are usually associated with other etiologies and require further work up (Table 2).

Progression of Hemorrhage, Edema Formation, and Local Ischemia

After the initial bleeding there can be expansion of the hematoma. Interestingly, this was essentially unknown until the advent of head CT scanning. Once CT scans were performed routinely and then progressively over the hospital course of patients with ICH, it was serendipitously realized that the hematoma can expand over time. In two studies, approx 20–25% of patients were found to have expansion of the hematoma within 1 h after initial head computed tomography (CT) *(34,35)*. It was partly on the basis of these findings that so much emphasis has been placed upon controlling blood pressure, the elevation of which is considered a risk factor for hematoma expansion *(see* below in the section on blood pressure management). In addition to elevated blood pressure, there is some evidence of a coagulopathy (perhaps acting locally) playing a role in continued bleeding *(36,37)*.

Around the hematoma itself brain parenchyma becomes edematous around 24–48 h after onset. Usually this edema persists for a few days, but there are reported cases of persistent edema up to 2 wk after an ICH *(38)*. The etiology of this edema appears to be multifactorial. Several animal studies have related edema to osmotic effects of proteins within the clot and the presence of thrombin along with classical mechanisms of edema formation in vasogenic and cytotoxic edema due to breakdown of the blood-brain barrier and neuronal cell death *(39–41)*. The prominent role of thrombin in edema formation has led to the use of intraclot thrombolytic therapy to reduce ICH size with mixed results *(see* below). It has also to be theorized that ischemic damage to brain tissue in the parenchyma bordering the hematoma occurs as a result of occlusion of nearby small vessels from compression by the hematoma *(42)*. However, more recent studies have determined this not to be the case *(38,43,44)*. Presently, available evidence, especially from animal studies, suggests that neuronal damage in the region around a hematoma is the result of secondary factors, such as plasma mediators, and possibly apoptosis-induced necrosis of neurons *(1)*.

CLINICAL PRESENTATION AND INITIAL CLINICAL PROGRESSION

The clinical presentation of ICH is not unlike that of other kinds of strokes. The location of the ICH determines the clinical effect, such as contralateral deficits in motor function if, say, there is disruption of the corticospinal tracts in the internal capsule. Brain stem ICH is known to produce

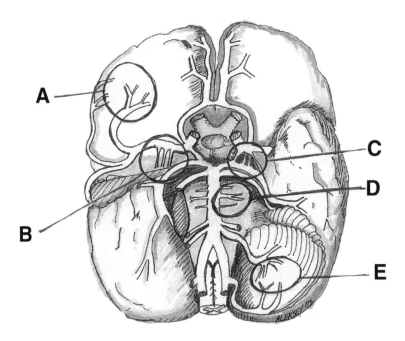

Fig. 1. Most common sites and sources of intracerebral hemorrhage: **(A)** Intracerebral hemorrhage involving the cerebral lobes most commonly originates from cortical branches of anterior, middle, and posterior cerebral arteries. **(B)** Lenticulostriate branches of the middle cerebral artery are the common source of basal ganglia hemorrhage. **(C)** Thalamogeniculate branches off the posterior cerebral artery are the source of thalamic hemorrhage. **(D)** Paramedian branches from the basilar artery are the source of hemorrhage in the pons. **(E)** Penetrating branches of posterior inferior, anterior inferior, and superior cerebellar arteries the source of cerebellar hemorrhage.

expected deficits in gaze and other motor functions, given the cranial nerve nuclei locations there. Cerebellar ICH classically produces ataxia and nystagmus *(45)*. Other clinical features typical of ICH include decreased level of consciousness, especially with large hematomas, because of the increased intracranial pressure (ICP) or as a consequence of disruption of the reticular activating system within the thalamus or brain stem *(46,47)*. Loss of higher cortical functions producing such deficits as aphasia and visual-spatial neglect, occur either with ICH into the appropriate cortex or possibly through a mechanism of diaschisis, when the ICH is in the subcortex. In this mechanism there appears to be functional suppression of a particular region of cortex through the disruption of the subcortical tracts stemming from that region *(48)*. In addition, ICH commonly produces headache and vomiting, which is often associated with the development of elevated ICP. Neck stiffness often occurs in the setting of ICH as well, especially if there is blood in the ventricular system *(45,49,50)*.

Qureshi et al. *(1,51)* and Mayer et al. *(52)* have identified several features of the clinical progression of ICH. Within the first 24 h after the onset of an ICH, approx 25% of patients who present in an alert state will experience a depressed level of consciousness. A large hematoma and blood within the ventricular system are factors that increase the odds of deterioration and mortality. Within the first 3 h after onset, the most common cause of deterioration is progression of bleeding. Beyond 24 h but up to 48 h after onset, edema also contributes to clinical deterioration.

DIAGNOSIS

Several factors may suggest the presence of ICH. The evidence of nausea and vomiting is usually an indication of mass effect and is seen in as much as 50% of ICH. These symptoms are rarely seen in

Table 2
Intracranial Hemorrhage Characteristics Regarding Location and Underlying Etiology

Location	Etiology
Putamen (28–42% of all cases)	Mostly hypertension (90%)
Thalamus (10–26% of all cases)	Mostly hypertension (90%)
Lobar (19–30% of all cases)	Usually arteriovenous malformations, coagulopathies, amyloid angiopathy (elderly), aneurysms, and hypertension (only 35%)
Cerebellum (8–15% of all cases)	Mostly hypertension (85%)
Brainstem (4–11% of all cases)	Mostly hypertension (70%)

patients with ischemic stroke. Often patients have a history of HTN and demonstrate markedly elevated blood pressure on admission. A history of anticoagulation or recent thrombolytics may suggest the diagnosis of hemorrhage. Certainly, the symptoms are acute in onset and may be anything from a headache to frank coma as mentioned previously. Abnormal clinical findings may be progressive, but their onset is generally acute in nature. Although ICH may be suspected it can only be verified with imaging as outlined below.

Head Computed Tomography Scanning

Head CT scanning is fast and effective at diagnosing acute blood, and remains the modality of choice *(53)* (*see* Chapter 7). Although it is important to quickly assess and diagnose ICH, patients with a Glasgow coma scale (GCS) score ≤ 8 or the inability to protect their airway should be intubated before diagnostic imaging is attempted. The CT should be obtained without contrast when suspecting hemorrhage because some contrast-enhancing tumors can have similar characteristics to acute blood. The addition of contrast agent can be made after the initial scan if a tumor is suspected, and may prove to be of benefit in some cases where it can demonstrate continued bleeding.

Acute Course

Acute blood appears hyperintense on CT, whereas infarcted brain will appear hypointense or isointense. Very rarely ICH can be isointense to the surrounding brain in severely anemic patients with a hematocrit of 20% or less *(53)*. An acute intracerebral clot is usually round and of homogeneous density. Typically there is little edema around a fresh clot, but there may be a fine rim of low density indicating clot retraction. Calcified and highly proteinaceous material can reach a similar density to fresh blood clot, but the clinical context usually suggests the diagnosis. ICH volume, which is important to determine outcome as outlined later, can be easily measured at the bedside *(54)*. It can be calculated by a quick ellipsoid method given by the following formula:

$$A \times B \times C / 2$$

Where A represents the largest diameter of the largest portion of ICH seen on CT; B is the diameter perpendicular to A; and C is the number of 10 mm-thick CT slices where ICH is appreciated (Fig. 2).

Time Course

Over the course of several days, an untreated hematoma becomes less radiodense, from the periphery towards the center, and therefore appears smaller. Vasogenic edema may develop in the surrounding white matter, and intravenous contrast medium given at this stage usually produces a ring of enhancement. After several weeks, the CT density of the blood products can be similar to that of the brain or cerebrospinal fluid (CSF).

Intraventricular Blood

In deep-seated or extensive intracranial hemorrhage, blood frequently leaks into the ventricles and may adhere to the ependyma or to the choroid plexus. Blood may sink to the most dependent part of

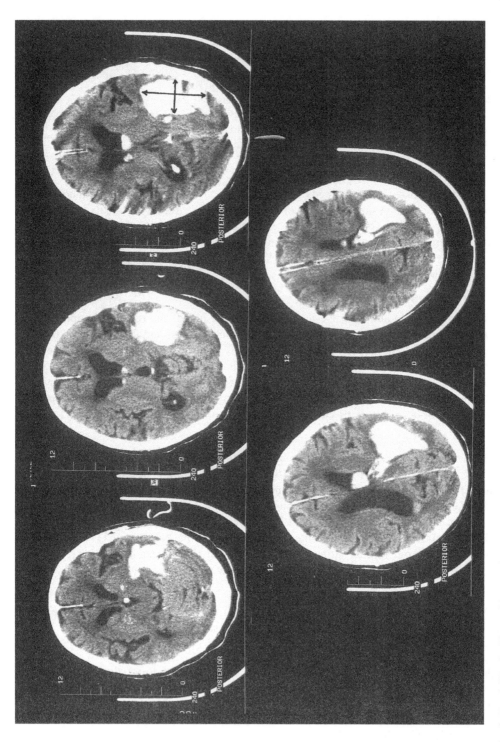

Fig. 2. Head CT of a 72-yr-old man who presented with sudden-onset global aphasia. Images reveal a moderate size left parietal-temporal ICH (38.4 cm³). The volume was calculated by the ellipsoid method as described in the text: A × B × C/2. The largest diameter A is depicted along with the perpendicular diameter B The number of 10-mm slices where ICH is appreciated is 5.

the ventricular system, usually the occipital horns, and form a ventricular fluid level (*see* Fig. 2). If blood is visualized within the third and fourth ventricles the patient is at risk of obstructing CSF outflow. This commonly causes hydrocephalus and may require urgent neurosurgical intervention to drain and reduce the pressure within the ventricles.

Magnetic Resonance Imaging

Magnetic resonance imaging (MRI) of the head is the method of choice to further evaluate for a possible neoplastic source, and for arteriovenous malformation. MRI of ICH follows a predictable time course, in which the presence of various hemoglobin degradation products and red blood cell lysis play important roles (55). As the hematoma ages, hemoglobin passes through a number of breakdown products, which include deoxyhemoglobin, methemoglobin and hemosiderin. This represents only an approximate guide and other factors contribute considerably to the MRI appearances, accounting for discrepancy.

Hyperacute Stage

MRI within the first few hours of ICH will reveal isointense or hypointense characteristics on T1-weighted imaging (T1), and slightly hyperintense on T2-weighted imaging (T2). This is based on the paramagnetic properties of oxyhemoglobin.

Acute Stage

Within the first several days of a hemorrhage, the hemoglobin within the clot has been converted mainly to deoxyhemoglobin. Signal characteristics on T1 and T2 will appear hypointense.

Subacute Stage

As time goes on and further ICH degradation occurs, deoxyhemoglobin is converted to methemoglobin. Based on whether the methemoglobin is intracellular or extracellular differentiates early subacute from late subacute. At 3–7 d, the majority of methemoglobin is intracellular and signal characteristics are hyperintense on T1 and hypointense on T2. As the balance shifts to an extracellular methemoglobin (1–4 wk) both T1 and T2 are hyperintense.

Chronic Stage

Breakdown of methemoglobin to hemosiderin occurs after approx 1 mo. At this stage, clots typically are homogeneously hyperintense on both T1 and T2 and have a pronounced low signal rim on T2.

Cerebral Angiography

Cerebral angiography should be performed in patients younger than 45 yr of age (especially if not known hypertensives), or patients with suspected aneurysm or AVM. Patients older than age 60 with HTN have a low probability of a revealing angiography. As discussed previously, lobar ICH or the presence of SAH should raise suspicion for secondary etiologies and these patients should be considered for further evaluation with cerebral angiography. Cavernous malformations have a typical "popcorn" appearance on MRI but do not appear on angiography.

MANAGEMENT

Initial Evaluation

Airway, breathing, and circulation are addressed first as discussed in Chapter 1. Initial management involves proper recognition of decreased level of consciousness. Patients with a GCS score of ≤8 or impaired gag reflexes should be intubated to protect their airway. Rapid sequence intubation is preferred (*see* Chapter 9). Muscle relaxants should not be maintained after intubation, but sedation with propofol can maintain comfort and prevent coughing and straining that are associated with subsequent ICP spikes. Sedation should be stopped for hourly neurologic examinations to assess for rebleeding and deterioration.

Blood Pressure Management

HTN is common and is present in most patients in the early period following ICH. It has been reported that average presenting pressures are systolic of 190 mmHg and diastolic of 100 mmHg within the first few hours after ICH *(56)*. The presence of higher blood pressure is most strongly associated with history of HTN and temporal proximity to the hemorrhage. The initial blood pressure on presentation should be treated with urgency. As discussed previously, it has been demonstrated that ICH is not a monophasic event and subsequent rebleeding can and does occur in the first 6–24 h after the initial event. Kazui et al. showed that about 36% of patients had expansion of their hematoma within the first 3 h of the initial scan and 16% within 3–6 h of first scan, but no enlargement in size after 24 h. They also demonstrated an improvement in 30-d mortality among those patients with controlled HTN (mean arterial pressure [MAP] <125 mmHg) vs uncontrolled (MAP >125 mmHg): 21% compared to 43%, respectively *(35)*. A goal reduction of 30% of initial presenting MAP to avoid hypotension and potential ischemia is usually recommended.

Studies have shown that autoregulation of cerebral vessels is shifted in hypertensive patients to a higher curve and thus they require higher MAP to maintain adequate cerebral perfusion pressures (CPP) *(56)*. It has been argued that MAP should be kept at relatively high values. However, the risk of reducing CPP is likely out weighed by the risk of increased ICP from continued HTN and clot expansion. Intravenous medications are fast acting and effective and are therefore first choice. Preferably short-acting and easily titratable agents should be used. Labetalol and enalaprilat are two medications that are not associated with elevation of ICP and are well tolerated. Hydralazine is an effective agent that should be considered second line, despite the theoretical risk of increasing ICP. Patients unresponsive to initial medications (i.e., systolic blood pressure >180 mmHg despite 60–150 mg of labetalol), or with extremely elevated pressures (systolic blood pressure > 220 mmHg or diastolic blood pressure >120 mmHg) should be started on a continuous intravenous drip, usually of nitroprusside, and subsequently weaned off over 12–24 h if possible (*see* Chapter 13).

Elevated Intracranial Pressure

Patients should be positioned with head of bed at 30–45 degrees to optimize venous drainage from the brain. Minimal stimulation should be performed and presedation should be given when suctioning, moving or cleaning patients. Signs of herniation should be treated acutely with hyperventilation and immediate mannitol treatment. After treatment with mannitol, serum osmolarity should be checked routinely. Mannitol treatments should not allow serum osmolarity to exceed 320 mOsm/L. Increasing the sedation of patients that are straining or coughing will help to reduce ICP, and if necessary paralytics can be used. Neurosurgical consultation may be required for further ICP concerns and external ventricular drainage (*see* Chapter 5 for detailed description of elevated ICP).

Other NSU Management

Other important considerations include prophylaxis for deep vein thrombosis and gastrointestinal ulcers (*see* Chapter 11). All patients should have sequential compression devices placed on both legs as standard precaution. These patients are at high risk for DVT, being bed-bound and often hemiparetic. The use of subcutaneous heparin should be avoided. There remains considerable controversy over when heparin can be started on patients with ICH. Conservative treatment is to wait 2–3 wk after ICH onset. However, some more current studies have addressed anticoagulation mostly after craniotomy, and found no increased risk of ICH when started as soon as 3 d after craniotomy *(57)*. High-risk patients or those in whom a DVT develops typically require an inferior vena cava filter to reduce the incidence of pulmonary embolism.

Surgical Management

All patients with ICH should have a neurosurgical evaluation early in their course. With that said, there are few surgical interventions that have shown any benefit in this patient population. Routine interventions include placing an ICP monitor in patients with large hemorrhage to help with ICP management, and placing a ventriculostomy in patients showing evidence of obstructive hydrocephalus. Surgical clot evacuation remains more controversial unless used as a lifesaving measure. The majority of ICH is related to hypertension, and is deep seeded within the parenchymal tissues of the basal ganglia and thalamus. Surgical evacuation of a clot requires a cortectomy, or incision in the cortex of the brain, and subsequent transection through white matter to remove hemorrhage. Few adequate trials have been performed to address the issue of when ICH removal is beneficial.

The STICH trial was a single center randomized clinical trial of surgical treatment for intracerebral hemorrhage, in which craniotomies were performed within 12 h of presentation vs best medical treatment. This study showed lower mortality at 1 mo but similar mortality at 6 mo in a group of 17 patients treated surgically and 17 treated medically (58). In this study, it was hypothesized that early surgical evacuation might produce better results, with lower mortality. In a follow up study, the same group performed craniotomies within 4 h of hemorrhage, and found a large proportion of rebleeding (40%) (59).

There remains little proven benefit to surgical evacuation of ICH to date, but it is still done routinely in many institutions. Certain factors should be considered when evaluating surgical candidacy of patients with ICH. Size and location may provide easy access for clot removal. More superficial clots, cortical or lobar, require less disruption of normal brain during the evacuation, while larger ones pose more risk of herniation and swelling. Certainly hemorrhage in the cerebellum benefits from evacuation, especially if showing signs of obstructive hydrocephalus or measures more than 3 cm in diameter, and must be addressed by a neurosurgeon. Patients with significant mass effect and impending herniation may benefit from emergent evacuation to prevent eminent death. However, patients with evidence of lost upper brainstem reflexes and extensor posturing likely obtain no benefit from surgery (60).

A number of surgical options are available at this time with mixed reports of success. Endoscopic approach provides the possibility of evacuating a clot with a minimal incision and less tissue disruption (61). An endoscopic approach in conjunction with thrombolytics or a high powered water jet are being investigated. Stereotactic approaches provide the possibility of placing a catheter into deep-seated clots and aspirating with or without the application of thrombolytics. There have been few studies to analyze the benefit of this application, but preliminary reports show that it is safe to apply thrombolytics. The safest and most effective time course for thrombolytic therapy remains to be seen. The administration of thrombolytics into hematomas via catheter placement remains the most promising surgical therapy on the horizon. Reports of intraventricular blood removed by thrombolysis have demonstrated some benefit; however, randomized and blinded studies need to be done (63). It has been suggested that the overall reduction of the clot material improves survival and reduces the subsequent swelling likely potentiated by release of vasogenic factors and breakdown products including thrombin as discussed before. Whether the removal of blood products can be done slowly, via catheter and thrombolytic, or should be done quickly, via surgical evacuation, remains to be seen.

PROGNOSIS

Short-Term Outcome

Overall outcome in ICH is poor. Mortality rates for spontaneous ICH generally remain in the 40% to 50% range. Broderick et al. found a 30-d mortality rate in these patients of 44% (54). In studies incorporating multivariate analysis volume of ICH, age, GCS score on admission, pulse pressure, and blood pressure on admission have all been demonstrated to be important independent predictors of survival. Volume of parenchymal hemorrhage is the single best prognostic indicator for all locations and age (54) (see Fig. 2). More recent studies have investigated and confirmed prior reports that the presence and degree of intraventricular extension and presence and degree of hydrocephalus are important independent predictors of outcome in spontaneous ICH in addition to parenchymal hemorrhage volume. These same variables have been shown to be predictive of poor outcome in thrombolysis-related ICH. Generally greater mean volume of hemorrhages related to thrombolysis or coagulopathy makes outcomes for these patients especially poor. Medical comorbidities, especially cardiopulmonary diseases, adversely affect outcome and are often exacerbated in the setting of acute ICH. We have proposed a grading scale that correlates with functional outcome at 30 d *(63)*. Using strength of association points are assigned to predictive factors: age $\geq$ 80 yr (1 point), admission GCS $\leq$ 8 (2 points), admission GCS 9–12 (1 point), ICH volume $\geq$ 30 cm^3 (2 points), presence of intraventricular hemorrhage (2 points), brainstem location (2 points), and supratentorial location (1 point). Patients with 0 points had no mortality and 75% good outcome, whereas those with 8 points had an 85.71% mortality rate and 0% good outcome. Grading scales such as this can potentially be used to design critical trials for newer therapies for ICH patients.

Long-Term Outcome

Overall, patients who regain functional independence after ICH have a risk of recurrence of 2–6% yearly, and this is highly correlated with old age. Men have a twofold higher risk than women and those placed on anticoagulation after their initial event triple their risk of recurrence *(64)*. However, as stated before some etiologies are associated with higher incidence of rebleeding than others.

CONCLUSION

ICH remains a devastating disease. However, newer and exciting research has shed light into several pathophysiologic mechanisms including ICH growth, edema formation, cerebral blood flow around the clot, and management of HTN. Clinical trials are desperately needed to evaluate various therapies for ICH such as intraclot thrombolysis, early surgical evacuation, and neuroprotective drugs.

REFERENCES

1. Qureshi AI, Tuhrim S, Broderick JP, Batjer, HH, Hondo H, Hanley DF. Spontaneous intracerebral hemorrhage. *N. Engl. J. Med.* 2001;344:1450–1460.
2. Diringer MN. Intracerebral hemorrhage: Pathophysiology and management. *Crit. Care Med.* 1993;21:1591–1603.
3. Dennis MS, Burn JP, Sandercock PA, Bamford JM, Wade DT, Warlow CP. Long-term survival after first-ever stroke: The Oxfordshire Community Stroke Project. *Stroke* 1993;24:796–800.
4. Foulkes MA, Wolf PA, Price TR, Mohr JP, Hier DB. The stroke data bank: design, methods, and baseline characteristics. *Stroke* 1988;19:547–554.
5. Vinters HV. Cerebral amyloid angiopathy: A critical review. *Stroke* 1987;18:311–324.
6. O'Donnell HC, Rosand J, Knudsen KA, et al. Apolipoprotein E genotype and the risk of recurrent lobar intracerebral hemorrhage. *N. Engl. J. Med.* 2000;342:240–245.
7. Passero S, Burgalassi L, D'Andrea P, Battistini N, et al. Recurrence of bleeding in patients with primary intracerebral hemorrhage. *Stroke* 1995;26:1189–1192.
8. Neau JP, Ingrand P, Couderq C, et al. Recurrent intracerebral hemorrhage. *Neurology* 1997;49:106–113.
9. Selman WR, Tarr RW, Ratcheson RA. Intracranial aneurysms and subarachnoid hemorrhage. In Bradley WG, Daroff RB, Fenichel GM, Marsden CD (eds). *Neurology in Clinical Practice*, 3rd ed. Boston: Butterworth-Heinemann, 2000, pp. 1185–1200.
10. Jane JA, Kassell NF, Tomer JC, Winn HR. The natural history of aneurysms and arteriovenous malformations. *J. Neurosurg.* 1985;62:321–323.
11. Mohr JP on behalf of the Arteriovenous Malformation Study Group. Arteriovenous malformations of the brain in adults. *N. Engl. J. Med.* 1999;340:1812–1818.
12. Robinson JR, Awad IA, Little, JR. Natural history of the cavernous angioma. *J. Neurosurg.* 1991;75:709–714.
13. Kondziolka D, Lunsford LD, Kestle JR. The natural history of cerebral venous malformations. *J. Neurosurg.* 1995;83:820–824.
14. Naff NJ, Wemmer J, Hoenig-Rigamonti K, Rigamonti D. A longitudinal study of patients with venous malformations. *Neurology* 1998;50:1709–1714.
15. Malik GM, Morgan JK, Boulos RS, Ausman JI. Venous angiomas: An underestimated cause of intracranial hemorrhage. *Surg. Neurol.* 1988;30:350–358.
16. Buxton N, McConachie NS. Amphetamine abuse and intracranial haemorrhage. *J. R. Soc. Med.* 2000;93:472–477.

17. Nolte KB, Brass LM, Fletterick CF. Intracranial hemorrhage associated with cocaine abuse: A prospective autopsy study. *Neurology* 1996;46:1291–1296.
18. McEvoy AW, Kitchen D, Thomas GT. Intracerebral haemorrhage and drug abuse in young adults. *Br. J. Neurosurg.* 2000;14:449–454.
19. Broderick JP, Brott T, Tomsick T, Huster G, Miller R. The risk of subarachnoid and intracerebral hemorrhages in blacks as compared with whites. *N. Engl. J. Med.* 1992;326:733–736.
20. Furlan AJ, Whisnant JP, Elveback LR. The decreasing incidence of primary intracerebral hemorrhage: a population study. *Ann. Neurol.* 1979;5:367–373.
21. Giroud M, Gras P, Chadan N, et al. Cerebral hemorrhage in a French prospective population study. *J. Neurol. Neurosurg. Psychiatry* 1991;54:595–598.
22. Suzuki K, Kutsuzawa T, Takita K, et al. Clinico-epidemiologic study of stroke in Akita, Japan. *Stroke* 1987;18:402–406.
23. Tanaka H, Ueda Y, Hayashi M, et al. Risk factors for intracerebral hemorrhage and cerebral infaction in a Japanese rural community. *Stroke* 1982;13:62–73.
24. Brott T, Thalinger K, Hertzberg V. Hypertension as a risk factor for spontaneous intracerebral hemorrhage. *Stroke* 1986;17:1078–1083.
25. Thrift AG, McNeil JJ, Forbes A, Donnan GA. Three important subgroups of hypertensive persons at greater risk of intracerebral hemorrhage. *Hypertension* 1998;31:1223–1229.
26. Qureshi AI, Suri MAK, Safdar K, Otenlips JR, Janssen RS, Frankel MR. Intracerebral hemorrhage in blacks: risk factors, subtypes, and outcome. *Stroke* 1997;28:961–964.
27. Hypertension Detection and Follow-up Program Cooperative Group. Five-year findings of the Hypertension Detection and Follow-up Program III. Reduction in stroke incidence among persons with high blood pressure. *JAMA* 1982;247:633–638.
28. SHEP Cooperative Research Group. Prevention of stroke by antihypertensive drug treatment in older persons with isolated systolic hypertension: Final results of the Systolic Hypertension in the Elderly Program (SHEP). *JAMA* 1991;265:3255–3264.
29. Klatsky AL, Armstrong MA, Friedman GD. Alcohol use and subsequent cerebrovascular disease hospitalizations. *Stroke* 1989;20:741–746.
30. Gorelick PB. Alcohol and stroke. *Stroke* 1987;18:268–271.
31. Iso H, Jacobs DR Jr. Wentworth D, Neaton JD, Cohen JD. Serum cholesterol levels and six-year mortality from stroke in 350,977 men screened for multiple risk factor intervention trial. *N. Engl. J. Med.* 1989;320:904–910.
32. Mutlu N, Berry RG, Alpers BJ. Massive cerebral hemorrhage: clinical and pathological correlations. *Arch. Neurol.* 1963;8:644–661.
33. Cole FM, Yates PO. Pseudo-aneurysms in relationship to massive cerebral hemorrhage. *J. Neurol. Neurosurg. Psychiatry* 1967;30:61–66.
34. Brott T, Broderick J, Kothari R, et al. Early hemorrhage growth in patients with intracerebral hemorrhage. *Stroke* 1997;28:1–5.
35. Kazui S, Naritomi H, Yamamoto H, Sawada T, Yamaguchi T. Enlargement of spontaneous intracerebral hemorrhage: Incidence and time course. *Stroke* 1996;27:1783–1787.
36. Olson JD. Mechanisms of homeostasis: effect on intracerebral hemorrhage. *Stroke* 1993;24:Suppl:I109–I114.
37. Kazui S, Minematsu K, Yamamoto H, Sawada T, Yamaguchi T. Predisposing factors to enlargement of spontaneous intracrerebral hematoma. *Stroke* 1997;28:2370–2375.
38. Zazulia AR, Diringer MN, Derdeyn CP, Powers WJ. Progression of mass effect after intracerebral hemorrhage. *Stroke* 1999;30:1167–1173.
39. Yang GY, Betz AL, Chenevert TL, Brunberg JA, Hoff JT. Experimental intracerebral hemorrhage: relationship between brain edema, blood flow, and blood-brain barrier permeability in rats. *J. Neurosurg.* 1994;81:93–102.
40. Wagner KR, Xi G, Hua Y, et al. Lobar intracerebral hemorrhage model in pigs: rapid edema development in perihematomal white matter. *Stroke* 1996;27:490–497.
41. Wagner KR, Xi G, Hua Y, Kleinholz M, de Courten-Myers GM, Myers RE. Early metabolic alteration sin edematous perihematomal brain regions following experimental intracerebral hemorrhage. *J. Neurosurg.* 1998;88:1058–1065.
42. Bullock R, Brock-Utne J, van Dellen J, Blake G. Intracerebral hemorrhage in a primate model: effect on regional cerebral blood flow. *Surg. Neurol.* 1988;29:101–107.
43. Qureshi AI, Wilson DA, Hanley DF, Traystman RJ. Pharmacological reduction of mean arterial pressure does not adversely affect regional cerebral blood flow and intracranial pressure in experimental intracerebral hemorrhage. *Crit. Care Med.* 1999;27:965–971.
44. Qureshi AI, Wilson DA, Hanley DF, Traystman RJ. No evidence for an ischemic penumbra in massive experimental intracerebral hemorrhage. *Neurology* 1999;52:2166–2172.
45. Ott KH, Kase CS, Ojemann RG, Mohr JP. Cerebellar hemorrhage: Diagnosis and treatment: A review of 56 cases. *Arch. Neurol.* 1974;31:160–167.
46. Mohr JP, Caplan LR, Melski JW, et al. The Harvard Cooperative Stroke Registry: A prospective registry. *Neurology* 1978;28:754–762

47. Andrews BT, Chiles BW, Olsen WL, Pitts LH. The effect of intracerebral hematoma location on the risk of brain-stem compression and on clinical outcome. *J. Neurosurg.* 1988;69:518–522.
48. Tanaka A, Yoshinaga S, Nakayama Y, Kimura M, Tomonaga M. Cerebral blood flow and clinical outcome in patients with thalamic hemorrhages: A comparison with putaminal hemorrhages. *J. Neurol. Sci.* 1996;144:191–197.
49. Ropper AH, Gress DR. Computerized tomography and clinical features of large cerebral hemorrhages. *Cerebrovasc. Dis.* 1991;1:38–42.
50. Melo TP, Pinto AN, Ferro JM. Headache in intracerebral hematomas. *Neurology* 1996;47:494–500.
51. Qureshi AI, Safdar K, Weil J, et al. Predictors of early deterioration and mortality in black Americans with spontaneous intracerebral hemorrhage. *Stroke* 1995;26:1764–1767.
52. Mayer SA, Sacco RL, Shi T, Mohr JP. Neurologic deterioration in noncomatose patients with supratentorial intracerebral hemorrhage. *Neurology* 1994;44:1379–1384.
53. Gaskill-Shipley M. Routine CT evaluation of acute stroke. *Neuroimaging Clin. North Am.* 1999;9:411–422.
54. Broderick JP, Brott TG, Grotta JC. Volume of intracerebral hemorrhage. A powerful and easy-to-use predictor of 30-day mortality. *Stroke* 1993;24:987–993.
55. Osborn AG. Intracranial hemorrhage. In: Osborn AG (ed). *Diagnostic Neuroradiology*. St Louis: Mosby, 1994:154–198.
56. Adams RE, Powers WJ. Management of hypertension in acute intracerebral hemorrhage. *Crit. Care Clin.* 1997;13:131–161.
57. Lazio BE, Simard JM. Anticoagulation in neurosurgical patients. *Neurosurgery* 1999;45:838–848.
58. Morgenstern LB, Fankowski RF, Shedden P, Pasteur W, Grotta JC. Surgical treatment for intracerebral hemorrhage (STITCH): A single-center, randomized clinical trial. *Neurology* 1998;51:1359–1363.
59. Morgentern LB, Demchuck AM, Kim DH, Frankowski RF, Grotta JC. Rebleeding leads to poor outcome in ultra-early craniotomy for intracerebral hemorrhage. *Neurology* 2001;56:1294–1299.
60. Rabinstein AA, Atkinson JL, Wijdicks EF. Emergency craniotomy in patients worsening due to expanded cerebral hematoma. To what purpose? *Neurology* 2002;58:1367–1372.
61. Auer LM, Deinsberger W, Niederkorn K, et al. Endoscopic surgery versus medical treatment for spontaneous intracerebral hemorrhage: a randomized study. *J. Neurosurg.* 1989;70:530–535.
62. Naff NJ, Carhuapoma JR, Williams MA, et al. Treatment of intraventricular hemorrhage with urokinase: Effects on 30-day survival. *Stroke* 2000;31:841–847.
63. Rodrigue TC, Suarez JI, Zaidat OO, et al. Prediction of functional outcome following spontaneous intracerebral hemorrhage in adults: a proposed grading system. *Stroke* 2003;34:319.
64. Vermeer SE, Algra A, Franke CL, Koudstaal PJ, Rinkel GJ. Long-term prognosis after recovery from primary intracerebral hemorrhage. *Neurology* 2002;59:205–209.

Nicholas C. Bambakidis and Warren R. Selman

INTRODUCTION

Although aneurysms of the intracranial circulation were first associated with hemorrhage of the subarachnoid space in the 17th and 18th centuries, it was Quincke in 1891 who first documented this with use of lumbar puncture. The development of cerebral angiography by Egas Moniz and its use in demonstrating the presence and location aneurysms in 1933 *(1,2)* heralded an age when effective treatment modalities could be developed for this heretofore uniformly fatal disease.

In 1937 Dandy became the first surgeon to definitively isolate an aneurysm from the circulation by applying a metal clip across its neck *(3)*. Tremendous advances since this monumental event include the development of the operating microscope and computed tomography imaging. Together with modern intensive care techniques and the recent use of endovascular occlusion of some types of aneurysms, neurosurgeons now have at their disposal many tools with which to ensure that patients have the best possible outcomes. Nevertheless, because of the consequences of hemorrhage in the subarachnoid space, these patients continue to pose significant challenges to the clinician in terms of their management in the intensive care unit setting.

EPIDEMIOLOGY

Incidence

The exact incidence of aneurysm formation is unknown, but most studies estimate it to be in the range of 0.2–10 per 100 *(1,4)*. A 30-yr review of the incidence of aneurysmal subarachnoid hemorrhage (SAH) in Olmstead County, Minnesota was calculated to be 6.9 per 100,000 *(5)*, while recent meta-analysis pooling relevant studies demonstrated an incidence of 10.5 per 100,000 person years *(6)*. Aneurysmal subarachnoid hemorrhage is exceedingly rare in neonates and unusual in children. The peak age of incidence is 55–60 yr, although approx 20% occur between the ages of 15 and 45 yr *(7–9)*. Overall there seems to be a clear female preponderance with the ratio of female to male patients ranging from 1.6–4.16:1 *(6,10)*. Recent evidence has demonstrated that there may be a higher risk in black people than whites *(11)*.

Risk Factors

Modifiable risk factors which have been implicated include hypertension, the use of oral contraceptives, atherosclerosis, cigarette smoking, and heavy alcohol consumption. An extensive analysis by Teunissen et al. *(12)* analyzing eight longitudinal and 10 case-control studies indicated that smoking, hypertension, and, to a lesser extent, alcohol abuse are significant risk factors for SAH. A more recent retrospective multivariate analysis by Qureshi et al. *(13)* demonstrates that the increased risk of SAH with smoking persists even after the cessation of smoking. Oral contraceptives also have

From: *Current Clinical Neurology*
Critical Care Neurology and Neurosurgery
Edited by: J. I. Suarez © Humana Press Inc., Totowa, NJ

been found to impart an increased risk of SAH in a meta-analysis by Johnston et al. *(14)*. Although collagen vascular disorders have been associated with SAH as well, including autosomal dominant polycystic kidney disease, Ehlers-Danlos disease IV, neurofibromatosis type I, and Marfan syndrome, these diseases are rarely found to be present in patients presenting with aneurysmal SAH *(15–17)*. Multiple studies have demonstrated an increased risk of SAH in first-degree relatives of patients, though the risk seems to drop off to that of the general population in second- degree relatives *(18–20)*.

DIAGNOSIS OF SUBARACHNOID HEMORRHAGE

The diagnosis of aneurysmal SAH can often be strongly suspected on purely clinical grounds. Classically, patients will present with a sudden onset of severe headache, which they will often describe as the worst headache of their lives. This may be accompanied by nausea, vomiting, neck pain, photophobia, and loss of consciousness in up to half of patients as well as the development of focal neurological findings *(21–23)*. In 30–60% of patients, headache may be the only presenting complaint and may clear completely within hours. This in fact is often retrospectively attributable to a sentinel hemorrhage from the aneurysm and is also referred to as a "warning leak." The average interval between this and a major hemorrhage has been estimated to be approx 3 wk *(24)*. Some patients may present without headache entirely, and instead demonstrate signs of mass effect, seizure, or with a confusional state. In these patients, SAH should still be considered in the differential, and the diagnosis can be confirmed with the appropriate imaging study *(25,26)*.

Physical Examination

The physical examination in these patients may be entirely normal, although many patients develop meningismus within 6 to 24 h of rupture as blood degrades within the subarachnoid space. Patients are often hypertensive, and up to 15% may demonstrate focal motor deficits or language disturbances *(1)*. Oculomotor nerve palsy is commonly associated with aneurysms arising from the posterior communicating artery, while monocular blindness may result from anterior communicating artery aneurysms *(27)*. Bilateral sixth cranial nerve palsies may occur as a direct result of a sustained increase in cerebrospinal fluid pressure. Up to 40% of patients have no localizing signs and may simply present in various degrees of coma. This is often multifactorial but commonly results from a combination of increased intracranial pressure as a result of hydrocephalus, damage to brain tissue from intraparenchymal hemorrhage, diffuse ischemia, or seizure *(28)*. Ocular hemorrhages occur in 20–40% of SAH patients because of direct effects of increased intracranial pressure on retinal veins *(29–31)*. Fundoscopic evidence of flame-shaped hemorrhage near the optic disc may be seen or extension of hemorrhage into the vitreous humor may develop. In these latter cases, patients should be observed for several months for development of increased intracocular pressure or retinal detachment *(32)*.

Radiological Studies

The development of computed tomography (CT) revolutionized the diagnosis of SAH. A high resolution CT scan without motion artifact will demonstrate high signal within the subarachnoid spaces in more than 95% of cases within 48 h of SAH (Fig. 1) *(1,32)*. CT also demonstrates ventricular size in assessing for hydrocephalus as well as the presence of intracerebral hemorrhage or subdural hematoma which may require emergent evacuation. It may predict aneurysm location, as posterior fossa aneurysms often rupture with extension into the third and fourth ventricles while blood within the interhemispheric or sylvian fissures is associated with anterior communicating and middle cerebral artery aneurysms respectively. These patterns are distinct from traumatic subarachnoid hemorrhage in which the blood is usually located over the cerebral convexities in association with a skull fracture or underlying contusion.

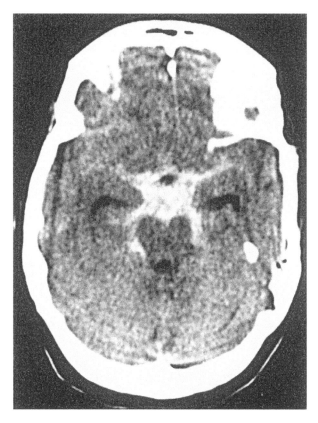

Fig. 1. Noncontrast-enhanced CT scan demonstrating diffuse subarachnoid hemorrhage in the basilar and ambient cisterns. There is also enlargement of the temporal horns indicative of hydrocephalus.

CT scanning is not without its limitations, however. Blood clears relatively quickly from the subarachnoid spaces from a radiographic perspective, so that the sensitivity of CT drops to 88% at 3 d and 50% at 7 d. Up to 55% of patients with warning leaks may have normal scans *(24,32)*. For this reason, lumbar puncture should be performed in patients with negative CT scans in whom the clinical picture suggests SAH (Fig. 2). Findings consistent with SAH include elevation of the opening pressure, an elevation of the red blood cell count that does not diminish with continued drainage, and an elevation of CSF protein due to red blood cell breakdown. All of these findings can be unreliable, and the most sensitive indicator is the presence of xanthochromia in the CSF supernatant. This may be seen within 6 h of hemorrhage, and a lumbar puncture done before this minimal time elapses must be carefully interpreted if negative *(33)*.

Magnetic resonance imaging (MRI) is generally not needed for the diagnosis of SAH. The difficulty in detecting acute blood with MRI renders this study less helpful in the acute setting. There is a role for MRI in preoperative planning for cases in which aneurysm size may not be accurately represented with angiography (e.g., when a large amount of intraluminal clot is present). MR angiography is a relatively new technique that as of yet has not been shown to possess the high degree of sensitivity for aneurysm detection that angiography does *(34)*. CT angiography is an alternative technique using spiral scanning and cine review of axial source images along with maximum intensity projection of the volume of interest *(35)*. Recent studies have demonstrated a sensitivity that approaches that of cerebral angiography, and in some cases operative therapy is performed without a conventional angiogram *(36,37)*.

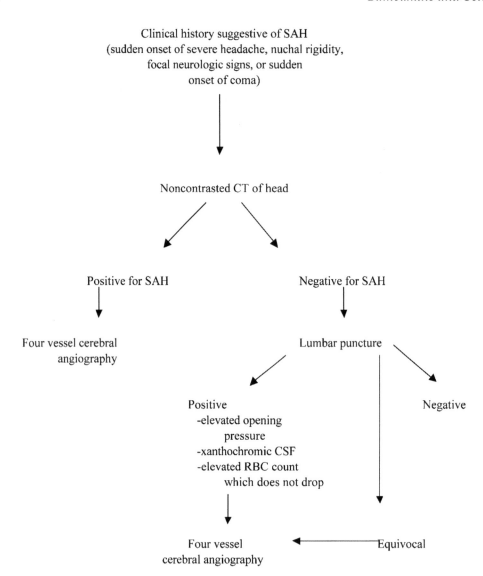

Fig. 2. Diagnostic algorithm for subarachnoid hemorrhage.

Cerebral angiography is the gold standard in aneurysm evaluation and demonstrates the source of SAH in 80–85% of cases. In all cases four-vessel angiography must be performed given that up to 15% of patients may harbor multiple aneurysms (Fig. 3) *(38)*. In these instances, determination of the offending aneurysm may be difficult. Localization of SAH on CT can be helpful as can the presence of aneurysm irregularity or focal vasospasm *(39)*.

When the workup for a documented case of SAH results in a negative angiogram one must consider nonaneurysmal etiologies in the differential diagnosis (e.g., angiographically occult vascular malformations or perimesencephalic nonaneurysmal SAH) *(40,41)*. Technical difficulties with the procedure itself or poor patient cooperation may be responsible as may obliteration of the aneurysm by hemorrhage or thrombosis. It is these latter possibilities, which prompt the general recommendation for Zrepeat angiography after 7–10 d in most cases *(42)*. In general, however, it should be recognized that these patients continue to be at risk for the complications of SAH and should be treated accordingly.

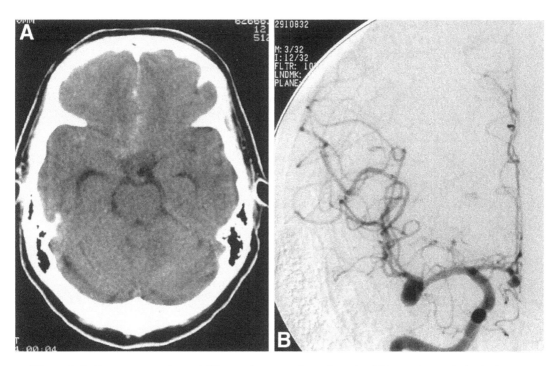

Figure 3. A: Noncontrast-enhanced CT scan demonstrating subarachnoid hemorrhage within the interhemispheric fissure. **B**: Anteroposterior view of a right internal carotid angiogram of the same patient showing aneurysms of both the anterior communicating and right middle cerebral arteries. Because of the location of the hemorrhage the anterior communicating artery aneurysm was felt to be the source, and this was confirmed at surgery, although both lesions were treated during the same operation.

GRADING OF ANEURYSMAL SUBARACHNOID HEMORRHAGE

Numerous methods of categorizing patients with SAH have been proposed. Most widely utilized is the Hunt and Hess classification *(43,44)*. It has five grades into which patients are assigned based on the presence or absence of various clinical signs and symptoms (Table 1), including the assessment of headache and neck stiffness.

In efforts to reduce interobserver variability and to better predict factors responsible for outcome other classification systems have been devised as well. The World Federation of Neurological Surgeons Scale (*see* Table 2) arose from findings from the Cooperative Study of Aneurysm Surgery, which concluded that the most important factors predicting outcome were level of consciousness and the presence of hemiparesis and/or aphasia. In the presence of normal consciousness, there was no relation between headache and neck stiffness and outcome. This grading scale uses the Glasgow coma scale score and the presence or absence of motor deficit *(45)*.

PATIENT MANAGEMENT

The initial concerns faced in treating patients with aneurysmal SAH are associated with the prevention of rebleeding as well as the prevention of complications associated with the initial hemorrhage, the most serious of which is vasospasm leading to the development of delayed ischemic deficits. The prognosis for patients who do suffer a second hemorrhage is quite poor, with a risk of permanent neurological morbidity and a mortality approaching 50% *(1,46,47)*.

The goal of treatment for aneurysmal SAH encompasses securing the aneurysm by isolating it from the normal intracranial circulation. Until this is accomplished, general measures are aimed at

Table 1
Hunt and Hess Grading Scale for Patients
With Subarachnoid Hemorrhage

Grade	Description
1	Asymptomatic or minimal headache and slight nuchal rigidity
2	Moderate-to-severe headache, nuchal rigidity, no neurologic deficit other than cranial nerve palsy
3	Drowsiness, confusion, or mild focal deficit
4	Stupor, moderate-to-severe hemiparesis, possible early decerebrate rigidity and vegetative disturbances
5	Deep coma, decerebrate rigidity, moribund appearance

Note: Patients are moved into the next worst category if they have vasospasm on angiography or serious systemic disease, such as hypertension, diabetes, atherosclerosis, or chronic lung disease. From ref. *43*.

minimizing factors which can predispose to rebleeding, such as seizures and hypertension. Patients are maintained in an environment with low levels of external stimulation, restricted visitation, and the absence of loud noises. Extreme hypertension is treated aggressively in the immediate posthemorrhagic period because there is little risk of cerebral ischemia from vasospasm until at least postbleed d 3. In general, short acting agents such as labetolol, hydralazine, or nitroprusside are utilized in conjunction with an arterial line. The ideal cutoff for blood pressure is controversial and must take into account the patient's baseline. In general, however, sustained systolic blood pressures above 160 mmHg are aggressively treated as noted above. Mild sedation with low doses of midzolam or phenobarbital and the use of analgesics such as codeine also aid in controlling hypertension as well as improving patient comfort. Low doses of dexamethasone may alleviate the symptoms of meningismus. If invasive procedures such as endotracheal intubation are required, then the administration of intravenous lidocaine is used to blunt any autonomic response.

Early aggressive fluid therapy is helpful in preventing vasospasm and cerebral salt wasting. Normal saline is administered at a rate of 140–150 mL/h. Phenytoin is generally used as a prophylactic anticonvulsant because a generalized seizure may be a devastating event in a patient with an unsecured aneurysm. Stool softeners and antiemetics are dispensed liberally, although phenothiazenes may lower the seizure threshold and are avoided.

Antifibrinolytic Agents

The use of antifibrinolytic agents has been controversial both in terms of their overall benefit and method and timecourse of administration. The beneficial effect of these agents, most commonly epsilon-aminocaproic acid or tranexamic acid, result from their ability to block the binding of plasminogen into fibrin thereby reducing the rate of rebleeding.

Many studies have demonstrated the efficacy of antifibrinolytic agents in lowering the rebleeding rate but have also demonstrated a marked increase in the incidence of cerebral ischemia with prolonged administration *(48–52)*. This seems to result in no change in patient outcome overall, even when maximal treatment for cerebral ischemia is enacted *(53)*. Nevertheless, antifibrinolytic agents are often used in the short term immediately after the onset of SAH for the prevention of rebleeding in this period

Table 2
World Federation of Neurological Surgeons Grading Scale
for Patients With Subarachnoid Hemorrhage

Grade	Description
1	Glasgow coma scale (GCS) score 15, no motor deficit
2	GCS score 13–14, no motor deficit
3	GCS score 13–14, with motor deficit
4	GCS score 7–12, with or without motor deficit
5	GCS score 3–6, with or without motor deficit

Cranial nerve palsies are not considered a motor deficit. From ref. *45.*

when the risk is highest, especially if definitive treatment must be delayed for 2–3 d. In these cases, a loading dose of 5 g of epsilon-aminocaproic acid is administered because therapeutic effects otherwise are not realized for 24–36 h. This is followed by a continuous infusion at a rate of 1.5 g/h.

Aneurysm Treatment Options

Surgical isolation of aneurysms from the remainder of the intracranial circulation has been the mainstay of treatment for decades. Controversy still exists regarding the optimal timing of surgery, specifically between proponents of "early" (defined as 48–96 h after SAH) and "late" surgery (generally 10–12 d after SAH). In general, the protection afforded by early surgery against rebleeding has fostered a recent trend toward this timing of treatment. This is despite the fact that early surgery is technically more difficult due to the presence of acute inflammation and edema, which necessitate retraction of brain which may be more friable. Although no studies have demonstrated a conclusive benefit for early surgery, there does seem to be a trend toward better outcomes *(54–57)*. The ability to more aggressively prevent and treat vasospasm with a secured aneurysm should also be considered when determining the timing of treatment. Patients also seem to do worse when surgery is performed during the peak period for vasospasm from day 4–10 *(58)*.

Endovascular treatment of aneurysms primarily consists of the placement of electrolytically detachable platinum coils within the aneurysm sac to promote thrombosis *(59–61)*. Originally utilized as an alternative to microsurgical clipping in poor grade patients or technically difficult aneurysms, its use has recently increased in frequency *(62)*. A recent meta-analysis reviewing 48 studies and approx 1383 patients estimated a complication rate of 3.7% with more than 90% occlusion of the aneurysm in approx 90% of patients *(63)*. Procedure-related perforation and ischemia are the most common complications. Long-term efficacy data are lacking, but at least 20% of patients with short follow-up needed retreatment in one study *(64)*. Direct comparisons between endovascular and surgical treatment is equivalent patients is not currently known *(65)*. The difficulty in achieving complete occlusion and the high incidence of the need for retreatment requires further scrutiny. Many centers consider microsurgical and endovascular techniques complementary and approach aneurysm treatment from a team-oriented perspective.

Alternative methods of treatment include proximal ligation, wrapping or coating the aneurysm, and trapping through occlusion of both proximal and distal arterial supply. As always, the exact method of treatment depends on aneurysm anatomy, patient condition, and the abilities and experience of the treating surgeon.

Hydrocephalus

Although the exact incidence of acute hydrocephalus is unknown and depends on the criteria used to define the condition, a reasonable estimate is that it occurs in approx 20% of patients *(66)*. Of these, anywhere from 30% to 60% of patients may be asymptomatic and require no treatment. In other cases alteration of consciousness necessitates placement of an external ventricular drain, which in most cases will result in prompt clinical improvement. Careful selection of patients in whom treatment is enacted is mandatory, however, since it is recognized that precipitous lowering of intracranial pressure may contribute to rebleeding *(67)*. For this reason, rapid pressure reduction is avoided and intracranial pressures are maintained in the range of 15–25 mmHg.

Hyponatremia

Hyponatremia is a relatively common complication of SAH and may be associated with natriuresis due to an increase in the level of atrial natriuretic factor (ANF). This may explain the frequency with which cerebral salt wasting is seen in these patients. Also common is the occurrence of inappropriate secretion of antidiuretic hormone (SIADH) although it is less common than cerebral salt wasting. Differentiating between the two entities is important because fluid restriction can increase blood viscosity as well as the risk of cerebral ischemia associated with vasospasm. Laboratory values may be identical in the two conditions and for this reason determination of central venous pressure (CVP) and/or pulmonary capillary wedge pressure (PCWP) are critical as these measurements are low in cerebral salt wasting and normal or elevated in SIADH. A negative salt balance is apparent in cerebral salt wasting and measurements of urinary sodium concentrations may be helpful. An elevation of serum potassium with hyponatremia is incompatible with the diagnosis of SIADH.

Treatment is geared towards the attainment of normovolemia and normalized sodium levels in the serum, and in general fluid restriction is avoided. Isotonic crystalloid is given if hypovolemia is present, and when sodium levels drop below 125 mEq/L, administration of hypertonic saline is the treatment of choice to prevent alteration in the level of consciousness or the onset of seizures. Fludrocortisone can be given in a dose of 0.2 mg intravenously (IV) or orally (PO) when natriuresis is a prominent sign but clinicians should recognize that this medication has been associated with pulmonary edema, hypertension, and hypokalemia. Correction of hyponatremia must also not be overly vigorous given the risk of central pontine myelinolysis, especially when administering hypertonic saline. In these cases fluids are generally begun at a rate of 25–50 mL/h. Serum sodium levels are checked frequently, and the maximum allowable correction rate is 1.3 mEq/L/h up to a total correction of 10 mEq/L in 24 h.

Vasospasm

By far the leading cause of morbidity and mortality in patients who survive the initial SAH is the development of cerebral ischemia due to vasospasm. The peak incidence of vasospasm is between the sixth and eighth days after hemorrhage, but it can rarely occur as early as day 3 or as late as day 17 *(58)*. Although the presence and location of thick collections of cisternal blood are thought to be predictive of the development and even severity of vasospasm *(68)*, the pathogenesis of its development is not completely understood. A requirement seems to be arterial blood at high pressure in contact with vessels located at the base of the brain. Pathologic changes include an infiltration of inflammatory cells in the acute stage followed by the development of muscle necrosis in the media of the vessel and interendothelial tight junction opening in the acute stage. This is later followed by smooth muscle proliferation and intimal thickening *(69)*. These changes seem to be triggered by breakdown products of hemoglobin. In 1980, Fisher et al. designed a grading system based on the amount of blood on CT based on his observations on 47 patients (Table 3) *(70)*. Vasospasm has not been shown to occur in perimesencephalic nonaneurysmal SAH and is rare in traumatic SAH or hemorrhage due to a ruptured arteriovenous malformation.

Although radiographic evidence of vasospasm is readily apparent in up to 70% of patients on angiography, symptomatic disease occurs in only 20–30% *(71)*. Symptoms range from headache, nausea, and vomiting to alterations in consciousness and focal neurologic deficit. The symptoms may be nonspecific and may be accounted for by alternative causes which must be ruled out (such as seizure, hydrocephalus, cerebral edema, hyponatremia, hypoxia, or sepsis). The diagnosis depends on the correlation of symptoms with radiographic regions of vasospasm on angiography. Transcranial Doppler sonography (TCD) can provide an early clue to the development of vasospasm by detecting elevations of blood flow velocity. Absolute values defining vasospasm are impossible to establish, however velocities less than 120 cm/s or greater than 200 cm/s are reasonably accurate in excluding or diagnosing vasospasm. Additionally, up to 60% of values will lie in the intermediate range *(72)*. Daily increases of more than 50 cm/s may be helpful in suggesting vasospasm. Any changes in daily measurements should be correlated with clinical changes in the patient's condition before alterations in therapy or further diagnostic studies are considered. Alterations in regional cerebral blood flow can be demonstrated with xenon CT, single photon-emission CT (SPECT) scans, or positron emission tomography (PET), although their roles continue to be evaluated.

Calcium Channel Blockers

The use of calcium channel blockers in preventing and treating secondary ischemia has been based on the belief that these agents reduce the incidence of vasospasm through direct relaxation of vascular smooth muscle. Several prospective randomized trials using the oral agent nimodipine have found that the drug consistently reduced poor outcome because of vasospasm although vessel caliber by angiography was not affected by treatment *(73)*. A recent meta-analysis of seven trials involving 1202 patients calculated that the odds of a good outcome were improved by 1.86:1, whereas the odds of deficit and/or mortality attributed to vasospasm and CT-assessed infarction rate were reduced by ratios of 0.46:1 to 0.58:1 *(74)*. These studies have focused on oral nimodipine given at a dose of 60 mg every 4 h for 21 d. Other agents included in clinical trials are intravenous nicardipine and AT877. However another recent review of all randomized controlled trials on these agents found that, when analyzed separately, only nimodipine demonstrated a significant reduction in the frequency of poor outcome *(75)*. Currently the use of nimodipine is a standard treatment in patients with aneurysmal SAH.

Free Radical Scavengers

Several agents have been studied based on their presumed effects. Tirilazad mesylate is a 21-aminosteroid that was found to improve outcome in a single subgroup of a single trial in a result that has since not been found to be reproducible *(18)*. Two other agents recently studied include N-propylenedinicotinamide (nicaraven) and ebselen. Conflicting results have alternately demonstrated either a decreased rate of cerebral ischemia without a change in 3-mo post-SAH outcomes or vice versa *(76,77)*.

Hyperdynamic Therapy

Also known as "triple H" therapy (for hypervolemia, hypertension, and hemodilution), hyperdynamic therapy is the most widely used treatment modality for vasospasm. In practice, hemodilution is not actively pursued but occurs passively in the face of hypervolemia. Clinical studies have not provided consistent results in favor of triple H therapy, however. Induced hypertension has been used since the 1960s, whether it be by expansion of circulating blood volume alone or by using pressor agents, with some reduction in the rates of cerebral ischemia but no clear reduction in overall morbidity or mortality *(78,79)*. The presumed mechanism of action is that, in the presence of abnormal cerebral autoregulation as may be the case in SAH, brain perfusion depends on systemic blood pressure. However the induction of hypertension and hypervolemia are themselves not without peril. Risks include rebleeding from an unclipped aneurysm, pulmonary complications and congestive heart failure, and increased hemorrhagic transformation or cerebral edema. A recent prospective study by Egge et al. compared prophylactic triple H therapy to a cohort who were treated with normovolemic fluid therapy with normotension. The authors found no significant differences between the two groups according to a variety of short- and long-term outcome measures *(80)*. Unfortunately the statistical power of this study was limited because of the small sample size (32 total patients), and the finding of

Table 3
Grading System of Fisher

Fisher group	Blood on computed tomography	No. of patients	Slight angiographic vasospasm	Severe angiographic vasospasm	Clinical vasospasm
1	No subaracnoid blood detected	11	2	2[a]	0
2	Diffuse or vertical layers[b] < 1 mm thick	7	3	0	0
3	Localized clot and/or vertical layer ≥ 1 mm	24	1	23	23
4	Intracerebral or intraventricular clot with diffuse or no SAH	5	2	0	0

[a]May actually be 0 since 1 patient was scanned late and 1 developed spasm only peripherally.
[b]"Vertical layer" refers to blood within the "vertical" subarachnoid spaces including the insular cistern, ambient cistern, and interhemispheric fissure.
   Measurements made in the greatest longitudinal and transverse dimension on a printed CT scan performed within 5 d of SAH. SAH, subarachnoid hemorrhage. From ref. *70.*

no difference between study groups, although suggestive, remains unproved. Nevertheless, the American Heart Association's evidence-based review *(73)* of the treatment of patients with SAH did not identify any controlled clinical trials that demonstrated the efficacy of hyperdynamic therapy but did recommend the use of this therapy on the basis of uncontrolled studies. In general, the use of hyperdynamic therapy is indicated to some degree in all patients with SAH pending the results of any future controlled studies.

   The exact level of treatment instituted must of course be tailored to each patient's clinical condition and risk factors for complications. In all cases, an arterial line and central line capable of measuring central venous pressure are placed. In patients who are at high risk for cardiopulmonary complications a pulmonary artery catheter is highly recommended. Volume expansion is maintained primarily with crystalloid (usually normal saline) totaling approx 3 L daily. Additional fluid boluses or administration of colloid as plasma fraction or 5% albumin are given to elevate the CVP to 8–12 cm H_2O or pulmonary capillary wedge pressure (PCWP) to 18–20 mmHg in most patients who are not at significant known risk for cardiopulmonary complications. In patients with symptomatic vasospasm and evidence of cerebral ischemia, hypervolemia is carefully maintained and cardiac output is optimized in high risk patients. In patients without evidence of underlying ischemic heart disease, pressors may be utilized as well. The endpoint of treatment is either the resolution of neurologic symptoms, maximum blood pressure of 160 mmHg in unclipped aneurysms, or any evidence of complications of therapy. Dopamine or phenylephrine are the preferred agents, while dobutamine is helpful in optimizing cardiac output. Bradycardia is treated with atropine as needed, while compensatory diuresis is managed with fludrocortisone or vasopressin in low doses. Ideally the hematocrit is kept between 30 and 35 to attain optimum blood rheology while maintaining adequate oxygen delivery.

Direct Vasodilatation

   Vasodilatation by the administration of intra-arterial papaverine (a calcium channel antagonist) has been used
   in an attempt to directly enhance cerebral perfusion in the face of vasospasm. There are no controlled trials available to demonstrate its efficacy, but uncontrolled trials have shown the effects to be short-lived *(81,82).* Moreover repeated administration increases the risk of complications, including changes in intracranial pressure, thrombocytopenia, and worsening rather than improving the vasospasm *(83).*

   Interventional angioplasty has also been reported to improve perfusion in uncontrolled studies *(84–86).* However, these procedures are also not without risk, including hyperperfusion injury or arterial occlusion or rupture. Distal cerebral vessels are also not accessible to this procedure. Further studies must be performed before a definitive recommendation can be made.

REFERENCES

1. Chyatte D. Diagnosis and management of aneurysmal subarachnoid hemorrhage. In: Tindall GT, Cooper PR, Barrow DL, eds. *The Practice of Neurosurgery*, 1st ed., vol. 2. Baltimore: Williams and Wilkins, 1996:1989–1995.
2. Moniz E. Aneuyrsme intra-cranien de la carotide interne droite rendu visible par l'arteriographie cerebrale. *Rev. Otoneurophthalmol.* 1933;11:746–748.
3. Dandy WE. Intracranial aneurysm of the internal carotid artery: Cured by operation. *Ann. Surg.* 1938;107:654–659.
4. Jellinger K. Pathology of intracerebral hemorrhage. *Zentrall. Neurochir.* 1977;38:29–42.
5. Menghini VV, Brown RD Jr, Sicks JD, O'Fallon WM, Wiebers DO. Incidence and prevalence of intracranial aneurysms and hemorrhage in Olmstead County, Minnesota, 1965 to 1995. *Neurology* 1998;51:405–411.
6. Linn FH, Rinkel GJ, Algra A, van Gijn J. Incidence of subarachnoid hemorrhage: role of region, year, and rate of computed tomography: A meta-analysis. *Stroke* 1996;27:625–629.
7. Longstreth WT Jr, Nelson LM, Koepsell TD, van Belle G. Clinical course of spontaneous subarachnoid hemorrhage: A population-based study in King County, Washington. *Neurology* 1993;43:712–718.
8. Lanzino G, Kassell NF, Germanson TP, et al. Age and outcome after aneurysmal subarachnoid hemorrhage: Why do older patients fare worse? *J. Neurosurg.* 1996;85:410–418.
9. Biller J, Toffol GJ, Kassell NF, et al. Spontaneous subarachnoid hemorrhage in young adults. *Neurosurgery* 1987;21:664–667.
10. Kassell NF, Torner JC, Haley EC Jr, et al. The international cooperative study on the timing of aneurysm surgery. Part I: Overall management results. *J. Neurosurg.* 1990;73:18–36.
11. Broderick JP, Brott T, Tomsick T, Huster G, Miller R. The risk of subarachnoid and intracerebral hemorrhage in blacks as compared with whites. *N. Engl. J. Med.* 1992;326:733–736.
12. Teunissen LL, Rinkel GJE, Algra A, van Gijn J. Risk factors for subarachnoid hemorrhage—a systematic review. *Stroke* 1996;27:544–549.
13. Qureshi AI, Suri MFK, Yahia AM, Suarez JI, et al. Risk factors for subarachnoid hemorrhage. *Neurosurgery* 2001;49:607–612.
14. Johnston SC, Colford JM Jr, Gress DR. Oral contraceptives and the risk of subarachnoid hemorrhage: A meta-analysis. *Neurology* 1998;51:411–418.
15. Schievink WI, Michels VV, Peipgras DG. Neurovascular manifestations of heritable connective tissue disorders. A review. *Stroke* 1994;25:889–903.
16. Pepin M, Schwarze U, Superti-Furga A, Byers PH. Clinical and genetic features of Ehlers-Danlos syndrome type IV, the vascular type. *N. Engl. J. Med.* 2000;342:673–680.
17. van den Berg JS, Limberg M, Hennekam RC. Is Marfan syndrome associated with symptomatic intracranial aneurysms? *Stroke* 1996;27:10–12.
18. van Gijn J, Rinkel GJ. Subarachnoid haemorrhage: Diagnosis, causes, and management. *Brain* 2001;124:249–278.
19. Schievink WI. Genetics of intracranial aneurysms. *Neurosurgery* 1997;40:651–662.
20. Bromberg JEC, Rinkel GJE, Algra A, Greebe P, et al. Subarachnoid hemorrhage in first and second degree relatives of patients with subarachnoid hemorrhage. *BMJ* 1995;311:288–289.
21. Sahs AL, Perret GE, Locksley HB, Nishioka H, eds. *Intracranial Aneurysms and Subarachnoid Hemorrhage: A Cooperative Study*. Philadelphia: Lippincott, 1969.
22. Linn FH, Rinkel GJ, Algra A, van Gijn J. Headache characteristics in subarachnoid hemorrhage and benign thunderclap headache. *J. Neurol. Neurosurg. Psychiatry* 1998;65:791–793.
23. Hop JW, Rinkel GJ, Algra A, van Gijn J. Initial loss of consciousness and risk of delayed cerebral ischemia after aneurysmal subarachnoid hemorrhage. *Stroke* 1999;30:2268–2271.
24. Leblanc R. The minor leak preceeding subarachnoid hemorrhage. *J. Neurosurg.* 1987;66:35–39.
25. Pinto AN, Canhao P, Ferro JM. Seizures at the onset of subarachnoid haemorrhage. *J. Neurol.* 1996;243:161–164.
26. Reijnveld JC, Wermer M, Boonman Z, van Gijn J, Rinkel GJ. Acute confusional state as presenting feature in aneurysmal subarachnoid hemorrhage: Frequency and characteristics. *J. Neurol.* 2000;247:112–116.
27. Chan JW, Hoyt WF, Ellis WG, Gress D. Pathogenesis of acute monocular blindness from leaking anterior communicating artery aneurysms: Report of six cases. *Neurology* 1997;48:680–683.
28. Ogilvy CS, Rordorf G. Mechanisms and treatment of coma after subarachnoid hemorrhage. In Bederson JP (ed). *Neurosurgical Topics*. Schaumburg, IL: The American Association of Neurological Surgeons, 1997:157–171.
29. Manschot WA. Subarachnoid hemorrhage: Intraocular symptoms and their pathogenesis. *Am. J. Ophthalmol.* 1954;38:501–505.
30. Pfausler B, Belcl R, Metzler R, Mohsenipour I, Schmutzhard E. Terson's syndrome in spontaneous subarachnoid hemorrhage: A prospective study in 60 consecutive patients. *J. Neurosurg.* 1996;85:392–394.
31. Frizzell RT, Kuhn F, Morris R, Quinn C, Fisher WS 3rd. Screening for ocular hemorrhages in patients with ruptured cerebral aneurysms: A prospective study of 99 patients. *Neurosurgery* 1997;41:529–533.

32. van der Wee N, Rinkel GJ, Hasan D, van Gijn J. Detection of subarachnoid hemorrhage on early CT: is lumbar puncture still needed after a negative scan? *J. Neurol. Neurosurg. Psychiatry* 1995;58:357–359.

33. Vermeulen M, van Gijn J. The diagnosis of subarachnoid hemorrhage [Review]. *J. Neurol. Neurosurg. Psychiatry* 1990;53:365–372.

34. Wardlaw JM, White PM. The detection and management of unruptured intracranial aneurysms [Review]. *Brain* 2000;123:205–221.

35. Velthius BK, van Leeuwen MS, Witkamp TD, Boomstra S, Ramos LM, Rinkel GJ. CT angiography: source images and postprocessing techniques in the detection of cerebral aneurysms. *AJR* 1997;169:1411–1417.

36. Velthius BK, Rinkel GJ, Ramos LM, et al. Subarachnoid hemorrhage: Aneurysm detection and preoperative evaluation with CT angiography. *Radiology* 1998;208:423–430.

37. Velthius BK, van Leeuwen MS, Witkamp TD, Ramos LM, van der Sprenkel JW, Rinkel GJ. Computerized tomography angiography in patients with subarachnoid hemorrhage: From aneurysm detection to treatment without conventional angiography. *J. Neurosurg.* 1999a;91:761–767.

38. Suzuki J. Multiple aneurysms: Treatment. In: Pia AW, Langmaid C. Zierski J (eds). *Cerebral Aneurysms: Advances in Diagnosis and Therapy*. Berlin: Springer, 1979:352–363.

39. Nehls DG, Flom RA, Carter LP, Spetzler RF. Multiple intracranial aneurysms: determining the site of rupture. *J. Neurosurg.* 1985;63:342–348.

40. Cioffi F, Pasqualin A, Cavazzoni P, et al. Subarachnoid hemorrhage of unknown origin: clinical and tomographic aspects. *Acta. Neurochir.* 1989;97:31–39.

41. Schwartz TH, Solomon RA. Perimesencephalic nonaneurysmal subarachnoid hemorrhage: review of the literature. *Neurosurgery* 1996;39:433–440.

42. Kaim A, Proske M, Kirsche E, et al. Value of repeat angiography in cases of unexplained subarachnoid hemorrhage. *Acta Neurol. Scand.* 1996;93:366–373.

43. Hunt WE, Hess RM. Surgical risk as related to time of intervention in the repair of intracranial aneurysms. *Neurosurgery* 1968;28:14–20.

44. Hunt WE, Kosnik EJ. Timing of perioperative care in intracranial aneurysm surgery. *Clin. Neurosurg.* 1974;21:79–89.

45. Drake CG. Report of World Federation of Neurological Surgeons committee on a universal subarachnoid hemorrhage grading scale. *J. Neurosurg.* 1988;68:985–986.

46. Hasan D, Lindberg KW, Wijdicks EF, et al. Effects of fludrocortisone acetate in patients with subarachnoid hemorrhage. *Stroke* 1989;20:1156–1161.

47. Kassell NF, Torner JC. Aneurysmal rebleeding: A preliminary report from the Cooperative Aneurysm Study. *Neurosurgery* 1983;13:479–481.

48. Roos YB, Rinkel GJE, Vermeulen M, et al. Antifibrinolytic therapy for aneurysmal subarachnoid haemorrhage. *Cochrane Database of Systematic Reviews* 2000; Issue 2. Oxford: Update Software.

49. Vermeulen M, Lindsay KW, Murray GD, et al. Antifibrinolytic treatment in subarachnoid hemorrhage. *N. Engl. J. Med.* 1984;311:432–437.

50. Ramirez-Lassepas M. Antifibrinolytic therapy in subarachnoid hemorrhage caused by ruptured intracranial aneurysm. *Neurology* 1981;31:316–322.

51. Kassell NF, Torner JC, Adams HP. Antifibrinolytic therapy in the acute period following aneurysmal subarachnoid hemorrhage: Preliminary observations from the Cooperative Aneurysm Study. *J. Neurosurg.* 1984;61:225–230.

52. Leipzig TJ, Redelman K, Horner TG. Reducing the risk of rebleeding before early aneurysm surgery: a possible role for antifibrinolytic therapy. *J. Neurosurg.* 1997;86:220–225.

53. Roos YB. Antifibrinolytic treatment in subarachnoid hemorrhage: a randomized placebo-controlled trial. STAR Study Group. *Neurology* 2000;54:77–82.

54. Ohman J, Heiskanen O. Timing of operation for ruptured supratentorial aneurysms: a prospective randomized study. *J. Neurosurg.* 1989;70:55–60.

55. Kassell NF, Torner JC, Jane JA, et al. The international cooperative study on the timing of aneurysm surgery. Part 2: surgical results. *J. Neurosurg.* 1990;73:37–47.

56. LeRoux PD, Elliott JP, Newell DW, et al. Predicting outcome in poor-grade patients with subarachnoid hemorrhage: a retrospective review of 159 aggressively managed cases. *J. Neurosurg.* 1996;85:39–49.

57. LeRoux PD, Elliott JP, Newell DW, et al. The incidence of surgical complications is similar in good and poor grade patients undergoing repair of ruptured anterior circulation aneurysms: a retrospective review of 355 patients. *Neurosurgery* 1996;38:887–897.

58. Weir B, Grace M, Hansen J, Rothberg C. Time course of vasospasm in man. *J. Neurosurg.* 1978;48:173–178.

59. Gugliemi G, Vinuela F, Dion J, et al. Electrothrombosis of saccular aneurysms via endovascular approach. Part 2: preliminary clinical experience. *J. Neurosurg.* 1991;75:8–14.

60. Gugliemi G, Vinuela F, Duckwiler G, et al. Endovascular treatment of posterior circulation aneurysms by electrothrombosis using electrically detachable coils. *J. Neurosurg.* 1992;77:515–524.

61. McDougall CG, Halbach VV, Dowd CF, et al. Endovascular treatment of basilar tip aneurysms using electrolytically detachable coils. *J. Neurosurg.* 1996;84:393–399.

62. Cognard C, Pierot L, Boulin A, et al. Intracranial aneurysms: Endovascular treatment with mechanical detachable spirals in 60 aneurysms. *Radiology* 1997;202:783–792.

63. Brilstra EH, Rinkel GJ, van der Graaf Y, et al. Treatment of intracranial aneurysms by embolization with coils: A systematic review. *Stroke* 1999;30:470–476.

64. Zubillaga A, Gugliemi G, Vinuela F, et al. Endovascular occlusion of intracranial aneurysms with electrically detachable coils: correlation of aneurysm neck size and treatment results. *AJNR* 1994;15:815–820.

65. Johnson SC, Dudley RA, Gress DR, et al. Surgical and endovascular treatment of unruptured cerebral aneurysms at University Hospitals. *Neurology* 1999;52:1799–1805.

66. Milhorat TH. Acute hydrocephalus after aneurysmal subarachnoid hemorrhage. *Neurosurgery* 1987;20:15–20.

67. Pare L, Delfino R, Leblanc R. The relationship of ventricular drainage to aneurysmal rebleeding. *J. Neurosurg.* 1992;76:422–427.

68. Kistler JP, Crowell RM, Davis KR, Heros R, et al. The relation of cerebral vasospasm to the extent and location of subarachnoid blood visualized by CT scan: A prospective study. *Neurology* 1983;22:424–436.

69. Sasaki T, Kassell NF, Zuccarello M, et al. Barrier disruption in the major cerebral arteries during the acute stage after experimental subarachnoid hemorrhage. *Neurosurgery* 1986;19:177–184.

70. Fisher CM, Kistler JP, Davis JM. Relation of cerebral vasospasm to subarachnoid hemorrhage visualized by CT scanning. *Neurosurgery* 1980;6:1–9.

71. Kassell NF, Sasaki T, Colohan ART, et al. Cerebral vasospasm following aneurysmal subarachnoid hemorrhage. *Stroke* 1985;16:562–572.

72. Vora YY, Suarez-Almazor M, Steinke DE, et al. Role of transcranial Doppler monitoring in the diagnosis of cerebral vasospasm after subarachnoid hemorrhage. *Neurosurgery* 1999;44:1237–1247.

73. Mayberg MR, Batjer JJ, Dacey R, et al. Guidlines for the management of aneurysmal subarachnoid hemorrhage. A statement for healthcare professionals from a sepcial writing group of the Stroke Council, American Heart Association. *Stroke* 1994;25:2315–2328.

74. Barker FG, Ogilvy CS. Efficacy of prophylactic nimodipine for delayed ischemic deficit after subarachnoid hemorrhage: A metaanalysis. *J. Neurosurg.* 1996;84:405–414.

75. Feigin VL, Rinkel GJE, Algra A, et al. Calcium antagonists for aneurysmal subarachnoid hemorrhage. *Cochrane Database of Systematic Reviews* 2000; Oxford: Update Software.

76. Asano T, Takakura K, Sano K, et al. Effects of a hydroxyl radical scavenger on delayed ischemic neurological deficits following aneurysmal subarachnoid hemorrhage: Results of a multicenter, placebo-controlled double-blind trial. *J. Neurosurg.* 1996;84:792–803.

77. Saito I, Asano T, Sano K, et al. Neuroprotective effect of an antioxidant, ebselen, in patients with delayed neurological deficits after aneurysmal subarachnoid hemorrhage. *Neurosurgery* 1998;42:269–277.

78. Kassell NF, Peerless SJ, Durward QJ, et al. Treatement of ischemic deficits from vasospasm with intravascular volume expansion and induced arterial hypertension. *Neurosurgery* 1982;11:337–343.

79. Awad IA, Carter LP, Spetzler RF, et al. Clinical vasospasm after subarachnoid hemorrhage: Response to hypervolemic hemodilution and arterial hypertension. *Stroke* 1987;18:365–372.

80. Egge A, Waterloo K, Sjoholm H, et al. Prophylactic hyperdynamic postoperative fluid therapy after aneurysmal subarachnoid hemorrhage: A clinical, prospective, randomized, controlled study. *Neurosurgery* 2001;49:593–606.

81. Kaku Y, Yonekawa Y, Tsukahara T, et al. Superselective intra-arterial infusion of papaverine for the treatment of cerebral vasospasm after subarachnoid hemorrhage. *J. Neurosurg.* 1992;77:842–847.

82. Elliot JP, Newell DW, Lam DJ, et al. Comparison of balloon angioplasty and papaverine infusion for the treatment of vasospasm following aneurysmal subarachnoid hemorrhage. *J. Neurosurg.* 1998;88:277–284.

83. Clyde BL, Firlik AD, Kaufmann AM, et al. Paradoxical aggravation of vasospasm with papaverine infusion following aneurysmal subarachnoid hemorrhage. Case report. *J. Neurosurg.* 1996;84:690–695.

84. Firlik AD, Kaufmann AM, Jungreis CA, Yonas H. Effect of transluminal angioplasty on cerebral blood flow in the management of symptomatic vasospasm following aneurysmal subarachnoid hemorrhage. *J. Neurosurg.* 1997;86:830–839.

85. Bejjani GK, Bank WO, Olan WJ, Sekhar LN. The efficacy and safety of angioplasty for cerebral vasospasm after subarachnoid hemorrhage. *Neurosurgery* 1998;42:979–986.

86. Eskridge JM, McAuliffe W, Song JK, et al. Balloon angioplasty for the treatment of vasospasm: results of first 50 cases. *Neurosurgery* 1998;42:510–516.

21

Cerebral Venous Sinus Thrombosis

Zeyad Marcos and Sophia Sundararajan

INTRODUCTION

With the advent and increasing availability of neuroimaging in the past few decades, cerebral venous thrombosis (CVT) has become a more easily recognized disease and appears to be more common than previously believed. Despite this, CVT remains a diagnostic and therapeutic challenge. The true incidence of CVT remains unclear. In the past the diagnosis of CVT was largely made at autopsy, leading many to believe that most cases were fatal. Early series based on angiographic diagnosis estimated mortality to be thirty to fifty percent [1,2]. More recent series, however, have estimated mortality at 6–33%. Improvement in magnetic resonance imaging (MRI) and magnetic resonance venography (MRV) techniques have led to an increase in premorbid diagnosis and it has become clear that CVT is more common than previously thought. More recent studies have found death rates ranging between 5 and 30% [3–7]. Furthermore, a wide range of disease symptomatology and severity may be present [3,5,8]. Although this may make CVT more difficult to diagnose, recent studies suggesting effective therapy underscore the importance of prompt recognition of this elusive, but treatable cause of neurologic deterioration

ANATOMY

To understand the pathophysiology of CVT, it is important to understand the venous circulation of the brain. The cerebral venous system can be divided into superficial and deep veins. The superficial veins serve the outer 2 cm of cerebral cortex and underlying white matter draining into the dural sinuses. These sinuses include the superior sagittal sinus, the inferior sagittal sinus, the lateral or transverse sinuses and the cavernous sinuses (Fig. 1). These sinuses in turn are drained by the internal jugular veins. The deep veins drain the choroidal plexus, cerebral hemisphere white matter, basal ganglia, and diencephalon. They empty into the paired internal cerebral veins, the basal veins of Rosenthal, and the great vein of Galen. These venous territories are rich in anastomostic vessels, allowing the development of collateral circulation. The dural sinuses lie between the periosteal and meningeal layers of dura matter, are devoid of valves, and do not collapse. They contain most of the arachnoid villi and granulations through which cerebrospinal fluid is absorbed.

There are anatomic variants that must be appreciated to correctly interpret imaging studies. The right lateral sinus is frequently larger than the left; the left lateral sinus does not opacify in approx 14% of normal angiograms [9]. Furthermore, Kaplan and his colleagues [10] showed that the anterior portion of the superior sagittal sinus is hypoplastic or atretic in 6–7% of the general population. Unlike the superficial venous system, the deep venous system of the brain is relatively constant with little anatomic variation [11,12].

From: *Current Clinical Neurology*
Critical Care Neurology and Neurosurgery
Edited by: J. I. Suarez © Humana Press Inc., Totowa, NJ

A

B

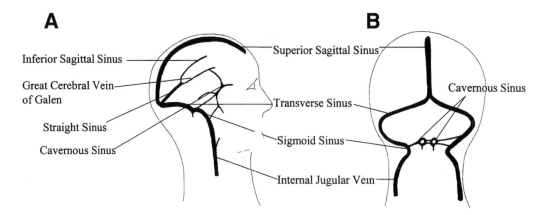

Inferior Sagittal Sinus

Great Cerebral Vein of Galen

Straight Sinus

Cavernous Sinus

Superior Sagittal Sinus

Transverse Sinus

Sigmoid Sinus

Internal Jugular Vein

Cavernous Sinus

Fig. 1. Anatomy of the cerebral dural sinuses. Anatomic drawing of the lateral view of the venous sinuses (**A**) and anteroposterior view of the venous sinuses (**B**).

DISTRIBUTION OF VENOUS STRUCTURE INVOLVEMENT

Sagittal Sinus Thrombosis

The superior sagittal sinus is the most common location of dural sinus venous thrombosis, represents 70–80% of CVT *(3,4,13)*, and is especially affected during puerperium. The superior sagittal sinus drains most of the cerebral cortex receiving diploic veins; those veins are connected via the emissary veins with the scalp, explaining the occurrence of superior sagittal sinus thrombosis after scalp infection or head trauma. Presentations of superior sagittal sinus thrombosis are varied and may be as dramatic as coma or limited to headache *(13)*. Some authors have suggested that up to 30% of patients with "benign intracranial hypertension" harbor occult sagittal sinus thrombosis *(14)*. Because the superior sagittal sinus drains cortical veins from both hemispheres, it may present with alternating focal motor or sensory signs.

Lateral Sinus Thrombosis

Lateral sinuses are the second most commonly involved sinuses. In the past an important cause of lateral sinus thrombosis was infectious mastoiditis *(2,3,15)*. The sigmoid portion of the lateral sinus lies adjacent to the mastoid air cells from which otologic infections can spread easily. Since the widespread use of antibiotics, the incidence of lateral sinus thrombosis has decreased. Men are more often affected than women. Patients usually present with a chronically infected ear, tenderness along the anterior border of the sternocleidomastoid and the mastoid, and a combination of temporal and cerebellar symtoms. These symptoms may include aphasia, agitation, visual defects, nystagmus, or gait ataxia.

Cavernous Sinus Thrombosis

Cavernous sinus thrombosis is a serious disease with high mortality. It is most commonly found following infections of the middle third of the face, and the sphenoid sinus. The walls of the sphenoid sinus are extremely thin. Occasionally the bone is absent, leaving adjacent structures separated from the sinus cavity by a thin mucosal barrier *(16)*. The most common organisms found in cavernous sinus thrombosis are *Staphylococcus aureus* and *Streptococcal pneumoniae*. However, with chronic infections, Gram-negative rods and fungi such as *Aspergillus* are more commonly isolated than Gram-positive organisms *(17)*. Because the abducens nerve is within the cavernous sinus, lateral gaze palsy may be an isolated early neurologic finding. Headache, papilledema, fever, ptosis, chemosis, proptosis, and weakness of extraocular muscles are seen frequently. Evidence of a systemic infection is found in 90% of cases and occlusion of the orbital vein may be present on orbital venography *(17)*.

Deep Venous System Occlusion

Deep cerebral venous thrombosis is defined as thrombosis of one or both internal cerebral veins and/or the vein of Galen. In most cases deep cerebral venous thrombosis is associated with dural sinus involvement. Thrombosis of these deep veins occurs more frequently in women, with a female-to-male ratio of 8.3:1. Deep cerebral venous thrombosis may be particularly difficult to diagnose. Sometimes it can be dramatic without obvious localizing signs. However, usually it presents with headache, nausea, vomiting, altered level of consciousness, and cortical dysfunction. Some patients may have decorticate or decerebrate posturing and seizures may occur. If unrecognized, death may occur within a few days. Partial syndromes exist and can be survived with surprisingly little residual *(3,18,19)*. Imaging studies may reveal bilateral hemorrhagic or nonhemorrhagic infarctions of the striatum, thalamus, hypothalamus, the ventral corpus callosum, the medial occipital lobe and the upper part of the cerebellum *(20)*. Computed tomography (CT) helps eliminate the possibility of hemorrhage as a potential etiology and may show hypodensity of the thalamus, basal ganglia, internal cerebral veins or the vein of Galen. Alternatively, if hemorrhage is present, hyperdensity will be present on CT. These imaging abnormalities can only be explained by thrombosis of all or portion of the deep cerebral venous drainage. Arterial ischemia will not show this pattern of change since these areas are well perfused by small branches from both the anterior and posterior circulations. Deep cerebral vein thrombosis remains a diagnostic challenge that must be suspected in patients presenting with headache, altered mental status, and bithalamic abnormalities on imaging studies.

Isolated Cortical Cerebral Vein Thrombosis

Cortical vein thrombosis without involvement of adjacent sinuses is extremely rare *(3,21)*. Cortical vein thrombosis causes venous infarction with or without hemorrhagic transformation. These patients tend to present with focal neurological signs and seizures, although headache and decreased level of consciousness may also be present.

PATHOPHYSIOLOGY

Cerebral venous thrombosis is a continuing process of disequilibrium between prothrombotic and thrombolytic mechanisms. Thrombus can form as a result of an abnormal coagulation cascade, increased blood viscosity as a result of dehydration, polycythemia or an ongoing inflammatory process within the vessel. After a thrombus completely obstructs the dural sinus, it may extend to involve cortical veins. Occlusion of these veins causes venous infarction. Blood is unable to drain adequately and pressure increases within the venous and capillary system leads to cerebral edema and perivascular hemorrhage. Furthermore, since thrombus within the dural sinuses obstructs arachnoid granulations, the normal flow of cerebral spinal fluid is impaired. As a consequence, intracranial pressure increases. Because of the rich anastomotic venous network in the brain, much of the tissue involved in venous infarction early on may be metabolically disturbed, but not irreversibly damaged *(22)*. This last fact underlines the importance of prompt therapeutic intervention.

ETIOLOGIES

Numerous conditions can predispose to CVT (Table 1). In an individual patient, multiple potential etiologies may be present, and a thorough workup is indicated, even in patients in whom the cause appears obvious. On the other hand, no risk factor is found in approx 20% of patients. Potential causes of CVT are discussed below.

Table 1
Cerebral Venous Sinus Thrombosis

Infection
  Local infection:
    Intracranial: abscess, subdural
      empyema, and meningitis
    Regional: otitis, sinusitis,
      tonsillitis, dental infections,
      orbital and cutaneous cellulitis
  Systemic infection:
    Bacterial
    Viral
    Parasitic
    Fungal
Hormonal
  Pregnancy; postpartum
  Oral contraceptive
  Androgens
Carcinoma
  Migratory thrombophlebitis
  Meningioma
  Cholesteatoma
  Jugular tumors
  Metastasis
Primary coagulopathy
  Factor deficiency
    Activated protein C resistance
      (factor V Leiden)
    Factor II (prothrombin) gene
      mutation (G20210A)
    Protein S deficiency
    Protein C deficiency
    Antithromboin III deficiency
    Antiphospholipid antibodies
      (anticardiolipin antibodies,
      lupus anticoagulant)
    Von Willebrand's disease
    5,10-methyl tetrahydrofolate
      reductase mutation
    Hyperhomocystinuria
Blood dyscrasia
  Thrombocytopenia
  Primary polythemia

Paroxysmal nocturnal
  hemoglobinuria
Iron deficiency anemia
Sickle cell disease
Disseminated intravascualar
  coagulopathy
After bone marrow
  transplantation
Polycythemia (primary or
  secondary)
Systemic illness
  Carcinoma
  Lymphoma
  Leukemia
  Nephrotic syndrome
  Inflammatory
  Systemic Lupus Erythematosus
  Bechet disease
  Ulcerative colitis
  Crohn's disease
  Wegener granulomatosis
  Giant cell arteritis
  Sarcoidosis
Medications
  Oral contraceptives
  E-Aminocarporic acid, L-asparaginase
  Corticorsteroids
  Dihydroerogotamine
  Androgens
  Ecstasy

Miscellaneous
  Severe dehydration
  Dural puncture: diagnostic lumbar
    puncture, epidural anesthesia,
    myelography, and intrathecal
    medications
  After neurosurery
  Any surgery (with or without deep vein
    thrombosis)
Head trauma (open or closed, with or
  without fracture)

Unknown causes approx 20%

Infections

Before the antibiotic era, CVT was divided between infectious and noninfectious etiologies. However, antibiotics have reduced the number of serious infection and most recent series show that infection accounts for only 10% of present-day CVT *(3)*. Superior sagittal thrombosis may complicate both bacterial meningitis and paranasal sinusitis *(15)*. Lateral sinus thrombosis is frequently secondary to otitis media and mastoiditis *(2,3,15)*. Infection increases acute-phase reactants that are involved in the coagulation cascade and shifts the equilibrium between prothrombotic and thrombolytic mechanisms toward thrombosis.

Hormonal Factors

Hormonal factors appear to play an important role in the balance of thrombotic and thrombolytic mechanisms. It is, therefore, not surprising that alterations in hormonal levels alter the risk of CVT. The incidence of CVT is higher in women, and risk further increases with oral contraceptive use, during pregnancy, and the first 2 wk postpartum. Oral contraceptives, even at low doses, significantly increase the risk of CVT. This is especially true if congenital thrombophilia is present, in which case, the risk increases more than 100-fold *(23)*. The US national hospital discharge survey shows a frequency of 11.4 cases of CVT per 100,000 deliveries. In India the incidence is considerably higher, 450 cases per 100,000 deliveries has been reported. CVT risk is higher with advanced maternal age *(24)* and in multiparous women *(25)*. Like most cases of CVT, the most common site for thrombosis in pregnant and postpartum women is the superior sagittal sinus. The high incidence of CVT during the puerperal period likely may be secondary to endothelial trauma occurring during labor, a hypercoagulable state and, in developing countries, dehydration and infection *(21,26)*.

Hormonal factors may also be important in males. Androgens potentiate platelet aggregation through either increased production of thromboxane A2 or decreased production of prostacyclin, and androgens predispose to thrombosis by increasing collagen and other fibrous proteins in arterial tissues and skin *(27)*. A case of venous thrombosis in a 31-yr-old man using androgens for bodybuilding has been reported *(28)*. Furthermore, superior sagittal sinus thrombosis developed in three of 27 patients with hypoplastic anemia treated with androgens *(29)*.

Carcinoma

Carcinoma may predispose to the development of CVT through multiple mechanisms. Adenocarcinoma of the pancreas, colon, or lung is associated with a hypercoagulable state and patients may present with migratory thrombophlebitis. This paraneoplastic syndrome has been dubbed "Trousseau's sign." Venous thrombosis appears spontaneously in one site, only to disappear and to be followed by thrombosis at other sites *(30)*. If the patient is known to have cancer, the thrombosis may not be appreciated because symptoms are attributed to the underlying malignancy *(31)*. Cranial neoplasms, either primary or metastatic, can invade or impinge on dural sinuses mechanically causing stasis and thrombosis.

Primary Coagulopathy

Abnormalities of several components of the coagulation cascade have been associated with CVT. The prevalence of mutation in the factor V Leiden gene is 15–20% in patients with CVT, and only 2–3% in normal control subjects. This abnormality is associated with a ninefold increased risk for CVT *(32,33)*. Another common inherited coagulopathy is a prothrombin gene mutation, *G20210A*, reported to be present in as many as 20% of patients with CVT *(34)*. Other coagulopathies that may contribute to CVT include deficiencies in protein S and protein C. Furthermore, plasminogen and antithrombin III levels may be depleted in nephrotic syndrome secondary to impaired urinary excretion and appear to predispose patients to thrombosis *(35,36)*. Abnormalities in coagulation factors are not uncommon and should be sought in all patients presenting with CVT regardless of whether other potential etiologies are present.

Systemic Inflammatory Diseases

Several systemic inflammatory diseases have been associated with increased risk of CVT. These diseases include inflammatory bowel disease. It is believed that the thromboembolic phenomena in inflammatory bowel disease are due to hypercoagulability, increased fibrinogen, elevations of factor V and VIII, thrombocytosis, and decreased antithrombin III *(37)*. Systemic lupus erythematousus has also been associated with CVT *(38)*. This association may be related to the development of nephrotic syndrome and urinary loss of coagulation factors *(39)*. However, anticardiolipin antibodies that develop in some lupus patients are also associated with a hypercoagulable state and CVT *(40)*. Behçet's disease, which is diagnosed on the basis of a triad of recurrent oral ulceration, genital ulcerations and relapsing eye inflammation, has also been implicated in the etiology of CVT. In one study from the Middle East, Behçet's disease actually accounted for 25% of CVT cases *(4)*. This high incidence is likely related to the prevalence of Beçhet's disease in the Middle East, which is many times what it is in the West *(41)*.

Lumbar Puncture

CVT is a rare complication of lumbar puncture and should be considered in the differential diagnosis of postdural puncture headache or peripartum postdural puncture headache, especially when no postural component is present. Aidi et al. reported two patients who underwent diagnostic lumbar puncture for suspected multiple sclerosis and were treated with high-dose intravenous methylprednisolone. Both developed a typical post-lumbar puncture headache with a postural component. However, within a few days the headache became constant and lost its postural component. Diplopia and bilateral papilledema developed; brain MRIs revealed CVT in the superior sagittal and lateral sinuses *(42)*. Furthermore, Stocks and colleagues have reported the case of a 20-yr-old woman with an accidental dural tear during epidural anesthesia who developed what was initially thought to be a "spinal headache." After two blood patches failed to relieve the headache and seizures and a decreased level of consciousness developed, it was recognized that the patient had CVT *(43)*.

CLINICAL FINDINGS

The clinical findings in CVT are variable and depend on the site of thrombosis, the etiology of thrombosis, and the premorbid condition of the patient. Clinical findings in superior sagittal sinus, or lateral sinus thrombosis may be limited to isolated intracranial hypertension. However, the usual presentation of cerebral cortical veins infarction is focal neurological signs. In most series, CVT is described as having an insidious onset characterized by headache, focal deficits, seizures, decreased alertness, and elevated intracranial pressure (Table 2). However, an "acute course" may be seen, especially associated with pregnancy, postpartum state and infectious etiologies.

Headaches

Headache is not only the most frequent symptom found in CVT, but is usually what prompts the patient to seek medical attention. It is present in over 80% of patients. The cause of the headache is multifactorial. Increased intracranial pressure, distension of the sinus wall by increased blood volume, irritation of the vessels by local inflammation, and leakage of blood on the surface of the brain all stimulate dural pain-sensitive fibers. There are no distinguishing features of the headache associated with CVT. The headache and the clinical picture may be similar to benign intracranial hypertension *(13)*. The headache can mimic the intermittent, unilateral features of migraine and can even be associated with aura *(44)*. Alternatively, the headache can be constant and accompanied by tearing and periorbital edema mimicking ophthalmic migraine *(17)*. The headache may even mimic subarachnoid hemorrhage. Several patients have been reported with acute severe headache with signs and symptoms suggestive of subarachnoid hemorrhage such as vomiting, photophobia and neck

Table 2
Frequency of Signs and Symptoms in Multiple Series of Cerebral Venous Sinus Thrombosis

Signs and symptoms	Cantu and Barinagarrementeria[a]		Ameri and Bousser[b] $n = 110$	Biousse and Bousser[c] $n = 160$
	Group 1, $n = 67$	Group 2, $n = 46$		
Headache	59 (88%)	32 (70%)	83 (75%)	131 (82%)
Papilledema	27 (40%)	24 (52%)	54 (49%)	81 (51%)
Focal signs	53 (79%)	35 (76%)	38 (34%)	62 (39%)
Seizures	40 (60%)	29 (63%)	41 (37%)	67 (42%)
Decreased level of consciousness	42 (62%)	27 (59%)	33 (30%)	49 (31%)

[a]Cantu and Barinagarrementeria *(21)*. Group 1 included 67 cases of CVT associated with pregnancy and puerperuim, and group 2 included 46 cases of CVT unrelated to obstetric events.

[b]Ameri and Bousser *(3)*. Total of 110 patients with CVT. Focal signs included motor and sensory symptoms. In addition, dysphasia was seen in 13 patients.

[c]Biousse and Bousser *(13)*. Total of 160 patients with CVT. Focal signs included motor and sensory symptoms as well as aphasia.

rigidity. In these cases, hyperdensity within the venous system was interpreted on CT to represent subarachnoid hemorrhage. However, further imaging including MRI and angiography revealed CVT. In summary, headache may occur in isolation and there are no distinguishing characteristics of the headache associated with CVT; therefore, special attention to the possibility that headache may represent CVT is required to make this diagnosis.

Papilledema

Papilledema is present in about half of patients. It is found more frequently among those with an acute presentation *(3,13,21)*. It is important to recognize papilledema and treat the underlying increased intracranial pressure because secondary optic atrophy may develop and lead to blindness. This atrophy is usually associated with infero-nasal quadrant visual field deficit and requires serial visual field follow-up examinations to monitor therapy *(13,45)*.

Focal Neurologic Signs and Symptoms

Focal neurologic signs and symptoms are present in approx half of CVT patients. The most frequent signs are motor or sensory deficits but others, including aphasia, ataxia, and agitation, may also be present. Focal neurological deficits may be associated with extension of thrombosis into cortical veins and may help localize the site of thrombosis. For example, an alternating paresis or parathesia may indicate a superior sagittal sinus thrombosis *(13,46)*, while a total opthalmoplegia suggests cavernous sinus thrombosis *(46,47)*. Fifth or sixth cranial nerve palsies are associated with petrosal sinus thrombosis *(46)* while ninth and tenth cranial nerve palsies are usually indicative of an internal jugular vein thrombosis *(47)*. We encountered three patients with chronic headache associated with hearing loss in one ear who were eventually diagnosed as having CVT involving the lateral sinus. Similar patients have been reported by others *(3,13)*.

Seizures

Seizures are relatively common in CVT. The incidence of seizures ranges 10 to 60% depending on the series *(3,21,25)*. Seizures are more likely to be of focal rather than generalized onset and imply focal injury or irritation of the underlying cortex. This injury is secondary to venous infarction, hemorrhage or dilated cortical veins *(13)*.

Decreased Level of Consciousness

Altered consciousness is rarely the initial symptom, but during the course of CVT is seen in 10–60% of patients *(3,4,21)*. In most cases, patients are lethargic or stuporous but may develop obtundation or coma. The latter may even be seen on presentation especially with thrombosis of the deep veins. Potential etiologies include increased intercranial pressure, seizures, mass effect secondary to infarction or hemorrhage or bilateral involvement of the medial thalami in deep venous occlusions.

DIAGNOSIS

In recent years it has become increasingly important to diagnose CVT because the potential benefits of anticoagulation have become clear. Patients suffering from venous thrombosis are often in the prime of life. In many cases, they are new mothers. Their disability and death is a tremendous burden to our society both in emotional and in economic terms. Recognizing that these previously healthy patients have this disorder is often complicated by the fact that patients may lack traditional risk factors for vascular disease. As mentioned previously CVT has diverse presentations. In some cases it may have a slow indolent course of headache, focal deficits, seizures, decreased alertness, and elevated intracranial pressure. Alternatively CVT may present fulminantly with thunderclap headache and coma mimicking subarachnoid hemorrhage. CVT should be suspected in any patient with unexplained neurologic symptoms, especially in the context of risk factors. To correctly diagnosis this entity, it is necessary to have a high index of suspicion and to understand which diagnostic tests are likely to demonstrate CVT.

Computed Tomography

CT is normal in 5–40% of cases *(4,7,21)*. It is the most frequently ordered brain-imaging test and is often performed in the emergency department when the patient first presents. Several abnormalities on this initial imaging study may point to the diagnosis of cerebral venous thrombosis. Rarely, non–contrast-enhanced head CT shows the cord or dense triangle sign. Acute clot within the venous system can be detected as hyperdensity within the venous system and depending on the location of the clot this may appear as a cord or triangle *(48,49)*. The cord sign disappears 1–2 wk after the onset of symptoms *(49,50)*. In addition the empty delta sign, which indicates mature clot within the dural covered sinuses may be present. This name refers to the fact that the thrombus does not enhance while the surrounding dura does *(48)*. The explanation for the enhancement of the dura is unclear but this enhancement may represent collateral venous circulation within the dura *(7)*. This sign takes approx 6–8 wk to disappear *(51,52)*. A "pseudo-delta sign" has also been reported in which a hyperdensity surrounds a hypodense sinus on an uncontrasted CT scan. When contrast is administered, the entire sinus enhances *(7)*. Additional findings on CT are not specific to CVT and are related to the consequences of venous thrombosis including small ventricles secondary to cerebral edema and cortically based hemorrhages or infarctions that do not conform to typical arterial distributions. In cases of deep cerebral venous thrombosis, hypodensity may be seen involving the basal ganglia and thalami. Severe edema with compression of the third ventricle may also be seen *(19)*.

The cord and empty delta sign are considered to be pathognomonic for CVT, however, not all patients will have these abnormalities on CT. Virapongse found that in a series of 76 patients the empty delta sign was the most frequently reported sign but was present in only 27% of patients. Among patients who died, the empty delta sign was the most common CT finding and was present in 37% of patients with a fatal outcome. Hemorrhagic infarction was present in 26% of patients with fatal outcome *(7)*.

While CT scans are helpful in making the diagnosis of cerebral infarction, the diagnosis should be confirmed with a more direct visualization of the venous circulation either through CT venography, MRI/MRV, or the venous phase of cerebral angiography.

Table 3
Stages of Cerebral Venous Sinus Thrombosis as Seen on Magnetic Resonance Imaging

	Normal sinus	CVT, first few days	CVT, 5–30 d	CVT, after 1 mo
T1-weighted	Hypointense	Isointense	Hyperintense	Isointense
T2-weighted	Hypointense	Hypointense	Iso then hyperintense	Isointense or Hyperintense
Pathophysiology		Oxy- then deoxyhemoglobin	Conversion to meth-hemoglobin	The venous sinus remained occluded partially or completely, or recanalized
Comments		Infrequent False-negative	The most frequently seen	They may persist for years and must not be confused with recurrence

CVT, cerebral venous sinus thrombosis.

Computed Tomography Venography

CT venography can be performed after non-contrasted CT using helical scans and a high dose of intravenous contrast. The source images are reconstructed to produce accurate detailed images of the venous system *(53)*. Unlike MRV, signal does not represent flow within the sinus; rather, images are produced by detecting contrast within the venous system. Compared to digital subtraction angiography, multiplanar reformatted images have a sensitivity of 95% and a specificity of 91% *(54)*. The examination is less invasive and less expensive than angiography and can be accomplished much more quickly than either angiography or MRI/MRV. This can be critical in patients that are either unable to cooperate or are critically ill. However, CT venography requires ionizing radiation and the administration of intravenous contrast agent (53). Therefore it is not the test of choice in pregnant patients or in patients unable to tolerate contrast. Additionally, reconstruction of the source images is operator-dependent and requires an understanding of venous anatomy. It has been suggested that this reconstruction should be performed by radiologists and not radiology technicians *(53)*, thus limiting the usefulness of this exam at times when these skilled personnel are not available.

Magnetic Resonance Imaging/Magnetic Resonance Venography

The combination of MRI and MRV currently is the most widely used method for both the diagnosis and follow-up of CVT *(1,3,55,56)*. MRI/MRV is less invasive than conventional angiography, is widely available, and allows direct visualization of thrombosis as well as a variety of parenchymal changes including early infarction, hemorrhage, and focal or diffuse edema (Table 3). However like all imaging modalities MRI and MRV have limitations. No abnormality may be seen if the study is performed in the extreme acute phase or if the cortical veins are incompletely thrombosed *(13)*. Furthermore, lack of flow may be due to normal anatomical variants such as a hypoplastic anterior superior sagittal sinus or lateral sinus and may cause false positive results. Both sagittal and axial T1 and T2-weighted images must be performed and analyzed to confirm whether the vein in question is truly occluded or hypoplastic.

Transcranial Doppler

Transcranial Doppler (TCD) provides a noninvasive and rapid technique for intracranial venous examination. Doppler studies may detect elevated mean blood velocities and/or microembolic signals *(57)*. Interestingly, microembolic signals decrease during adequate heparin therapy and increase during inadequate heparin therapy *(58)*. The main disadvantage of TCD is the need for arterial landmarks to locate venous structures and the difficulty reliably insonating dural sinuses. In addition, the quality of TCD studies is highly operator-dependent. Stolz and colleagues studied the use of transcranial color-coded Doppler sonography, in 75 healthy volunteers and eight patients with CVT. They found that this technique allowed reliable evaluation of deep venous structures but not the anterior and mid-portion of the superior sagittal sinus. Furthermore, they correlated clinical recovery with decreasing blood flow velocities. The authors concluded that transcranial color-coded Doppler sonography may be a useful method to monitor therapy at the bedside of critically ill patients.

Cerebrospinal Fluid

Lumbar puncture must be performed only after CT of the head has shown no evidence of mass effect and an open ventricular system. Lumbar puncture may be needed to rule out meningitis or subarachnoid hemorrhage in patients presenting with nonspecific symptoms that may be suggestive of these diseases. In cases with isolated intracranial hypertension and papilledema, lumbar puncture may be therapeutic lowering intercranial pressure and protecting vision. Lumbar puncture reveals an increased opening pressure and elevated protein in approximately half of cases. Leukocytosis and evidence of hemorrhage may also be present in one third and two thirds of cases, respectively *(13)*.

Conventional Angiography

Historically angiography has been one of the most common techniques used to diagnose cerebral venous thrombosis. Thrombosed sinuses or deep cortical vein appear as empty channels devoid of contrast and surrounded by dilated collateral venous channels. A thrombosed cortical vein may be recognized by a cord-like collection of contrast that hangs in space and represents decreased flow in the area just proximal to the thrombosis *(59)*. Visualization of the venous phase is best accomplished by examining at least two projections *(13)* with the head filmed in a slightly oblique position. Additional views of the neck may be necessary to show whether the jugular bulb and vein are thrombosed.

MANAGEMENT

As our ability to diagnosis CVT improves, it becomes more important to develop clear guidelines for management. In recent years several trials have addressed the therapeutic efficacy of thrombolytic and anticoagulation in CVT and while most investigators agree that these treatments are of value, some controversy remains.

Anticoagulation

Because the underlying pathology of CVT is abnormal thrombosis within the venous system, heparin seems to be a logical therapy. Unfortunately, CVT is often accompanied by intracranial hemorrhage and so the use of heparin has been controversial. Evidence from retrospective and prospective trials accumulated over the years, however, show that heparin is both safe and effective even when hemorrhage is present *(1,3,5,60,61)*. In 1967, Krayenbuhl *(2)* noted that CVT patients treated with heparin and antibiotics have a mortality rate of 7%, compared with 37% in those treated only with antibiotics, and 70% in those treated with neither.

The first randomized clinical trial was prematurely stopped after enrolling only 20 patients due to dramatically different outcomes in the two treatment groups *(62)*. Eight patients in the heparin-treated group and only one patient in the placebo group had full recovery. Furthermore, there were no deaths in the heparin-treated group and three deaths in the placebo-treated group. However this study attracted considerable criticism. First of all the difference in the death rate between the two groups, while dramatic, was not statistically significant. In addition, the grading system used in the trial counted patients in the placebo group with mild sequelae as having poor outcomes while more serious sequelae such as aphasia and visual loss were not scored *(63)*. Therefore, a second randomized placebo controlled trial was undertaken. Sixty patients with CVT were randomized to receive either low-molecular-weight heparin or placebo. Even though there was no significant difference statistically, there was a trend toward improved outcome in the heparin treated group and no evidence of clinical worsening attributable either to new or an enlarged cerebral hemorrhage in those randomized to heparin. This included 15 patients who had hemorrhagic infarction on head CT.

De Bruijn conducted a meta-analysis of the two trials and found an absolute risk reduction in mortality of 14% and in death or dependency of 15%, with relative risk reductions of 70% and 56%, respectively. These differences, however, do not reach statistical significance and have a wide confidence interval *(64)*. To realize a statistical difference between the two groups of patients, it is estimated that three hundred patients would need to be enrolled in a trial. It is unlikely that such a trial will be realized in the near future and given the suggested benefit and lack of evidence to suggest harm from anticoagulation, the use of anticoagulation with heparin in the treatment of CVT is advocated *(65)*.

Local Thrombolytic Therapy

More recently, the idea of using local thrombolytic therapy to treat CVT has been proposed. Several anecdotal cases and small case series are in the literature. Many of the initial cases used urokinase. However, recombinant tissue plasminogen activator (r-tPA) has been used in more recent cases (Fig. 2). The largest series of patients thus far reported (12 patients) found that recanalization occurred in one half of the patients. Flow restoration was rapid (on average 29 h) and five of 12 patients had complete functional recovery *(66)*. Significantly, of the seven patients in the series with hemorrhage on imaging studies, two experienced extension of their hemorrhage and associated clinical deterioration *(66)*. Given these data, treatment with thrombolytic does not appear to be safe in the setting of existing hemorrhage, however, in patients without hemorrhage, the therapy may be useful when clinical status does not improve with heparin alone.

Anticonvulsant Drugs

Anticonvulsant agents should be used in every patient with seizures. Some controversy remains as to whether all patients should receive anticonvulsants regardless of presence of seizure. Furthermore, it is not clear how long patients should continue to receive anticonvulsants once they have been started. There are no studies that have addressed these issues, however, long-term epilepsy following CVT is uncommon. It is reasonable to begin anticonvulsants only in patients known to have experienced seizures and to taper them after 1 year in patients with a normal electroencephalogram *(13)*.

Management of Intracranial Hypertension

Intracranial hypertension is commonly seen in CVT and carries a poor prognosis because of the risk of brain herniation and the risk of blindness secondary to papilledema and optic nerve atrophy. When herniation is not a risk, repeated lumbar puncture may be beneficial. Alternatively, acetazolamide, steroids, mannitol, and water restriction may help avoid blindness. By improving venous flow, heparin may be sufficient to reduce increased intracranial pressure. If these measures are insufficient, it may be necessary for the patient to undergo a shunting procedure or optic nerve fenestration *(13)*.

Treatment of Underlying Pathology

It is imperative that the cause of CVT be determined. In many cases, the cause of CVT may be multifactorial and a thorough workup is indicated, even in cases where an obvious risk factor, such as a postpartum state, is present. Underlying infection must be looked for and treated with either antibiotics or surgical debridement. One must assure that the patient is not dehydrated and correct hydration status promptly. In fact, aggressive hydration to maintain central venous pressures between 6

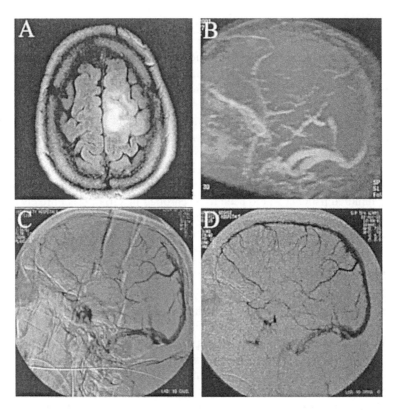

Fig. 2. Radiographic images of a 52-yr-old man with superior sagittal thrombosis. He underwent a decompressive L2-L5 laminectomy at an outside hospital, which was complicated by cerebrospinal fluid leak requiring wound revision. In the recovery room following wound revision, he was noted to have a right-sided hemiplegia and thought to have suffered a stroke. Head CT scan at the outside hospital soon after the development of hemiplegia was normal and the patient was thought to have suffered an arterial stroke and was transferred to our institution. MRI showed increased T2 signal in the left hemisphere adjacent to the superior sagittal sinus **(A)**. MRV at this time demonstrates thrombosis of the superior sagittal sinus **(B)**. Cerebral angiogram performed the same day also shows absence of flow within the superior sagittal sinus **(C)**. r-tPA was infused in the thrombosis for 24 h and the patients clinical examination improved. Repeat cerebral angiograms 1 wk after thrombolytic infusion shows complete resolution of superior sagittal thrombosis **(D)**.

and 12 mmHg is commonly instituted in this patient population. Patients should be screened for malignancies and systemic inflammatory disease. Finally, all patients should be screened for hypercoagulable states, and family counseling may be necessary in cases of hereditary hypercoagulability.

OUTCOME

Although the outcome of CVT is much better than that of arterial stroke, it remains highly unpredictable. Patients that are deeply comatose may have a rapid recovery without sequelae. Alternatively, patients presenting with only headache may develop serious sequelae, such as hemiplegia or visual loss. Recovery is usually between 50% and 70% of cases, disabling sequelae occur in about ten percent of patients and the overall mortality rate appears to be between 6% and 33% *(3–7)*. Death is usually related to the cerebral consequences of CVT, most often massive cerebral hemorrhagic infarction. However, complications such as status epilepticus, pulmonary embolism, and underlying sepsis or malignancy may contribute to mortality *(1,67)*. Potential sequelae of CVT include blindness from intercranial hypertension, focal neurological deficits, seizures and arteriovenous malformations *(1,68)*, and recurrent CVT.

Poor prognostic factors in CVT include very young or advanced age, rapid clinical course, focal deficits, coma, underlying infectious etiology, and hemorrhagic infarction *(69)*. Location of venous thrombosis, however, is also an important factor since deep cerebral vein and cerebellar vein thromboses are associated with higher mortality than thrombosis of superficial veins *(1)*. It is important to note that CVT associated with the postpartum state has a particularly good prognosis with one series recently reporting a 90% survival *(1)*.

REFERENCES

1. Bousser M, Russell R. *Cerebral Venous Thrombosis*, vol 1. London: WB Saunders, 1997.
2. Krayenbuhl H. Cerebral venous and sinus thrombosis. *Clin. Neurosurg.* 1967;14:1–24.
3. Ameri A, Bousser M. Cerebral venous thrombosis. *Neurol. Clin.* 1992;10:87–111.
4. Daif A, Awada A, Al-Rajeh S, Abduljabbar M, et al. Cerebral venous thrombosis in adults: A study of 40 cases from Saudi Arabia. *Stroke* 1995;26:1193–1195.
5. Bousser M, Chiras J, Bories J, Castaigne P. Cerebral venous thrombosis: A review of 38 cases. *Stroke* 1985;16:199–213.
6. Thron A, Wessel K, Linden D, Schroth G, Dichgans J. Superior sagittal sinus thrombosis: Neuroradiological evaluation and clinical findings. *J. Neurol.* 1986;233:283–288.
7. Virapongse C, Cazenave C, Quisling R, Sarwar M, Hunter S. The empty delta sign: Frequency and significance in 76 cases of dural sinus thrombosis. *Radiology* 1987;162:779–785.
8. Tsai F, Wang A, Matocich V, et al. MR staging of acute dural sinus thrombosis: Correlation with venous pressure measurements and implications for treatment and prognosis. *Am. J. Neuroradiol.* 1995;16:1021–1029.
9. Mas J, Meder J, Meary E, Bousser M. Magnetic resonance imaging in lateral sinus hypoplasia and thrombosis. *Stroke* 1990;21:1350–1356.
10. Kaplan H, Browder J. Atresia of the rostral superior sagittal sinus: substitute parasagittal venous channels. *J. Neurosurg.* 1973;38:602–607.
11. Huber P. *Cerebral Angiography*. New York: Thieme, 2001.
12. Meder J, Chiras J, Roland J, Guinet P, Bracard S, Bargy F. Venous territories of the brain. *J. Neuroradiol.* 1994;21:118–133.
13. Biousse V, Bousser M. Cerebral venous thrombosis. *Neurologist* 1999;5:326–349.
14. Tehindrazanarivelo A, Evard S, Schaison M, Mas J-L, Dormaont D, Bousser M. Prospective study of cerebral sinus thrombosis in patients presenting with benign intracranial hypertension. *Cerebrovasc. Dis.* 1992;2:22–27.
15. Southwick F, Richardson EJ, Swartz M. Septic thrombosis of the dural venous sinuses. *Medicine* 1986;65:82–106.
16. Lew D, Southwick F, Montgomery W, Weber A, Baker A. Sphenoid sinusitis. A review of 30 cases. *N. Engl. J. Med.* 1983;309:1149–1154.
17. DiNubile M. Septic thrombosis of the cavernous sinuses. *Arch. Neurol.* 1988;45:567–572.
18. Baumgartner R, Landis T. Venous thalamic infarction. *Cerebrovasc. Dis.* 1992;2:353–358.
19. Haley E, Brashear H, Barth J, Cail W, Kassell N. Deep cerebral venous thrombosis: Clinical, neuroradiological, and neuropsychological correlates. *Arch. Neurol.* 1989;46:337–340.
20. Ur Rahman N, Al Tahan A. Computed tomographic evidence of an extensive thrombosis and infarction of the deep venous system. *Stroke* 1993;24:744–746.
21. Cantu C, Barinagarrementeria F. Cerebral venous thrombosis associated with pregnancy and puerperium. Review of 67 cases. *Stroke* 1993;24:1880–1884.
22. Villringer A, Mehraein S, Einhaupl K. Pathophysiological aspects fo cerebral sinus venous thrombosis (SVT). *J. Neuroradiol.* 1994;21:72–80.
23. Bousser M, Kittner S. Oral contraceptives and stroke. *Cephalalgia* 2000;20:183–189.
24. Lanska D, Kryscio R. Stroke and intracranial venous thrombosis during pregnancy and puerperium. *Neurology* 1998;51:1622–1628.
25. Srinivasan K. Cerebral venous and arterial thrombosis in pregnancy and the puerperium. A study of 135 patients. *Angiology* 183;34:731–746.
26. Mas J, Lamy C. Stroke in pregnancy and the puerperium. *J. Neurol.* 1998;245:305–313.
27. Wilder-Smith E, Kothbauere-Margreiter I, Lammle B, Sturzenegger M, Ozdoba C, Hauser S. Dural puncture and activated protein C resistance: risk factors for cerebral venous sinus thrombosis. *J. Neurol. Neurosurg. Psychiatry* 1997;63:351–356.
28. Jaillard A, Hommel M, Mallaret M. Venous sinus thrombosis associated with androgens in a healthy young man. *Stroke* 1994;25:212–213.
29. Shiozawa Z, Yamada H, Mabuchi C, Hotta T, Saito M, Sobue I et al. Superior sagittal sinus thrombosis associated with androgen therapy for hypoplastic anemia. *Ann. Neurol.* 1982;12:578–580.
30. Crawford J, Cotran R. The pancreas. In: Cotran R, Kumar V, Collins T, eds. *Pathologic Basis of Disease*. Philadelphia: WB Saunders, 2001:902–929.

31. Hickey W, Garnick M, Henderson I, Dawson D. Primary cerebral venous thrombosis in patients with cancer—a rarely diagnosed paraneoplastic syndrome. Report of three cases and review of the literature. *Am. J. Med.* 1982;73:740–750.
32. Zuber M, Toulon P, Marnet L, Mas J. Factor V leiden mutation in cerebral venous thrombosis. *Stroke* 1996;27:1721–1723.
33. Martinelli I, Landi G, Merati G, Cella R, Tosetto A, Mannucci P. Factor V gene mutation is a risk factor for cerebral venous thrombosis. *Thromb. Haemost.* 996;75:393–394.
34. Martinelli I, Sacchi E, Landi G, Taioli E, Duca F, Mannucci P. High risk of cerebral vein thrombosis in carriers of a prothrombin-gene mutation and in users of oral contraceptives. *N. Engl. J. Med.* 1998;338:1793–1797.
35. Lau S, Tkachuck M, Hasegawa D, Edson J. Plasminogen and antithrombin III deficiencies in the childhood nephrotic syndrome associated with plasminogenuria and antithrombinuria. *J. Pediatr.* 1980;96:390–392.
36. Lau S, Bock G, Edson J, Michael A. Sagittal sinus thrombosis in the nephrotic syndrome. *J. Pediatr.* 1980;97:948–950.
37. Markowitz R, Ment L, Gryboski J. Cerebral thromboembolic disease in pediatric and adult inflammatory disease: case report and review of the literature. *J. Pediatr. Gastroenterol. Nutr.* 1989;8:413–420.
38. Vidaihet M, Piette J, Wechsler B, Bousser M, Brunet P. Cerebral venous thrombosis in systemic lupus erythematosus. *Stroke* 1990;21:1226–1231.
39. Laversuch C, Brown M, Clifton A, Bourke B. Cerebral venous thrombosis and acquired protein S deficiency: an uncommon cause of headache in systemic lupus erythematous. *Br. J. Rheumatol.* 1995;34:572–575.
40. Carhuapoma J, Mitsias P, Levine S. Cerebral venous thrombosis and anticardiolipin antibodies. *Stroke* 1997;28:2363–2369.
41. Sakane T, Takeno M, Suzuki N, Inaba G. Behcet's disease. *N. Engl. J. Med.* 1999;341:1284–1291.
42. Aidi S, Chaunu M, Biousse V, Bousser M. Changing pattern of headache pointing to cerebral venous thrombosis after lumbar puncture and intravenous high-dose corticosteriods. *Headache* 1999;39:559–564.
43. Stocks G, Wooller D, Young J, Fernando R. Postpartum headache after epidural blood patch: investigation and diagnosis. *Br. J. Anesth.* 2000;85:498–499.
44. Newman D, Levine S, Curtis V, Welch K. Migraine-like visual phenomena associated with cerebral venous thrombosis. *Headache* 1989;29:82–85.
45. Purvin V, Trobe J, Kosmorsky G. Neuro-opthalmic features of cerebral venous obstruction. *Arch. Neurol.* 1995;52:880–885.
46. Caplan L. *Posterior Circulation Disease: Clinical Findings, Diagnosis, and Management.* Cambridge, MA: Blackwell Science, 1996.
47. Kuehnen J, Schwartz A, Neff W, Hennerici M. Cranial nerve syndrome in thrombosis of the transverse/sigmoid sinuses. *Brain* 1998;121:381–388.
48. Bouonanno F, Moody D, Ball M, Laster D. Computed cranial tomographic findings in cerebral sino-venous occlusion. *J. Comput. Assist. Tomogr.* 1978;2:281–290.
49. Patronas N, Duda E, Mirfakhraee M, Wollmann R. Superior sagittal sinus thrombosis diagnosed by computed tomography. *Surg. Neurol.* 1981;15:163–170.
50. Kim D, Walczak T. Computed tomography of deep cerebral venous thrombosis due to high-altitude polycythemia: Case report. *J. Comput. Assist. Tomogr* 1986;10:148–150.
51. Zilkha A, Stenzler S, Lin J. Computed tomography of the normal and abnormal superior sagittal sinus. *Clin. Radiol.* 1982;33:415–425.
52. Brant-Zawadzki M, Chang G, McCarty G. Computed tomography in dural sinus thrombosis. *Arch. Neurol.* 1982;39:446–447.
53. Casey S, Alberico R, Patel M, Jimenez J, Ozsvath R, Maguire W et al. Cerebral CT venography. *Radiology* 1996;198:163–170.
54. Wetzel S, Kirsch E, Stock K, Kolbe M, Kaim A, Radue E. Cerebral vein: comparative study of CT venography with intraarterial digital subtraction angiography. *Am. J. Neuroradiol.* 1999;20:249–255.
55. Mas J, Meder J, Meary E, Bousser M. Magnetic resonance imaging in lateral sinus hypoplasia and thrombosis. *Stroke* 1990;21:1350–1356.
56. Perkin G. Cerebral venous thrombosis: developments in imaging and treatment. *J. Neurol. Neurosurg. Psychiatry* 1995;59:1–3.
57. Valdueza J, Hoffmann O, Weih M, Mehraein S, Einhaupl K. Monitoring of venous hemodynamics in patients with cerebral thrombosis by transcranial doppler ultrasound. *Arch. Neurol.* 1995;56:229–234.
58. Valdueza JM, Harms L, Doepp F, Koscielny J, Einhaupl KM. Venous microembolic signals detected in patients with cerebral sinus thrombosis. Stroke 1997; 28:1607–1609.
59. Osborn A. Stroke. *Diagnostic Neuroradiology.* St. Louis: Mosby, 1994:330–400.
60. Brucker M, Vollert-Rogenhofer H, Wagner M, et al. Heparin treatment in acute cerebral sinus venous thrombosis: a retrospective clinical an MR analysis of 42 cases. *Cerebrovasc. Dis.* 1998;8:331–333.
61. Einhaupl K, Masuhr F. Cerebral venous and sinus thrombosis: an update. *Eur. J. Neurol.* 1994;1:109–126.
62. Einhaupl K, Villringer A, Meister W, Mehracin S, Garner C, Pelkofer M et al. Heparin treatment in sinus venous thrombosis. *Lancet* 1991;338:597–600.
63. Stam J, Lensing A, Vermeulen M, Tijssen J. Heparin treatment in sinus venous thrombosis. *Lancet* 1991;338:1154.
64. de Bruijn S, Stam J, for the Cerebral Venous Sinus Thrombosis Study Group. Randomized, placebo controlled trial of anticoagulant treatment with low-molecular-weight heparin for cerebral venous thrombosis. *Stroke* 1999;30:484–488.

65. Bousser M. Cerebral venous thrombosis: nothing, heparin or local thrombolysis. *Stroke* 1999;30:481–483.
66. Frey J, Muro G, McDougall C, Dean B, Jahnke H. Cerebral venous thrombosis: combined intrathrombus rtPA and intravenous heparin. *Stroke* 1999;30:489–494.
67. Diaz J, Schiffman J, Urban E, Maccario M. Superior sagittal thrombosis and pulmonary embolism: a syndrome rediscovered. *Acta. Neurol. Scand.* 1992;86:390–396.
68. Houser O, Campbell J, Campbell R, Sundt T. Arteriovenous malformation affecting the transverse dural venous sinus. An acquired lesion. *Mayo Clin. Proc.* 1979;54:651–661.
69. Kalbag R, Woollf A. *Cerebral Venous Thrombosis*, vol 1. London: Oxford University Press, 1967.

22

Traumatic Head Injury

Sandra Kuniyoshi and Jose I. Suarez

INTRODUCTION

The role of neuroscience intensive care in the patient with traumatic brain injury (TBI) has advanced rapidly over the past few decades. Injury induced by trauma is not limited to vascular distributions of the brain or anatomically discrete regions. As our understanding of the biochemical and pathophysiologic mechanisms of ischemia, seizure, and neurodegenerative disease has evolved so has our recognition that the mechanism of damage in TBI probably encapsulates similar cellular mechanisms of injury. The penumbra at risk for secondary injury in severe TBI is often larger than a vascular distribution and the course more progressive, requiring rapid and often multiple levels of acute neurosurgical and neurologic care. With the advent of neuroscience critical care units (NSUs), these needs are being systematically addressed. In this chapter we will review the primary aspects of TBI, including its epidemiology, mechanisms of injury, early management, monitoring, and prognosis.

EPIDEMIOLOGY

The Centers for Disease Control and Prevention reports estimate that each year 1.5 million Americans will sustain a TBI. Approximately 230,000 will be hospitalized and 50,000 will die as a consequence of TBI. Eighty to ninety thousand will sustain significant long-term disability. Currently, 5.3 million people (2% of the US population) are living with permanent deficits associated with TBI *(1–4)*. One study in 1985 estimated the annual cost of TBI to the United States to be upwards of 37.8 billion *(5)*.

TBI in the US has a bimodal distribution, with a peak incidence in young adults aged 15–24 yr and a second smaller peak in the elderly (>60 yr old). Men are twice as likely as women to sustain and three times as likely to die from a TBI.

Transportation-related events remain the leading cause of TBI. In the past decade, the mortality rates of TBI in transportation related events have decreased from 11.1/100,000 to 6.9/100,000; whereas they have increased for events involving violence and use of a firearm (from 7.2/100,000 to 8.4/100,000). Thus in a decade the leading cause of mortality associated with TBI has changed from transportation-related events to violent events with firearms. Falls remain the predominant cause of TBI and mortality in the elderly (men older than 85 yr; women older than 75 yr) *(4)*.

Mortality rates overall attributed to TBI have decreased 20% (from 24.7/100,000 in 1985 to 19.4/100,000 in 1994) in the past decade. The decline in mortality rate is more dramatic (40%) in women and in children younger than 15 in whom the leading cause of TBI-associated death remains transport related injury. Increased usage of seat belts, car seats for children, and fewer drunk drivers have been suggested as contributory factors to this decline. The development of trauma centers, triage protocols, and neurosciences critical care units (NSU) with an emphasis on efficient prehospital and criti-

From: *Current Clinical Neurology*
Critical Care Neurology and Neurosurgery
Edited by: J. I. Suarez © Humana Press Inc., Totowa, NJ

cal care resuscitation and maintenance are also factors associated with the decrease in TBI mortality rate. Curiously, hospitalization rates for TBI have decreased 50%, suggesting that rapid triage with discharge of the less critical patients remains a priority in a medical society more cognizant of its limited resources *(3–5)*.

MECHANISMS OF INJURY

Several publications have dealt with the possible mechanisms of cell damage in TBI. Although it has been described in Chapter 1 of this book, recognition of primary and secondary brain injury is of utmost importance if treating physicians are to impact upon clinical outcome in this patient population. In Table 1, we describe the key mechanisms of injury and their influence on brain pathology. In Table 2, we present a summary of clinical and management aspects of these mechanism of injury.

Scalp Injury

The scalp has five layers. The subcutaneous layer contains the vasculature. Anteriorly, the supraorbital and supratrochlear arteries, branches of the ophthalmic arising from the internal carotid artery, perfuse the scalp. Posteriorly and laterally, the scalp is fed primarily by arterial branches derived from the external carotid artery. A scalp laceration or avulsion may hemorrhage profusely, resulting in hypovolemic shock. Hemostasis should be obtained and tissue cleaned and kept hydrated for immediate or delayed repair *(6)*.

Skull Fractures

Linear Skull Fractures

The presence of a linear skull fracture has been cited as a risk factor for the development of delayed epidural hematoma. However, other clinical signs are more sensitive regarding prognosis and should be reviewed in conjunction, in determining triage and management.

Depressed Skull Fracture

Depressed skull fractures commonly occurs with injuries involving objects with a high kinetic energy. Closed fractures refer to fractures that do not have overlying scalp lacerations or avulsions. Those with avulsed or lacerated scalp continuous with the fracture are referred to as compound or open *(7)*. Closed fractures are not associated with a high rate of infection. Depressed compound fractures are associated with infections in 2.5–10.6% *(7)*.

Basal Skull Fractures

Most basal skull fractures are extensions of fractures through the cranial vault. Linear fractures in the basal skull associated with disrupted dura places the central nervous system (CNS) in contact with the paranasal sinuses predisposing the patient to the development of fistulas and meningitis. Fistulas occur in 5–10% of the patients with basal skull fractures *(8)*. Immunofixation of beta-2-transferrin can be detected to differentiate cerebrospinal fluid (CSF) from other bodily secretions *(9)*. Antibiotic prophylaxis is not warranted in patients without fistulas, and it is unclear whether it is beneficial in patients with fistulas but without meningitis *(10)*.

Focal Brain Injury

Epidural Hemorrhage

Epidural hematomas (EDH) occur in approx 1.5% of head injuries. The peak occurrence is in the second and third decades of life. EDH occurs because of trauma to the skull and underlying vessels, rather than to the brain itself. Skull fractures are present in the majority of cases (80–97%) *(11)*. Hydraulic force from the torn meningeal artery (50–85%) into an area of dural separation dissects the

Table 1
Intracranial Consequences of Traumatic Brain Injury

Extension of injury	Mechanism of injury	Imaging findings	Pathologic correlate
Focal brain injury			
EDH	Injury to bone, torn middle meningeal artery (85%) with blood dissecting the dura from the inner table. 15% middle meningeal vein or dural sinus source	80–97% manifest skull fracture identifiable on CT skull films; 85% biconvex high density mass adjacent to the dura	Hemorrhage and mass effect
SDH	Tearing of surface bridging veins secondary to acceleration-deceleration or accumulation around parenchymal laceration.	Acute: hyperdense lesion less uniform and concave over parenchyma Subacute (4 d–3 wk): isodense Chronic (3 wk–4 mo): hypodense	Hemorrhage, edema, mass effect, contact of hemorrhage with parenchyma may induce inflammation/ necrosis
ICH	Rapid deceleration causing impact of brain on bony prominences of inner table Essentially bleeding into a contusion—similar mechanism	Hyperdense globular lesion commonly in temporal, frontal, occipital white matter	Hemorrhage, necrosis, ischemia
Contusion	Rapid deceleration causing brain to impact bony prominences	Low or high density on CT depending upon hemorrhagic component (high)	Similar to ICH with less hemorrhage component
Diffuse brain injury			
Concussion	Acceleration-deceleration injury	Little or no CT/MRI findings	Little or no microscopic abnormalities—may be associated with mild reticular cell drop out or axonal damage
Diffuse axonal injury	Acceleration/deceleration injury causing a differential of force between gray and white matter→shear injury	Severe: may be associated with small cortico-medullary hemorrhages, or hemorrhagic/hypodense foci in the corpus callosum and brainstem	Diffuse axonal swelling (<1–3 h)→ Axonal retraction balls (>3–6 h)

EDH, epidural hematoma; SDH, subdural hematoma; ICH, intracranial hemorrhage; CT, head CT; MRI, head MRI.

Table 2
Clinical and Management Features of Common Intracranial Pathology after TBI

Pathology	Clinical presentation	Management	Prognosis
Linear skull fracture	Similar to EDH, history of trauma	Determine the presence of EDH	Good, but presence of a linear skull fracture not an appropriate prognostic tool
Depressed skull fracture	Evidence of a crush injury on the cranium, symptoms dependent on the degree of intraparenchymal involvement	Determine whether the injury is closed/open Open or compound fracture may require immediate exploration and elevation, as 4.5–10.6% associated with infection	Dependent on the associated complications, >48 h delay in elevation associated with increased infectious complications
Basal skull fracture	Hemotympanum, laceration of external auditory canal, periorbital ecchymosis (raccoon eyes) Postauricular ecchymosis (Battle's sign) later in the course Involvement of CN I, II, VII, and VIII Rhinorrhea/otorrhea	Avoid placement of NG tube or nasal intubation if suspect basal skull fracture Immunofixation test for β2 transferrin for otorrhea/rhinorrhea Prophylactic use of antibiotics Absolute indication for repair include herniation of brain into sinus, bone spicule invading brain or meningitis	80% of fistulas close spontaneously Prognosis excellent if complications such as meningitis avoided antibiotics
EDH	Classical presentation of brief loss of consciousness followed by a lucid interval lasting several hours occurs in less than 10–27% Deterioration typically occurs in hours	In most cases EDH is a surgical condition Medical management may be considered if: the size is < 1cm maximal thickness in a chronic/subacute SDH with minimal neurologic symptoms and no evidence of hematoma However prolonged hospitalization and close observation is required	Prognosis is worse in those without a lucid interval and those who develop symptoms early after trauma Mortality ranges from 5 to 55% Surgical mortality in noncomatose patients is minimal

(continued on next page)

398

	Clinical presentation	Treatment	Outcome
SDH	Clinical presentation depends on size. 50% remain unconscious from onset of injury. Clinical suspicion should be entertained when patient has a declining level of consciousness	Rapid surgical evacuation is the treatment of choice. Some studies suggest that prognosis is improved if surgery occurs within the first 4 h	Mortality is 50–90%. Outcome correlates with GCS on admission inversely with age and ICP
ICH	Clinical presentation reflects that ICH reaches maximal size in 84% of patients within 12 h > 50% rendered unconscious on impact of initial injury 19% have a lucid interval and 30% never lose consciousness	2/3 will require surgical evacuation within 48 h	
DAI	Clinically manifest as significant loss of consciousness (< 6 h), and significant amnesia, which lasts greater than a few hours	As with other mechanisms of severe TBI evaluate and aggressively treat elevated ICP and hypotension	15–65% will have a good outcome

EDH, epidural hematoma; SDH, subdural hematoma; GCS, Glasgow coma scale; ICP, intracranial pressure; ICH, intracranial hematoma; DIA, diffuse axonal injury.

dura further in a positive feedback loop. Venous (diploic, meningeal veins) or venous sinus (<10%) origin EDH must bleed into a region of significant prior dural stripping *(12)*.

Nine to 10% of patients may present with delayed EDH. Patients initially have a normal computed tomography (CT) scan followed by a CT scan with evidence of EDH. Skull fracture may be a risk factor *(13)*.

Subdural Hematoma

Acute subdural hematomas (SDHs) occur in approx 0.5–5% of head injuries. Although traffic trauma is responsible for the majority of TBI, assaults and falls are more likely to be the culprit in SDH. The mean age of patients is 41–42 yr. Acceleration of the brain sagittally results in a stretching and tearing of the surface bridging veins that drain into the dural venous sinuses *(14)*.

SDH commonly occurs following trauma but may occur with minimal or no history of trauma in patients who are on anticoagulation therapy or who have bleeding dyscrasias. SDH may also be associated with aneurysm rupture *(15)*.

Intraparenchymal/Intracerebral Hemorrhage

The incidence of intraparenchymal/intracerebral hemorrhage (ICH) is reported as 4–23% in TBI. Acceleration of the brain as it slides over the irregularities of the inner table is the most common mechanism *(16,17)*. Penetrating missiles and crush injuries associated with depressed skull fractures can also cause ICH. Most of these (80–90%) occur in the white matter of the temporal and frontal lobes. ICH is often accompanied by other pathologies of TBI. Signs and symptoms often mimick other presentations, particularly infarction. Over 50% are rendered unconscious with the impact of initial injury, 19% may have a lucid interval, and approx 30% never lose consciousness. Two thirds will require surgery within 48 h. ICH reaches its maximum size in 84% of the patients in 12 h *(16,17)* (Fig. 1).

Delayed ICH as delayed EDH, is characterized by a CT that is initially negative for hemorrhage and subsequently found to have ICH. It is reported in 1.7–7% of head injury patients and may occur in the region of a contusion. Eighty percent present in the first 48 h after injury, but they may be delayed for longer than 1 wk *(18)*.

Contusion

Contusions occur in a large percentage of TBI (89% in one postmortem study) *(19)*. Head CT scans are less sensitive than pathologic studies, but contusions remain the most commonly identified lesions in TBI (23–56%) *(20)* (*see* Fig. 1). MRI is more sensitive (98% of contusions identified in one study) *(21)*. Contusion refers most commonly to the injury that occurs after sudden deceleration impacts the brain with the bony prominences of the inner table. The resultant countercoup (distant from impact) ischemia, necrosis, edema, and hemorrhage predominantly appear in the frontal and temporal poles, as they are proximal to the frontal and middle fossa *(22)*. Contusions can also occur in the medial brain with acceleration of the falx against the brain *(22)*. Contusions in isolation seldom result in loss of consciousness. Focal neurologic deficits associated with the site of the lesion are most common in the acute phase. Rapid deterioration may indicate hemorrhage into the contusion with increasing mass effect. Multiple contusions (tripolar/tetrapolar), predispose the patient to diffuse cerebral edema and elevated intracranial pressure (ICP) *(22)*. Temporal lobe (pole/lateral) contusions provide a special hazard because they are proximal to the incisura and midbrain; herniation may occur without increased ICP or evidence of severe mass effect on scans. Overall mortality rate for contusions is reported as ranging from 25% to 60% *(23)*.

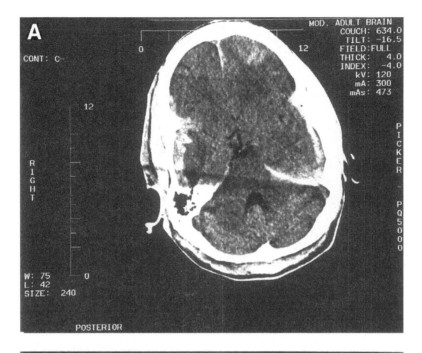

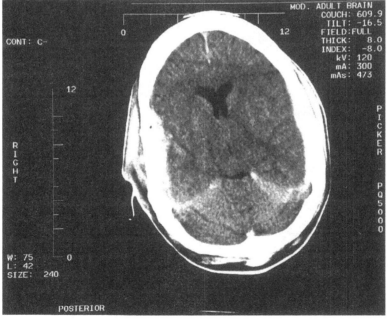

Fig. 1. Head CT scan without contrast of a 36-yr-old male with severe TBI. (**A**) initial scan performed in the emergency department shows mild left frontal and right temporal contusions with a right acute subdural hematoma (SDH).

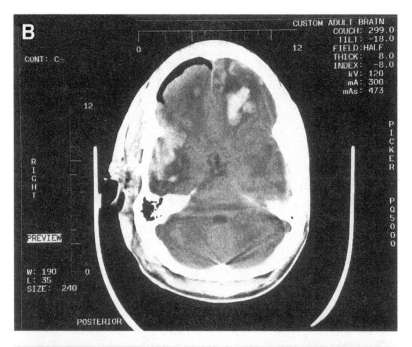

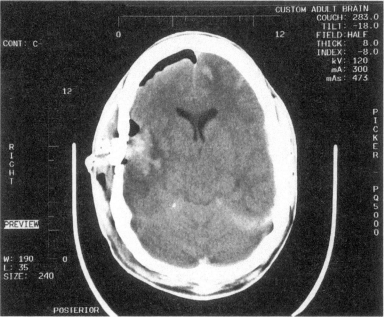

Fig. 1B. Head CT scan 8 h after admission: the patient deteriorated 3 h after scan A and underwent emergent right craniotomy with evacuation of SDH and right temporal contusion. Also note cerebral edema in the involved lobes and enlargement of left frontal lobe contusion.

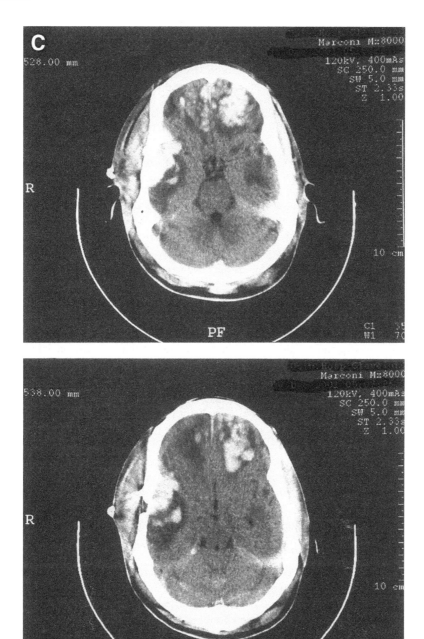

Fig. 1C. Head CT scan 5 d after admission: the patient was treated for elevated ICP and cerebral edema and level of consciousness improved by d 4. This scan reveals final size of bifrontal and right temporal contusion with improved basal cistern compression.

Diffuse Brain Injury

Acceleration-deceleration, particularly rotatory acceleration, is associated with a host of diffuse brain injuries. This mechanism of injury currently describes a continuum of clinical presentations. Concussion is the mild end of the spectrum. Diffuse axonal injury refers to the severe end.

Concussion

Concussion is clinically described by a transient alteration in consciousness, with confusion and amnesia. Concussion is on a clinical continuum with diffuse axonal injury (DAI). Pathologic correlates will be discussed under DAI.

Diffuse Axonal Injury

DAI refers to the disruption of intracerebral axons caused by the effect of angular acceleration on the viscoelastic brain, resulting in a differential of force between gray and white matter and subsequent shear injury *(24)*. Clinically, the syndrome is differentiated from concussion by a loss of consciousness that lasts longer than 6 h, significant amnesia lasting more than a few hours and a 3-mo good outcome that ranges from 15% to 65% as opposed to concussion patients who have 100% good outcome *(25)*.

Neuropathological evidence of destroyed axonal cytoskeleton and retraction bulbs were considered pathognomonic for the diagnosis of DAI. In DAI, within 15 min of injury, the axon is disrupted, followed by a structural change in the microtubules. Within 6 h, the neurofilaments compact and the side arms collapse. Subsequently, Calpain, a calcium-activated protease, is activated; the neurofilament disintegrates and the axotomy is accomplished *(26)*. This time dependent model of axonal injury, suggests that interventions may be possible. Postmortem examination of patients who died 1 h vs 3 d postinjury confirmed the time-dependent pathology. The former do not manifest the retraction bulbs but manifest only diffuse axonal swelling while the latter manifests both *(27)*.

CELLULAR MECHANISMS OF INJURY

Our understanding of the multiple abnormal biochemical reactions unleashed by TBI has significantly been enhanced by the publication of various animal and human studies in the past 10 yr. Knowledge of these cellular mechanisms of secondary injury is of the utmost importance because further improvement in clinical outcome will most likely be derived from early intervention and modification of these pathophysiologic processes.

Cerebral Blood Flow in Traumatic Brain Injury

The literature on cerebral blood flow (CBF) after TBI remains controversial. However, there are some features that can be summarized here (*see* Chapters 3 and 4). A decrease in CBF has been reported within the first hours after TBI *(28)*. However, arterio-venous oxygen differences ($AVDO_2$) reveal that this drop in CBF still exceeds metabolic requirements in most patients during this stage and may not translate into cerebral ischemia *(28–30)*. The available reports point out that about one third of TBI patients will have cerebral ischemia as determined by low CBF (< 20 mL/100 g/min) and abnormal $AVDO_2$ *(28–32)*. Contrary to this early diminution in CBF, an increase is seen in the first few days after TBI. This has been called hyperemia or "luxury perfusion" *(28)*. This reflects an uncoupling of CBF and cerebral metabolism as determined by changes in $AVDO_2$ and cerebral metabolic rate for oxygen ($CMRO_2$) *(28)* (*see* Chapter 4). Of all patients with elevated ICP during the first few days after TBI, the majority (approx 80%) will experience hyperemia, whereas the rest will have decreased CBF *(28)*. Taking all this into consideration, it has been proposed that TBI patients should be classified into three groups based on CBF measurements: low CBF (< 33 mL/100 g/min), relative hyperemia (33–55 mL/100 g/min), and absolute hyperemia (> 55 mL/100 g/min) *(28)*. TBI patients with low CBF will be more prone to developing cerebral ischemia secondary to hypotension, whereas those with hyperemia will be more likely to have elevated ICP. This latter group could also have cerebral ischemia if ICP remains untreated.

Disruption of the Electron Transport System and Ion Homeostasis

The biochemical mechanisms of secondary neuronal injury in TBI mirrors that described for ischemia. Decreased cerebral perfusion pressure (CPP) and/or hypoxia results in failure of the electron transport system (ETS), and oxidative phosphorylation, which requires oxygen as the final electron acceptor *(33)*. This disruption of the mitochondrial membrane potential results in the depletion of the adenosine triphosphate (ATP) required to maintain the neuronal membrane potential. Moreover, disruption of the ETS results in production of oxygen radicals and oxidative enzymes, which directly damages the phospholipid bilayer of the neuron. Anaerobic metabolism results in increased levels of lactate, CO_2, and K^+ lowering the pH and initiating cellular edema and preventing repolarization further exacerbating the depletion of ATP and the destructive cycle *(34–36)*.

Excitotoxic Neurotransmitters

Reduced CBF (<20 cc/mL/100 g/min) stimulates, in a threshold pattern, the release of excitatory amino acids. CSF concentrations of glutamate, glycine, and aspartate increase two- to eightfold following a TBI *(37,39)*. The elevation is present for up to one week and the peak level correlated with Glascow Outcome Scale score in one study *(39)*. Glutamate in the synapse through activation of NMDA receptors opens Ca^{2+} channels. Excessive levels of intracellular Ca^{2+} activates multiple enzymatic processes resulting in the further uncoupling of the oxidative phosphorylation process and production of free radicals. Glutamate reuptake mechanisms are also disrupted as they resemble the mechanism for K^+ homeostasis *(37,39)*.

The Immune Response

The immunologic response to TBI is multifaceted *(40)*. Suppression of the proliferative ability and the concentration of T cells, IgG/M, and IL-2 responsive cells has been found in the immediate post-trauma period. This correlates with a higher number of infectious complications occurring within the first 4 d of injury *(41,42)*.

Increased cytokine production has been documented. Cytokines can be inhibitory or stimulatory to inflammatory cascades. Elevated levels of inhibitory IL-10 and excitatory IL-6, IL-8 as well as tumor growth factor-beta (TGF-β) and tumor necrosis factor (TNF) have been reported. Many of these factors have been shown to have a direct effect on the dysfunction of the blood brain barrier and the release of growth factors *(43–45)*. Hypothermia induces depression of IL-6 in TBI patients. Correlation of good outcome has been found in those patients who sustain low levels of IL-6 after rewarming *(43)*.

Activated microglia release factors that stimulate the production of adhesion molecules, which allow migration of leukocytes into the tissue promoting further inflammatory response. The concentration of the soluble intercellular adhesion molecules (sICAM) has been found to correlate with the injury severity and outcome *(46)*.

Brain Trauma Proteins

Brain trauma-specific tau proteins have been identified by monoclonal antibodies developed from hybridoma screening of head trauma vs control patients. Enzyme-linked immunosorbent assay (ELISA) testing confirmed a more than 1000-fold increase in head trauma patients vs controls, normal pressure hydrocephalus and multiple sclerosis patients. The level of specific CSF tau correlated inversely with recovery. The brain trauma specific isoforms were found to retain the microtubule binding domain *(47)*. The amyloid peptide has been shown to accumulate in neurons with traumatic injury *(48,49)*.

EARLY EVALUATION AND MANAGEMENT

The initial triage of a TBI patient by medical personnel occurs typically in the emergency department. Evaluation of the ABCs (airway, breathing, and circulation) should be accomplished and their stability secured before pursuing more complex examinations. Tracheal intubation is indicated in patients who have a Glasgow Coma Scale (GCS) score less than 8, inability to protect their airway, or inability to maintain adequate ventilation *(50)*. Fluid resuscitation with isotonic saline, and immobilization of the spine, if indicated, should be accomplished. Spinal injury is a complication in 10–15% of head injury patients. Patients should be immobilized (spine board, cervical collar, spine bags) and spine radiographs obtained (anteroposterior and lateral; open- mouth odontoid if patient is stable) *(50)*.

Assessment of pupillary responsivity, level of consciousness and GCS score should occur in rapid sequence *(51,52)*. These parameters have been shown to have a good correlation with outcome in TBI. GCS scoring has been used to rapidly classify the patients into categories of mild GCS scores of 13–15, moderate TBI to 9–12, and severe to less than 8 *(52)*. Severe patients, as indicated previously, are candidates for intubation and admission to an NSU. They also warrant evaluation for emergent surgical intervention. Obtaining an accurate history is critical including mechanism of injury and other medical conditions, medications, allergies, and illicit substance exposure. A proficient neurologic examination should be obtained early. Often the prehospital triage and treatment of patient care will compromise the initial GCS and neuroexamination (i.e., administration of paralytics and sedatives). The European Brain Injury consortium found that a full GCS score was unobtainable 44% of the patients, nearly half of all admissions to the neurosurgery ward *(50)*. There is also considerable variation in the scoring and assessment of intubated patients. The Traumatic Coma Data Bank arbitrarily scores the verbal aspect of all patients who arrive intubated as 1.1. Others score the GCS without regard to the patients' intubated status or recent administration of paralytics. Some score only the motor and eye examination when the patient is intubated. Not surprisingly, the predictive value is much better 88% vs 65% for poor outcome with testable GCS scores of 3–5 vs those arbitrarily assigned verbal scores of 1 while intubated *(52,53)*. Following this, head and neck imaging should be accomplished in a timely manner in these patients.

Hospital admissions for TBI have decreased 50% in the past decade, *vida infra*. Some suggest that it is the managed care ideology of limited resources that has decremented the number of patients admitted although that remains to be proven. White published a review on TBI, which included a classification that ranks patients into low, moderate, or high risk *(54)*. Moderate or high risk patients warrant hospitalization. Low risk patients include those patients who are asymptomatic or have predominantly scalp lacerations, abrasions, or contusions with no moderate- or high-risk criteria. Nonprogressive headache and nonvertiginous dizziness may occur. Moderate risk is characterized by a change in the level of consciousness at any time during or since the injury, post traumatic seizure or amnesia, vomiting, signs of skull fracture or depressed skull fracture, basilar fracture, multiple trauma, serious facial trauma, alcohol or drug intoxication, unreliable or inadequate history, younger than 2 yr old children/infants with more than very trivial history and presentation and/or suspected child abuse. High-risk patients are defined as those with depressed level of consciousness not attributable to alcohol or drug exposure or metabolic derangement or postictal state. This category also includes patients with focal neurologic signs, palpable depressed skull fracture, or penetrating skull injury.

Sedation

Light sedation is indicated for the anxious patient with TBI. In patients with severe TBI, who require mechanical ventilation, deep sedation may be beneficial. Sedation can decrease the $CMRO_2$. Various maneuvers common to ICU management can cause considerable anxiety and increase metabolic rate by 15–20% *(55)*. Respiratory distress can increase metabolic rate from 24 to 50% *(53–55)*. Sympathetic response in agitated patients can elicit constriction of peripheral vasculature, hyperdynamic cardiac response, and increases in mean arterial pressure (MAP), CPP, and ICP. Combativeness and agitation can elevate ICP considerably and rapid management may necessitate the usage of sedation with morphine (2–4 mg IV every hour), fentanyl/propofol (1–2 mL/h) or benzodiazepines, midazolam/lorazepam as an IV bolus or drip (0.01–0.08 mg/kg/h) and finally paralytic agents (vecuronium 8–10 mg IV) *(56,57)*. The obvious disadvantage in deeply sedated and pharmaceutically paralyzed patients is the loss of the neurologic examination and the risks of pneumonia and infection associated with deep sedation. Hypotension can be an adverse effect in opioidergic sedation. In sedatives without known hypotensive adverse effects, loss of sympathetic tone unmasks hypovolemia and severe hypotension can result *(see also* Chapter 21).

PREVENTION OF SECONDARY INJURY

Secondary injury refers to the sequelae of complications following primary TBI. Prognosis in TBI is primarily dependent upon the ability to escape secondary injury. Nonmedical preventative laws regarding restraints and helmets may be effective in preventing primary TBI. Secondary injury prevention is the goal of emergency medical services, triage, and medical personnel. The NSU is designed to rapidly identify, record, treat and where possible prevent the development of secondary injury. The role of multimodality monitoring has been discussed elsewhere in this book *(see* Chapter 6).

Hypoxia

Resuscitation of the patient with TBI necessitates administration and maintenance of adequate oxygenation. Pragmatic attention to adequate airway, ventilation, and perfusion encompass a significant proportion of the initial triage of the patient and continue to a be primary consideration in the subsequent management. There is considerable evidence that efficient vigilant treatment of hypoxia improves the prognosis of the patient with TBI *(58)*.

An immediate goal of patients with TBI is adequate cerebral oxygenation. Jugular venous oxygen saturation ($SvjO_2$) is a purported measure of the global oxygen delivery to the brain. An infrared catheter allows continuous monitoring of global cerebral oxygenation *(59,60)*. The mechanics and specificities regarding utilization and monitoring are discussed in detail elsewhere *(see* Chapter 6). Values of 65% are considered normal for $SvjO_2$, levels of more than 50% are considered satisfactory for patients with TBI. Continuous monitoring of $SvjO_2$ appears to be a useful indicator of progressive cerebral ischemia *(59,60)*. However, the degree of loss of metabolic and pressure autoregulation differ between patients and sensitivity to small changes in oxygenation, pressure, carbon dioxide level, may vary markedly. The difficulty of monitors, which fluctuate in response to multiple factors, is interpretation of the recordings. One study, which did find a benefit in prognosis and management with $SvjO_2$ monitoring, used an algorithm that considered multiple etiologies for a sustained decrease in $SvjO_2$ less than 50%. This included evaluation for hypoxia ($SaO_2 < 90\%$), hemoglobin concentration (anemia, hemoglobin < 9 g/dL), systolic blood pressure (hypotension, SBP < 90 mmHg), ICP, and carbon dioxide (hypocarbia, $PaCO_2$ <28 mmHg) levels were assessed and resuscitated. The effectiveness of the resuscitation was verified by improving saturation. This suggests that continuous monitoring that fluctuates back to baseline with corrections of insult may provide the indications needed to more effectively and efficiently respond to fluctuating ischemia.

Measurements of CBF, $AVDO_2$, oxygen extraction ratio (OER), and $CMRO_2$ have been used to help determine coupling of supply and demand of brain tissue in TBI patients with the hope of avoiding cerebral ischemia *(see* Chapter 4). The major criticism to using these metabolic indices is that they are affected by anemia, which is very common in TBI patients. Because of this, measurement of cerebral oxygen extraction (COE) has been recommended (normal values: 24–42%). This is easily calculated as the difference between systemic arterial oxygen saturation (SaO_2) and $SvjO_2$ *(61)*.

Hypotension

CPP is contingent upon the MAP. It is formally calculated as the difference between the MAP and the ICP. There is considerable evidence, that poor prognosis and increased mortality is associated with prehospital as well as in NSU hypotension (SBP < 90 mmHg) *(62,63)*. Early resuscitation of hypotension is strongly associated with a good outcome *(63)*. Vigilant maintenance of adequate MAP remains one of the only evidenced based treatments that is consistently found to be associated with decreased mortality and morbidity. Liebert describes it as one of the five most powerful predictors of outcome and it is the only one that is subject to medical manipulation *(63)*. The "ideal" MAP to maintain an "ideal" CPP has not been clearly determined. However, most studies imply that CPP greater than 55–60 mmHg is adequate. Increasing CPP to values greater than 70 mmHg is associated with increased incidence of systemic complications such as acute respiratory distress syndrome (ARDS), which may negate any significant favorable impact on neurologic outcome *(64,65)*.

Elevated Intracranial Pressure

Considerable research and engineering have been invested in the technology of accurately measuring and treating increased ICP, in the interest of arresting and reversing the associated secondary injury. Refractory elevated ICP has been associated with increased mortality and poor prognosis *(see also* Chapter 5).

Head Position

Simple measures such as raising the head of the bed 30–45° (reverse Trendelenberg) have been cited as initial therapy to reduce ICP. This maneuver has been associated with decreased ICP concomitant with decreased MAP, while CPP/CBF is unchanged. Positioning of the head at midline will prevent kinking of jugular veins. Another study has advocated positioning the patients' head in Trendelenberg, flat, and reversed Tredelenberg to determine which head position is associated with the best ICP or $SvjO_2$. They discovered that although the majority of patients had better ICP readings in the reverse Tredelenberg position, a significant percentage (<30%), had better results in the Trendelenberg position *(66)*.

Mannitol Therapy

Mannitol therapy, through multiple mechanisms, has been found to be effective in reducing elevated ICP. It acts as both an osmotic agent, a rheologic agent—reducing viscosity, as well as a free radical scavenger. Doses of 0.25 g–1.5 g/kg bolus injection followed by 0.25 g or more every 6 h are recommended to keep serum osmolarity between 300 and 320 osm/L *(67,68)*. Disadvantages associated with the usage of mannitol include reverse osmolarity and renal failure. Multiple boluses (more than three to four) or continuous infusion of mannitol increases the risk of these adverse effects. Reverse osmolarity refers to the accumulation of mannitol in the brain after multiple doses, causing a reverse osmotic shift. Contraindications for mannitol include hypovolemia and hypotension, renal failure, although paradoxically, because of its rheologic properties, including increasing venous return, it has been used for hypovolemic resuscitation *(67)*.

Hypertonic Saline Therapy

Hypertonic saline has a higher reflection coefficient than mannitol, suggesting it might have a better tonicity. Hypertonic saline (2.7–29.2%) has been used after extensive animal data had reported beneficial effects on elevated ICP. It has been reported to be effective in cases resistant to mannitol without the adverse effects of renal insufficiency *(69,70)*. However, this treatment is still undergoing investigation in humans.

Table 3
Goals of Treatment in Patients With Severe TBI

Variable	Goal
ICP	<20 mmHg
CPP	>60 mmHg
$SvjO_2$	<50%
SaO_2	<97%
COE	24–42%
Temperature	<37.5°C
Blood glucose	100–150 mg/dL

TBI, traumatic brain injury; ICP, intracranial pressure; CPP, cerebral perfusion pressure; $SvjO_2$, Jugular venous saturation of oxygen; SaO_2, Arterial saturation of oxygen; COE, Cerebral oxygen extraction.

Hyperventilation

Mild hyperventilation to hypocarbia ($PaCO_2$ 30–35 mmHg) has also been found to be transiently effective in reducing ICP. The Joint Section on Neurotrauma and Critical Care recommends that it not be used during the first 5 d of TBI *(71)*. Decreased $PaCO_2$ decreases the pH and causes constriction of the cerebral vasculature, thereby decreasing ICP and CBF. Constriction of the cerebral vasculature could place the penumbra at increased risk of ischemia indicating a small window of therapeutic potential. There is also the risk of losing autoregulatory control of the pressure. Tachyphylaxis associated with the reflexive drop in CSF pH has been reported, reverting the brain back to its acidotic state with dilated vasculature once hyperventilation has been discontinued. Other studies have suggested that although the CBF is decreased the metabolic rate is also decreased in TBI patients and the expected ischemia may not occur *(72)*.

Barbiturate Coma

Pentobarbital or barbiturate coma induction has been utilized effectively to lower ICP in a fraction of patients refractory to other therapies. Barbiturates can reduce the $CMRO_2$ by more than 50% (approx 55%). This correlates with a decrease in CBF of approx 48%. The maximum decrease in $CMRO_2$ is associated with a burst suppression pattern on electroencephalography (EEG). Recommended doses are 10 mg/kg as an IV bolus, followed by a continuous infusion of 0.5 to 2 mg/kg/h titrated to EEG burst suppression *(73,74)*.

Comparison of Techniques

Curiously, statistical data does not rigorously support one form of treatment regarding lowering ICP over another *(75)*. Therapeutics that are recognized to be necessary and the standard of care are no longer measured against placebo. In addition, comparison studies have not had the statistical power to show a significant advantage of one therapy over another. Most of the therapies also have significant therapeutic window and a relative optimal period of effectiveness vs risk of detrimental effects, with few monitoring devices to determine the optimal range and doses. The development of continuous monitoring devices such as $SvjO_2$ allows rapid resuscitation in the event of adverse effects from treatment on multiple levels. It also forces us to consider the nonlinear nature of neuronal pathology and approaches to treatment.

The use of cerebral metabolic monitoring to guide management of patients with severe TBI has been advocated. However, this is not widely practiced. In Table 3, we present some general recommendations for the most commonly used parameters in this patient population. If we are to manage severe TBI patients based on cerebral metabolic parameters then the following proposed guidelines by Cruz appear to integrate many of the discussed modalities *(61)*:

1. Group 1: this includes patients with normal ICP, CPP, and COE. In this situation no specific therapeutic maneuvers are indicated and patients should be maintained in same supportive measures.
2. Group 2: patients with elevated ICP but normal CPP and COE. In this case sedation and neuromuscular blockade should be maximized followed by mannitol and finally controlled hyperventilation.
3. Group 3: patients with normal ICP and CPP but increased COE ("oligemic cerebral hypoxia"). If patients have a $PaCO_2$ <30 mmHg and normal basal cisterns as determined by head CT, then $PaCO_2$ should be normalized. However, when $PaCO_2$ <30 mmHg and basal cisterns are compressed, sedation should be optimized followed by mannitol.
4. Group 4: patients with elevated ICP and COE but with normal or diminished CPP. These patients should receive mannitol. Once ICP is normalized and if COE remains elevated, then controlled hyperventilation should be instituted.
5. Group 5: patients with elevated ICP, low COE and normal CPP ("relative hyperperfusion" or "luxury perfusion"). These patients should be treated with controlled hyperventilation.

Whether following these recommendations will result in better long-term clinical outcome remains to be confirmed by further prospective clinical studies.

Craniectomy

The use of decompressive craniectomy in severe TBI patients has been reported *(76–79)*. This therapy appears to decrease mortality in patients with elevated ICP refractory to medical therapy. However, the timing of surgery may be important since not all the studies have found similar encouraging results *(78)*. Further investigations including randomized clinical trials are needed before decompressive craniectomy is widely recommended.

Hyperglycemia

Few appreciate the considerable role of hyperglycemia on outcome in secondary ischemic injury. Emphasis is placed on resuscitation from hypoxia and hypotension, which have continuous monitoring. Hyperglycemia is a major prognostic factor in the outcome of patients with an ischemic penumbra. Hyperglycemia increases the metabolism of the neuron, inducing rapid conversion to anaerobic metabolism, accelerating the oxidative stress on the cell. Early hyperglycemia is a frequent component of the stress response to severe TBI, thus indicating the severity of injury, and is a reliable predictor of poor clinical outcome *(80)*. Prompt regulation of blood glucose to within normoglycemic range (90–150 mg/dL), has been shown to prevent further ischemic insult, seizures, and mortality *(80,81)*.

Seizures

A significant percentage (22% in one study) of patients with moderate to severe TBI develop seizure activity *(82)*. Seizure prophylaxis with phenytoin or other anti epileptics is indicated. Risk factors which suggest seizure prophylaxis include new cortical-subcortical lesions identified on MRI, hemorrhage involving cortex, prolonged (>24 h) amnesia or change in mental status, and early seizure activity. One study found that 11% of those patients who presented in coma were discovered to have subclinical status epilepticus. The threshold for EEG monitoring of TBI patients who present with change in mental status or coma should be low. However, because of the absence of evidence of improved outcome or decrement of late onset seizures prophylactic treatment of seizure activity in patients with and without risk factors is not recommended for longer than 7 d in patients without evidence of seizure activity clinically or on EEG *(83,84)*.

Hyperthermia

Substantial evidence exists regarding the potential therapeutic role of hypothermia in traumatic injury *(85,86)*. Therefore, normothermia and/or mild hypothermia (temperature < 37.5°C) should be obtained with both pharmacologic and cooling therapy. The main mechanism is thought to involve suppression of the inflammatory response (*see* immune reaction under cellular mechanism *vida supra*). However, simple cooling techniques used in clinical trials have not shown the dramatic improvement in outcome (vs controls) expected *(87)*. Rapid initiation of more efficient cooling techniques in a larger more stratified study may be required to determine which patients benefit from hypothermia *(85,86)*.

Infection

Infection, fever, and respiratory difficulties all increase the metabolic rate and exacerbate neuronal ischemia. Prophylactic treatment of hyperthermia may mask a brewing infectious process. TBI patients have been shown to have depressed lymphocyte proliferation activity and an increased incidence of infection (in one study 60%), mortality and morbidity because of the infection *(39,40)*. Patients are particularly vulnerable in the first 4 d after TBI, although the lymphocyte activity does not normalize for 3 wk *(41,42)*. Appropriate critical care monitoring and antimicrobial therapy should be initiated early in the patient suspected of an infectious process to avoid devastating sequelae.

Deep Venous Thrombosis and Pulmonary Embolism

Patients with TBI are at significant risk for deep venous thrombosis (DVT) and subsequent pulmonary emboli (PE) (*see* Chapter 11). Appropriate prophylactic measures should be instituted, including sequential compression devices, thigh-high elastic stockings hose, and subcutaneous heparin, these measures have been found to be synergistic in preventing DVT *(88)*.

Nutrition

Patients with severe TBI have increased metabolic requirements *(89–92)* (*see* Chapter 14). This patient population may lose up to 15% of their body weight within 1 wk and can easily become malnourished and infected *(89)*. There is sufficient evidence to support institution of early nutrition in these patients (within 7 d after TBI). Enteral feedings are preferred because of a lower rate of complications compared to parenteral routes. Early enhanced nutrition therapy (start feeding that meet estimated energy and nitrogen requirements from day 1) is associated with improved clinical outcome and reduced in-hospital infection rates compared to standard treatment (gradual increase in feeding from 15 mL/h up to estimated caloric needs) *(89)*.

Vasospasm Prophylaxis

The risk of vasospasm in patients with TBI is significant, reported as ranging from 20 to 35% in transcranial Doppler ultrasound studies of moderate and severe TBI patients *(93)*. This has provoked investigations into the prophylactic use of calcium channel blockers *(94,95)*. The Cochrane database post hoc analysis seems to indicate that in the case of a subarachnoid hemorrhage (SAH) prophylactic usage of calcium channel blockers may improve outcome. However, adverse effects were also noted suggesting that further testing be warranted for optimum period of treatment and patient subgroup *(93,96)*. We recommend that patients with vasospasm after TBI should be treated in a similar fashion as patients with SAH (*see* Chapters 20 and 24).

PROGNOSIS IN TRAUMATIC BRAIN INJURY

The National Trauma Coma Data Bank studies revealed that the two most important factors in determining outcome in brain trauma were time spent with ICP more than 20 mmHg and time spent with systolic blood pressure less than 80 mmHg. Other factors which have been consistently found to be prognostically important include age of the patient, clinical indices evaluating the severity of injury (the depth and duration of coma [GCS and pupillary response]) and imaging studies indicating the type of injury (SAH, SDH, ventricular hemorrhage, etc.) *(96,97)*. Other factors reported to have prognostic significance are blood glucose level, body temperature, cerebral lactate concentration and platelet count *(97)*.

The decrease in mortality and morbidity of patients with severe TBI has been attributed to the recognition of the need to prevent secondary injury or ischemia. Emphasis has been placed on the rapid evacuation of hematomas and control of ICP to improve neurologic outcome. Review of the outcome studies has shown that vigilant attention to oxygenation and hypotension are of equal importance to outcome as the treatment of mass and mass effect *(96–98)*. Other factors shown to be of prognostic significance (blood glucose, body temperature, etc.) had been previously recognized as significant in predicting outcome in cerebral vascular ischemia. Recognition of the overlap in cellular and biochemical mechanisms of injury of the patient with TBI and the patient with more widely investigated areas of research such as vascular ischemia and neurodegenerative disease may facilitate more effective treatment protocols and investigations.

The quality-of-life issues and the neuropsychological toll on the patient and the family of the patient with TBI are often onerous. Patients with TBI may have delayed symptoms of chronic headache, memory difficulties, a decline in the ability to perform activity of daily living and an overall decrement in quality of life, resulting in loss of income, occupation, and social supports such as family. Those factors predictive of mortality do not translate easily into morbidity and neuropsychological outcome. GCS score and pupillary response have been reported to be fair predictors of neuropsychological outcome and quality of life as tested by SIP (sickness impact profile). While ICP, blood glucose, CT observations failed to show a significant relationship with morbidity as assessed by the SIP, GOS (Glasgow Outcome Scale) and the neuropsychological testing. Other studies suggest that APACHE (acute physiology age and chronic health evaluation) II and III scores may be better predictors of late mortality (15 d after admission). APACHE III score was found to be the best predictor of morbidity or functional outcome as assessed by the index of ADL (index of independence of activity of daily living) *(99)*.

CONCLUSION

TBI is the leading cause of death and disability in children and young adults. There is no sine que non with which to identify a patient with TBI, therefore, it has been called the invisible epidemic. The mechanisms of severe TBI are varied and numerous and the prognosis after the initial event depends on the ability to prevent secondary injury. The 22% decline in the severe TBI mortality within the past decade indicates that early resuscitation and prevention of secondary injury can have a dramatic effect on outcome. Many of the principles of resuscitation of hypoxia and hypotension as well as effect of hyperglycemia have been previously investigated in studies in vascular ischemia. The long term post-trauma effects on memory, intellectual behavior, communication, and overall quality of life are difficult to quantitate but may parallel in an advanced rate the effects seen in neurodegenerative disease. TBI, the invisible epidemic, may provide the microcosm in which the proposed therapies for neurodegenerative disease may be found effective as the victims often do not have the premorbid risk factors of advanced age or comorbid diseases. Clearly, more research needs to be accomplished with this population in mind.

REFERENCES

1. Sosin DM, Sniezek JE, Thurman DJ. Incidence of mild and moderate brain injury in the United States, 1991. *Brain Injury* 1996;10:47–54.
2. Centers for Disease Control and Prevention, National Center for Injury Prevention and Control. Unpublished analysis of data from the 1994 National Hospital Discharge Survey, 1998.
3. Sosin DM, Sniezek JE, Waxweiler RJ. Trends in death associated with traumatic brain injury, 1979 through 1992. *JAMA* 1995;273:1778–1780.
4. Centers for Disease Control and Prevention, National Center for Injury Prevention and Control. Unpublished analysis of data from Multiple Cause of Death Public Use Data, 1997.

5. Max W, MacKenzie EJ, Rice DP. Head injuries: costs and consequences. *J. Head Trauma Rehabil.* 1991;6:76–91.

6. Tremolada C, Candiani P, Signorini M, Vigano M, Donati L. The surgical anatomy of the subcutaneous fascial system of the scalp. *Ann. Plast. Surg.* 1994;32:8–14.

7. Braakman R. Depressed skull fracture: Data, treatment, and follow-up in 225 consecutive cases. *J. Neurol. Neurosurg. Psychiatry* 1972;35:395–402.

8. Brawley BW, Kelly WA. Treatment of basal skull fractures with and without cerebrospinal fluid fistulae. *J. Neurosurg.* 1967;26:57–61.

9. Fransen P, Sindic CJ, Thauvoy C, Laterre C, Stroobandt G. Highly sensitive detection of beta-2 transferrin in rhinorrhea and otorrhea as a marker for cerebrospinal fluid (C.S.F.) leakage. *Acta Neurochir. (Wien)* 1991;109:98–101.

10. Einhorn A, Mizrahi EM. Basilar skull fractures in children. The incidence of CNS infection and the use of antibiotics. *Am. J. Dis. Child.* 1978;132:1121–1124.

11. Ford LE, McLaurin RL. Mechanisms of extradural hematomas. *J. Neurosurg.* 1963;20:760–769.

12. Ganz JC, Zwetnow NN. Analysis of the dynamics of experimental epidural bleeding in swine. *Acta. Neurochir. (Wien)* 1988;95:72–81.

13. Piepmeier JM, Wagner FC Jr. Delayed post-traumatic extracerebral hematomas. *J. Trauma* 1982;22:455–460.

14. Stone JL, Rifai MH, Sugar O, Lang RG, Oldershaw JB, Moody RA. Subdural hematomas. I. Acute subdural hematoma: Progress in definition, clinical pathology, and therapy. *Surg. Neurol.* 1983;19:216–231.

15. Servadei F. Prognostic factors in severely head injured adult patients with acute subdural haematomas. *Acta Neurochir.* 1997;139:279–285.

16. Jamieson KG, Yelland JD.Traumatic intracerebral hematoma. Report of 63 surgically treated cases. *J. Neurosurg.* 1972;37:528–532.

17. Baratham G, Dennyson WG. Delayed traumatic intracerebral haemorrhage. *J. Neurol. Neurosurg. Psychiatry* 1972;35:698–706.

18. Alvarez-Sabin J, Turon A, Lozano-Sanchez M, Vazquez J, Codina A. Delayed posttraumatic hemorrhage. "Spatapoplexie." *Stroke* 1995;26:1531–1535.

19. Lindenberg R, Freytag E.The mechanism of cerebral contusions: A pathologic-anatomic study. *Arch. Pathol.* 1960;69:440–469.

20. Dublin AB, French BN, Rennick JM. Computed tomography in head trauma. *Radiology* 1977;122:365–369.

21. Hesselink JR, Dowd CF, Healy ME, Hajek P, Baker LL, Luerssen TG. MR imaging of brain contusions: A comparative study with CT. *AJR* 1988;150:1133–1142.

22. Gurdjian ES. Cerebral contusions: re-evaluation of the mechanism of their development. *J. Trauma* 1976;16:35–51.

23. Schonauer M, Schisano G, Cimino R, Viola L. Space occupying contusions of cerebral lobes after closed brain injury: considerations about 51 cases. *J. Neurosurg. Sci.* 1979;23:279–288.

24. Misra JC, Chakravarty S. A study of rotational brain injury. *J. Biomech.* 1984;17:459–466.

25. Report of the ad hoc committee to study head injury nomenclature: Proceedings of the Congress of Neurological Surgeons in 1964. *Clin. Neurosurg.* 1966;12:386–394.

26. Fitzpatrick MO, Dewar D, Teasdale GM, Graham DI. The neuronal cytoskeleton: An insight for neurosurgeons. *Br. J. Neurosurg.* 1996;10:483–487.

27. Yamaki T, Murakami N, Iwamoto Y, et al. Pathological study of diffuse axonal injury patients who died shortly after impact. *Acta Neurochir.* 1992;119:153–158.

28. Bouma GJ, Muizelaar JP, Choi SC, Newlon PG, Young HF. Cerebral circulation and metabolism after severe traumatic brain injury: the elusive role of ischemia. *J. Neurosurg.* 1991;75:685–693.

29. DeSalles AA, Kontos HA, Becker DP, et al. Prognostic significance of ventricular CSF lactic acidosis in severe head injury. *J. Neurosurg.* 1986;65:615–624.

30. Obrist WD, Langfitt TW, Jaggi JL, Cruz J, Gennarelli TA. Cerebral blood flow and metabolism in comatose patients with acute head injury. Relationship to intracranial hypertension. *J. Neurosurg.* 1984;61:241–253.

31. Langfitt TW, Marshall WJ, Kassell NF, Schutta HS. The pathophysiology of brain swelling produced by mechanical trauma and hypertension. *Scand. J. Clin. Lab. Invest. Suppl.* 1968;102:XIV:B.

32. Muizelaar JP, Ward JD, Marmarou A, Newlon PG, Wachi A. Cerebral blood flow and metabolism in severely head-injured children. Part 2: Autoregulation. *Neurosurgery* 1989;71:72–76.

33. Lee SM, Wong MD, Samii A, Hovda DA. Evidence for energy failure following irreversible traumatic brain injury. *Ann. NY Acad. Sci.* 1999;893:337–340

34. Goodman JC, Valadka AB, Gopinath SP, Uzura M, Robertson CS. Extracellular lactate and glucose alterations in the brain after head injury measured by microdialysis. *Crit. Care Med.* 1999;27:1965–1973.

35. Reinert M, Hoelper B, Doppenberg E, Zauner A, Bullock R. Substrate delivery and ionic balance disturbance after severe human head injury. *Acta. Neurochir. Suppl.* 2000;76:439–444.

36. Hovda DA, Becker DP, Katayama Y. Secondary injury and acidosis. *J. Neurotrauma* 1992;9 Suppl 1:S47–S60.

37. Palmer AM, Marion DW, Botscheller ML, Bowen DM, DeKosky ST. Increased transmitter amino acid concentration in human ventricular CSF after brain trauma. *Neuroreport* 1994;6:153–156.

38. Hong Z, Xinding Z, Tianlin Z, Liren C. Excitatory amino acids in cerebrospinal fluid of patients with acute head injuries. *Clin. Chem.* 2001;47:1458–1462.

39. Obrenovitch TP, Urenjak J. Is high extracellular glutamate the key to excitotoxicity in traumatic brain injury? *J. Neurotrauma* 1997;14:677–698.

40. Allan SM. The role of pro- and antiinflammatory cytokines in neurodegeneration. *Ann. NY Acad. Sci.* 2000;917:84–93.

41. Quattrocchi KB, Frank EH, Miller CH, et al. Suppression of cellular immune activity following severe head injury. *J. Neurotrauma* 1990;7:77–87.

42. Wolach B, Sazbon L, Gavrieli R, Broda A, Schlesinger M. Early immunological defects in comatose patients after acute brain injury. *J. Neurosurg.* 2001;94:706–711.

43. Aibiki M, Maekawa S, Ogura S, Kinoshita Y, Kawai N, Yokono S. Effect of moderate hypothermia on systemic and internal jugular plasma IL-6 levels after traumatic brain injury in humans. *J. Neurotrauma* 1999;16:225–232.

44. Csuka E, Morganti-Kossmann MC, Lenzlinger PM, Joller H, Trentz O, Kossmann T. IL-10 levels in cerebrospinal fluid and serum of patients with severe traumatic brain injury: Relationship to IL-6, TNF-alpha, TGF-beta1 and blood-brain barrier function. *J. Neuroimmunol.* 1999;101:211–221.

45. Kossmann T, Stahel PF, Lenzlinger PM, et al. Interleukin-8 released into the cerebrospinal fluid after brain injury is associated with blood-brain barrier dysfunction and nerve growth factor production. *J. Cereb. Blood Flow Metab.* 1997;17:280–289.

46. McKeating EG, Andrews PJ, Mascia A. The relationship of soluble adhesion molecule concentrations in systemic and jugular venous serum to injury severity and outcome after traumatic brain injury. *Anesth. Analg.* 1998;86:759–765.

47. Zemlan FP, Rosenberg WS, Luebbe PA, et al. Quantification of axonal damage in traumatic brain injury: Affinity purification and characterization of cerebrospinal fluid tau proteins. *J. Neurochem.* 1999;72:741–750.

48. Raby CA, Morganti-Kossmann MC, Kossmann T, et al. Altered expression of amyloid precursors proteins after traumatic brain injury in rats: in situ hybridization and immunohistochemical study. *J. Neurotrauma* 2000;17:123–134.

49. Spiegel K, Kuo YM, Roher AE, Emmerling MR. Traumatic brain injury increases beta-amyloid peptide 1-42 in cerebrospinal fluid. *J. Neurochem.* 1998;71:2505–2509.

50. Murray GD, Teasdale GM, Braakman R, et al. On behalf of the European Brain Injury Consortium The European Brain Injury Consortium survey of head injuries. *Acta. Neurochir. (Wien.)* 1999;141:223–236.

51. Sakas DE, Bullock MR, Teasdale GM. One-year outcome following craniotomy for traumatic hematoma in patients with fixed dilated pupils. *J. Neurosurg.* 1995;82:961–965.

52. Teasdale G, Jennett B. Assessment of coma and impaired consciousness: A practical scale. *Lancet* 1974;2:81–84.

53. Gale JL, Dikmen S, Wyler A, Temkin N, McLean A. Head injury in the Pacific Northwest. *Neurosurgery* 1983;12:487–491.

54. White RJ, Likavec MJ. The diagnosis and initial management of head injury. *N. Engl. J. Med.* 1992;327:1507–1511.

55. Mazzeo AJ. Sedation for the mechanically ventilated patient. *Crit. Care Clin.* 1995;11:937–955.

56. Durbin CG Jr. Sedation of the agitated, critically ill patient without an artificial airway. *Crit. Care Clin.* 1995;11:913–936.

57. Angelini G, Ketzler JT, Coursin DB. Use of propofol and other nonbenzodiazepine sedatives in the intensive care unit. *Crit Care Clin.* 2001;17:863–880.

58. Robertson CS, Cormio M. Cerebral metabolic management. *New Horiz.* 1995;3:410–422.

59. Sheinberg M, Kanter MJ, Robertson CS, Contant CF, Narayan RK, Grossman RG Continuous monitoring of jugular venous oxygen saturation in head-injured patients. *J. Neurosurg.* 1992;76:212–217.

60. Robertson CS, Gopinath SP, Goodman JC, Contant CF, Valadka AB, Narayan RK. SjvO$_2$ monitoring in head-injured patients. *J. Neurotrauma* 1995;12:891–896.

61. Cruz J, Minoja G, Mattioli C, et al. Severe acute brain trauma. In: Cruz J, ed. *Neurologic and Neurosurgical Emergencies.* Philadelphia: WB Saunders, 1998, pp. 405–436.

62. Chesnut RM. Secondary brain insults after head injury: Clinical perspectives. *New Horiz.* 1995;3:366–375.

63. Liebert M. Hypotension. *J. Neurotrauma* 2000;17:591–595.

64. Contant CF, Valadka AB, Gopinath SP, Hannay HJ, Robertson CS. Adult respiratory distress syndrome: a complication of induced hypertension after severe head injury. *J. Neurosurg.* 2001;95:560–568.

65. Robertson CS, Valadka AB, Hannay HJ, et al. Prevention of secondary ischemic insults after severe head injury. *Crit. Care Med.* 1999;27:2086–2095.

66. Feldman Z, Kanter MJ, Robertson CS, et al. Effect of head elevation on intracranial pressure, cerebral perfusion pressure, and cerebral blood flow in head-injured patients. *J. Neurosurg.* 1992;76:207–211.

67. Bullock R. Mannitol and other diuretics in severe neurotrauma. *New Horiz.* 1995;3:448–452.

68. Miller JD, Piper IR, Dearden NM. Management of intracranial hypertension in head injury: matching treatment with cause. *Acta Neurochir. Suppl* 1993;57:152–159.

69. Qureshi AI, Suarez JI. Use of hypertonic saline solutions in treatment of cerebral edema and intracranial hypertension. *Crit. Care Med.* 2000;28:3301–3313.

70. Suarez JI, Qureshi AI, Bhardwaj A, et al. Treatment of refractory intracranial hypertension with 23.4% saline. *Crit. Care Med.* 1998;26:1118–1122.

71. The Brain Trauma Foundation. The American Association of Neurological Surgeons. The Joint Section on Neurotrauma and Critical Care. Hyperventilation. *J. Neurotrauma* 2000;17:513–520.
72. Diringer MN, Videen TO, Yundt K, et al. Regional cerebrovascular and metabolic effects of hyperventilation after severe traumatic brain injury. *J. Neurosurg.* 2002;96:103–108.
73. Kassell NF, Hitchon PW, Gerk MK, Sokoll MD, Hill TR. Alterations in cerebral blood flow, oxygen metabolism, and electrical activity produced by high dose sodium thiopental. *Neurosurgery* 1980;7:598–603.
74. Rea GL, Rockswold GL. Barbiturate therapy in uncontrolled intracranial hypertension. *Neurosurgery* 1983;12:401–404.
75. Roberts I, Schierhout G, Alderson P, Absence of evidence for the effectiveness of five interventions routinely used in the intensive care management of severe head injury: A systematic review. *J. Neurol. Neurosurg. Psychiatry* 1998;65:729–733.
76. De Luca GP, Volpin L, Fornezza U, et al. The role of decompressive craniectomy in the treatment of uncontrollable post-traumatic intracranial hypertension. *Acta Neurochir. Suppl* 2000;76:401–404.
77. Meier U, Zeilinger FS, Henzka O. The use of decompressive craniectomy for the management of severe head injuries. *Acta Neurochir. Suppl* 2000;76:475–478.
78. Munch E, Horn P, Schurer L, Piepgras A, Paul T, Schmiedek P. Management of severe traumatic brain injury by decompressive craniectomy. *Neurosurgery* 2000;47:315–322.
79. Coplin WM, Cullen NK, Policherla PN, et al. Safety and feasibility of craniectomy with duraplasty as the initial surgical intervention for severe traumatic brain injury. *Trauma* 2001;50:1050–1059.
80. Rovlias A, Kotsou S. The influence of hyperglycemia on neurological outcome in patients with severe head injury. *Neurosurgery* 2000;46:335–342.
81. Lam AM, Winn HR, Cullen BF, Sundling N. Hyperglycemia and neurological outcome in patients with head injury. *J. Neurosurg.* 1991;75:545–551.
82. Vespa PM, Nuwer MR, Nenov V, et al. Increased incidence and impact of nonconvulsive and convulsive seizures after traumatic brain injury as detected by continuous electroencephalographic monitoring. *J. Neurosurg.* 1999;91:750–760.
83. The Brain Trauma Foundation. The American Association of Neurological Surgeons. The Joint Section on Neurotrauma and Critical Care. Role of antiseizure prophylaxis following head injury. *J. Neurotrauma* 2000;17:549–553.
84. Annegers JF, Hauser WA, Coan SP, Rocca WA. A population-based study of seizures after traumatic brain injuries. *N. Engl. J. Med.* 1998; 338:20–24.
85. Markgraf CG, Clifton GL, Moody MR. Treatment window for hypothermia in brain injury. *J. Neurosurg.* 2001 95:979–983.
86. Clifton GL, Choi SC, Miller ER, et al. Intercenter variance in clinical trials of head trauma—experience of the National Acute Brain Injury Study: Hypothermia. *J. Neurosurg.* 2001;95:751–755.
87. Clifton GL, Miller ER, Choi SC, et al. Lack of effect of induction of hypothermia after acute brain injury. *N. Engl. J. Med.* 2001 344:556–563.
88. Kamran SI, Downey D, Ruff RL.Pneumatic sequential compression reduces the risk of deep vein thrombosis in stroke patients. *Neurology* 1998;50:1683–1688.
89. Taylor SJ, Fettes SB, Jewkes C, Nelson RJ. Prospective, randomized, controlled trial to determine the effect of early enhanced enteral nutrition on clinical outcome in mechanically ventilated patients suffering head injury. *Crit. Care Med.* 1999;27:2525–2531.
90. Yanagawa T, Bunn F, Roberts I, Wentz R, Pierro A. Nutritional support for head-injured patients. *Cochrane Database Syst. Rev.* 2000;2:CD001530.
91. The Brain Trauma Foundation. The American Association of Neurological Surgeons. The Joint section on Neutrotrauma and Critical Care. Nutrition. *J. Neurotrauma* 2000;17:539–547.
92. Pepe JL, Barba CA. The metabolic response to acute traumatic brain injury and implications for nutritional support. *J. Head Trauma Rehabil.* 1999;14:462–474.
93. Zubkov AY, Pilkington AS, Parent AD, Zhang J. Morphological presentation of posttraumatic vasospasm. *Acta Neurochir. Suppl* 2000;76:223–236.
94. Kaspera W, Majchrzak H, Zientek A. Dynamics of cerebral circulation on the basis of transcranial Doppler ultrasonography evaluation in patients with moderate and minor head injury. *Neurol. Neurochir. Pol.* 2001;35:261–279.
95. Langham J, Goldfrad C, Teasdale G, Shaw D, Rowan K. Calcium channel blockers for acute traumatic brain injury. *Cochrane Database Syst. Rev.* 2000;2:CD000565.
96. Peter B. Letarte, Neurotrauma care in the new millennium. *Surg. Clin. North Am.* 1999;79:1449–1455.
97. The Brain Trauma Foundation. The American association of neurological surgeons. The Joint Section on Neurotrauma and Critical Care. Age. *J. Neurotrauma* 2000;17:573–581.
98. Lannoo E, Van Rietvelde F, et al. Early predictors of mortality and morbidity after severe closed head injury. *J. Neurotrauma* 2000;17:403–414.
99. Ghajar J. Traumatic brain injury. *Lancet* 2000;356:923–929.

23

Spinal Cord Injury and Related Diseases

Joy Derwenskus and Osama O. Zaidat

INTRODUCTION

Acute spinal cord injury (SCI), whether traumatic or nontraumatic in etiology, has a tremendous cost not only for patients and families, but also for society as a whole. The incidence of SCI in the United States is estimated to be 30–40 cases per 1 million inhabitants. However, an exact incidence is difficult to ascertain because SCI is not reportable and there have not been large prospective and comprehensive studies done since the 1970s (1–4). There are 8000–10,000 new cases of acute SCI a year. It does appear, however, that despite the currently available acute and emergency care as well as the preventive measures the incidence of SCI and disorders and the resulting disabilities have remained stable. Approximately 183,000–230,000 people are living today with SCI (1–4).

The resultant life-long disability is devastating for the patients, particularly since the most commonly affected individuals are young adults. The average age of acute SCI is 31.8 yr and 80% of those affected are male. Contrary to common belief SCI is not only associated with severe disability, but also with increased mortality in this population. It has been estimated that the SCI and disorders are the fourth leading cause of death after ischemic heart disease, cancer and stroke in the United States. Besides, beyond the emotional impact, the financial one is very significant. The annual cost of caring for SCI patients in 1995 was estimated at $7.736 billion US (1).

The survival following acute SCI has improved because of recent advances in understanding and treating patients' suffering from this debilitating injury. Better trained emergency personnel, more rapid transportation and immobilization, and the availability of specialized neurosciences critical care units (NSU) are likely to further reduce the secondary damage in acute SCI and improve the survival rate following this devastating event.

ETIOLOGY

Traumatic Spinal Cord Injury

The most common causes of traumatic SCI include motor vehicle accident (MVA), motorcycle accidents (MCA), and falls (Table 1). Other causes are work-related injuries, recreation, and sports activities such as diving injuries, and penetrating injuries secondary to knife or gunshot wounds. Percentages of these injuries vary in different studies, but overall recreation or sporting injuries have declined due to education and preventive measures to 10%, while the rate of penetrating or violent injuries is on the rise.

The most common location of SCI is the cervical spine (C5–C6 level) followed by the thoracolumbar junction, thoracic, and lumbar spine (5) (Table 2). Lap belt injuries are associated with thoracolumbar flexion distraction injury. Multiple level injuries occur in as high as 20% of the cases. Associated traumatic brain injuries (TBI) are common but are usually mild. Severe TBI may occur in

From: Current Clinical Neurology
Critical Care Neurology and Neurosurgery
Edited by: J. I. Suarez © Humana Press Inc., Totowa, NJ

Table 1
Etiology of Traumatic Spinal Cord Injury

Etiology	Incidence
Motor vehicle accident	20–25%
Motorcycle accidents	25–30%
Recreational and sports	10–15%
Work-related injuries	10–15%
Falls	20–25%
Violence injuries	10–15%

Table 2
Frequency of Traumatic Spinal Cord Injury According to the Level of Injury

Level of injury	Frequency (%)
Cervical spine; most common C5–6	50–55
Thoracic spine	10–15
Thoracolumbar	15–20
Lumbosacral	10
Sacral	<10
Multiple levels	20
Associated head injury	
Mild	40–50
Severe	2–3

only 2–3% of SCI cases *(5,6)* *(see* Table 2). The mechanism of injury usually accounts for the differing levels of involvement. For instance, gun shot wounds are more likely to involve the thoracic spine *(7)*. The spinal canal becomes progressively narrower in the lower cervical and thoracic regions. Thus, SCI is more likely to be a complete injury in these regions *(8)*. The thoracolumbar spine is frequently injured due to the transition in this region from the more rigid upper thoracic spine to the more mobile lower thoracic and upper lumbar spine *(5)*.

Neurologic damage varies with location of the injury. Atlanto-occipital dislocations are associated with extreme hyperflexion or extension-avulsion injury that frequently has a fatal neurologic outcome. A C1 or Jefferson fracture is caused by compressive forces forcing the ring of the atlas to burst. Frequently there is no neurologic damage with this fracture. Diving into shallow water or the head hitting the roof or windshield of the car are examples of injuries causing a Jefferson fracture. C2 fractures commonly include either the odontoid process or the pedicles (hangman's fracture). Fortunately, due to sufficient space in the upper cervical canal, no neurological damage results from these injuries. The most frequent injury of thoracolumbar junction occurs due to compressive forces causing compression or burst fractures of the vertebral body. There are also dislocations in this region. The injury often occurs during falls from varying heights or MVA. Again the increased space in the lower thoracic and lumbar region limits neurological damage, but bone fragments or a disk may impinge upon and cause compromise of the spinal cord *(5,6,8)*.

SCIWORET/SCIWBA

Acute SCI can also occur without evidence of trauma referred to as "spinal concussion" or SCIWORET (spinal cord injury without radiologic evidence of trauma) *(9)*. SCI without bony abnormality (SCIWBA) is typically described in children with neurological deficits despite no abnormality

Table 3
Etiology of the Nontraumatic Spinal Cord Injury

Acute	Subacute–chronic	Chronic
Acute transverse myelitis	Spinal cord tumor	Syringomyelia
Spinal epidural abscess	Primary	Multiple sclerosis
Spinal epidural hematoma	Secondary	Lumbar canal stenosis
Spinal cord infarction	Radiation myelopathy	Cervical spondylosis
Functional (conversion or	Vascular malformation (AVM)	Amyotrophic lateral
hysterical)	Infectious:	sclerosis
	Syphilis	
	Tuberculosis	
	Acquired Immunodeficiency	
	Syndrome	
	Nutritional: vitamin B_{12}	
	deficiency	

seen on imaging studies. This injury may be the result of ligament laxity (9). This condition is usually associated with good prognosis and recovery, but long-term sequelae may occur in some patients.

Nontraumatic Spinal Cord Injury

Nontraumatic etiologies leading to an acute SCI include various bacterial, viral, fungal, or parasitic infections; tumors or other compressive lesions of the spinal cord; vascular events such as infarction; demyelinating lesions in spinal multiple sclerosis; toxins; autoimmune disorders; or nutritional deficiencies such as pernicious anemia (Table 3) *(10)*.

Infectious

An acute myelopathic presentation occurs with various infections, and a common etiology is spinal epidural abscess. Its incidence is 0.2–1.2 per 10,000 admissions and appears to be increasing. It occurs most commonly in 50–70-yr-old men. Risk factors for development of spinal epidural abscess include intravenous drug use, spinal procedures, immunosuppression, diabetes mellitus, degenerative joint disease, and inflammatory bowel disease. The most common site of infection is the thoracic spine followed by lumbar and cervical regions. The abscess is usually located posteriorly, but can be anterior especially in the cervical spine *(10–12)*. Approximately 50% of epidural abscesses are hematogenously spread from distant sites such as skin infections, urinary tract infections, pneumonia, pharyngitis, dental sources, and bacterial endocarditis *(10–12)*. These patients often present with fever, back pain, and a radicular or myelopathic picture. The most common infectious organism is *Staphylococcus aureus* followed by *Streptococcus* and Gram-negative bacilli. Other agents include: *Mycobacterium tuberculosis, Salmonella, Listeria, Brucella, Actinomyces, Norcardia, Cryptococcus neoformans, Aspergillus* species, *Mucorales, Coccidiodes immitis, Blastomyces dermatitidis, Taenia solium* (cysticerci), *Echinococcus,* and *Schistosoma.*

A variety of viral, fungal, and parasitic infections of the spinal cord occur more commonly in patients afflicted with acquired immunodeficiency syndrome (AIDS). Myelopathy has been reported with varicella zoster (VZV), herpes simplex virus (HSV), cytomegalovirus (CMV), and *Toxoplasma gondii* in these patients.

Other rare causes of spinal cord infection in otherwise healthy individuals include measles, mumps, poliovirus, VZV, Epstein-Barr virus (EBV), rabies, human T-cell leukemic virus (HTLV) I and II, and spirochetes as in syphilis and Lyme disease. Often a history of recent viral symptoms and general constitutional symptoms can be elicited in these patients. Herpes simiae (monkey B virus) has caused myelopathy in laboratory workers *(10,13)*.

Spinal Cord Tumors

Tumors can affect the spinal cord by external compression or invasion of the cord itself. Tumors are divided by location into extradural, intradural, or intramedullary. Extradural tumors are more commonly due to metastases than primary tumors. Myeloma is the only primary tumor invading the spine in adults. Lung, breast, and prostate are common epidural metastases. Typically symptoms of extradural involvement are more slowly progressive. However, occasionally there is a more rapid progression over a few days resulting in paraparesis, sensory loss below the level of the lesion, and the loss of sphincter control. Symptoms of intradural involvement such as meningioma, neurofibroma, or schwannoma are typically more chronic and would not present in the setting of acute SCI. Similar to intradural, the intramedullary tumors are slow-growing and more chronic in their presentation. These consist of ependymomas, benign or malignant astrocytomas, or metastases from lung, breast, lymphoma, colorectal, head and neck, and renal cancers *(10)*.

Vascular Events

Spinal cord ischemia is an important etiology of nontraumatic SCI causing devastating myelopathy. Infarction of the spinal cord occurs with spontaneous aortic dissections, especially with types I and III. Type I dissections involve the ascending and part of the descending aorta. Type III dissections involve the aorta distal to the left subclavian artery. These patients typically present with sudden onset of sharp, crushing chest or abdominal pain with paraplegia. Spinal cord ishemia is a known complication of cardiovascular surgery usually involving aneurysm repair of the thoracic aorta. Hypotension and prolonged clamp times must be avoided as these have devastating and deleterious effect on the spinal cord and are powerful predictors of postoperative paraplegia. Iatrogenic etiologies related to epidural or spinal anesthesia have occurred. Rare reports of syphilitic arteritis causing spinal vessel occlusion and myelopathy occur today. Vascular malformations including spinal cord arteriovenous malformations (AVM) or spinal dural arteriovenous fistulas also may cause acute myelopathy due to sudden hemorrhage, but commonly they present slowly due to mass effect and steal phenomenon *(13)*.

Acute Spinal Multiple Sclerosis

Multiple sclerosis (MS) is typically a chronic, progressive demyelinating disease of the central nervous system. The number of patients with only spinal cord involvement is not known. Patients may develop an acute myelopathy as an initial presentation or some may have discounted prior symptoms *(10)*. Lhermitte's sign, a shock-like sensation into the spine or extremities with flexion of the neck, may be more prominent in acute spinal involvement of MS *(13)*. Typically, spinal MS progresses slowly causing an asymmetrical spastic paraparesis with sensory changes. Devic's syndrome is an MS variant with spinal cord involvement and optic neuritis.

Others

Paraneoplastic involvement of the spinal cord occurs. Patients may develop a rapidly progressing myelopathy associated with systemic carcinoma. Tumor antibodies are suspected to cross-react with spinal cord tissue and cause necrosis of the tracts *(10)*. Lung, prostate, renal, and ovarian cancers can be associated with paraneoplastic syndromes. Vitamin B_{12} deficiency occurs in strict vegetarians, patients with prior gastric and ileal resections, or in pernicious anemia due to intrinsic factor deficiency. These patients manifest dorsal column sensory loss and weakness of extremities. Other toxic causes of acute myelopathy include intrathecal injections of chemotherapeutic agents such as methotrexate or cytosine arabinoside. Rarely, acute myelopathy occurs postimmunization *(10)*.

CLINICAL FEATURES

The extent of spinal cord damage is determined by the complete neurological examination (Table 4). Incomplete injury is the preservation of some sensory or motor function below the injury

Table 4
Clinical Presentation of Spinal Cord Injury

Clinical syndromes	Key clinical features
Central cord syndrome	Arm weakness in disproportion to legs
Anterior cord syndrome	Sparing position and vibratory senses
Posterior cord syndrome	Loss of vibratory and position senses
Brown-Sequard syndrome	Ipsilateral motor and contralateral pain and temperature sensory loss
Complete cord transection	Complete loss of motor, sensory and autonomic functions below the level of injury
Spinal shock	Initial areflexic hypotonia
Cord concussion	Transient neurologic deficit
Incomplete cord transection	Scattered presentation
Cauda equina syndrome	Flaccid areflexic paraparesis or paraplegia
Conus medullaris syndrome	Deep tendon reflexes may be preserved
Mixed cauda-conus syndrome	Mixed

level and around the sacral area whereas a complete injury involves loss of all sensory or motor function. There is a zone of partial preservation described in complete injuries below the lesioned level due to partially innervated dermatomes and myotomes. Tetraplegia (preferred to quadriplegia) is the loss of motor or sensory function in the cervical region of the spinal cord whereas paraplegia is the loss of motor or sensory function from the thoracic, lumbar, or sacral regions of the spinal cord *(14–16)*. The involvement of extremities may be somewhat asymmetrical especially with nontraumatic spinal cord involvement.

There are several common spinal cord syndromes seen with incomplete or partial SCI: central cord syndrome, anterior spinal artery syndrome, Brown-Sequard syndrome, and spinal shock. Of all the clinical signs, spasticity and dysautonomia represent important problems and will be discussed separately below. The central cord syndrome (CCS) occurs after cord contusion, usually in elderly patients with degenerative joint spine disease. CCS lead to greater upper extremity weakness compared to the lower extremity. This injury occurs almost exclusively in the cervical region and has a good prognosis. Anterior spinal artery syndrome (ASAS) results from retropulsion of bony or disc material impinging upon the blood supply of the anterior cord. The injury causes loss of all motor and sensory functions below the level of injury with exception of the dorsal column functions. Therefore, these patients will have intact joint position and vibratory sensation. Recovery from ASAS is often poor. Brown-Sequard Syndrome (BSS) results from spinal fracture or penetrating injury. BSS is the result of a hemisection of the cord with ipsilateral loss of motor function and dorsal column sensation and contralateral loss of pain and temperature. These patients often have good recovery *(15)*. After an acute SCI, spinal shock (SS) supervenes and typically lasts from 2 to 6 wk. During this time, everything below the level of the lesion is hypofunctioning. There is marked decrease in muscle tone throughout, including the urinary bladder and loss of deep tendon reflexes. The pathophysiology of SS remains poorly understood. The amount of recovery from SCI must typically be assessed once SS resolves.

Spasticity refers to the velocity dependent increase in muscle tone related to upper motor neuron (UMN) injury. This develops over time as SS is resolving. Its underlying pathophysiology is not known, but is thought to be secondary to motor neurons forming new connections after loss of supraspinal input. Other UMN symptoms include hyperreflexia, clonus, spasms, postural abnormalities, weakness, fatigue, and pain. One of the most important clinical features encountered in patients with SCI is dysautonomia, with sympathetic over activity and subsequent elevation of the systemic

Table 5
General Measures of Management of Acute Spinal Cord Injury Patients

Measures	Key note
Airway	Careful oxygenation, with attention to spine mobility
Breathing	Nasotracheal intubation and avoidance of neck extension
Circulation	Volume, and vasopressors as needed
Immobilization	Hard collars with block, strapping, and hard board
Transportation	Immediate transport to a specialized trauma/SCI center
Clinical examination	ASIA score and FIM score
Radiologic examination	Five views plain radiographs

ASIA, American Spinal Injury Association; FIM, functional independence measure.

blood pressure. It usually presents with severe headache, skin changes, such as flushing and sweating. Early following SCI fluctuating and labile blood pressure is common whereas episodes of autonomic dysreflexia (ADR) may supervene later. Immediate identification of the life-threatening ADR and its prompt treatment is crucial as discussed below.

MANAGEMENT

General Measures

Initial management of SCI patients consists of establishing airway, breathing, and circulation (ABCs) (Table 5) (*see* Chapter 1). If endotracheal intubation is required, the nasotracheal approach with a fiberoptic bronchoscope is preferred to minimize damage with hyperextension of the neck. After trauma, any region of the spine suspicious for injury must be immobilized at the scene. A combination of rigid cervical collar and supportive blocks with backboard with straps is sufficient. Sandbags and tapes are not recommended. The immediate aim of treatment is to prevent the secondary damage to the spinal cord and nerve tissue. Anything that can hinder circulation or oxygenation to the cord can lead to further damage such as hypotension, hypoxia, hypoxia, hyperpyrexia, or compression from bony fragments *(14,15)*.

Once the patient enters the hospital, it is critical that an initial neurological assessment be made. The exam should be comprehensive enough to allow for proper identification of patients according to the American Spinal Injury Association (ASIA) standard classification of SCI (Fig. 1 and Table 6) and obtain the initial functional independence measure score (FIM score) (usually performed after the emergent evaluation and treatment) (Table 7). The former includes sensory examination with light touch and pin prick of 28 areas as well as strength testing of 10 upper and lower extremity muscles using a 0–5 score for complete loss to normal strength *(14,16)*. After completing the examination using the ASIA criteria, the injury is determined to be either complete or incomplete. SCI is deemed complete when there is no motor or sensory function preserved below the level of injury or in the sacral segment (S4–5) (*see* Table 6). The level of injury is the most caudal level intact on examination *(16)*.

The type of radiographic examination is determined from the evaluation of the injuries. With a cervical injury, the initial films should include anteroposterior (AP) and lateral (LAT) views of the entire cervical spine including visualization of T1. Open mouth films should also be obtained for visualization of the odontoid process of C2. If C7 and T1 are not clearly visualized, then a swimmers view should be obtained. We present a normal cervical spine radiograph in Fig. 2. CT scans have improved the detection of fractures that may have otherwise been missed with plain radiography and should be considered when plain radiographs are of insufficient quality. Magnetic resonance imaging (MRI) provides additional information of surrounding soft tissues, ligaments, and the spinal cord itself which may contribute to the management of the patient with SCI *(14,17)*. Frequently, the entire

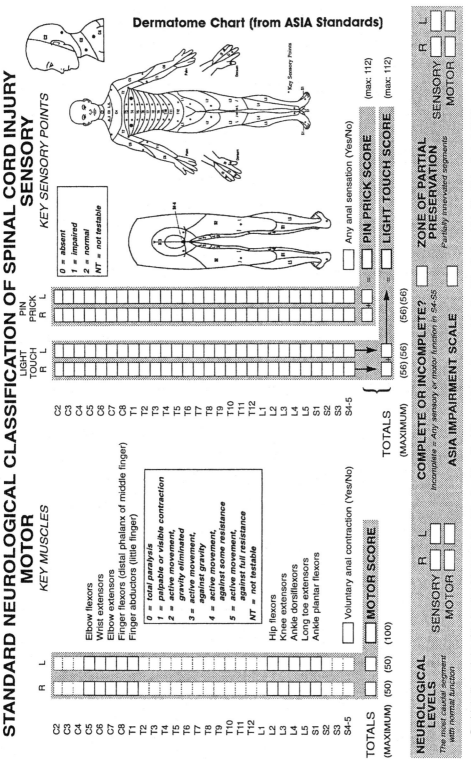

Fig. 1. Standard neurologic classification of spinal cord injury. Reproduced with permission of the Spinal Injury Association.

Table 6
ASIA Impairment Scale

Classification	Explanation
Complete (ASIA A)	No motor or sensory function is preserved in the sacral segment (S4–5)
Incomplete (ASIA B)	Only sensory function is preserved below the neurological level including the S4–5 segments
Incomplete (ASIA C)	Motor function is preserved below the neurological level and MORE than half of the muscles have a motor strength grade of 3 or more
Incomplete (ASIA D)	Motor function is preserved below the neurological level and AT LEAST half of the key muscle have a motor strength grade of 3 or more
Normal (ASIA E)	Motor and sensory function is normal

Table 7
FIM SCORE for Daily Activities (Self-Care, Sphincter Control, Mobility, Locomotion, Communications, and Social Cognition)

Explanation	Score in points
Complete independence	7
Modified independence (device) without supervision	6
Supervision by helper (No assist)	5
Minimal assist (25% or less by helper)	4
Moderate assist (50% by helper)	3
Maximal assist (75% by helper)	2
Total assist (100% by helper)	1

spine is imaged so as not to miss a second fracture, which occurs in 5% of patients *(17)*. MRI is a vital part of imaging when concerns about tumor, infection, vascular, or demyelinating process arise *(18)*. In traumatic SCI patients who are awake and alert without abnormal neurological findings on examination, no neck tenderness, and no significant associated injuries, imaging studies are not warranted.

Intensive care management in a specialized neurosciences critical care unit (NSU) plays an important role in SCI patients. While in the NSU aggressive monitoring of heart rate, blood pressure, oxygenation, temperature, and hourly neurological assessments can be performed and any changes in these can be quickly addressed. In addition every system is monitored including neurologic, cardiovascular, respiratory, urologic, gastrointestinal, metabolic, and infectious (Table 8). This aggressive care is also necessary for prevention of medical complications such as pressure ulcers, deep venous thrombosis (DVT), and various infections. It has been demonstrated that SCI patients frequently do better and have a shorter length of stay when treated in centers specialized to provide such care.

Neurociences Critical Care Unit Management of Spinal Cord Injury Patients

Cardiovascular System

Cardiovascular effects can be very pronounced especially with upper SCI above the mid-thoracic region. The higher the lesion the more pronounced the dysfunction of the sympathetic nervous system (SNS) is. These patients can have "low resting blood pressure, orthostatic hypotension, autonomic dysreflexia, reflex bradycardia and cardiac arrest, limited vascular responses to exercise, and

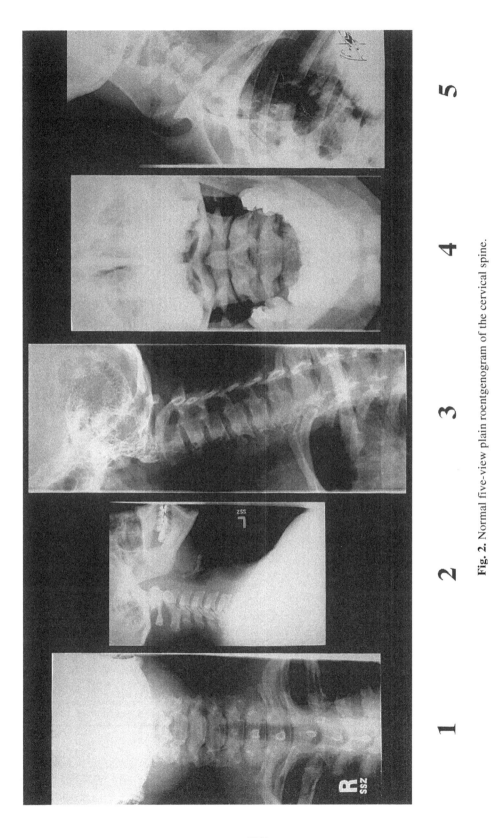

Fig. 2. Normal five-view plain roentgenogram of the cervical spine.

Table 8
Systemic Manifestations of Spinal Cord Injury and Recommended Management

Manifestations	Management
Cardiovascular:	
Hypoptension	Aggressive hydration, vasopressors
Bradycardia	Atropine, theophylline, pacemaker
Acute coronary syndrome	Nitroglycerin, antiplatelets
Autonomic dysreflexia	Avoid triggers, nifidipine and nitroglycerine
Pulmonary:	
Atelectasis	Aggressive pulmonary toilet
Collapse/mucus plugging	As above, cough stimulator
Aspiration pneumonia	As above, antibiotics if fever present
Gastrointestinal:	
Gastroesophageal reflux	Avoid flat position, motility agents
Pepticulcer	Prophylaxis with proton pump inhibitor or H2-blocker
Ileus	Bowel rest, correct electrolytes, consider total parenteral nutrition
Bowel Obstruction	Same as above; surgery if no improvement
Fecal impaction	Bowel care program, scheduled laxatives
Genitourinary:	
Neurogenic bladder	Intermittent cathetrization
Nephrolithiasis	Urinary acidification, hydration, surgery
Urinary tract infection	Urinary acidification, hydration, antibiotics
Vascular:	
Deep venous thrombosis	Sequential compression devices, subcutaneous heparin, warfarin, green field filter
Pulmonary embolism	Intravenous heparin, warfarin, possibly thrombolysis
Neurological:	
Pain	Nonsteroidal agents, tricylcic, codeine, morphine
Spasticity	Baclofen, diazepam, tizanidine, dantrolene
Contracture	Botox injection, nerve blocks, surgery
Integument:	
Skin pressure ulcer	Prevention: avoid friction, pressure relief, turning, ointment to maintain moisture. Active: dressing (wet to dry), debridement (medical or surgical), skin graft or flap
Osteomyelitis	Antibiotics and surgical treatment

likely changes to the skin microcirculation" *(19)*. The mechanism of SNS dysfunction is not definitively known but is thought to be the loss of supraspinal regulatory control, reduced sympathetic activity, morphologic changes in sympathetic preganglionic neurons, and peripheral alpha-adrenoreceptor hyperresponsiveness *(19)*. The risk of hypotension and bradycardia are greatest early after injury. Therefore, these patients must be closely monitored in the NSU. Aggressive hydration with intravenous fluids should be given. Those with severe cervical injuries are more likely to require atropine or temporary transvenous pacing for marked bradycardia and hemodynamic instability. Theophylline may also be used since it can produce both bronchodilation and tachycardia. Dopamine in small doses 3–8 µg/kg/min may be beneficial to augment both the heart rate as well as the blood pressure early on after SCI. In addition to the above measures; turning, suctioning or clapping may trigger arrhythmia; such triggers should be avoided with enough analgesia and preoxygenation prior to performing them. The different vasoactive drugs used to treat hemodynamic instability are reviewed in Chapter 8.

ADR is a mild to life-threatening reaction in patients with SCI above the sixth thoracic segment due to uninhibited sympathetic system over-discharges in response to a stimulus. ADR usually occurs as the SS resolves, and the vasomotor tone returns, but may be seen during the acute period. Signs and symptoms typically consist of a significant increase in blood pressure to 250–300/200–210 mmHg (although even an increase of 20–40 mmHg over the baseline blood pressure can be an indicator), bradycardia, throbbing occipital or bifrontal headache, sweating above the level of the lesion, initially pallor followed by flushing above the lesion level, the sensation of needing to void, nasal congestion, blurred vision, and anxiety *(19–21)*. There are numerous triggering factors for ADR and they usually occur below the level of the lesion. The bladder or bowel are the organs most frequently causing ADR via urinary tract infection, bladder distension, nephrolithiasis, bowel distension, bowel impaction, gastric ulcers, gastroesophageal reflux, and gallstones. Additional triggers include: sunburns, ingrown toenails, pressure sores, pain, coitus, cystoscopy, pregnancy especially during labor and delivery, DVT, pulmonary embolism (PE), and fractures. Treatment involves removing any of the possible triggering factors and also symptomatic. The patient should be placed in the upright, seated position especially if the blood pressure is elevated. The blood pressure and pulse must be closely monitored and if systolic blood pressure is greater than 150 mmHg it should be treated. Most frequently nifedipine or nitrates are used for blood pressure control. It is also important to look for urinary retention and fecal impaction. This should be done after instilling lidocaine jelly if possible so as to eliminate worsening of the ADR by inserting a catheter or performing a rectal examination *(20,21)*. ADR is a medical emergency and can result in seizures, myocardial infarction, or intracerebral hemorrhage if not aggressively treated.

Pulmonary System

Respiratory function must be closely monitored, as respiratory embarrassment is the most common cause of morbidity and mortality in SCI patients. During the initial examination the respiratory rate, oxygen saturation, and the vital capacity should be recorded in addition to obtaining a chest radiograph. Patients with C1-C3 injury are usually apneic after injury and require mechanical ventilation. In patients not requiring instant intubation, the vital capacity should be recorded several times daily. If vital capacity decreases to less than 15 mL/kg ideal body weight along with increasing respiratory rate, decreasing oxygen saturation, and decreasing negative inspiratory force to less than 20 cm H_2O then the patient should be intubated for impending respiratory failure (*see* Chapter 9). The most frequent respiratory complications include atelectasis, pneumonia, pulmonary edema, and respiratory failure. The treatment goal is to prevent these complications. Several methods including aggressive pulmonary toilet, intermittent positive pressure ventilation (IPPV), intrapulmonary percussion, cough stimulation (with vibration using vest or vibrator, or cough stimulators), and postural drainage (via clapping, position changes, or special positioning beds) are used for prevention. Despite these measures, SCI patients often have reduced cough and increased secretions, which may require mechanical ventilation. Tracheostomy should be considered in patients during the first one to two weeks even if the patient is considered a candidate for weaning in the future *(22)*.

Genitourinary System

Urological complications were significant causes of morbidity and mortality in the past, but this is declining with improving current genitourinary care. Initial workup after SCI should include a baseline blood urea nitrogen and creatinine, urine analysis, and urine culture. The patient may have an indwelling foley catheter after SCI. During this period of SS, the urinary bladder is atonic. This usually lasts 6–8 wk as mentioned previously, but may extend up to 1 yr. When the patient is medically stable, intermittent catheterization should begin. Routinely this is done every 4 h, but should be done more frequently for increased fluid intake or when residual volumes are greater than 500 cc for two consecutive measurements. Nurses may measure the urinary bladder residual noninvasively with bladder scan at the bedside. Urodynamic studies including external sphincter electromyogram and water cystometrogram are done once the patient has reflex bladder function in between the intermittent catheterizations. The final bladder pattern whether normal, acontractile, hypercontractile, or hypercontractile with sphincter dyssynergia cannot be determined during the initial hospitalization. Often an anticholinergic agent such as oxybutinin or propantheline is added to lower bladder pressure *(23)*.

Frequent urological complications include urinary tract infection, pyelonephritis, renal nephrolithiasis, and renal failure. These patients frequently have chronic bacteruria, but should only be treated if symptoms of fever, flank pain, purulent urine, or hematuria develop. Periodic urine cultures should be obtained, so rapid treatment with the proper antibiotic can be initiated if the patient becomes symptomatic. The best preventative measure is good hydration. Other methods for prevention of infection such as chronic low dose antibiotic, intravesical instillation of antibiotic, or the acidification of urine with vitamin C have not proven to be beneficial, but still are used as standard of care in SCI patients. Once aggressive medical management fails, then alternate surgical options should be explored *(23)*.

Gastrointestinal System

Gastrointestinal manifestations such as gastro-esophageal reflux (GERD), delayed gastric emptying, altered colonic motility with increased transit time, severe constipation, prolonged bowel evacuation times, abdominal distension, and hemorrhoids are common after SCI. Some of these complications have dramatic psychosocial implications for the patient. GERD and delayed gastric emptying occur with tetraplegia *(24)*. Ileus commonly occurs a few days after SCI and occurs more frequently with complete lesions. The anal sphincter tone varies with the level of injury. Lesions above T12 cause the anal sphincter to be spastic and patients retain reflex bowel emptying while in lesions below T12, the sphincter is flaccid and both voluntary and reflex emptying are lost *(24)*.

Adequate diet and fluid intake are important aspects of maintaining normal bowel function. Although not proven, eating a diet comprised of at least 15 g of fiber is likely beneficial to increase the stool bulk. Too much fiber has actually been demonstrated to prolong colonic transit time. Fluids are extremely important for stool consistency. Two to 3 L of daily fluid intake is recommended. If proper diet and fluid intake is not enough to maintain bowel function, then pharmacological agents can be added. These agents include stool softeners such as docusate; bulk formers like calcium polycarbophil, methylcellulose, psyllium, or lactulose; peristaltic stimulants and prokinetic agents such as senna; and contact irritants like bisacodyl or glycerin suppositories. Stool softeners and bulking agents are helpful to maintain stool consistency *(24)*. A bowel program should be started soon after the injury once the patient is medically stable. This program should be consistent, but unique for each patient depending upon the level of injury, lifestyle, plans to return to work/school, and availability of caregiver. Patients with incomplete lesions may not require any special modifications. After the initial injury, the rectum is usually flaccid (lower motor neuron bowel) because of SS. During this time, manual removal of stool from the rectum is required daily to maintain bowel function. Patients with cervical or thoracic lesions have reflexive bowel function in which evacuation of stool results from digital stimulation of the rectum.

Vascular System

DVT and PE are common medical complications occurring in SCI patients. Even with prophylaxis the incidence of DVT can be as high as 60% *(25,26)*. Studies have demonstrated that early prophylaxis with pneumatic sequential compression devices (SCD) and gradient elastic stockings greatly reduce development of DVT *(25,26)*. These should be included as part of the therapeutic regimen from admission. If prophylaxis is not begun within 72 h of injury, a venous Doppler of the lower extremities should be obtained to rule out DVT prior to instituting prophylaxis that could lead to PE. If subcutaneous heparin or low molecular heparin is not contraindicated, one of these agents should also be added for prophylaxis. The use of SCDs, stockings, and heparin are more effective than using either alone and may be used up to 3 mo following the acute SCI and during rehabilitation *(25,26)* (*see* Chapter 11). It is thought that metabolic changes in the blood vessels along with adaptations to inactivity and resultant atrophy lead to thrombosis *(25,26)*.

Integument

Proper skin care is also a very important consideration for the SCI patient. The skin should be examined daily for any early signs of pressure ulcers. Prevention is the key because it is more difficult to heal them medically or even surgically. Patients should be positioned so as to avoid pressure on bony prominences (pressure relief training). The bottom sheet needs to be tight and kept dry. A frequent and regimented turning schedule must be followed at least every 2 h (*see* Chapter 33). The skin should be kept moist and caregivers should avoid sliding the patient as this may cause friction. There are several special beds now available that greatly reduce the development of pressure ulcers.

There are four stages of skin ulcers: stage I refers to erythema of intact skin; stage II represents partial thickness skin loss; stage III is characterized by full-thickness skin loss which may extend into fascia; and stage IV is defined as full thickness skin loss extending into underlying muscle or bone. Most hospitals now have a wound care team participating and making recommendations of the various types of topical therapies and dressings. Once a stage III or IV ulcer develops, surgical staff should become involved for debridement, skin graft, or flap placement or other surgical modalities of treatment *(27)*.

Spasticity

The increased tone is beneficial for some activities such as sitting, standing, and even coughing, but proves to be a hindrance for mobility during rehabilitation, activities of daily living, and sleep. Initial treatment includes stretching of the limbs and physical therapy. The next step involves adding pharmacologic agents. The most common medications used are baclofen 10–200 mg daily in four divided doses, diazepam 4–60 mg daily in three divided doses, dantrolene 25–400 mg daily in three divided doses, clonidine 0.05 mg twice daily to 0.4 mg daily, or tizanidine 2–36 mg daily. If the above medications fail, injections are attempted such as peripheral nerve blocks, botulinum toxin, or motor point blocks. Intrathecal baclofen can be delivered via an implanted pump. If these therapeutic modalites fail, then other surgical options are explored. The most common surgical procedure in SCI patients is dorsal root entry zone lesions (DREZ-otomy) during which the lateral small pain fibers are destroyed reducing the pain and spasticity *(14,28)*.

Pain Management

Pain plays an important role early in the course of SCI and can be encountered in the NSU setting. It is crucial to manage SCI patients with adequate pain control while they are still in the NSU. Pain may be a trigger for serious central bradycardia or life-threatening ADR. Sources of pain can be related to the primary trauma and the neuronal injury, or may be secondary and related to the various types of management approaches. Patients may not be able to communicate with the treating team their pain due to physical barriers such as being intubated or sedated. Attention should be paid to the vital signs including blood pressure and heart rate. Elevation of the blood pressure with or without tachycardia may be an occult manifestation of pain. Adequate immobilization and positioning may be sufficient to ease patients' discomfort but more often pain control with non-steroidal agents or narcotics such as morphine sulfate or codeine parenterally is needed. Sleep control may also be a contributing factor and should be managed accordingly with mild sedating agents at bedtime. Prior to initiating pain treatment or embarking on increasing pain medications, underlying medical complications should be ruled out such as urinary tract infection, pneumonia, DVT, and PE among others.

Specific Measures

Surgical Intervention

Surgical treatment is often necessary for decompression and stabilization of the spine. Immediate surgical intervention is warranted if the spine is unstable or evidence of cord compression exists with an incomplete injury. Otherwise, the timing of intervention remains controversial. The intent is to maintain an environment for optimal recovery of the cord. Early surgery can remove bony fragments or herniated disc material and stabilize the spine with severe ligamentous injury, which may cause impingement upon the cord despite immobilization. In theory, early surgery is done before worsening symptoms related to edema or hematoma occur. The argument for late surgery (more than 7 d after injury) is to allow time for medical management such as treatment of autonomic instability while at the same time letting swelling subside (14,15,29,30). Patients undergoing early intervention often worsen neurologically in the post-operative period related to swelling. The current available evidence suggests favorable outcome for surgeries that are performed within 25 h or after 200 h of the acute SCI (14,15,29,30). However, there are no studies of hyperacute SCI surgeries (i.e., within 6 h of symptom onset) (14,15,29,30).

Traction may be required to decompress the malaligned spine if early surgical intervention is not desired. Care must be taken to avoid further injury with too much traction. MRI of the spine before and after traction is recommended. In some cases the patient may heal without an operation and these patients should be stabilized in a hard collar or halo vest allowing for early mobilization and rehabilitation (14).

Rarely is there any improvement after a complete SCI making surgery at any time controversial. Penetrating SCI from a knife, bullet, or other foreign object frequently does not require surgery. Infection and the development of cerebrospinal fluid fistulae would favor surgical exploration and possible debridement of the foreign body tract. Broad-spectrum antibiotics such as a third generation cephalosporin should be given for 2 wk after injury regardless of surgical intervention (30).

Methylprednisolone Therapy

Methylprednisolone was demonstrated to be an effective therapy for acute SCI in the National Acute Spinal Cord Injury Study (NASCIS) 2 (31–33). The NASCIS 1 failed to demonstrate improvement after a single dose of methylprednisolone, but this dose was much lower. Patients in NASCIS 2 were treated with a bolus of 30 mg/kg body weight over 15 min and followed by infusion of 5.4 mg/kg of body weight for 23 h. Only the patients started on treatment within 8 h of injury had improvement in both motor and sensory functioning. If therapy was begun more than 8 h after SCI, then there was no statistically significant improvement (31–33). The NASCIS 3 demonstrated improvement if the duration of methylprednisolone therapy was increased to 48 h for those patients started between 3 and 8 h after injury (31–33). The prior treatment regimen of 24 h should be continued in those patients started on therapy within 3 h (32). Despite these trials, the practice of giving high-dose steroids remains controversial as a result of increased morbidity and early mortality (33).

Other Experimental Neuroprotective Therapies

Neuroprotective measures are used as prevention of secondary injury in SCI. There are numerous mechanisms of secondary injury including vascular changes, electrolyte shifts, free radical release, endogenous opoid release, edema, inflammation, and metabolic changes. Various interventions are under investigation to prevent this injury including nimodipine, growth factors, and naloxone (34,35). Other therapeutic agents are being tried experimentally to improve recovery of neurons. In a small study, monosialotetrahexosylganglioside (GM-1) given intravenously for 18–32 doses demonstrated improvement of neurological functioning 1 yr after injury *(34)*. In addition, cellular transplantation of stem cells, schwann cells, macrophages, and fibroblasts have been tested in animals *(35)*.

Nontraumatic Spinal Cord Injury Therapies

Treatment of spinal epidural abscess is surgical drainage, laminectomy, and typically 3–4 wk of intravenous antibiotics. The length of antimicrobial therapy is increased in the setting of osteomyelitis. The regimen should include ceftriaxone and vancomycin until the specific organism is identified. If the patient is on steroids, ceftriaxone and rifampin is used instead. Once identification and sensitivities are obtained, the antibiotics can be tailored for the specific organism *(10,12)*. Tumors frequently require surgical decompression and may be responsive to radiation therapy. Vascular malformations of the spinal cord are defined by angiography and repaired via endovascular embolization or surgical resection. Spinal cord infarcts result from a variety of etiologies. The goal of therapy is to reduce progression of insult. Anticoagulation is used for suspected embolic disease. High dose steroids have demonstrated some improvement in outcome. Acute onset of spinal multiple sclerosis is also treated with high dose corticosteroids.

REFERENCES

1. American Society of Paraplegia. Spinal cord injury: Facts and figures at a glance. *J. Spinal Cord Med.* 2000;23:153–155.
2. Marshall L. Epidemiology and cost of central nervous system injury. *Clin. Neurosurg.* 2000;46:105–112.
3. Burney R, Maio R, Maynard F, Karunas R. Incidence, characteristics, and outcome of spinal cord injury at trauma centers in North America. *Arch. Surg.* 1993;128:596–599.
4. Tator CH, Duncan EG, Edmonds VE, et al. Changes in epidemiology of acute spinal cord injury from 1947 to 1981. *Surg. Neurol.* 1993;40:207–215.
5. Meyer PR, Cybulski GR, Rusin JJ, Haak MH. Spinal cord injury. *Neurol. Clin. North Am.* 1991;9:625–661.
6. Marion DW. Head and spinal cord injury. *Neurol. Clin. North Am.* 1998;16:485–502.
7. Farmer JC, Vaccaro AR, Balderston RA, et al. The changing nature of admissions to a spinal cord injury center: Violence on the rise. *J. Spinal Disord.* 1998;11:400–403.
8. Meyer PR, Sullivan DE. Injuries to the spine. *Emerg. Med. Clin. North Am.* 1984;2:313–329.
9. Koyanagi I, Iwasaki Y, Hida K, et al. Acute cervical cord injury without fracture of dislocation of the spinal column. *J. Neurosurg. (Spine 1)* 2000;93:15–20.
10. Adams RD, Salam-Adams M. Chronic nontraumatic diseases of the spinal cord. *Neurol. Clin. North Am.* 1991;9:605–623.
11. Pruitt AA. Infections of the nervous system. *Neurol. Clin. North Am.* 1998;16:419–447.
12. Yin KS, Wang C, Lucero Y. Myelopathy secondary to spinal epidural abscess: Case reports and a review. *J. Spinal Cord Med.* 1998;21:348–354.
13. Dawson DM, Potts F. Acute nontraumatic myelopathies. *Neurol. Clin. North Am.* 1991;9:585–603.
14. Belanger E, Levi A. The acute and chronic management of spinal cord injury. *J. Am. Coll. Surg.* 2000;190:603–618.
15. Fenstermaker RA. Acute neurologic management of the patient with spinal cord injury. *Urol. Clin. North Am.* 1993;20:413–421.
16. Maynard FM, Bracken MB, Creasey G, et al. International standards for neurological and functional classification of spinal cord injury. *Spinal Cord* 1997;35:266–274.
17. Corr P, Govender S. The role of magnetic resonance imaging on spinal trauma. *Clin. Radiol.* 1999;54:629–635.
18. Greenberg, JO. Neuroimaging of the spine. *Neurol. Clin. North Am.* 1991;9:679–704.
19. Teasell RW, Arnold MO, Krassioukov A, Delaney GA. Cardiovascular consequences of loss of supraspinal control of the sympathetic nervous system after spinal cord injury. *Arch. Phys. Med. Rehab.* 2000;81:506–516.
20. Karlsson AK. Autonomic dysreflexia. *Spinal Cord* 1999;37:383–391.
21. American Society of Paraplegia. Acute management of autonomic dysreflexia: Adults with spinal cord injury presenting to health-care facilities. *J. Spinal Cord Med.* 1997;20:284–308.
22. Lanig IS, Peterson WP. The respiratory system in spinal cord injury. *Phys. Med. Rehab. Clin. North Am.* 2000;11:29–43.
23. Wheeler JS, Walter JW. Acute urologic management of the patient with spinal cord injury. *Urol. Clin. North Am.* 1993;20:403–411.
24. Chen D, Nussbaum SB. The gastrointestinal system and bowel management following spinal cord injury. *Phys. Med. Rehab. Clin. North Am.* 2000;11:45–56.
25. Winemiller MH, Stolp-Smith KA, Silverstein MD, et al. Prevention of venous thromboembolism in patients with spinal cord injury: Effects of sequential pneumatic compression and heparin. *J. Spinal Cord Med.* 1999;22:182–191.
26. Miranda AR, Hassouna HI. Mechanisms of thrombosis in spinal cord injury. *Hematol. Oncol. Clin. North Am.* 2000;14:401–416.

27. Frost F. APS Recommendations for skin care of hospitalized patients with acute spinal cord injury. *J. Spinal Cord Med.* 1999;22:133–138.
28. Kirshblum S. Treatment alternatives for spinal cord injury related spasticity. *J. Spinal Cord Med.* 1999;22:199–217.
29. Vaccaro AR, Daugherty RJ, Sheehan TP, et al. Neurologic outcome of early versus late surgery for cervical spinal cord injury. *Spine* 1997;22:2609–2613.
30. Amar AP, Levy ML. Surgical controversies in the management of spinal cord injury. *J. Am. Coll. Surg.* 1999;188:550–566.
31. Bracken MB, Shepard MJ, Collins WF, et al. A randomized, controlled trial of methylprednisolone or naloxone in the treatment of acute spinal cord injury. *N. Engl. J. Med.* 1990;322:1405–1411.
32. Bracken MB, Shepard MJ, Holford TR, et al. Administration of methylprednisolone for 24 or 48 hours or tirilazad mesylate for 48 hours in the treatment of acute spinal cord injury. *JAMA* 1997;277:1597–1604.
33. Short DJ, El Masry WS, Jones PW. High dose methylprednisolone in the management of acute spinal cord injury—A systematic review from a clinical perspective. *Spinal Cord* 2000;38:273–286.
34. Geisler FH, Dorsey FC, Coleman WP. Recovery of motor function after spinal cord injury—A randomized, placebo-controlled trial with gm-1 ganglioside. *N. Engl. J. Med.* 1991;324:1829–1838.
35. Tator CH. Experimental and clinical studies of the pathophysiology and management of acute spinal cord injury. *J. Spinal Cord Med.* 1996;19:206–214.
36. Barami K, Diaz FG. Cellular transplantation and spinal cord injury. *Neurosurgery* 2000;47:691–700.

24

Postoperative Management in the Neurosciences Critical Care Unit

Tina Rodrigue and Warren R. Selman

INTRODUCTION

Caring for the postoperative neurosurgical patient presents unique challenges to the critical care physician. Not only does the clinician need to be comfortable with routine postsurgical concerns, but he or she also requires specialized knowledge about the functioning of the central nervous system. There is a wide variety of central nervous system (CNS) pathology requiring surgical intervention, and treatments appropriate for one type of brain injury may prove to be detrimental to patients with a different disease process. It is essential to understand these differences, to institute proper treatment. In addition, the physician must always keep in mind that patients in the neurosciences critical care unit (NSU) may have problems not only within the central nervous system, but also of various other organ systems. Preoperative medical conditions often profoundly complicate postoperative management. It is important to understand the effects of neurologic interventions on normal body homeostasis and vice versa in order to provide effective care to patients in the NSU. This chapter attempts to cover most of the topics that face the clinician working with neurosurgical patients, starting with general issues and moving on to specific neurologic disease entities and their distinctive concerns. Basic clinical management, emergent treatment, early diagnosis and anticipation of potential complications will be addressed. The goal of this chapter is to provide a practical and precise overview of critical care for postoperative neurosurgical patients.

GENERAL POSTOPERATIVE CONSIDERATIONS

General Note

Of critical importance in the NSU is prompt recognition of neurologic deterioration, and timely diagnosis and management of postoperative complications. Many complications of neurologic disease result from cerebral ischemia or increased intracranial pressure. Depending on their causes, these processes may be reversible, but only with timely management. The fact is, delays in detection of treatable problems can lead to permanent neurologic injury. It is not appropriate to wait several hours to evaluate a patient, or to delay definitive imaging studies for the sake of convenience. Uncal herniation and permanent brainstem damage can occur over a matter of minutes, and oftentimes by the time the pupil dilates, the patient has already suffered irreversible damage (1). Therefore, concerns about a patient's neurologic status need to be evaluated immediately, starting with a complete bedside evaluation by a physician.

From: *Current Clinical Neurology*
Critical Care Neurology and Neurosurgery
Edited by: J. I. Suarez © Humana Press Inc., Totowa, NJ

Immediate Postoperative Evaluation

Perhaps the most important first step in the care of any neurosurgical patient is a thorough evaluation as soon as he or she is admitted to the NSU. Because of the urgency in making diagnoses and instituting therapy for neurologic problems, it is crucial to have a good baseline exam as early as possible in the course of therapy. Ideally, this would encompass a preoperative examination by all treating physicians. Often this is not possible, and the preoperative neurologic examination documented by the neurosurgeon's office note is all that is available. Any changes in the neurologic examination need to be evaluated in the immediate postoperative period. Some deficits may be expected due to the region of surgical intervention; therefore, it is important that the neurointensivist has a good grasp of neuroanatomy, and of the surgical procedure performed on any given patient. For example, a person who has just undergone resection of an occipital glioma may be fully expected to have a visual field cut. Pupillary sluggishness or slow awakening may be seen for approx 1 h following general anesthetic and narcotic administration *(2)*. However, certain deficits should not be written off as a result of normal surgical intervention. Lethargy, unresponsiveness, or focal deficits such as hemiparesis and aphasia are often clues pointing to mass effect and increased intracranial pressure in the postoperative period. Most patients in whom a postoperative intracranial hematoma develops do so within 6 h of surgery; therefore, an immediate postoperative neurologic examination and close monitoring in the NSU is crucial for rapid detection of this complication *(3)*. The neurologic examination should be detailed, and include documentation of cranial nerve function, level of consciousness, speech, motor, and visual systems. It is useful for the nurse who will be caring for the patient in the postoperative period to be present during the initial bedside examination, so that he or she is familiar with the patient's postoperative baseline.

The postoperative evaluation also needs to include evaluation of cardiac and respiratory parameters. As soon as the patient enters the NSU, he or she should be connected to continuous cardiac and respiratory monitors. Continuous electrocardiography (EKG), pulse oximetry, and arterial blood pressure monitors are typically used. Often the patient may have additional monitors, such as a ventriculostomy or intracranial pressure (ICP) monitor, or possibly even a central venous line or Swan-Ganz catheter. The neurointensivist needs to be familiar with all of these devices. Many patients may remain mechanically ventilated in the immediate postoperative period, and these parameters need to be evaluated and optimized. Any patient with a cardiac history or with intraoperative arrhythmia or blood pressure instability also deserves a formal 12-lead EKG upon arrival to the NSU. Most postoperative neurosurgical patients should get laboratory studies checked as well, including hematocrit, electrolytes, coagulation parameters, anticonvulsant levels, and blood gases.

Cardiovascular System

Many of the cardiovascular issues facing the neurosurgical patient are no different from those facing any surgical patient. Hemorrhage, hypovolemia, myocardial infarction, and heart failure are all problems that need to be cared for, as they would be for any intensive care unit (ICU) patient. However, there are several problems that are peculiar to the neurosurgical patient.

Strict Blood Pressure Control

Perhaps more than any other type of postoperative patient, blood pressure parameters in neurosurgical patients need to be strictly monitored and corrected when necessary. Almost all craniotomy patients should have an arterial line as well as intermittent noninvasive blood pressure monitoring. In most cases, normotension is advisable, which means within a range similar to the patient's baseline systolic blood pressure. It is important to avoid hypertension in order to reduce the risk of hemorrhage into the surgical bed. Conversely, hypotension must also be avoided, to reduce the risk of hypoperfusion and ischemia to surrounding edematous brain. Often, patients tend to be slightly hypertensive in the postoperative period with respect to baseline. Adequate pain control should be en-sured and treatment with antihypertensives should be used as needed (*see also* Chapters 12 and 13). Most patients are successfully managed using intermittent treatment with beta blockers. Occasionally, continuous intravenous (IV) infusion of nitroprusside is necessary in the short term to maintain systolic blood pressure within a safe range. However, this should not be maintained more than 24 h because of the risk of thiocyanate toxicity *(4)*. In certain cases controlled hypertension may be required to minimize the risk of vasospasm and hypoperfusion, such as following intracerebral aneurysm clipping or revascularization procedures *(5)*.

Volume Resuscitation

There is a great deal of controversy surrounding the appropriate IV resuscitation and fluid management of postoperative neurosurgical patients, in an attempt to achieve the optimal balance between adequate tissue perfusion and minimization of cerebral edema. Most neurosurgical patients do not have problems with hypovolemia, because the third-spacing and fluid shifts that are so common during intra-abdominal and thoracic cases are not seen. If a neurosurgical patient requires volume resuscitation, it should be given as aggressively as necessary to maintain normovolemia, adequate cardiac output, and tissue perfusion. Isotonic IV fluids are the appropriate choice for most patients. Most neurosurgeons choose to use normal saline for routine IV fluid replacement. Hypotonic saline and lactated ringer's (LR) solution are generally not used in postoperative neurosurgical patients, because in experimental animals, they have been found to increase total brain water and intracranial pressure *(6)*. It is important to realize, however, that postoperative neurosurgical patients cannot be assumed to have an intact blood–brain barrier (BBB). Because of the interruption of the BBB at the surgical site, the normal regulatory mechanisms of cerebral blood flow, ICP, and brain water are disrupted, and many interventions are therefore less effective. Several studies have revealed that the injured BBB is unable to maintain either an oncotic or osmotic gradient, and that the amount of cerebral edema around the site of brain injury is unaffected by the type of IV fluid administered *(7)*. Fluid restriction following ischemic brain injury has not been demonstrated to significantly reduce cerebral edema *(8)*. Rats which were under-resuscitated following hemorrhagic shock were actually found to have a higher cerebral water content than rats who were adequately resuscitated with either isotonic or hypertonic IV fluids *(9)*. Using hypertonic saline or dextran as resuscitation fluids has been touted because of their ability to both rapidly restore intravascular volume and decrease brain water *(10)*. However, again, this effect on cerebral water content relies on an intact BBB with the ability to maintain an osmotic gradient, and dextran can potentially worsen cerebral edema by increasing cerebral blood flow. It seems that cerebral edema will occur to some extent in most postoperative neurosurgical patients. Therefore, the most reasonable approach to IV fluid use should be an attempt to maintain normovolemia, with normal serum osmolality. Normal saline should generally be used, to avoid the potential complications associated with the other IV fluids mentioned previously.

Arrhythmia

Most neurosurgical patients who have an arrhythmia usually have an underlying cardiac problem that can be elicited through history and physical examination (*see also* Chapter 8). Based on the patient's history and admission EKG, appropriate therapy should be instituted regardless of his or her neurologic disease. Cardiac enzymes should be checked on any neurosurgical patient with sustained abnormalities on EKG to rule out acute myocardial ischemia. Myocardial ischemia needs to be treated aggressively, to preserve cardiac function and adequate tissue perfusion. Sometimes the practitioner will see a patient whose intracranial pathology directly affects his or her cardiac status. Patients who present with subarachnoid hemorrhage (SAH) sometimes suffer characteristic EKG changes and sudden arrhythmias. Usually, these changes occur shortly after the initial hemorrhage, and may include ventricular tachycardia, ventricular fibrillation and torsades de pointes *(11)*. It is believed that these arrhythmias may be responsible for some cases of sudden death following aneurysm rupture *(12)*. Of those who present to medical attention, EKG changes may be transiently seen in up to 50% of SAH patients, and may include inverted T-waves, S-T segment abnormalities, or Q-T prolongation *(13)*. If these cardiac abnormalities become life threatening, they should be treated symptomatically using standard accepted protocols as described elsewhere in this book. Usually, however, the EKG changes resolve spontaneously over several days.

Respiratory System

Neurosurgical patients are often prone to respiratory difficulties, usually due to decreased level of consciousness and/or lack of mobility. Physicians caring for these patients need to be familiar with endotracheal intubation techniques and ventilator management *(see* Chapter 9). Nurses and respiratory therapists play important roles in prevention of respiratory problems, as well as their treatment.

Pneumonia

Pneumonia is extremely common in the NSU. The intensivist should always be vigilant for this complication, and aggressive in its treatment. Most commonly, pneumonia results either from aspiration or inability to clear secretions. Patients with brain injury are extremely prone to aspiration. Patients with high spinal cord injury may be unable to produce a strong cough or breathe deeply. Protection of a patient's airway is foremost in preventing pneumonia. Awake patients should be mobilized as quickly as is feasible. Patients who cannot be mobilized require frequent changes in position, chest physiotherapy, and suctioning. Treatment with broad-spectrum antibiotics should be instituted if there is clinical evidence of pneumonia, such as fever, infiltrate on chest roentgenogram, elevated peripheral leukocytosis, copious secretions, and positive sputum cultures as described in Chapter 11.

Tracheostomy

Patients with brain injury or postoperative neurologic deficits may require aggressive pulmonary care for several weeks to months, and may be very difficult to wean from the ventilator. The decision to pursue tracheostomy should come from careful evaluation not only of the patient's pulmonary status, but also of their prognosis for neurologic recovery. The timing of elective tracheostomy is often questioned. Several studies demonstrate that early tracheostomy (within the first week after injury) shortens ICU stays and reduces the frequency of pneumonia *(14,15)*. In addition, the probability of successful extubation decreases with time. In patients with infratentorial lesions, only 5.8% of surviving patients are able to be successfully extubated after 8 d of endotracheal intubation *(16)*. A good recommendation is to plan for tracheostomy after 7–10 d of intubation and mechanical ventilation in patients who have a significant neurologic deficit but not a terminal diagnosis.

Neurogenic Pulmonary Edema

This is an extremely rare complication of severe neurologic damage, usually associated with head injury or subarachnoid hemorrhage. The mechanism underlying the rapid and massive pulmonary edema that occasionally follows neurologic injury is poorly understood. Treatment is supportive, with positive-pressure ventilation and diuretics as needed.

Positive End-Expiratory Pressure

Positive end-expiratory pressure, or PEEP, is useful in patients with low lung compliance with risk of alveolar collapse, such as patients with adult respiratory distress syndrome (ARDS). The use of PEEP has been debated in patients with the potential for increased ICP, because of the theoretical risk of transmitting the higher pulmonary venous pressure into the cerebral vasculature. However, levels of PEEP up to 10 cm H_2O do not cause clinically significant increases in ICP, and can be used safely *(17)*.

Infectious Complications

Postoperative patients, are susceptible to many infectious complications. As in the case of pneumonia mentioned previously, lack of mobility is one reason for this, and the prolonged use of invasive devices also puts the neurosurgical patient at risk. Foley catheters should be changed regularly, and other invasive catheters, such as central lines, arterial lines, subarachnoid pressure monitors, and ventriculostomies need to be evaluated regularly for signs of infection, and removed or replaced if needed *(18)*.

Antibiotic Prophylaxis

Most postoperative infections result from contamination with skin flora, namely, staphylococcus, and sometimes streptococcus (*see also* Chapter 29). Various antibiotic regimens have been suggested for perioperative prophylaxis. However, neurosurgical procedures carry, for the most part, a fairly low risk of infection, and general principles of antibiotic prophylaxis are applicable *(19)*. Cefazolin has been demonstrated to have therapeutic levels in brain tissue after intravenous administration, and is active against the most common postoperative infecting organisms *(20)*. Given immediately preoperatively and in the 24 h following incision, it has been shown to reduce the risk of infection in patients without foreign implants, and has a low risk of side effects *(21)*. For invasive catheters including ventriculostomies, central venous lines, ICP monitors, and arterial lines, most institutions use some sort of antibiotic prophylaxis, although there is no definitive study to support its necessity. Duration of placement of these catheters relates most importantly to rate of infection. Cerebrospinal fluid (CSF) infection is four times more likely to occur if a ventriculostomy is required for more than 5 d, whether antibiotics are administered or not *(22)*. Most institutions have their own preferred prophylactic antibiotic regimen, that should be followed in the NSU.

Postoperative Infections

A patient who has undergone a craniotomy is at risk for many infectious complications, including meningitis, cerebritits, or brain abscess. Patients most at risk include those who are immunosuppressed, those with foreign implants, or those who have undergone prolonged surgery with hypothermia *(23)*. Patients may develop fever, elevated peripheral white blood cell count, increasing headache, meningismus, decreased level of consciousness, or focal neurologic deficits. If concern about an intracranial infection arises, a patient should undergo imaging with administration of intravenous contrast to rule out any large masses or obviously enhancing fluid collections. In the postoperative period, meningeal enhancement is common and should not be considered by itself as evidence of infection *(24)*. If imaging rules out any large intracranial masses, the patient should undergo lumbar puncture to obtain CSF cultures prior to institution of antibiotics. A lumbar puncture in someone with bacterial meningitis usually demonstrates neutrophilia, increased protein and decreased glucose, and the gram stain may be positive. Broad-spectrum antibiotics, usually a combination of a cephalosporin, vancomycin, and gentamycin, are commonly begun as soon as CSF cultures are obtained. Antibiotic coverage is narrowed once the offending organism is identified. Untreated intracranial infections can lead to loss of neurologic functioning or even death, and so should be treated promptly, without waiting for final cultures. It is important to realize that the meningitis seen in the postoperative setting is usually fairly indolent and caused by staphylococcus, and that it does not have the infectious capacity of community-acquired bacterial meningitis. Therefore, no special isolation needs to be undertaken. Postoperative meningitis should be treated with antibiotics for 7–10 d, depending on the organism and response to treatment *(25)*. If an abscess or subdural empyema is seen on imaging, the treatment is surgical—exploration and debridement, with drainage of the purulent material and often also removal of the bone flap. Again, broad-spectrum antibiotics should be started once a sample is obtained, and the regimen refined based on culture sensitivities. Abscesses, post-surgical or not, are usually treated with at least 6 wk of antibiotics.

Spinal Epidural Abscess

This is a rare postoperative complication; it most commonly presents spontaneously, either through direct extension of a disc space infection or through hematogenous spread from a remote site. People with diabetes, and people who use intravenous substances are particularly vulnerable. It is mentioned here because of the need for emergent surgical intervention. If a patient presents with severe back pain and tenderness, fever, and leukocytosis, that patient should undergo an emergent spinal MRI with and without contrast to rule out epidural abscess. Neurologic deterioration with this condition can be rapid, and once it occurs, is usually irreversible *(26)*. It is believed that neurologic compromise is the result of venous thrombosis and infarction, rather than simple compression of the spinal cord; hence, the low chance for recovery of function *(27)*. Spinal epidural abscess should be treated by emergent surgical drainage followed by aggressive IV antibiotics.

Aseptic Meningitis

This is not a true infection, as it is usually caused by some chemical meningeal irritation. The most common causes following surgery include use of chemotherapeutic wafers, reaction to the contents of an epidermoid tumor, or reaction to a bovine pericardial dural graft *(28)*. The symptoms are similar to those associated with bacterial meningitis: fever, headache, nausea, meningismus. Aseptic meningitis is a diagnosis of exclusion and the clinician must rule out bacterial meningitis before accepting it as the diagnosis. A lumbar puncture in someone with aseptic meningitis usually demonstrates lymphocytosis, elevated protein a normal glucose level, and negative bacterial culture results *(29)*. Steroids are the treatment of choice for aseptic meningitis; usually starting with intravenous dexamethasone, and continuing a taper after discharge for approx 2 wk.

Endocrine System

Syndrome of Inappropriate Antidiuretic Hormone Secretion

SIADH is sometimes seen in the NSU, usually as a result of trauma or intracranial infection, namely meningitis *(see also* Chapter 11). The name of this syndrome is descriptive: there is an oversecretion of anti-diuretic hormone, regardless of serum osmolar stimulation. The hallmark features of this syndrome are hyponatremia (<134 mEq/L), low serum osmolality (<280 mOsm/L), and a high ratio of urine to serum osmolality (usually >1.5:1) *(30)*. The definitive test for making the diagnosis is a water-load test, in which the patient is given a large oral water load, and subsequent urine output is monitored *(31)*. In the NSU it is not usually advisable to proceed with this type of testing, as the risk of worsening hyponatremia exists. Clinical diagnosis is usually sufficient. Patients usually present with confusion and lethargy, and they may progress to seizure and coma if the hyponatremia becomes severe (<125 mEq/L). Treatment for SIADH is usually simple fluid restriction to less than 800 cc/da in most adults, with absolutely no free water to be given. In severe, symptomatic cases, hypertonic saline may be administered judiciously *(32)*. In an adult, it is possible to start intravenous 3% NaCl (513 mEq/L) at a rate of 25–50 cc/h to help correct severe hyponatremia. It is important to monitor serum sodium frequently (every 4–6 h), and to maintain a rate of correction not exceeding approx 1.3 mEq/L/h. The reason behind this relatively slow correction of severe hyponatremia is that there is a risk of developing central pontine myelinolysis (CPM) with too rapid a correction. CPM is a disorder in which the pontine white matter becomes demyelinated, producing flaccid quadraparesis and cranial nerve deficits, and is most often seen in people who suffer from malnourishment or alcoholism *(33)*. Because CPM is such a devastating complication, many clinicians are hesitant to use hypertonic saline in the correction of hyponatremia; however, the risk of CPM is extremely low with a carefully measured rate of correction.

Diabetes Insipidus

This hormonal abnormality can be thought of as the opposite of SIADH. In central diabetes insipidus (DI), patients do not secrete sufficient antidiuretic hormone (ADH). There also exists a peripheral form of DI that is rare, in which the kidneys become unresponsive to ADH. In patients with severe brain injury, or damage to the hypothalamic-pituitary axis, central DI is frequently seen. Patients with DI present with a high output of dilute urine, and serum hypernatremia. A sustained urine output of >250 cc/h in an adult, or >3 cc/kg/h in a child, should prompt workup for DI. The urine osmolarity in DI is usually less than 150 mOsm/L, and the specific gravity is less than 1.005 *(34)*. Serum sodium and osmolarity may initially be normal, however, with continued loss of free water these values become elevated. If the patient is awake, he or she will complain of terrible thirst, and will exhibit polydipsia to compensate for the loss of water in the urine. The diagnosis is usually made based on these clinical signs and laboratory values. It is possible to do a water deprivation test to prove the diagnosis of DI; however, this is not advisable because of the risk of worsening existing hypernatremia. If a patient has been treated with an osmotic diuretic such as mannitol, urinary osmolarity cannot be relied on to help make the diagnosis, and serum sodium is a more reliable measure. It is in the unconscious patient that DI can become life-threatening, because these patients are unable to take in a sufficient amount of water to maintain a normal serum sodium and osmolarity. Often, patients in the NSU require IV replacement of free water losses, and careful urine output monitoring is necessary to achieve euvolemia. Most cases of DI are self-limiting, lasting 12–36 h following a neurosurgical procedure. Patients who have undergone resection of a pituitary adenoma are most at risk because there is often retraction injury to the pituitary stalk. In most of these transient cases, free access to water and frequent serum sodium checks is all that is needed for postoperative management. In those cases which seem to be prolonged, or in which it is difficult to keep up with the loss of water in the urine, it may become necessary to treat patients with exogenous vasopressin to reduce urine output. Intranasal desmopressin (DDAVP®) can be used in awake patients, while subcutaneous (SC) or IV formulations can be used in patients who are intubated or have decreased mentation. Intravenous aqueous vasopressin (Pitressin®) is most frequently used in the setting of brain death. Patients who suffer brain death often exhibit refractory DI with profound fluid losses, secondary to the cessation of ADH production by the hypothalamus. If the patient is a candidate for organ donation, it may become necessary to control severe DI with Pitressin® to prevent dehydration. A solution of one unit of Pitressin in 1000 cc of hypotonic IV fluid (D5 water or 0.45% NaCl) is usually infused to match urine output in these cases until hypernatremia is corrected.

Cerebral Salt Wasting

This is most commonly seen following subarachnoid hemorrhage. In this syndrome, there is loss of sodium through the urine, with concomitant fluid loss. Patients present with symptoms of hyponatremia, usually with confusion and lethargy. Patients also have decreased plasma volume, and may show signs of dehydration. Laboratory values demonstrate hyponatremia, and it can sometimes be difficult to differentiate SIADH from cerebral salt wasting. Often, it is necessary to directly evaluate intravascular volume by using a central venous pressure measurement in order to differentiate between the two, as patients with SIADH should have normal plasma volume, while patients with cerebral salt wasting are hypovolemic. The treatment for cerebral salt wasting is repletion of salt and fluid, usually by IV administration of normal saline. Misdiagnosing cerebral salt wasting as SIADH may be disastrous, as fluid restriction in cerebral salt wasting will result in rapid worsening of hyponatremia. Sometimes, IV fludrocortisone acetate can be used to help promote retention of sodium in the renal tubule, in patients who do not seem to respond solely to normal saline treatment *(35)*.

Hematological Disorders

Deep Venous Thrombosis

This is a relatively frequent complication in the neurosurgical patient. The routine use of compression stockings decreases the incidence of DVT, and should be instituted immediately before induction of anesthesia and continued postoperatively until the patient is ambulating *(36)*. There is evidence that heparin, 5000 SC twice daily, can be safely given to neurosurgical patients starting postoperative day 1 with a significant decrease in the incidence of DVT and pulmonary embolus. Frim et al. reported that in none of 138 postoperative neurosurgical patients given SC heparin, thromboembolic complications or intracranial hemorrhage developed while in 3.2% of control patients DVT or pulmonary embolus (PE) developed. An important caveat, however, is that the patient must not have active hemorrhage or bleeding diathesis *(37)*. See a more detailed discussion in Chapter 11.

A common question facing the clinician involves the timing of institution of full anticoagulation in the postcraniotomy patient. In patients who require chronic anticoagulation, such as those with atrial fibrillation, known DVT, mechanical heart valves, peripheral vascular disease or past stroke secondary to carotid stenosis, the risk of hemorrhage versus the risk of thromboembolic complications must be weighed. In general, if the person is at low risk of thromboembolic complications, intravenous heparin and warfarin can be restarted 7–14 d after craniotomy. If, however, the patient is considered to be at high risk, it may become necessary to begin anticoagulation as early as 3–5 d postcraniotomy. In any case, full anticoagulation should not be started in a craniotomy patient for at least 24–48 h postoperatively because the risk of hemorrhage into the surgical bed is highest at that time *(38)*.

Coagulopathy

Patients with massive intracranial trauma can present with disseminated intravascular coagulopathy (DIC), which presents as profound thrombocytopenia, prolonged PT/PTT, low fibrinogen, and elevated fibrin degradation products *(see also* Chapter 11). These patients should be treated with FFP and platelets as needed to keep coagulation parameters as normal as possible, however, they are often refractory to treatment and may require repeated transfusions until the condition resolves *(39)*. Thrombocytopenia may also occasionally be seen in response to treatment with ranitidine, heparin or phenytoin, and these drugs may need to be discontinued in patients with an otherwise unexplained low platelet count.

Gastrointestinal System

The major concern with the gastrointestinal (GI) system in neurosurgical patients is gastric stress ulceration. There is a high rate of stress ulcers in the critically ill neurosurgical population, and patients most at risk include those with severe head injury or those taking a prolonged course of steroids. It is imperative that these patients receive some sort of GI prophylaxis. Most commonly, an acid-reducing agent such as ranitidine is used, and this is effective in reducing the incidence of hemorrhage secondary to gastric ulcers *(40)*. However, there is some concern that by reducing the acidity of the gastric contents, bacterial colonization of the stomach can occur, worsening the risk of aspiration pneumonia *(41)*. Sucralfate is also effective at reducing the risk of stress ulceration, does not significantly change gastric pH, and can be safely used in most neurosurgical patients.

Pain Control and Sedation

Sometimes it is difficult to balance the comfort of the patient against the necessity of obtaining a reliable neurologic examination. Pain medication should be given to maintain a level of comfort acceptable to the patient, while attempting to avoid over-medication with narcotics. Fortunately, most craniotomy patients report less postoperative pain compared with other postsurgical patients, and treatment with acetaminophen and low-dose morphine or codeine is usually adequate *(42)*. In unconscious or aphasic patients, signs such as agitation or hypertension may indicate inadequate pain control. Most neurosurgeons avoid treating craniotomy patients with NSAIDs in the immediate postoperative period, to reduce the risk of platelet dysfunction and hemorrhage. Patients who have a history of alcoholism require prophylaxis against delirium tremens (DT), regardless of neurologic examination. The risk of seizures and death with DT is much higher than the risk of over-sedating these patients, and the small, intermittent doses of benzodiazepine used to prevent DT usually have no appreciable effect on the patient's neurologic examination.

SPECIFIC NEUROSURGICAL DIAGNOSES

Immediate Postoperative Complications

Most postoperative complications that will require surgical reintervention will occur in the first 6 h following craniotomy *(3)*. These include postoperative subdural, epidural, or intraparenchymal hematomas. Therefore, it is crucial that postoperative craniotomy patients be observed closely during this time period in an ICU setting. Close neurologic monitoring in an ICU following craniotomy has been associated with a decrease in morbidity and mortality following neurosurgical procedures *(43)*.

Intracranial Hypertension

Elevated ICP is a fairly common complication seen in the NSU, and can be caused by a variety of disparate pathologies, each requiring different treatment (*see* Chapter 5). Patients with increased ICP present with headache, nausea, emesis, decreased level of consciousness, and occasionally with focal findings such as sixth cranial nerve palsy and hemiparesis. The "Cushing response," considered to be the classical presentation for patients with increased ICP, consists of hypertension, respiration irregularity, and bradycardia *(44)*. Normal ICP should be roughly equivalent to central venous pressure, usually between 5 and 15 mmHg at rest.

In the case of the postoperative neurosurgical patient, the most common causes of increased ICP include hydrocephalus, cerebral edema, or mass effect from a tumor or hematoma. It is important to rapidly determine the underlying cause of increased ICP, to institute proper treatment. An emergent head CT should be obtained in any patient suspected of having increased ICP. Emergent treatment of the patient with increased ICP should be commenced even before getting definitive imaging, especially if the patient is beginning to show signs of brainstem dysfunction. Patients should be quickly intubated and hyperventilated to achieve a PCO_2 of 30–35. It is usually safest to sedate and paralyze the patient before intubation to prevent coughing which may worsen ICP. Hyperventilation is only useful for short periods, and should not be continued past 24 h after initiation. An osmotic diuretic such as mannitol (0.5–1 g/kg) should be rapidly infused, as this helps to reduce total brain water and can significantly reduce ICP in the short run. The patient's head should be elevated above the level of the heart, to improve venous return *(44)*. Once these temporary control measures have been instituted, definitive imaging needs to be obtained to determine the cause of the elevated ICP. Acute hydrocephalus should be treated with bedside ventriculostomy. Mass lesions secondary to traumatic or postoperative hematoma usually require urgent surgical evacuation in order to control ICP. Cerebral edema, either focal or generalized, can be more difficult to treat. Often, the edema surrounding brain tumors is very responsive to high-dose steroids, and these may be all that are necessary to improve the patient's examination. If they are not sufficient, surgical tumor resection should be undertaken, if possible. Generalized edema following head trauma, if severe enough to produce a decrease in consciousness, often requires placement of a subdural ICP monitor to provide clinicians with a measurement to tailor treatment. The goal of such treatment is to maintain a cerebral perfusion pressure of 60–70 mmHg *(45)*. Cerebral perfusion pressure is defined as the difference between mean arterial pressure and ICP, and in normal patients is usually within the range of 70–95 mmHg *(46)*. Patients should be treated with intermittent mannitol to keep a serum osmolarity of approx 300–310 mEq/L, with head elevation, and with sedation and paralytics as needed to keep ICP, and CPP, within reasonable limits. Increasing the serum osmolarity above 310 has little benefit, in terms of reducing ICP, and greatly increases the patient's risk of renal failure. Chapter 5 of this text contains more details on the pathophysiology and treatment of cerebral edema.

Seizures and Status Epilepticus

Recognition and management of seizure activity is a basic part of practice in the NSU. Most seizures are self-limited, and should be simply observed, and the patient made safe from injury. For focal seizures, observation and treatment with standard anticonvulsants is usually all that is necessary. However, generalized seizures lasting more than 1–2 min in the NSU should be treated aggressively. Any seizure in a patient who has never before had a history of seizures should be worked up with imaging, as well as with laboratory evaluation for electrolyte abnormalities. In the postoperative patient with seizure, the immediate concern is for postoperative hematoma. This should be quickly evaluated with an uncontrasted head CT once the seizure activity has ceased. Another major cause of seizures in the postoperative patient is infection; either because of abscess or meningitis. These possibilities need to be considered and treated if found. Emergent treatment of generalized seizures and status epilepticus includes the following: (1) protection of the patient from injury, and airway protection, including intubation if necessary; (2) administration of an IV benzodiazepine, such as lorazepam, 2–4 mg, every 5 min for three doses or until the seizures stop; (3) IV load with phenytoin, 20 mg/kg at a rate not to exceed 50 mg/min. If these measures do not result in cessation of seizure activity, an IV load of phenobarbital (20 mg/kg) or valproic acid (20 mg/kg) can also be added *(47) (see also* Chapter 25*).* If seizure activity continues despite these aggressive measures, general anesthesia with pentobarbital may need to be instituted.

Prevention of seizure activity is preferable to treatment, in the postoperative neurosurgical patient. Most patients undergoing craniotomy are placed on prophylactic phenytoin, with serum levels maintained between 10 and 20 µg/dL. Patients with supratentorial tumors or subarachnoid or intraparenchymal hemorrhage are usually also given prophylactic anticonvulsant therapy. Patients with head trauma have been shown to have a decreased risk of posttraumatic seizures if given phenytoin for a short time following head injury *(48)*. However, extending treatment past 1–2 wk following the initial trauma in a patient who has never seized has not been shown to provide additional benefit. Patients who undergo craniotomy for infratentorial lesions do not need to be treated prophylactically, as they are at extremely low risk for seizure.

Vasospasm

Vasospasm is a complication seen almost exclusively in patients who have suffered SAH, and it describes a phenomenon in which cerebral vessels become reduced in caliber with resultant restriction of blood flow. SAH is described in more detail in Chapter 20. Vasospasm is a potentially dangerous problem, in that cerebral infarction may occur. Radiographic evidence of vasospasm may be seen in as many as 70% of patients following SAH, however, only about 20% of patients have clinical evidence of vasospasm *(49)*. The risk of vasospasm begins usually about 3 d after the initial hemorrhage, and is greatest within the first 7–10 d, although it can frequently be seen as late as 21 d after subarachnoid hemorrhage *(50)*. The risk of vasospasm is associated with the patient's Fisher grade on admission. It is important to understand that vasospasm is a result of the initial subarachnoid hemorrhage, and has little to do with any surgical or endovascular intervention used to obliterate the aneurysm. Therefore, regardless of which, if either, modality is used to treat the patient, vasospasm remains a possibility. All patients with SAH should be started on nimodipine, a calcium-channel blocker that has been demonstrated to improve the outcome of patients with SAH *(51)*. The effects of vasospasm can be reduced by employing a series of treatments intended to increase cerebral blood flow, using manipulations to produce a state of hemodilution, hypertension, and hypervolemia or "triple H therapy" *(52)*. Once an aneurysm has been secured, a patient is begun on high-volume intravenous fluid therapy, usually twice maintenance volume, as well as intermittent fluid boluses with the goal of maintaining a central venous pressure of 10–12 mmHg, or a wedge pressure of 18–20 mmHg. This helps to achieve a hypervolemic status and reduces the patient's hematocrit to some degree; both of these interventions help improve blood flow through potentially spastic vessels. A Swan-Ganz catheter is usually placed in patients with a previous history of cardiac disease to help manage congestive heart failure, should it occur. In other patients a central venous line is used to monitor volume status. In patients in whom symptoms of vasospasm never develop, maintaining the increased level of fluids for 7–10 d post-hemorrhage may be all the treatment that is needed. However, in patients in whom clinical vasospasm is suspected, induction of controlled hypertension may also become necessary to help force blood past the spastic vessels. Usually, either phenylephrine or norepinephrine is used to maintain a systolic blood pressure approx 15–20% above the patient's baseline, usually between 140 and 160 mmHg. If the patient is normally hypertensive, he or she is permitted to remain so. Dopamine is not usually as effective as the other two pressors in this setting, and it has the drawback of potentially increasing natriuresis and therefore, urine output. This is at odds with the desire to maintain a high plasma volume. Duration of "triple H therapy" is variable. In patients who never demonstrate any symptoms, hypervolemic therapy can usually be stopped 7–10 d after the hemorrhage, and the patient observed for another 1–2 d before discharge. In patients with symptoms, therapy must be continued until the symptoms have resolved, or there is no longer any angiographic evidence of vasospasm. Some institutions use daily transcranial Doppler measurements in order to help dictate the course of treatment. During the period of vasospasm, the blood velocity is noted to increase in spastic vessels, sometimes as much as two to three times baseline. Once the trend comes back down to normal, one can assume that the period of vasospasm is ending, and that it is safe to begin weaning therapy. One point about hyperdynamic therapy which needs to be kept in mind is that it should only be instituted in patients whose ruptured aneurysms have been secured. Increasing blood flow and blood pressure past a ruptured, unsecured aneurysm may increase the risk of rerupture, and is not recommended.

Any neurologic deterioration in a patient with subarachnoid hemorrhage should be evaluated quickly with a head CT. If neither recurrent hemorrhage nor hydrocephalus is obvious on the imaging, vasospasm needs to be considered as the cause. Because vasospasm can lead to cerebral infarction, treatment needs to be instituted immediately. Following the head CT, patients should be taken for an urgent cerebral angiography, not only to confirm the diagnosis of vasospasm, but also for potential endovascular intervention. Balloon angioplasty of spastic vessel segments or infusion of papaverine may help to relieve the degree of vasospasm and improve blood flow *(53)*. Of course, if a large area of infarction is seen on CT scan, these interventions are contraindicated because of the risk of reperfusion hemorrhage. Once a patient has evidence of clinical vasospasm he or she should be treated for at least 14 d with triple-H therapy, or until the symptoms have resolved and there is no angiographic evidence of vasospasm.

Arteriovenous Malformation

Arteriovenous malformations (AVMs) alter cerebral hemodynamics both within the nidus of the malformation and in the surrounding brain parenchyma. The autoregulation of blood flow is believed to be abnormal, demonstrating chronically low perfusion pressure in the parenchyma surrounding AVMs *(54)*. This disordered blood flow can be evaluated both preoperatively and postoperatively using stable xenon-enhanced computed tomography or single-photon emission tomography (SPECT). Following surgical resection of an AVM, the blood flow in the surrounding parenchyma increases and there may be increased risk of cerebral edema and hemorrhage. This phenomenon, known as "normal perfusion pressure breakthrough," is believed to be a result of the disordered autoregulation of blood flow surrounding AVMs. Large, high-flow AVMs may be more prone to normal perfusion pressure breakthrough, and some advocate staged endovascular treatment of these lesions to allow for more gradual changes in surrounding cerebral blood flow *(55)*. In the NSU, it is important to maintain strict normotension for at least 24–48 h postoperatively, in order to minimize the risk of hemorrhage. Although hemorrhage can occur by normal perfusion pressure breakthrough, the most common cause of postoperative hemorrhage is actually incomplete excision of the AVM. A postoperative angiogram is mandatory to evaluate for remaining abnormal blood vessels at the surgical site.

Cerebrospinal Fluid Leak

CSF leak is not a particularly common complication in neurosurgical patients. It is important to recognize, however, because it can lead to further complications such as meningitis and cerebral abscess. Three populations of patients are particularly at risk: patients with basilar skull fractures, patients who have undergone a transsphenoidal operation, and patients who have undergone a posterior fossa craniotomy with dural opening.

Patients who have suffered trauma, which results in a fracture through the temporal bone or the cribiform plate, are at risk for CSF otorrhea or rhinorrhea. These patients will present with frank CSF flowing from the ear or nose, or may complain of a salty-sweet taste in their mouths. Often,1 CSF rhinorrhea can be demonstrated by having the patient sit up and hang his head between his knees. If in doubt, the fluid can be collected and tested for glucose. Normal nasal secretions should not contain a significant amount of glucose, while CSF will have a glucose level approx 60% of the serum glucose. The patient presenting with CSF otorrhea or rhinorrhea as a result of traumatic skull fracture usually has a good prognosis. Patients should be managed with bed rest, with a head elevation between 0 and 30 degrees. Most patients (<90%) will be able to seal the leak within 5–7 d without further intervention. Prophylactic antibiotics are not recommended because they do not reduce the rate of meningitis, and they tend to select for more virulent organisms *(56)*. Patients with a persistent CSF leak after 5–7 d should then have a lumbar subarachnoid drain placed, and CSF drained from that at a rate of 5–15 cc/h. By providing a lower-resistance path for CSF, the flow through the skull fracture is reduced, allowing for sealing of the leak. If, after another 5–7 d of lumbar drainage, the patient continues to have a CSF leak, he or she will most likely require surgical exploration and repair of the dural defect *(57)*.

Patients in whom a CSF leak develops following a transsphenoidal approach to the sella or posterior fossa craniotomy may have a more difficult course. Several factors may predispose patients to poor healing and CSF leak following surgery: diabetes, chronic steroid use, and placement of dural allograft are some of these. CSF leaks following a transsphenoidal approach to the sella may be very difficult to treat, and if a repeat exploration and repacking of the sella and sphenoid does not rectify the problem, the patient may need to undergo a formal craniotomy for intracranial visualization and repair of the dural defect. Some patients may develop an inflammatory reaction to the bovine pericardium often used to patch the dural defect in a posterior fossa craniotomy *(58)*. This "chemical meningitis" leads to an increase in ICP, which may worsen leakage of CSF through the dural suture line.

Psuedomeningoceles are not common following posterior fossa surgery, however if they occur and are large, or if there is leakage through the incision, aggressive treatment needs to be undertaken. Usually, patients who develop CSF leak after surgery require lumbar drainage immediately, as they do not usually heal spontaneously. Once the drain is placed, the CSF should be checked for evidence of infection, and this should be treated if found. If evidence of chemical meningitis is noted, the patient should be started on steroids to reduce the inflammatory reaction. If after 5–7 d of lumbar drainage the patient shows no sign of cessation of the CSF leak, or if the surgical wound appears infected or is not healing well, the patient will need to go back to surgery for exploration, debridement, and closure of the dural defect.

Head Injury

Traumatic brain injury (TBI) frequently requires admission to the NSU. Although a detailed description of TBI is presented in Chapter 22, a brief discussion is needed because this patient population frequently requires neurosurgical intervention. Any trauma patient should have his or her neurologic status quickly evaluated in the emergency room using a brief neurologic examination as well as the Glasgow Coma Scale (GCS, Table 1). If there is a history of TBI or the neurologic examination

Table 1
Glasgow Coma Scale

Points	Best motor response	Best verbal response	Best eye opening
1	None	None	None
2	Extensor posturing	Incomprehensible	To pain
3	Flexor posturing	inappropriate	To speech
4	Withdraws to pain	Confused	Spontaneous
5	Localizes pain	Oriented	
6	Obeys commands		

Teasdale G, Jennett B. Assessment of coma and impaired consciousness. A practical scale.
Lancet 1974;2:81–84.

is not completely intact, the patient should be taken for a noncontrasted head CT scan as soon as the initial evaluation and hemodynamic stabilization is completed. Mass lesions such as subdural or epidural hematomas should be surgically evacuated immediately. Open skull fractures or penetrating trauma may also require surgical intervention, depending on their severity. There are many types of closed head injury that do not require surgical intervention but warrant careful ICU monitoring and support. Contusions, traumatic subarachnoid hemorrhage, and diffuse axonal injury may all be seen following head injury. The most important concern for the neurointensivist is monitoring the patient's neurologic examination. If on admission the patient has a GCS of less than 8 with an unremarkable CT scan, the patient should have a subarachnoid bolt placed for measurement of ICP, and this should be treated as necessary *(44)*. Any deterioration in exam requires re-imaging because contusions can blossom in the first 24–48 h, and sometimes become large enough to require surgical decompression. Sedation and pain medication should be used only as necessary to maintain patient comfort. Sedatives should be short acting, so that an accurate neurologic exam can be obtained every 1–2 h. Once any necessary surgical intervention has been completed, and the patient's neurologic examination has stabilized, supportive care is necessary. The patient may require ventilatory and nutrition support, as well as physical therapy. Prognosis is variable, depending on the severity of the initial injury. GCS rating on admission along with head CT scan findings is most predictive of long-term outcome *(59)*.

Brain Death

One of the most difficult tasks facing the neurointensivist is declaring death by reason of cessation of cerebral function (*see also* Chapter 16). Most states consider brain death to be legally equivalent to death due to cardiopulmonary arrest, and have specific criteria for the diagnosis of brain death. A sample of brain death criteria is found in Table 2. Usually, two brain death exams need to be performed at least 6 h apart to declare death. However, in the case of patients who are hemodynamically unstable and unable to tolerate an apnea test, other confirmatory tests can be used. Transcranial Doppler, cerebral angiography, or nuclear medicine cerebral perfusion studies can confirm cessation of cerebral blood flow. Electroencephalography (EEG) can demonstrate a lack of cerebral electrical activity. Explaining brain death to a family can be the most daunting of tasks. It can be difficult to explain how a patient can be dead while retaining cardiac activity, and difficult to discuss the option of organ donation. It is often helpful to have a representative of the local organ procurement team present during these discussions. It is important, once the decision to donate organs is made, to support the patient as aggressively as possible, to maintain euvolemia and normal blood pressure. The patient may develop refractory diabetes insipidus requiring intravenous vasopressin, and may require pressor support to maintain perfusion to the heart, liver, and kidneys. The process of organ donation

Table 2
Sample Brain Death Criteria

I. Absence of brainstem reflexes
    a. Fixed pupils
    b. Absent corneal reflexes
    c. Absent oculocephalic reflexes
    d. Absent gag reflex
    e. Absent cough reflex
II. Apnea (No respiratory function despite serum $PCO_2 > 60$ mmHg)
III. No response to pain
IV. No complicating factors
    a. No hypothermia ($<32.2°C$)
    b. No significant hypotension (SBP< 90 mmHg)
    c. No intoxication with alcohol, sedatives, or paralytic
       medication

From Practice parameters for determining brain death in adults (summary statement). The Quality Standards Subcommittee of the American Academy of Neurology. *Neurology* 1995;45:1012–1014.

usually takes 10–16 h, and continuous aggressive support is often needed to maintain tissue perfusion during this time.

CONCLUSION

Care of patients in the NSU presents unique challenges to the caregivers. The rapidity with which neurologic injury can occur, and the devastating consequences of such injury, requires constant vigilance as well as diligence to perform timely evaluations and aggressive treatments. Many postoperative complications can be avoided, or their morbidity lessened, with quality neuroscience intensive care.

REFERENCES

1. Qureshi AI, Romergryko GG, Suarez JI, et al. Long term outcome after medical reversal of transtentorial herniation in patients with supratentorial mass lesions. *Crit. Care Med.* 2000;28:1556–1564.
2. Rosenberg H, Clofine R, Bialik O. Neurologic changes during awakening from anesthesia. *Anesthesiology* 1981;54:125–130.
3. Taylor WAS, Thomas NWM, Wellings JA, et al. Timing of postoperative intracranial hematoma development and implications for the best use of neurosurgical intensive care. *J. Neurosurg.* 1995;82:48–50.
4. Ram Z, Spiegelman R, Findler G, Hadani M. Delayed postoperative neurological deterioration from prolonged sodium nitroprusside administration. Case report. *J. Neurosurg.* 1989;71:605–607.
5. Qureshi AI, Suarez JI, Bhardwaj A, Yahia AM, Tamargo RJ, Ulatowski JA. Early predictors of outcome in patients receiving hypervolemic and hypertensive therapy for symptomatic vasospasm after subarachnoid hemorrhage. *Crit. Care Med.* 2000;28:824–829.
6. Tommasino C, Moore S, Todd MM. Cerebral effects of isovolemic hemodilution with crystalloid or colloid solutions. *Crit. Care Med.* 1988;16:862–868.
7. Sutin KM, Ruskin KJ, Kaufman BS. Intravenous fluid therapy in neurologic injury. *Crit. Care Clin.* 1992;8:367–408.
8. Morse ML, Milstein JM, Haas JE, Taylor E. Effect of hydration on experimentally induced cerebral edema. *Crit. Care Med.* 1985;13:563–565.
9. Smith SD, Cone JB, Bowser BH, Caldwell FT Jr. Cerebral edema following acute hemorrhage in a murine model: the role crystalloid resuscitation. *J. Trauma* 1982;22:588–590.
10. Berger S, Schurer L, Hartl R, Messmer K, Baethmann A. Reduction of post-traumatic intracranial hypertension by hypertonic/hyperoncotic saline/dextran and hypertonic mannitol. *Neurosurgery* 1995;37:98–107.
11. Andreoli A, Di Pasquale G, Pinelli G, et al. Subarachnoid hemorrhage: frequency and severity of cardiac arrhythmias. *Stroke* 1987;18:558–564.
12. Di Pasquale G, Andreoli A, Lusa AM, Urbinati S, Biancoli S, Cere E, Borgatti ML, Pinelli G. Cardiologic complications of subarachnoid hemorrhage. *J. Neurosurg. Sci.* 1998;42s:33–36.

13. Harries AD. Subarachnoid hemorrhage and the electrocardiogram: A review. *Postgrad. Med.* 1981;57:294–296.

14. Koh WY, Lew TW, Chin NM, et al. Tracheostomy in a neuro-intensive care setting: indications and timing. *Anaesth. Intensive Care* 1997;25:365–368.

15. Kluger Y, Paul DB, Lucke J, et al. Early tracheostomy in trauma patients. *Eur. J. Emerg. Med.* 1996;3:95–101.

16. Qureshi AI, Suarez JI, Parekh PD, et al. Prediction and timing of tracheostomy in patients with infratentorial lesions requiring mechanical ventilatory support. *Crit. Care Med.* 2000;28:1383–1387.

17. Cooper KR, Boswell PA, Choi SC. Safe use of PEEP in patients with severe head injury. *J. Neurosurg.* 1985;63:552–555.

18. Hagley MT, Martin B, Gast P, Traeger SM. Infectious and mechanical complications of central venous catheters placed by percutaneous venipuncture and over guidewires. *Crit. Care Med.* 1992;20:1426–1430.

19. Kaiser AB. Antimicrobial prophylaxis in surgery. *N. Engl. J. Med.* 1986;315:1129–1138.

20. Frame PT, Watanakunakorn C, McLaurin RL. Penetration of nafcillin, methicillin, and cefazolin into human brain tissue. *Neurosurgery* 1983;12:142–147.

21. Young RF, Lawner PM. Perioperative antibiotics for prevention of postoperative neurosurgical infection. *J. Neurosurg.* 1987;66:701–705.

22. Rebuck JA, Murry KR, Rhoney DH, Michael DB, Coplin WM.Infection related to intracranial pressure monitors in adults: analysis of riskfactors and antibiotic prophylaxis. *J. Neurol. Neurosurg. Psychiatry* 2000;69:381–384.

23. Kurz A, Sessler DI, Lenhardt R. Perioperative normothermia to reduce the incidence of surgical-wound infection and shorten hospitalization. Study of Wound Infection and Temperature Group. *N. Engl. J. Med.* 1996;334:1209–1215.

24. Knauth M, Aras N, Wirtz CR, Dorfler A, Engelhorn T, Sartor K. Surgically induced intracranial contrast enhancement: Potential source of diagnostic error in intraoperative MR imaging. *AJNR* 1999;20:1547–1553.

25. Kim YS, Pons VG.Infections in the neurosurgical intensive care unit. *Neurosurg. Clin. North Am.* 1994; 5:741–754.

26. Hlavin ML, Kaminski HJ, Ross JS, Ganz E. Spinal epidural abscess: A ten-year perspective. *Neurosurgery* 1990;27:177–184.

27. Russell NA, Vaughan R, Morley TP. Spinal epidural infection. *Can. J. Neurol. Sci.* 1979;6:325–328.

28. Carmel PW, Greif LK. The aseptic meningitis syndrome: A complication of posterior fossa surgery. *Pediatr Neurosurg.* 1993;19:276–280.

29. Forgacs P, Geyer CA, Freidberg SR. Characterization of chemical meningitis after neurological surgery. *Clin. Infect. Dis.* 2001;32:179–185.

30. Kroll M, Juhler M, Lindholm J. Hyponatraemia in acute brain disease. *J. Intern. Med.* 1992;232:291–297.

31. Harrigan MR. Cerebral salt wasting syndrome. *Crit. Care Clin.* 2001;17:125–138.

32. Lauriat SM, Berl T. The hyponatremic patient: practical focus on therapy. *J. Am. Soc. Nephrol.* 1997;8:1599–1607.

33. Ayus JC, Krothapalli RK, Arieff AI. Changing concepts in treatment of severe symptomatic hyponatremia. Rapid correction and possible relation to central pontine myelinolysis. *Am. J. Med.* 1985;78:897–902.

34. Thibonnier M. Antidiuretic hormone: regulation, disorders, and clinical evaluation. In: Barrow DL, Selman W, (eds). *Neuroendocrinology. Concepts in Neurosurgery*, vol. 5. Baltimore: Williams and Wilkins, 1992:19–30.

35. Hasan D, Lindsay KW, Wijdicks EF, Murray GD, Brouwers PJ, Bakker WH, van Gijn J, Vermeulen M. Effect of fludrocortisone acetate in patients with subarachnoid hemorrhage. *Stroke* 1989;20:1156–1161.

36. Black PM, Baker MF, Snook CP. Experience with external pneumatic calf compression in neurology and neurosurgery. *Neurosurgery* 1986;18:440–444.

37. Frim DM, Barker FG 2nd, Poletti CE, Hamilton AJ. Postoperative low-dose heparin decreases thromboembolic complications in neurosurgical patients. *Neurosurgery* 1992;30:830–832.

38. Lazio BE, Simard JM. Anticoagulation in neurosurgical patients. *Neurosurgery* 1999;45:838–847; discussion 847–848.

39. Goodnight SH, Kenoyer G, Rapaport SI, Patch MJ, Lee JA, Kurze T. Defibrination after brain-tissue destruction: A serious complication of head injury. *N. Engl. J. Med.* 1974;290:1043–1047.

40. Lu WY, Rhoney DH, Boling WB, Johnson JD, Smith TC. A review of stress ulcer prophylaxis in the neurosurgical intensive care unit. *Neurosurgery* 1997;41:416–425; discussion 425–426.

41. Cook DJ, Reeve BK, Guyatt GH, Heyland DK, Griffith LE, Buckingham L, Tryba M. Stress ulcer prophylaxis in critically ill patients. Resolving discordant meta-analyses. *JAMA* 1996;275:308–314.

42. Dunbar PJ, Visco E, Lam AM. Craniotomy procedures are associated with less analgesic requirements than other surgical procedures. *Anesth. Analg.* 1999;88:335–340.

43. Warme PE, Bergstrom R, Persson L. Neurosurgical intensive care improves outcome after severe head injury. *Acta. Neurochir. (Wien.)* 1991;110:57–64.

44. Bullock R, Chestnut RM, Clifton G, et al. Guidelines for the management of severe head injury. The Brain Trauma Foundation, the American Association of Neurological Surgeons, and the Joint Section of Neurotrauma and Critical Care. *J. Neurotrauma* 1996;13:641–734.

45. Rosner MJ, Rosner SD, Johnson AH. Cerebral perfusion pressure: Management protocol and clinical results. *J. Neurosurg.* 1995;83:949–962.

46. Kelly DF. Neurosurgical postoperative care. *Neurosurg. Clin. North Am.* 1994;5:789–810.

47. Treatment of convulsive status epilepticus. Recommendations of the Epilepsy Foundation of America's Working Group on Status Epilepticus. *JAMA* 1993;270:854–859.

48. Haltiner AM, Newell DW, Temkin NR, Dikmen SS, Winn HR. Side effects and mortality associated with use of phenytoin for early posttraumatic seizure prophylaxis. *J Neurosurg.* 1999;91:588–592.
49. Kassell NF, Sasaki T, Colohan AR, Nazar G. Cerebral vasospasm following aneurysmal subarachnoid hemorrhage. *Stroke* 1985;16:562–572.
50. Weir B, Grace M, Hansen J, Rothberg C. Time course of vasospasm in man. *J. Neurosurg.* 1978;48:173–178.
51. Barker FG 2nd, Ogilvy CS. Efficacy of prophylactic nimodipine for delayed ischemic deficit after subarachnoid hemorrhage: a metaanalysis. *J. Neurosurg.* 1996;84:405–414.
52. Kassell NF, Peerless SJ, Durward QJ, Beck DW, Drake CG, Adams HP. Treatment of ischemic deficits from vasospasm with intravascular volume expansion and induced arterial hypertension. *Neurosurgery* 1982;11:337–343.
53. Zubkov YN, Nikiforov BM, Shustin VA. Balloon catheter technique for dilatation of constricted cerebral arteries after aneurysmal SAH. *Acta. Neurochir. (Wien.)* 1984;70:65–79.
54. Spetzler RF, Wilson CB, Weinstein P, et al. Normal perfusion pressure breakthrough theory. *Clin. Neurosurg.* 1978;25:651–672.
55. Tarr RW, Johnson DW, Horton JA. Impaired cerebral vasoreactivity after embolization of arteriovenous malformations: assessment with serial acetazolamide challenge xenon CT. *Am. J. Neuroradiol.* 1991;12:417–423.
56. Klastersky J, Sadeghi M, Brihaye J. Antimicrobial prophylaxis in patients with rhinorrhea or otorrhea: a double-blind study. *Surg. Neurol.* 1976;6:111–114.
57. Dagi TF, George ED. Surgical management of cranial cerebrospinal fluid fistulas. In: Schmidek HH, Sweet WH, (eds). *Operative Neurosurgical Techniques*, 3rd ed., vol. 1. Philadelphia: WB Saunders, 1995:117–131.
58. Parizek J, Mericka P, Husek Z, Suba P, Spacek J, Nemecek S, Nemeckova J, Sercl M, Elias P. Detailed evaluation of 2959 allogeneic and xenogeneic dense connective tissue grafts (fascia lata, pericardium, and dura mater) used in the course of 20 years for duraplasty in neurosurgery. *Acta. Neurochir. (Wien.)* 1997;139:827–838.
59. Ono J, Yamaura A, Kubota M, Okimura Y, Isobe K. Outcome prediction in severe head injury: analyses of clinical prognosticfactors. *J. Clin. Neurosci.* 2001; 8:120–123.

25

Status Epilepticus

Dakshin Gullapalli and Thomas P. Bleck

INTRODUCTION

Status epilepticus (SE) is a life-threatening neurologic emergency with high mortality and morbidity. Although it was recognized many centuries ago, it was not until the middle of the nineteenth century that complications from continuous or prolonged seizures were first well described *(1)*. Initially these recurring convulsive seizures were called "etat de mal epileptique" referring to repeated generalized motor seizures *(2)*. Subsequently the term "status epilepticus" was used. Since then there have been numerous clinical descriptions and definitions of SE. Clinical research into this condition began an upsurge with Berger's invention of the electroencephalogram (EEG), and the recognition of seizure as a clinical manifestation or "outward manifestation of a disordered rhythm of brain potentials" *(3)*. Henri Gastaut led the first meeting devoted to status epilepticus in 1962 at the tenth Marseilles Colloquium. Over the past few decades, our understanding of SE has progressed through experimental and human research. The implications of prolonged seizures on the brain are increasingly understood. Progressive research into the neurochemical bases of SE has helped promote novel therapies to treat this life-threatening problem. Information obtained from recent experimental studies and antiepileptic drug trials recommend changes from the previous treatment algorithms and incorporation of new approaches in the management of SE patients. We will review the salient pathophysiologic, clinical, and therapeutic aspects of SE, which is a common entity in those patients admitted to the neurosciences critical care unit (NSU).

EPIDEMIOLOGY

SE accounts for 1–8% of all hospital admissions for epilepsy *(4)*, and in the United States is estimated to afflict between 50,000 and 152,000 patients per year *(4–6)*. As many as 50,000 deaths per year may be associated with this condition. Nonconvulsive status epilepticus (NCSE) is reported to be rare, although arguably under recognized, with an annual incidence of one per million for absence and 35 per million for complex partial SE *(5)*. Approximately 44% of adults admitted to an urban San Francisco hospital with status epilepticus had no history of seizures *(7)*. Between one-tenth and one-third of adults with new-onset seizures present with status epilepticus *(4,8)*. Age-related incidence of status epilepticus shows two peaks, the first at less than 1 yr of age and the second in adulthood *(6)*.

CLASSIFICATION AND DEFINITIONS

Recurrent or continuous seizures can occur with any seizure type. Categories of SE include generalized convulsive, simple partial, myoclonic, and nonconvulsive (NCSE). However, the term *status*

From: *Current Clinical Neurology*
Critical Care Neurology and Neurosurgery
Edited by: J. I. Suarez © Humana Press Inc., Totowa, NJ

epilepticus generally refers to generalized convulsive seizures, unless otherwise specified. NCSE encompasses multiple seizure types including absence, complex partial, and atonic. Kaplan proposes classifying NCSE into three broad categories as follows: NCSE of generalized epilepsies, NCSE of localization-related epilepsies (subclassified based on EEG features), and undetermined form of NCSE *(2)*.

There has been debate regarding the definition of SE. In the 1962 Marseilles conference SE was defined as an "enduring epileptic state" *(9)*. The International League against Epilepsy defined it as a seizure persisting for sufficient length of time to produce such an enduring state, or repeated seizures occurring frequently without recovery between attacks *(10)*. Subsequent definition of SE as seizures lasting 20–30 min was related to the approximate time needed to result in cerebral injury *(5,11,12)*. For a long time, this definition of 30 min of continuous seizure activity or repetitive seizures without recovery between them has been used in studies and treating patients. However, this definition causes some practical difficulties with management, because aggressive management specific to SE cannot be delayed for 20–30 min in order to achieve success and prevent brain injury. Control of SE becomes progressively difficult with time. A typical secondarily generalized tonic-clonic seizure generally stops by 3 min and almost always by 5 min *(13)*. These seizures may last somewhat longer in children, but a seizure in a child that has lasted 12 min is unlikely to terminate spontaneous within the next 30 min *(13a)*. Prolonged or repetitive seizures reach a point when they are unlikely to end spontaneously. Any seizure that is prolonged is capable of causing brain injury. Hence, defining SE should be based on knowledge about the timing of neuronal damage in relation to a prolonged seizure type and the point at which a seizure has less chance of ending spontaneously. In view of these reasons, subsequent operational definitions suggested "seizure lasting more than five to seven minutes or recurrent seizures with poor recovery of consciousness between attacks irrespective of duration" *(13–16)*. This lack of uniform definition may generate variable results in outcome studies.

PATHOPHYSIOLOGY

There are mechanisms within the brain to stop an ongoing seizure. However, in SE, these mechanisms are lost resulting in persistent seizure activity. This occurs either due to increased neuronal excitatory state *(17)* or loss of normal inhibitory pathways. A number of recent advances have helped our understanding of the pathophysiology of SE *(18,19)*. Also information on the role of neuroanatomic structures in the development of SE is improving. However, there are many unanswered questions. We will summarize some of these advances.

Experimentally, induction of reverberating seizure activity between cerebral sites has been shown *(20,21)*. Also, some excitatory neurotransmitters have been implicated as playing a major role in SE including glutamate, aspartate, and acetylcholine with the main inhibitory neurotransmitter being γ-aminobutyric acid (GABA) *(22)*. N-methyl-D-aspartate (NMDA) linked calcium channels appear to be particularly involved in the pathogenesis of SE *(17)*. Dantrolene, a muscle relaxant, has been shown to be effective in reducing release of calcium pool induced by NMDA receptor activation and thus may have a role in neuroprotection in SE *(23)*. The first evidence supporting increased excitatory state in humans was recognized during an outbreak of toxic encephalopathy with SE after ingestion of mussels contaminated with domoic acid (an analogue of glutamic acid, which is the principal excitatory amino acid in the brain) *(24,25)*. Experimentally both NMDA and non-NMDA receptor antagonists control SE. Reduction of redox sites has been proposed as a mechanism in increasing endogenous potentiation of NMDA receptor function that can facilitate epileptogenesis and SE *(19)*. Another important piece of information is the fact that proconvulsants like penicillin can precipitate SE by inhibiting the inhibitory neurotransmitter GABA *(20)*. Inhibition of GABA-A receptors, which are postsynaptic ionotropic receptors linked to chloride channels, can cause SE. Several experimental drugs such as bicucullin, picrotoxin, and pentylenetetrazol are inhibitors of GABA-A receptors capable of precipitating SE. Anticonvulsants like benzodiazepines and phenobarbital act through GABA-A receptors to terminate SE. The role of GABA-B receptors, which are postsynaptic metabotropic receptors linked to G protein, in SE is unclear. There are data to support that prolonged seizure activity would also tend to alter the functional properties of GABA-A receptors causing failure of inhibition of seizure activity *(26)*. Moreover, there is some evidence that heat shock proteins are induced during SE, which may have some protective role *(22)*.

Cerebral injury occurs from prolonged seizures independent of systemic disturbances *(27–29)*. Pathological changes are seen after an episode of SE, and although the underlying mechanisms are not completely understood at this time, they are beginning to be elucidated. This primary neuronal injury appears to be secondary to excitotoxicity through glutamate and increased metabolic demands from excessive neuronal activity. Glutamate binds to the NMDA receptors allowing calcium entry into the cell, which in turn activates proteases and lipases and these along with intracellular second messenger systems cause mitochondrial dysfunction and cell death. The upregulation of glial metabotropic glutamate receptors has been proposed as a mechanism in the SE-induced epileptogenesis *(19)*. Recently, nerve growth factor and other neurotrophins have been suggested as having specific protective role against excitotoxic cell stress *(18)*. Susceptibility for neuronal injury is less in younger patients. A possible explanation for better outcome in younger individuals with SE is less calcium accumulation demonstrated in immature animal brain *(18)*. Serine proteases are thought to play a role in glial sclerosis, brain edema, seizures and neuronal death after acute brain insult including SE *(19)*. Zinc is shown to have a role in seizure spread and predisposition of certain brain areas to seizure induction *(18)*. Neuronal injury can be prevented if SE is controlled promptly. In addition, effects of secondary systemic influences in the form of hyperthermia, hypoxia, and hypotension contribute to the neuronal insult *(30–32)*.

Lothman very well described the sequential clinical, biochemical, electrophysiological, and systemic changes that occur during the course of SE (Table 1) *(17)*. During the initial phases, recurrent isolated or continuous clinical seizures are accompanied by discrete electrographic seizures. There is evidence for sympathetic overactivity with raised blood pressure. Blood lactate and glucose concentrations increase with reduced pH secondary to metabolic acidosis and some times secondary to respiratory acidosis. Brain parenchymal oxygenation is impaired during seizure. At this stage, brain glucose metabolism, oxygen utilization and cerebral blood flow (CBF) increase acutely because of increased metabolic demand. Brain lactate levels are also increased. Despite these changes, no significant brain injury is notable in these initial stages. However, with persistence of SE beyond 30–60 min, clinical seizure manifestations become subtle, resembling focal myoclonic twitches followed by complete disappearance of motor manifestations despite persistence of ongoing electrographic seizures akin to electromechanical dissociation in the heart. On the electroencephalogram (EEG), discrete seizures are seen initially corresponding to the clinical seizures. Subsequently, merging electrographic seizures followed by continuous ictal activity is seen. With time, either periodic lateralizing epileptiform discharges (PLEDS) or continuous epileptiform activity interrupted by flat periods is seen *(32)*. Hypotension sets in along with persistent systemically increased lactate, hypoglycemia, hyperthermia and respiratory compromise. Cerebral autoregulation is impaired with decreased CBF related to systemic hypotension. Cerebral glucose and oxygenation are also reduced *(33)*. Brain lactate concentration falls during and after prolonged SE. Brain damage occurs progressively with persistence of seizures. Cerebral edema occurs due to vasogenic causes with prolonged seizures. This in turn compromises CBF and contributes to further brain injury in the face of increased metabolic demands, systemic hypotension, hypoxia and disregulated cerebral autoregulation. Similar evidence for brain injury is reported in animal experimental studies of NCSE. However, there is considerable debate on the risk of brain injury from NCSE in humans *(34)*.

Table 1
Sequential Changes Occurring During the Course of Status Epilepticus

	Early SE: initiation phase	Late SE: self-sustaining phase
Clinical manifestations	Generalized convulsions	Subtle motor manifestations; myoclonus
EEG manifestations	Discrete seizures	Continuous seizures; recurrent seizures; periodic discharges
Systemic effects	↑ BP, lactate, pH, temp, glucose, catecholamines	BP, lactate, pH normal or ↓; glusose ↓; rhabdomyolysis
CNS effects	↑ cerebral blood flow and parenchymal oxygenation	Cerebral blood flow inadequate for demand
Brain damage	subtle	Significant and may increase with seizure duration
Spontaneous remission	25% lasting 5 min or more stop spontaneously	7% lasting > 30 min stop spontaneously
Treatment	GABA agonist usually terminate seizures	GABA agonists often fail; NMDA antagonists more effective (?)
30-d mortality	2.6% for seizures between 10 and 29 min	27.8% for seizures > 30 min

From Lothman EW. The biochemical basis and pathophysiology of status epilepticus. *Neurology* 1990;40:Suppl 2:13–23.

COMPLICATIONS

SE is associated with the following multiple neurologic and systemic complications, which contribute to mortality and morbidity:

Cerebral

Cerebral injury from seizures
Cerebral anoxia/hypoxia
Cerebral edema
Cerebral venous thrombosis
Intracranial hemorrhage

Cardiovascular

Arrhythmias
Impaired contractility
Hypertension/hypotension

Respiratory

Hypopnea/apnea
Respiratory failure
Aspiration pneumonia
Pulmonary edema
Pulmonary hypertension

Metabolic

Metabolic/respiratory acidosis
Electrolyte disturbances
Hepatic dysfunction
Pancreatitis
Acute tubular necrosis and renal failure
Dehydration

Other

Rhabdomyolysis and myoglobinuria
Disseminated intravascular coagulation
Fractures
Hyperthermia
Infections

Many of these complications can occur simultaneously and interact to lead to brain damage. Hypoxia may result from impaired ventilation, increased upper respiratory secretions, aspiration, and increased oxygen demands. Cerebral and systemic hypoxia is the primary mechanism for many complications from SE. Hypoxia is associated directly or indirectly with reduced adenosine triphosphate, brain glucose *(35)*, high brain lactate concentration, and low intracellular pH *(36)*. Hypoxia in conjunction with seizures and acidosis causes disturbances of cardiac contractility with reduced output and hypotension, which further compromises neuronal and tissue cellular function. About half of patients may have potentially fatal cardiac dysrhythmias *(37)*. Metabolic acidosis is primarily due to impaired tissue oxygenation in the face of increased metabolic demands. Respiratory acidosis also common and may be due to impaired ventilation from convulsive seizures, aspiration, and excess production of carbon dioxide from increased metabolic activity. Myoglobinuria from rhabdomyolysis secondary to repeated convulsions could lead to acute tubular necrosis and acute renal failure. Patients with SE are also prone to respiratory failure either from aspiration due to poor airway protection or neurogenic pulmonary edema. Raised intracranial pressure may also occur from increased CBF, loss of cerebral autoregulation, acidosis, vasogenic edema, and possibly from the underlying causes such as tumor, infection and stroke. SE-associated cytotoxic edema has also been demonstrated on the brain with magnetic resonance imaging (MRI) *(38)*.

CLINICAL MANIFESTATIONS

Recognizing convulsive SE is not difficult unlike NCSE. As discussed previously, patients with SE have level of consciousness ranging from impaired responsiveness to deep comatose state between convulsions. Initially these patients show either continuous or repeated generalized tonic-clonic seizures. Subsequently, the seizures are not obvious and become subtle in the form of focal twitches of either extremities, face or nystagmoid jerks *(39,40)*. With persistent SE, clinical manifestations of seizures gradually become less perceptible with continuation of electrical seizure activity and require EEG monitoring to be recognized *(40)*. This, electroclinical dissociation should be always considered in cases of poor recovery of responsiveness after control of clinical seizures. The possibility of electrical seizures without clinical seizure manifestations was recognized to be more common than was originally thought in intensive care unit (ICU) patients *(41)*. Similarly, it is mandatory to perform EEG monitoring in patients who have received neuromuscular junction blockers for intubation during treatment of status epilepticus for these patients can no longer manifest clinical motor aspects of seizures.

Diagnosis of NCSE is intriguing because of varied clinical features. Diagnosis is difficult and delayed because of ambiguous clinical features and varied underlying causes *(42)*. Almost all patients need EEG for confirmation of diagnosis. In many, the diagnosis may be an incidental finding on EEG. In one study 8% of patients referred for evaluation of coma had evidence of NCSE *(43)*.

Table 2
Etiology of Status Epilepticus

Cause	%
AED noncompliance	26
Ethanol related	24
Drug toxicity	10
CNS infection	8
Refractory epilepsy	5
Trauma	5
Tumor	6
Stroke	4
Metabolic	4
Anoxia	4
Other	4

Adapted from Lowenstein DH. Status epilepticus: An overview of the clinical problem. *Epilepsia* 1999;40(Suppl 1):S3–S8.

Complex partial SE patients clinically show fluctuation of level of consciousness between confusional states, periods of staring, automatisms to complete unresponsiveness *(2,44)*. The proposed diagnostic criteria for NCSE include (1) period of behavioral change from baseline, (2) EEG evidence of epileptic activity, and (3) response to antiepileptic medication *(2)*. No single EEG pattern is typical for complex partial SE, except for lateralization of epileptiform activity at onset *(2)*. EEG patterns could include recurrent focal spikes, spike and wave, or spike and slow wave discharges *(1)*. Complex partial NCSE generally occurs in people with prior history of epilepsy and that occurring de novo suggests underlying structural brain pathology *(2)*. There is a lack of clarity on the potential of NCSE of complex partial seizures for cerebral injury *(45)*. Recent evidence suggests that recurrent complex partial seizures (but not absence status) can result in brain injury in animal experiments if sufficiently prolonged, but human morbidity secondary to direct brain injury from NCSE is debated and argued to rather be due to comorbidity *(34)*.

Absence NCSE occurs as a part of a generalized epileptic syndrome. Similar to complex partial NCSE, clinical features may vary in depth and diversity. In absence SE, the EEG shows continuous bursts of bilaterally synchronous, symmetric rhythmic or arrhythmic 3-Hz spike and waves (some times the frequency can vary from 2 to 6 Hz) *(46)*. The EEG patterns can vary from moment to moment or between episodes.

Finally, simple partial SE is rare. It can present with behavioral symptomatology (fear, depression, anger), oculovisual features (epileptic nystagmus, visual hallucinations), vegetative problems (rising epigastric sensation), language disturbances, or focal muscle twitches *(2)*. The origin of epilepsia partialis continua is controversial, but there is some evidence to support cortical origin *(18)*.

CAUSES OF STATUS EPILEPTICUS

SE can occur either due to an overwhelming acute insult to the brain or in situations with prior underlying chronic brain injury with superimposed acute processes. SE can be precipitated de novo in patients with no history of seizures due to acute metabolic or structural injury to the brain (Table 2). Antiepileptic noncompliance or withdrawal is by far the most common precipitating cause of SE, followed by alcohol-related SE. Acute electrolyte disturbances, renal failure, sepsis, neuroinfections, stroke, toxicity from medications, hypoxic conditions, and head trauma are also among the common causes of SE. These latter acute insults are associated with poorer outcome and are usually difficult to treat *(7,48)*. On the other hand, SE in patients with preexisting epilepsy occur usually due to poor compliance of tapering of medications. In this situation and in other etiologies including ethanol abuse, cerebral tumors, late epilepsy following strokes, there is usually good response to treatment. The leading causes in children include infection, congenital malformation, anoxia, metabolic dysfunction and tapering or discontinuation of antiepileptics.

MANAGEMENT

The following discussion of management applies to SE of generalized motor seizure type. The management of complex partial NCSE is also similar because of the potential for brain injury. However, absence NCSE is approached less aggressively. There is no data to support that simple partial status epilepticus causes significant injury. Less vigorous efforts are also recommended since these seizures are remarkably resistant to treatment and efforts to completely abolish them generally result in medication-induced side effects.

There are five principles of management of SE as follows: general supportive care, termination of SE, prevention of recurrence of seizures, correction of precipitating causes, and prevention and treatment of complications. Aggressiveness of treatment should reflect the seriousness of brain injury and systemic complications with prolonged convulsive SE. Early initiation of therapy is critical for a favorable outcome. This is especially difficult in situations wherein the SE occurs outside of hospital. Emergency personal must be trained to recognize and initiate the treatment as soon as possible. Initiation of the protocols for the management is generally not difficult in hospital setting, especially if the patient is in the NSU.

General Supportive Care

Initial therapy does not differ significantly from general principals of any emergency medical condition in the way of airway, breathing, and circulation (ABCs). There are, however, some special precautions and difficulties specific to SE. Airway management is very critical to avoid hypoxia, which may exacerbate the adverse effects of SE. To further complicate the situation, airway management is particularly difficult in patients with ongoing seizures. In those patients with spontaneous adequate breathing, airway patency should be maintained by either oral or nasopharyngeal devices supplemented by 100% oxygen. The practice of tongue blade and oral padding has fortunately fallen out of vogue. Intubation with mechanical ventilation is required in those with evidence of respiratory compromise. This should be undertaken even before respiratory compromise once the decision is made to treat with high-dose benzodiazepines, barbiturates or anesthetic agents, which tend to cause respiratory depression. Patients with SE generally need neuromuscular blocking agents to facilitate intubation. It is important to remember to use very short acting neuromuscular blocker (e.g., vecuronium, 0.1 mg/kg) during intubation, as this would lead to cessation of motor activity, making difficult to follow seizure activity clinically. One can consider reversing the neuromuscular blockade with neostigmine (50–70 µg/kg). Use of succinylcholine for neuromuscular paralysis should be avoided due to the risk of severe hyperkalemia associated with this drug in neurologic patients.

Secure intravenous access is essential for blood draws, management of fluid and electrolyte states and for administration of medications. Cardiac monitoring is important to recognize and treat potentially life-threatening arrhythmias, a common occurrence in these patients. If patients are hypotensive, physicians should begin volume replacement and consider vasoactive agents. On the other hand, if patients are hypertensive, it is wise to withhold controlling the blood pressure, since termination of SE usually corrects it. Besides, most medications used in SE are associated with systemic hypotension. With prolonged SE, NSU admission is essential. In cases of severe hypotension and neurogenic pulmonary edema, central venous access may become necessary for fluid management. If blood glucose measurements are unavailable, 50 mL of 50% dextrose (or 1 mL/kg) along with thiamine 100 mg should be administered intravenously because hypoglycemia is a common precipitant of seizures. Hypoglycemia can also occur as a complication of prolonged seizures. Maintenance intravenous fluids should be administered to avoid dehydration.

Routine laboratory workup should include complete blood cell count, blood chemistries including serum glucose, electrolytes, liver and renal function tests, arterial blood gas analysis, determination of serum anticonvulsant concentration, urine analysis, and toxicology. Treatment, however, should not be delayed waiting for these results. Abnormalities of the tests would help in understanding the underlying etiology and identifying complications of SE. Clinical history and examination findings would, in a similar way, help elucidate the underlying precipitating factors. Head CT scanning would exclude major underlying structural lesions of the brain accounting for the seizures. Lumbar puncture should always be considered as infections of the central nervous system (CNS) can lead to SE.

The role of EEG in the management of SE cannot be understated. An EEG is imperative in those without improving responsiveness, in those receiving neuromuscular blocking agents, and in patients with refractory SE. Persistent electrographic seizures without clinical manifestation after control of visible signs were seen in 20% of the patients in the VA cooperative study *(49)* and in approx half in the study by DeLorenzo et al *(50)*. NSUs are generally equipped with facilities for continuous EEG monitoring.

Termination of Status Epilepticus and Prevention of Recurrence of Seizures

Anticonvulsants should be used with the goal of termination of both clinical and electrographic seizures. Selection of anticonvulsant is usually based on ease of administration, speed of action, efficacy, and side effect profile. None of the currently available anticonvulsants have the properties of an ideal anticonvulsant for SE. Most of these tend to cause cardiorespiratory disturbances. In many situations, timing, route and adequacy of the medications are more important than the choice of the drug. Early initiation of treatment is crucial in managing these patients. Animal and human experiments show that seizures in SE become progressively refractory to anticonvulsants with increasing duration *(51)*. In an experimental model, SE induced by lithium and pilocarpine, the dose of diazepam required to control seizure more than doubled after the second seizure, compared to the dose required following the first seizure *(52)*. Lowenstein and Alldredge showed that SE can be terminated in 80% of patients if treatment was begun within 30 min of onset vs less than 40% success if treatment was delayed for 2 h or more *(7)*.

The intramuscular route cannot be relied upon for drug administration in SE due to erratic bioavailability, unpredictable serum concentration, and delayed effect. Drugs should be given intravenously. However, in critical situations and in children, rectal route can be used as an alternative for diazepam, paraldehyde, thiopental and valproate to achieve adequate serum concentration *(53)*. Midazolam given buccal route was also shown to be effective in controlling acute recurrent seizures *(54)*. Various anticonvulsants and anesthetic agents are effective in the management of SE (Table 3).

Benzodiazepines

Lorazepam has smaller area of distribution due to lower lipid solubility and longer duration of action than diazepam. These are distinct advantages of the former over the latter. The slight delay in brain uptake of lorazepam compared to diazepam is not clinically significant. It is metabolized by the liver into an inactive metabolite. There is no significant difference in the respiratory depression between the two drugs *(55)*. Lorazepam should be diluted in an equal volume of the solution vehicle, as it is very viscous. Diazepam can be given rectally. This is especially useful in children with recurrent seizures or status epilepticus. Given this route, however, the bioavailability is less than intravenous administration. Midazolam is also highly lipophilic and rapidly metabolized by the liver and hence has a very short half-life requiring continuous infusion rather than single bolus doses. Continuous intravenous administration has been shown to be successful in refractory SE *(56)*. Like other benzodiazepines, tolerance develops requiring titration of the dose. Cardiovascular depression is relatively less common compared to barbiturates. Side effects related to benzodiazepines include impaired consciousness (20–60%), hypotension (<2%), and respiratory depression (3–10%) *(55–58)*.

Table 3
Antiepileptic Medications Used in the Management of Status Epilepticus

Drug	Route	Loading dose (mg/kg)	Maintenance dose
Diazepam	IV, ET	0.2–0.5 at 2–4 mg/min	None
Lorazepam	IV, ET	0.05–0.1 at 2 mg/min	9 mg/h
Midazolam	IV	0.05–2 at <4 mg/min	0.75–10 µg/kg/min
Phenytoin	IV	18–20 at 50 mg/min or 1 mg/kg/min	5 mg/kg/d
Fosphenytoin	IV	18–20 at 150 mg/min or 3 mg/kg/min	None
Phenobarbital	IV	15–20 at 2 mg/kg/min or 50–75 mg/min	1–4 mg/kg/h
Thiopental	IV	12 mg over seconds	250 mg/min
Pentobarbital	IV	5–12 at 0.2–0.4 mg/kg/min or over 1 h	0.5–5 mg/kg/h
Etomidate	IV	0.3	30 mg/s
Propofol	IV	2–5 mg/kg	1–15 mg/kg/h
Paraldehyde	IM, PR	60–150 or 0.07–0.35 mL/kg (1 g/mL)	1 mg/min
Lidocaine	IV, ET	2–3 mg/kg at <50 mg/min	1–3 mg/kg/h or 100 mg/min
Valproate	IV	20–40 at 3–6 mg/kg/min	—
Isoflurane	Inhalant	—	—
Ketamine	IV	? 1–4.5 mg/kg	10–50 µg/kg/min

Phenytoin

Phenytoin is lipid soluble. Parenteral forms contain 40% propylene glycol, 10% ethanol, and sodium hydroxide with pH 12. It has unpredictable and poor absorption when given intramuscularly and rectally. Peak brain concentration of phenytoin reaches about 6 minutes from completion of infusion *(59)*. Because the infusion of the loading dose takes approx 20–25 min, clinical effect may not be seen until after its completion. Phenytoin is metabolized in the liver by hydroxylation. Cardiovascular risks with loading doses of phenytoin are hypotension and cardiac arrhythmias *(60,61)*. These are due to both phenytoin itself and the diluent (propylene glycol) used in the preparation of the parenteral form; slowing or stopping the infusion generally corrects these complications *(61)*. Phenytoin infusion also carries the risk of subcutaneous extravasation, especially with poor intravenous access, which can lead to thrombophlebitis and soft tissue necrosis.

Fosphenytoin

Fosphenytoin is a water-soluble prodrug of phenytoin, the phosphate ester group of which is rapidly removed by phosphatases once it is in the blood stream. It does not require propylene glycol and ethanol diluent at pH 12, as required for phenytoin. Fosphenytoin can be given at a faster intravenous rate (150 mg/min) than phenytoin. Taking into consideration for its conversion to phenytoin, free phenytoin level of 2 µg/mL is achieved in 15 min. Fosphenytoin is distributed in phenytoin equivalent doses, hence no calculations are required in converting the dose from phenytoin. The advantages with fosphenytoin, when used as a loading dose alternative to phenytoin, include faster rate infusion, no requirement for dextrose solution as vehicle of infusion, and fewer infusion-site reactions. At the recommended rates of administrations, incidence of hypotension requiring intervention is uncommon (1% for fosphenytoin and 9% for phenytoin) *(62)*. Infusion site reactions are significantly reduced with fosphenytoin (86% for phenytoin vs 11% with fosphenytoin) except for increased pruritis (49%) compared with phenytoin (5%). Another advantage of fosphenytoin is the ability to be given intramuscularly, but the peak plasma concentrations would take 1–2 h. Although it is more expensive, it is suggested to be cost effective in the treatment of acute seizures *(63)*.

Phenobarbital

Phenobarbital is lipophilic reaching therapeutic brain concentration in 3 min following administration and much faster during seizure activity *(64)*. Half-life of phenobarbital ranges from 50 to 150 h after a loading dose with a wide range of serum concentration obtained after this bolus *(65)*. Sedation, hypotension and respiratory depression are common side effects following a loading dose. Dose adjustments are required in patients with hepatic or renal failure. The recommended loading dose of phenobarbital is 20 mg/kg to be given at a rate of 50–75 mg/min.

Thiopental and Pentobarbital

Thiopental is a much faster acting barbiturate with peak brain concentration obtained within 30 s. Like phenytoin, extravasation into subcutaneous tissue during infusion can cause tissue necrosis. Because of the high lipophilic nature of the drug, it tends to accumulate in the fatty tissues when given for long periods resulting in delayed clearance. It is metabolized in the liver to pentobarbital, which is an active anticonvulsant. Rare hypersensitivity reactions can occur once in 30,000 people. It tends to cause significant hypotension and respiratory depression and hence the need for pressor agents and intubation with mechanical ventilation. Pentobarbital has a shorter half-life. It is a much more preferred barbiturate anesthetic due to fewer side effects compared to thiopental.

Propofol

Propofol is a very short-acting intravenous anesthetic, highly lipid soluble, metabolized in the liver and requires continuous infusion. It is originally approved for rapid inductions and maintenance of anesthesia. It is a GABA-A receptor agonist with additional possible mechanisms of action. Prolonged administration can result in marked hyperlipidemia, metabolic acidosis, and Gram-negative sepsis.

Other Medications

Isoflurane is a volatile anesthetic, eliminated through ventilation. The advantages with this drug are little risk of hepatotoxicity, less cardiac suppression, although hypotension may develop, which requires pressors. Finally, Isoflurane is safe in patients with porphyria, where most other medications are contraindicated. However, the use of this anesthetic requires facilities for inhalational anesthesia and gas scavenging in the NSUs. Etomidate is an intravenous anesthetic agent shown to be effective in controlling refractory status epilepticus *(66)*. However, it causes adrenal suppression after prolonged administration, requiring corticosteroid supplementation. Paraldehyde is a cyclic polymer of paraldehyde with a foul odor and unpleasant taste. It is metabolized in the liver but approx one third is excreted by the lungs. Its advantages are that it can be given rectally, intramuscularly or intravenously, but it is not freely available in the United States. Paraldehyde has to be used only in glass syringes as it reacts with plastic and rubber, and cannot be exposed to light to prevent conversion to acetic acid. Lidocaine is a short acting anticonvulsant in the recommended doses, but can be proconvulsant in higher doses. The advantages are lower risk of cardiorespiratory depression or sedation. Ketamine, generally used as general (dissociative) anesthesia, also appears to be effective in the treatment of SE. The optimum dose in refractory SE is uncertain. The anesthetic doses are 1–4.5 mg/kg with supplements of 0.5–2.5 mg/kg every 30–45 min or 10–50 μg/kg/min.

Recently a parenteral form of valproate was introduced. Valproate has broader antiepileptic activity with efficacy in several seizure types. Given its broad antiepileptic activity, ease of administration, lack of significant cardiorespiratory depression, and less sedation, it can be a very useful alternative in the treatment of SE.

Medication Selection

Based on the recent evidence from antiepileptic trials, there is a need for change in the approach to the drug selection and treatment algorithm for SE (Fig. 1). Algorithmic approach appears to result in better clinical outcome in these patients *(67)*.

For a long time intravenous diazepam was the first drug of choice in SE. In the past few years, it has been replaced by lorazepam as preferred first drug because of its relative longer duration of action (12–24 h for lorazepam vs 15–30 min for diazepam). However, both drugs were shown to have equal speed of action (2 min for diazepam vs 3 min for lorazepam) and efficacy (79% with diazepam vs 89% for lorazepam) *(55)*. Lack of response to lorazepam after 5 min of administration, is usually considered a failure. There is no substantial evidence to support repeating the dose if the first dose fails. Outside the hospital setting, rectal diazepam appears to be safe and an effective choice, especially for serial repetitive seizures in children *(68)*. Following benzodiazepine administration, follow up with another anticonvulsant with prolonged duration of action is required to prevent recurrence of seizures. Generally phenytoin is the preferred second line of drug in SE.

The VA Status Epilepticus Cooperative Study has addressed very essential elements of drug selection in the initial treatment of SE *(49)*. In this study, patients were divided into "overt" and subtle" SE. Subtle SE patients had less intense clinically obvious convulsive activity, and these patients responded poorly to therapy, irrespective of the drug choice. The "overt SE" group, where the clinical seizures were obvious, were randomized into lorazepam (0.1 m/kg) alone, diazepam (0.15 mg/kg) followed by phenytoin (18 mg/kg), phenytoin alone, and phenobarbital (15 mg/kg) alone. Successful treatment was defined as complete cessation of clinical and electrographic seizures within 20 min of therapy. Patients failing the first drug were given a second drug choice, and if necessary, a third choice. The success rates are presented in Table 4. There were no statistically significant differences among the different drugs, except for significantly better outcome with lorazepam over phenytoin. Similarly lorazepam was shown to be effective in termination of seizures in 85% of SE in another study *(55)*. However, in this study only clinical cessation of seizures were taken into consideration. VA study indicated that approx 20% of patients with clinical control of seizures were shown to have ongoing electrographic seizures *(49)*.

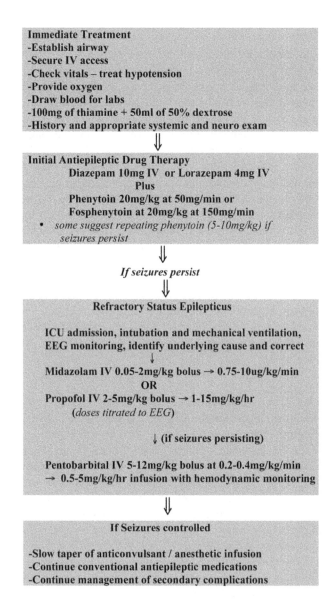

Fig. 1. Suggested treatment of status epilepticus in adults.

Preliminary data from the VA trial reportedly showed that if one drug fails, successful termination of SE becomes progressively difficult with the subsequent choice of drugs (Table 5) *(69)*. However, the consensus among many neurologists is to try phenytoin or fosphenytoin as a second line drug. The advantage of this approach is that if SE can be controlled with this second drug, one can avoid intubation and prolonged NSU admission. On the other hand, since phenytoin infusion and its maximal effect takes approx 20–25 min (12–15 min in the case of fosphenytoin), it may delay a more aggressive and likely effective treatment. Physicians should use clinical judgment in deciding between these alternatives, depending on the clinical situation and knowledge of the likelihood of response of SE to therapy. An example would be the situation in which SE has begun outside of hospital setting with several minutes or hours elapsed before definitive treatment is initiated, which dimin-

Table 4
Treatment Results for First-Line Agents in the VA Cooperative Study

Agent	Overt SE success rate (%)	Subtle SE success rate (%)
Lorazepam	64.9	17.9
Phenobarbital	58.2	24.2
Diazepam + phenytoin	55.8	8.3
Phenytoin alone	43.6	7.7

ishes the chance of responsiveness of SE to conventional drugs. The recommended loading dose of phenytoin is 20 mg/kg infused at a rate of 50 mg/min to avoid cardiac side effects. Maximal clinical effect following a loading dose takes approx 20–25 min from the start of infusion (infusion takes approx 30 min in an individual weighing 75 kg) *(70)*. This time reflects time required for maximal brain concentrations *(60)*. With the advent of fosphenytoin, water-soluble prodrug of phenytoin, some of the complications associated with phenytoin loading are reduced. However, cost of fosphenytoin is few times more than phenytoin, but the associated convenience in administration, fewer complications appear to offset the higher price, as mentioned previously.

Phenobarbital traditionally was considered after phenytoin in SE *(71)*. However, the unpublished data from the VA study suggest less likelihood of a third conventional antiepileptic drug being effective if the first two drugs fail *(69)*. Moreover, phenobarbital tends to cause cardiorespiratory and CNS depression, which is more common after an initial benzodiazepine administration *(72)*.

After the recent development of a parenteral form, there is emerging evidence for an important role of valproate in SE. There is some experimental data to suggest that a serum concentration of 250 μg may be required in SE *(73)*. Doses of 20–40 mg/kg given at 3–6 mg/kg/min may achieve these concentrations while effectively controlling SE and eliminating the respiratory and cardiovascular depression of most other antiepileptics *(69,74,75)*. In one study of 41 children with persistent SE despite a trial of one of the first-line anticonvulsants (diazepam, phenytoin, phenobarbital), administration of valproate with a loading dose of 20–40 mg/kg given over 1–5 min followed by intravenous infusion of 5 mg/kg/h, resulted in control of SE in 78% of patients *(76)*. It was well tolerated with no significant systemic or local side effects. It appears to be safe in the elderly even with cardiovascular instability and hypotension. However, in a recent review of the literature on the role of valproate in SE, the authors concluded that there is limited data to support its use as a first-line drug in SE, but can be considered as third- or fourth-line medication if others have failed or are contraindicated *(77)*.

At this stage, if patients continue to have seizures, SE should be considered refractory and one or more aggressive therapies should be planned.

Refractory Status Epilepticus

SE not responding to the initial two or more anticonvulsants should be considered refractory and aggressive approach is required. These patients are generally in coma, have respiratory and cardiovascular compromise, and have associated systemic complications. Hence, these individuals are best managed in an NSU setting, as these therapies, although effective in controlling seizures, frequently are associated with significant cardiovascular and respiratory compromise and risk of infections. Patients should be intubated with mechanical ventilation for adequate ventilation as well as protection of airway. Hypotension should be corrected and some patients will need central line placement for hemodynamic monitoring. Chest radiography, urine output, routine blood cell counts, and chemistries should be monitored to detect and treat systemic complications. Once patients reach the stage of refractory SE, following the clinical seizures become difficult and continuous EEG monitoring is required both to identify ongoing electrographic seizures and to adjust anticonvulsant dosing. Agents

Table 5
Response to Treatment

	Overt SE	Subtle SE
% Responding to	$N = 384$	$N = 134$
First agent	55.5	14.9
Second agent	7.0	3.0
Third agent	2.3	4.5
Any other agent	23.2	27.6
Not responding	11.7	50.0

available in the treatment of refractory SE include high dose barbiturates (pentobarbital, thiopental, and phenobarbital), high-dose benzodiazepines (midazolam, lorazepam), propofol, ketamine and other anesthetics. There are limited head-to-head comparisons of these drugs in refractory SE.

There has been recent preference for midazolam and propofol as first line of medications in refractory SE. Midazolam is administered as 0.2 mg/kg bolus followed by 2–40 µg/kg/min. Advantages of midazolam are rapid onset, greater water solubility, avoidance of metabolic acidosis from propylene glycol vehicle of benzodiazepines and barbiturates. Like other benzodiazepines, its major disadvantage is tachyphylaxis. Several reports have demonstrated its efficacy in refractory SE *(78–80)*. However, it is unclear how midazolam terminates SE when the other benzodiazepines have failed. In one study, high dose lorazepam was used successfully in treating refractory SE when used up to a dose of 9 mg/h *(81)*.

Propofol has gained popularity recently in the treatment of refractory SE. It can be given as 2–5 mg/kg bolus followed by 1–15 mg/kg/h infusion *(82)*. Onset of action is 3–5 min, and activity persists only for 5–10 min after the drug has been stopped. Potential side effects are respiratory suppression, hypotension, and infections with prolonged infusions. Adjustments of dietary calories should be considered to prevent overfeeding because propofol is delivered in lipid vehicle. There was some concern about its proconvulsant role. However, this is probably myoclonus rather than seizures. It has been shown to be effective in terminating refractory SE *(83)*. Rapid discontinuation should be avoided, as it may precipitate withdrawal seizures *(84)*. The advantages of propofol include less tachyphylaxis than midazolam, and less hypotension than phenobarbital *(85)*. Both midazolam and propofol are more expensive than high dose barbiturates.

The role of propofol and midazolam were compared recently in a retrospective study of 20 patients with refractory SE with continuous EEG monitoring *(86)*. Overall mortality was higher with propofol (57% with propofol vs 17% with midazolam). However, this was not statistically significant. There does not seem to be significant cost differences between the two drugs. If patients fail one of these drugs, the other should be tried before considering high-dose barbiturates or other anesthetics.

Thiopental and pentobarbital have been used frequently to treat refractory SE. Their use in refractory SE has fallen out of favor as initial agents in the past few years since demonstration of efficacy of midazolam and propofol. Although anesthesia with these barbiturates is effective in controlling seizures, they are associated with severe hypotension, requiring vasopressor agents. Thiopental has added disadvantages including accumulation in lipoid tissues with prolonged infusions, saturable metabolism with conversion to pentobarbital, an active metabolite *(5)*. Pentobarbital is favored over thiopental and is administered with a loading dose of 5–12 mg/kg infused in 1 h, followed by 1–10 mg/kg/h *(87)*. High-dose barbiturates are potentially immunosuppressive, and extra care is needed to prevent and treat nosocomial infections *(88)*. In a recent retrospective analysis of about 28 studies involving use of either propofol, midazolam or pentobarbital, the authors noted lower frequency of treatment failure and breakthrough seizures with pentobarbital relative to the other two agents, but increased incidence of hypotension and no difference in mortality *(89)*.

Ketamine has been recently shown to be effective in controlling prolonged refractory SE in rat animal model and in a human case report *(90,91)*. Irrespective of seizure control there is suggestion from animal models that ketamine may have neuroprotective role *(92)*.

The above mentioned medications need to be titrated to the desired effects. Generally propofol and midazolam are titrated to cessation of clinical and electrographic seizures, whereas pentobarbital use has been targeted for burst-suppression pattern on the EEG. However, debate persists as to what activity on EEG should be taken as the goal to be considered as successful termination of SE *(93)*. Although some neurologists prefer to achieve burst-suppression pattern with general anesthetic agents, there are no prospective data supporting requirement or efficacy of this EEG activity. The one reason for preferring this goal is due to the fact that this is an easily recognized pattern even by non-neurology intensive care physicians. SE can be controlled in many patients with evidence of slowing of background activity along with cessation of clinical seizures and hence one can avoid the medication-induced higher risks in achieving burst-suppression pattern. To further complicate the controversy, some patients may have seizures emerging out of a burst-suppression pattern. This may be one situation, where one might consider achieving very long periods of suppression or even a "flat" EEG, using higher doses of medications. The lack of continuous EEG may force one to rely on intermittent samples of EEG resulting in under- or overtreatment.

Despite recent advances in the development of many effective newer antiepileptic agents, none of them so far have shown to be effective in SE. Parenteral lamotrigine did not show significant anti-SE effect in a cobalt-homocysteine–induced SE rat model *(94)*. In animal models, vigabatrin and tiagabine but not carbamazepine has shown to prevent brain damage and behavioral deterioration *(18)*. Experimental pharmacological studies suggest future role for felbamate, nefiracetam, L-arginine and isoflurane (more than other inhalant anesthetic agents) *(19)*. There is ongoing search for agents with neuroprotectant role in SE. There is not yet convincing evidence for a role of the newer antiepileptic agents in SE.

Once control of SE is achieved with one or more of the above medications, the infusions are maintained for another 12–24 h, if hemodynamic status is maintained. At the same time, maintenance doses of traditional anticonvulsants should be continued to facilitate withdrawal of high dose antiepileptic/anesthetic drug infusions. If there is no evidence for recurrence of seizures, the infusions can be tapered and patients observed for further seizure activity. If there is recurrence of seizures on tapering the infusions or if the underlying precipitating cause of SE is still active, patients should be further continued on these infusions for longer periods before considering tapering once again. These patients generally require higher than usual maintenance doses. Selection of the dose and drug for maintenance depends upon the underlying cause and antiepileptic medication history. If the precipitating event is corrected, patients can be restarted on their previous regimen. On the other hand, if the seizures are of new onset with ongoing epileptogenic stimuli, high dose anticonvulsants are generally needed.

Treatment of Complications

Hyperthermia, which is seen in 28–79% of patients, occurring after the onset of SE, is generally due to effect of seizures *(95,96)*. However, this needs to be treated to avoid exacerbation of cerebral injury. In rare cases, cool peritoneal lavage or extracorporeal blood cooling may be required. Pentobarbital may have poikilothermic effect in some patients. Metabolic acidosis that follows seizures generally resolves with control of seizures. However, in extreme situations, sodium bicarbonate can be used *(95,96)*. Myoglobnuria should be treated with saline infusion, and alkaline diuresis. Cerebral edema could be secondary to both vasogenic edema from seizures and underlying cause of SE. It is important to control seizures, correct underlying neurological causes and systemic complications to reduce the edema. In some life threatening situations, general measures directed primarily at reducing intracranial pressure including mannitol, hyperventilation and even steroids are indicated.

OUTCOME

SE has great potential for significant mortality and morbidity, even with treatment, especially if delayed. The mortality from SE is approx 20% within 30 d of onset *(5,6,49)*. In the VA study, higher mortality (65%) was noted in the 'subtle SE' group, which included patients with less obvious clinical manifestations of seizures at presentation. The mortality rate increases with age in adults and is lower in the pediatric population *(6,97)*. In a recent population-based retrospective study of long-term mortality following SE, there was a threefold increase in the mortality among survivors from SE at 10 yr compared to the general population. Myoclonic SE, prolonged SE beyond 1 h and those with symptomatic SE had higher mortality *(98)*. An episode of SE also increases the risk of subsequent epilepsy even in those with no history of seizures. However, arguably both acute SE and chronic epilepsy could be secondary to a common primary brain insult *(5,19)*. Outcome is usually a reflection of the underlying etiology rather than a direct effect of the episode of SE. On analysis of 12 case series of SE, Shorvon noted that a major factor determining death was underlying cause in 89% of cases and only 2% of the deaths were directly related to the SE itself *(5)*. Outcome is also poor in those patients with prolonged SE lasting longer than 1 h (32% vs 2.7% in adults) *(97)* and with concomitant severe systemic disturbances. SE secondary to noncompliance or discontinuation of antiepileptics, alcohol withdrawal, and head trauma has good outcome in 90% of patients, whereas etiologies such as stroke, acute metabolic dysfunction and anoxia have a poorer outcome *(7)*. Presence of electrocardiographic changes also has been shown to predict poorer prognosis *(99)*. Patients with poorer outcomes were noted to have increased cerebrospinal fluid lactate, but not beta-endorphin *(100)*.

Prolonged complex partial SE also has been shown to be associated with increased morbidity and mortality *(101)*, but there is some controversy as to whether this reflects a consequence of NCSE or associated comorbidity *(34)*. Shneker and Fountain studied 71 patients with NCSE, of whom 12 died and in these, a medical problem was the etiology of NCSE in nine *(102)*.

Causes of death include primary underlying cause of SE; cerebral injury; trauma; and cardiac, respiratory, and systemic complications. In children, one review reported neurological abnormalities in 29% among infants younger than 1 yr of age, 11% among children ages 1–3 yr, and 6% in children older than 3 yr of age *(103)*. The mortality rate was only 3%. Approximately one third of patients developed subsequent chronic epilepsy. Infants were noted to have more risk for neurologic sequelae than older children, possibly reflecting increased frequency of severe neurologic insults in this age group *(104)*.

CONCLUSION

SE is a serious neurologic emergency that demands an early and aggressive therapeutic approach. It is associated with significant mortality and both systemic and neurologic morbidity. Knowledge of general supportive care, pharmakokinetics and side effects of anticonvulsants and facilities for intensive care are essential in the management of these patients.

If intervention can be initiated early and the underlying precipitating cause is reversed, SE can be effectively treated with decreased mortality and morbidity. The findings from experimental and clinical studies suggest that SE necessitates prompt attempts at termination of seizures to provide protection from secondary neuronal injury. A coherent understanding of the various pathophysiological processes observed in SE, is still unclear. Precise mechanisms involved in the initiation and termination of SE are yet to be uncovered. Refractory SE, which is generally due to delay in treatment or underlying overwhelming cause, requires more intensive care, requiring intravenous anesthetic agents, continuous monitoring, intubation with mechanical ventilation, and a multidisciplinary approach. Recently, newer medications with fewer side effects have been used effectively. Large, randomized, controlled multicenter trials are needed to improve our knowledge in selection of appropriate antiepileptic regimen. Despite major advances in our understanding of pathophysiology and experience in the management of SE, there is still a need for greater comprehensive knowledge of this life threatening neurologic emergency to improve and develop more effective anti-SE and neuroprotective therapies.

REFERENCES

1. Payne TA, Bleck TP. Status epilepticus. *Crit. Care Clin.* 1997;13:17–38.
2. Kaplan PW. Nonconvulsive status epilepticus. *Semin. Neurol.* 1996;16:33–40.
3. Gibbs FA, Gibbs EL, Lennox WG. Epilepsy: A paroxysmal cerebral dysrhythmia. *Brain* 1937;60:377–389.
4. Hauser W. Status epilepticus: Epidemiologic considerations. *Neurology* 1990;40(suppl 2):9–13.
5. Shorvon S. *Status Epilepticus: Its Clinical Features and Treatment in Children and Adults.* Cambridge, England: Cambridge University Press, 1994.
6. DeLorenzo RJ, Pellock JM, Towne AR, Boggs JG. Epidemiology of status epilepticus. *J. Clin. Neurophysiol.* 1995;12:316–325.
7. Lowenstein DH, Alldredge BK. Status epilepticus at an urban public hospital in the 1980s. *Neurology* 1993;43:483–488.
8. Sung C-Y, Chu N-S. Status epilepticus in the elderly: Etiology, seizure type and outcome. *Acta. Neurol. Scand.* 1989;80:51–56.
9. Gastaut H. Classification of status epilepticus. *Adv. Neurol.* 1983;34:15–35.
10. Proposal for revised clinical and electroencephalographic classification of epileptic seizures: From the Commission on Classification and Terminology of the International League against Epilepsy. *Epilepsia* 1981;22:489–501.
11. Treatment of convulsive status epilepticus: Recommendations of the Epilepsy Foundation of America's Working Group on Status Epilepticus. *JAMA* 1993;270:854–859.
12. Bleck TP. Convulsive disorders: status epilepticus. *Clin. Neuropharmacol.* 1991;14:191–198.
13. Theodore WH, Porter RJ, Albert P, et al. The secondarily generalized tonic-clonic seizure: a videotape analysis. *Neurology* 1994;44:1403–1407.
13a. Shinnar S, Berg AT, Moshe SL, Shinnar R. How long do new-onset seizures in children last? *Ann. Neurol.* 2001;49:659–664.
14. Gastaut H, Broughton R. *Epileptic Seizures: Clinical and Electrographic Features, Diagnosis and Treatment.* Springfield, Ill.: Charles C Thomas, 1972:25–90.
15. Lowenstein H, Alldredge BK. Status epilepticus. *N. Engl. J. Med.* 1998;338:970–976.
16. Lowenstein DH, Bleck TP, Macdonald RL. It's time to revise the definition of status epilepticus. *Epilepsia* 1999;40:120–122.
17. Lothman EW. The biochemical basis and pathophysiology of status epilepticus. *Neurology* 1990;40(Suppl 2):13–23.
18. Kim J, Treiman D. New developments in the treatment of seizures and status epilepticus. *Curr. Opin. Crit. Care* 1997;3:101–109.
19. Treiman DM. Therapy of status epilepticus in adults and children. *Curr. Opin. Neurol.* 2001;14:203–210.
20. Lothman EW, Bertram EH III, Stringer JL. Functional anatomy of hippocampal seizures. *Prog. Neurobiol.* 1991;37:1–82.
21. Treiman DM, Walton NY, Wickboldt C, DeGiorgio C. Predictable sequence of EEG changes during generalized convulsive status epilepticus in man and three experimental models of status epilepticus in the rat. *Neurology* 1987;37(suppl 1):244–245.
22. Wasterlain CG, Fujikasw DG, Penix L, et al. Pathophysiological mechanisms of brain damage from status epilepticus. *Epilepsia* 1993;34(suppl 1):37.
23. Mody I, MacDonald JF. NMDA receptor-dependent excitotoxicity: the role of intracellular Ca^{++} release. *Trends Pharmacol. Sci.* 1995;16:356–359.
24. Perl TM, Bedard L, Kosatsky T, Hockin JC, Todd ECD, Remis RS. An outbreak of toxic encephalopathy caused by eating mussels contaminated with domoic acid. *N. Engl. J. Med.* 1990;322:1775–1780.
25. Teitelbaum JS, Zatorre RJ, Carpenter S, et al. Neurological sequelae of domoic acid intoxication due to the ingestion of contaminated mussels. *N. Engl. J. Med.* 1990;322:1781–1787.
26. Kapur J, Macdonald RL. Rapid seizure-induced reduction of benzodiazepine and Zn^{2+} sensitivity of hippocampal dentate granule cell $GABA_A$ receptors. *J. Neurosci.* 1997;17:7532–7540.
27. Corsellis JAN, Bruton CJ. Neuropathology of status epilepticus in humans. In: Delagado-Escueta AV, Wasterlain CG, Treiman DM, Porter RJ (eds). *Advances in Neurology.* Vol. 34. *Status Epilepticus: Mechanisms of Brain Damage and Treatment.* New York: Raven Press, 1983:129–139.
28. Sloviter RS. "Epileptic" brain damage in rats induced by sustained electrical stimulation of the perforant path. I. Acute electrophysiological and light microscopic studies. *Brain Res. Bull.* 1983;10:675–697.
29. Meldrum BS. Metabolic factors during prolonged seizures and their relationship to nerve cell death. *Adv. Neurol.* 1983;34:261–275.

30. Meldrum BS, Brierley JB. Prolonged epileptic seizures in primates: Ischemic cell change and its relation to ictal physiological events. *Arch. Neurol.* 1973;28:10–17.

31. Meldrum BS, Vigouroux RA, Brierley JB. Systemic factors and epileptic brain damage: prolonged seizures in paralyzed, artificially ventilated baboons. *Arch. Neurol.* 1973;29:82–87.

32. Treiman DM, Walton NY, Kendrick C. A progressive sequence of electroencephalographic changes during generalized convulsive status epilepticus. *Epilepsy Res.* 1990;5:49–60.

33. Kreisman NR, Lamansa JC, Rosenthal M, et al. Oxidative metabolic responses with recurrent seizures in rat cerebral cortex: Role of systemic factors. *Brain Res.* 1981;218:175–188.

34. Kaplan PW. Assessing the outcomes in patients with nonconvulsive status epilepticus: Nonconvulsive status epilepticus is underdiagnosed, potentially overtreated, and confounded by comorbidity. *J. Clin. Neurophysiol.* 1999;16:341–52.

35. Sapolsky RM, Stein BA. Status epilepticus: Induced hippocampal damage is modulated by glucose availability. *Neurosci. Lett.* 1989;97:157.

36. Young RS, Briggs RW, Yagel SK, et al. 31P Nuclear magnetic resonance study of the effect of hypoxemia on neonatal status epilepticus. *Pediatr. Res.* 1986;20:581.

37. Boggs JG, Painter JA, DeLorenzo RJ: Analysis of electrocardiographic changes in status epilepticus. *Epilepsy Res.* 1993;14:87–94.

38. Hisano T, Ohno M, Egawa T, et al. Changes in diffusion-weighted MRI after status epilepticus. *Pediatr. Neurol.* 2000;22:327–329.

39. Simon RP, Aminoff MJ. Electrographic status epilepticus in fatal anoxic coma. *Ann. Neurol.* 1986;20:351–355.

40. Lowenstein DH, Aminoff MJ. Clinical and EEG features of status epilepticus in comatose patients. *Neurology* 1992;42:100–104.

41. Jordan KG. Continuous EEG and evoked potential monitoring in the neuroscience intensive care unit. *J. Clin. Neurophysiol.* 1993;10:445–475.

42. Kaplan PW. Nonconvusive status epilepticus in the emergency room. *Epilepsia* 1996;37:643–650.

43. Towne AR, Waterhouse EJ, Boggs JG, Garnett LK, Brown AJ, Smith JR Jr, DeLorenzo RJ. Prevalence of nonconvulsive status epilepticus in comatose patients. *Neurology* 2000;54:340–345.

44. Treiman DM, Delgado-Escueta AV. Complex partial status epilepticus. *Adv. Neurol.* 1983;34:69–81.

45. Cockerell OC, Walker MC, Sander JWAS, Shorvon SD. Complex partial status. *Neurology* 1996;47:307–308.

46. Gaustaut H, Tassinari C. Status epilepticus. In: Redmon A (ed). *Handbook of Electroencephalography and Clinical Neurophysiology*. Amsterdam: Elsevier, 1975:35–45.

47. Lowenstein DH. Status epilepticus: An overview of the clinical problem. *Epilepsia* 1999;40(Suppl 1):S3–S8.

48. Towne AR, Pellock JM, Ko D, DeLorenzo RJ. Determinants of mortality in status epilepticus. *Epilepsia* 1994;35:27–34.

49. Treiman DM, Meyers PD, Walton NY, et al. A comparison of four treatments for generalized convulsive status epilepticus. Veterans Affairs Status Epilepticus Cooperative Study Group. *N. Engl. J. Med.* 1998;339:792–798.

50. DeLorenzo RJ, Waterhouse EJ, Towne AR, Boggs JG, Ko D, DeLorenzo GA, Brown A, Garnett L. Persistent nonconvulsive status epilepticus after the control of convulsive status epilepticus. *Epilepsia* 1998;39:833–840.

51. Walton NY, Treiman DM. Rational polytherapy in the treatment of status epilepticus. *Epilepsy Res.* 1996;11:S123–S139.

52. Walton NY, Treiman DM. Response of status epilepticus induced by lithium and pilocarpine to treatment with diazepam. *Exp. Neurol.* 1988;101:267–75.

53. Hanhan UA, Fiallos MR, Orlowski JP. Status epilepticus. *Pediatr. Clin. North Am.* 2001;48:683–694.

54. Scott RC, Besag FM, Neville BG. Buccal midazolam and rectal diazepam for treatment of prolonged seizures in childhood and adolescence: A randomized trial. *Lancet* 1999;353:623–626.

55. Leppik IE, Derivan AT, Homan RW, Walker J, Ramsay RE, Patrick B. Double-blind study of lorazepam and diazepam in status epilepticus. *JAMA* 1983;249:1452–1454.

56. Kumar A, Bleck TP. Intravenous midazolam for the treatment of refractory status epilepticus. *Crit. Care Med.* 1992;20:483–488.

57. Nicol CF, Tutton JC, Smith BH. Parenteral diazepam in status epilepticus. *Neurology* 1969;19:332–343.

58. George KA, Dundee JW. Relative amnesic actions of diazepam, flunitrazepam and lorazepam in man. *Br. J. Clin. Pharmacol.* 1977;4:45–50.

59. Ramsay RE, Hammond EJ, Perchalsli RJ, et al. Brain uptake of phenytoin, phenobarbital, and diazepam. *Arch. Neurol.* 1979;36:535–539.

60. Wilder BJ, Ramsay RE, Willmore LJ, Feussner GF, Perchalski RJ, Shumate JB Jr. Efficacy of intravenous phenytoin in the treatment of status epilepticus: Kinetics of central nervous system penetration. *Ann. Neurol.* 1977;1:511–518.

61. Cranford RE, Leppik IE, Patrick B, Anderson CB, Kostick B. Intravenous phenytoin: clinical and pharmacokinetic aspects. *Neurology* 1978;28:874–880

62. Ramsey RE, Philbrook B, Fischer JH, et al. Safety and pharmacokinetics of fosphenytoin (Cerebyx) compared with Dilantin following rapid intravenous administrations. *Neurology* 1996;46(suppl 2):A245.

63. Graves N. Pharmacoeconomic considerations in treatment options for acute seizures. *J. Child Neurol.* 1998;13(suppl 1):S27–S29.

64. Walton NY, Treiman DM. Phenobarbital treatment of status epilepticus in a rodent model. *Epilepsy Res.* 1989;4:216–221.
65. Treiman DM, Gunawan S, Walton NY, et al. Serum concentrations of antiepileptic drugs following intravenous administration for the treatment of status epilepticus. *Epilepsia* 1992;33(suppl 3):3–4.
66. Yeoman P, Hutchinson A, Byrne A, et al. Etomidate infusions for the control of refractory status epilepticus. *Intensive Care Med.* 1989;15:255–259.
67. Gilbert KL. Evaluation of an algorithm for treatment of status epilepticus in adult patients undergoing video/EEG monitoring. *J. Neurosci. Nurs.* 2000;32:101–107.
68. Dreifuss FE, Rosman NP, Cloyd JC, et al. A comparison of rectal diazepam gel and placebo for acute repetitive seizures. *N. Engl. J. Med.* 1998;338:1869–1875.
69. Bleck TP. Management approaches to prolonged seizures and status epilepticus. *Epilepsia* 1999;40 (suppl 1):S59–S63.
70. Wilder BJ. Efficacy of phenytoin in treatment of status epilepticus. In: Delgado-Escueta AV, Wasterlain CG, Treiman DM, Porter RJ (eds). *Advances in Neurology.* Vol. 34. *Status Epilepticus: Mechanisms of Brain Damage and Treatment.* New York: Raven Press, 1983:441–446.
71. Treiman DM. Status epilepticus. *Baillieres Clin. Neurol.* 1996;5:821–839.
72. Goldberg MA, McIntyre HB. Barbiturates in the treatment of status epilepticus. In: Delgado-Escueta AV, Wasterlain CG, Treiman DM, Porter RJ (eds). *Advances in Neurology.* Vol. 34. *Status Epilepticus: Mechanisms of Brain Damage and Treatment.* New York: Raven Press, 1983:499–503.
73. Walton NY, Treiman DM. Valproic acid treatment of experimental status epilepticus. *Epilepsy Res.* 1992;12:199–205.
74. Venkataraman V. Wheless JW. Safety of rapid intravenous infusion of valproate loading doses in epilepsy patients. *Epilepsy Res.* 1999;35:147–153.
75. Sinha S. Naritoku DK. Intravenous valproate is well tolerated in unstable patients with status epilepticus. *Neurology* 2000;55:722–724.
76. Uberall MA, Trollmann R, Wunsiedler U, et al. Intravenous valproate in pediatric epilepsy patients with refractory status epilepticus. *Neurology* 2000;54:2188–2189.
77. Hodges BM. Mazur JE. Intravenous valproate in status epilepticus. *Ann. Pharmacother.* 2001;35:1465–1470.
78. Igartua J, Silver P, Maytal J, et al. Midazolam coma for refractory status epilepticus in children. *Crit. Care Med.* 1999;27:1982–1985.
79. Lal Koul R, Raj Aithala G, Chacko A, et al. Continuous midazolam infusion as treatment of status epilepticus. *Arch Dis. Child.* 1997;76:445–448.
80. Rivera R, Segnini M, Baltodano A, et al. Midazolam in the treatment of status epilepticus in children. *Crit. Care Med.* 1993;21:991–994.
81. Labar DR, Ali A, Root J. High-dose intravenous lorazepam for the treatment of refractory status epilepticus. *Neurology* 1994;44:1400–1403.
82. Stecker MM, Kramer TH, Raps EC, O'Meeghan R, Dulaney E, Skaar DJ. Treatment of refractory status epilepticus with propofol: clinical and pharmacokinetic findings. *Epilepsia* 1998;39:18–26.
83. Brown LA, Levin GM. Role of propofol in refractory status epilepticus. *Ann. Pharmacother.* 1998;32:1053–1059.
84. Finley GA, MacManus B, Sampson SE, Fernandez CV, Retallick R. Delayed seizures following sedation with propofol. *Can. J. Anaesth.* 1993;40:863–865.
85. Huff JS, Bleck TP. Propofol in the treatment of refractory status epilepticus [Letter]. *Acad. Emerg. Med.* 1996;3:179.
86. Prasad A. Worrall BB. Bertram EH. Bleck TP. Propofol and midazolam in the treatment of refractory status epilepticus. *Epilepsia* 2001;42:380–386.
87. Bleck TP. Seizures in the critically ill. In: Parrillo JE, Bone RC (eds). *Critical Care Medicine: Principles of Diagnosis and Management.* Chicago: Mosby-Year Book, 1995:1217–1233.
88. Devlin EG, Clarke RS, Mirakhur RK, McNeill TA. Effect of four i.v. induction agents on T-lymphocyte proliferations to PHA in vitro. *Br. J. Anaesth.* 1994;73:315–317.
89. Claassen J, Hirsch LJ, Emerson RG, Mayer SA. Treatment of refractory status epilepticus with pentobarbital, propofol, or midazolam: A systematic review. *Epilepsia* 2002;43:146–153.
90. Borris DJ, Bertram EH, Kapur J. Ketamine controls prolonged status epilepticus. *Epilepsy Res.* 2000;42(2–3):117–122.
91. Sheth RD, Gidal BE. Refractory status epilepticus: response to ketamine. *Neurology* 1998;51(6):1765–1766.
92. Fujikawa DG. Neuroprotective effect of ketamine administered after status epilepticus onset. *Epilepsia* 1995;36:186–195.
93. Bleck TP. Electroencephalographic monitoring. In: Tobin MR (ed). *Principles and Practice of Intensive Care Monitoring.* New York: McGraw Hill, 1998:1035–1046.
94. Walton NY, Jiang OB, Hyun B, Treiman DM. Lamotrigine vs phenytoin for treatment of status epilepticus: comparison in an experimental model. *Epilepsy Res.* 1996;24:19–28.
95. Aminoff MJ, Simon RP. Status epilepticus: Causes, clinical features and consequences in 98 patients. *Am. J. Med.* 1980;69:657–666.
96. Simon RP. Physiologic consequences of status epilepticus. *Epilepsia* 1985;26(Suppl 1):S58–S66.
97. DeLorenzo RJ, Towne AR, Pellock JM, et al. Status epilepticus in children, adults, and the elderly. *Epilepsia* 1992;33(suppl 4):S15–S25.

98. Logroscino G, Hesdorffer DC, Cascino GD, Annegers JF, Bagiella E, Hauser WA. Long-term mortality after a first episode of status epilepticus. *Neurology* 2002;58:537–541.
99. Boggs JG, Painter JA, DeLorenzo RJ. Analysis of electrocardiographic changes in status epilepticus. *Epilepsy Res.* 1993;14:87–94.
100. Calabrese VP, Gruemer HD, James K, et al. Cerebrospinal fluid lactate levels and prognosis in status epilepticus. *Epilepsia* 1991;32:816–821.
101. Krumholz A, Sung GY, Fisher RS, et al. Complex partial status epilepticus accompanied by serious morbidity and mortality. *Neurology* 1995;45:1499–1504.
102. Shneker B, Fountain NB. Etiology-specific morbidity and mortality of nonconvulsive status epilepticus. *Epilepsia* 2000;41(suppl 7):251.
103. Maytal J, Shinnar S, Moshe SL, et al. Low morbidity mortality of status epilepticus in children. *Pediatrics* 1989;83:323–331.
104. Lombroso CT. Prognosis in neonatal seizures. *Adv. Neurol.* 1983;34:101.

26

Myasthenic Crisis

Nazli Janjua and Stephan A. Mayer

INTRODUCTION

Epidemiology

Myasthenia gravis (MG) is an autoimmune disorder caused by antibodies directed against the acetylcholine receptor (AchR) of skeletal muscle (1,2). The disease carries a 2:1 female to male predominance and follows a bimodal age distribution, peaking before age 50 among women and again in late midlife among men (3,4). Older cases of newly diagnosed myasthenia are more commonly associated with thymoma. Myasthenic crisis, defined as respiratory failure requiring mechanical ventilation, is a potentially life-threatening complication that occurs in approx 15–20% of patients (2,5). An even greater percentage of all patients affected with the disease experience some degree of respiratory muscle weakness (2,5,6).

Approximately one third of patients who survive their first crisis will later experience a second crisis (2). Although crisis can occur in any patient with myasthenia, thymoma appears to be an important risk factor because it is generally associated with a more aggressive disease course (7–9), and is identified twice as often among patients in crisis (approx 30%) (9) than among myasthenics in general (approx 15%) (1,10,11).

Mechanisms of Disease

Anatomically, the pathology of MG occurs at the postsynaptic neuromuscular junction. Although classically described as an antibody-mediated immune disease, the epitope being the acetylcholine receptor, there does appear to be some role of cell mediated immune mechanisms in antigen presentation, cytokine proliferation, and augmentation of the immune response (12–19).

PRECIPITATING FACTORS

Infection

Myasthenic crisis is most often precipitated by infection (40%); the most common causes are bacterial pneumonia, viral upper respiratory tract infections, aspiration pneumonitis, and bronchitis (2,20–22). Accordingly, a thorough search for infection should be performed in every patient admitted for crisis (Table 1). However, it is probably wisest to avoid full-course empiric antibiotics in patients with viral infections or simple aspiration pneumonia, in order to minimize the risk of *Clostridium difficile* colitis, which can have a devastating effect on the course of illness (2).

Medications

Other important precipitants of crisis include changes in medications such as withdrawal (or initiation) of steroids or withdrawal of anticholinesterase medication (2). Aside from drugs used in the

Table 1
Precipitating Factors in 73 Episodes of Myasthenic Crisis

Factor	Primary precipitant	
	N	*%*
Infection	28	38
Bacterial pneumonia	12	16
Viral URI	6	8
Bacterial URI	4	5
Sepsis	3	4
Other	3	4
No obvious precipitant	22	30
Aspiration pneumonia	7	10
Medication related	6	8
Steroid administration	2	2
Steroid withdrawal	2	2
Pyridostigmine withdrawal	1	1
Aminoglycoside use	1	1
Pregnancy/postpartum	3	4
Upper airway obstruction	3	4
Surgery	2	2
Other	2	2

URI, upper respiratory infection. Adapted from Thomas *(2)*.

treatment of MG, there is a wide range of medications known to worsen myasthenia, of which the neurointensivist should be well aware. When any myasthenic is admitted to the hospital, it is important to identify and avoid such provoking factors (Table 2). In addition, α-interferon and D-penicillamine, used in the treatment of rheumatoid arthritis, may induce *de novo* immune-mediated disease in a patient without a previously established diagnosis *(3)*.

Medical Comorbidities

Other medical comorbidities such as anemia, or concomitant exacerbations of other autoimmune diseases such as systemic lupus erythamotosis, and even normal physiologic functions such as menstruation, pregnancy, and parturition *(23)* can trigger crises. Hyperthyroidism, usually in the form of Graves' disease, has an increased association with MG *(24)*. Thyrotoxicosis may lead to a hypermetabolic state causing increased total body CO_2 and producing excessive work of breathing *(25)*. Furthermore, treatment of a hyperthyroid state with beta adrenergic blocking agents may precipitate crisis in a patient with MG *(24)*. In a full 30% of patients, no precipitating factor is identified, and the exacerbation of myasthenic weakness appears to be spontaneous *(2,20)*.

DIFFERENTIAL DIAGNOSIS

Disease Mimickers

Occasionally, a patient presenting with new onset generalized weakness and respiratory failure presents a diagnostic challenge. Other causes of ocular or oropharyngeal weakness and respiratory failure to be considered in the differential diagnosis of MG include organophosphorus poisoning, Lambert-Eaton syndrome, Guillain-Barré syndrome, botulism, tick paralysis, polymyositis, critical illness myopathy, mitochondrial myopathy, motor neuron disease, diphtheria, Graves disease, and

Table 2
Drugs That Can Exacerbate Weakness in Myasthenia Gravis

Antibiotics
    Aminoglycosides (gentamycin, streptomycin, others)
    Peptide antibiotics (polymyxin B, Colistin)
    Tetracyclines (tetracycline, doxycycline, others)
    Erythromycin
    Clindamycin
    Ciprofloxacin
    Ampicillin
Antiarrhythmics
    Quinidine
    Procainamide
    Lidocaine
Neuromuscular junction blockers (vecuronium, pancuronium, others)
Quinine
Steroids
Thyroid hormones (thyroxine, levothyroxine, and so forth)
Beta-blockers (propranolol, timolol, others)
Phenytoin
D-penicillamine*
Alpha-interferon*

*May induce autoimmune MG, *see* text. Adapted from Mayer *(6)*.

brainstem vascular lesions (e.g., aneurysm, arteriovenous malformation) *(1,3,5,6)* (*see also* Chapters 27, 28, and 31). Even classic central nervous system diseases such as multiple sclerosis may mimic MG in its propensity for oculobulbar involvement, symptom variability, and late-day fatigability (Table 3).

Cholinergic Crisis

"Cholinergic crisis" is a controversial entity. In prior decades, depolarizing blockade from standard acetylcholinesterase inhibitors such as pyridostigmine had been thought to play a major role in precipitating crisis in a large subset of patients *(6,21,26–28)*. The diagnosis is supported by skeletal muscle weakness associated with excessive secretions, diarrhea, sweating, bradycardia, fasciculations, and improvement after discontinuation of anticholinesterase medication. Key in the differentiation between myasthenic crisis and crisis due to excessive cholinergic depolarization is examination of the pupil size, which should be small or pinpoint in the latter condition. In our experience, cholinergic overstimulation rarely plays a role in exacerbating myasthenic weakness *(6)*.

CLINICAL PRESENTATION AND PATHOPHYSIOLOGY

Life-threatening respiratory compromise develops in myasthenic patients through two mechanisms of equal importance: (1) respiratory muscle weakness (diaphragm and intercostals), which leads to impaired lung expansion, hypoventilation, and a weak cough; and (2) oropharyngeal weakness, which leads to aspiration of secretions and inability to clear the upper airway. Although crisis is usually associated with generalized weakness, 20% do not have limb weakness at the time of intubation *(2)*. Neuromuscular respiratory failure in MG resembles a vicious cycle. With progressive respiratory muscle weakness, the ability to maintain normal lung expansion is lost, and the force of coughing is diminished, which prevents adequate clearing of the airway. Patients are often asymptomatic in the early stages, but as weakness progresses (vital capacity < 30 mL/kg), atelectasis, reduced lung com-

Table 3
Differential Diagnosis of Myasthenic Crisis

Central nervous system
    Multiple sclerosis
    Motor neuron disease
    Brainstem vascular lesions
Peripheral nervous system
    Neuromuscular junction
        Lambert-Eaton syndrome
        Botulism
        Organophosphorus poisoning/ cholinergic crisis
    Nerve roots, peripheral nerves
        Guillain-Barré syndrome
        Tic paralysis
        Diphtheria
    Myopathies
        Polymyositis
        Critical illness myopathy
        Mitochondrial myopathy
        Thyroid myopathy/Graves' disease

pliance, ventilation-perfusion mismatch, and hypoxia develop. This leads to a further increase in the work of breathing, and as vital capacity approaches 15 mL/kg, rapid shallow breathing and hypercapnia develop. At this stage, the situation can rapidly and unexpectedly deteriorate once muscle fatigue develops and the patient can no longer compensate with increased respiratory effort *(6)*.

DIAGNOSTIC TESTING

An attempt to establish a diagnosis is done by one of the following means: direct assay of circulating antibodies, edrophonium (Tensilon®) administration, and electrical testing. Each method has its limitations.

Antibody Testing

A variety of antibodies modulating the acetylcholine receptor (AchR Abs) have been identified. The most commonly tested include binding antibodies, blocking antibodies, and modulating antibodies. Patients who are negative for AchR Abs, may harbor less widely assayed antibodies such as those directed against striational muscle and muscle specific tyrosine kinase (MuSK) *(3,29,30)*. There is also growing work on the presence of antititin antibodies, particularly among patients with thymomas *(11,31–33)*. Thus, apparently seronegative patients may still test positive to other less routine antibodies associated with the disease.

Although AchR binding antibodies may be as high as 80% in patients with generalized MG, they are found in only 50% of ocular myasthenics *(3)*. Therefore if the diagnosis of myasthenic crisis is highly suspected in a seronegative patient, treatment should not be withheld.

Edrophonium Testing

The interpretation of response to edrophonium, a rapid onset, short-acting cholinesterase inhibitor, is highly subjective unless clear ptosis or other unequivocal changes in extraocular movement are present. In a patient presenting in myasthenic crisis, a more relevant measure may be to follow changes in the forced vital capacity before edrophonium or neostigmine and at several intervals afterward, beginning at 2 min after administration. Occasionally patients may acutely suffer bradyarrhythmias following administration of cholinesterase inhibitors *(3)* and thus should always be under direct supervision, including cardiac monitoring until the duration of action of the drug is complete (in the case of edrophonium approx 10 min). A 1- to 2-mg dose is first administered, and if tolerated the remaining 8 mg is pushed over 60 s.

Electromyography and Nerve Conduction Velocity Studies

The utility of electrical testing in diagnosing MG is dependent on examiner and center expertise, and careful thought to the nerves and muscles tested. Single-fiber electromyography (EMG) and repetitive nerve stimulation, usually offered in academic centers, enhance the sensitivity of neurophysiologic testing in MG. Increased time from stimulation to muscle contraction (jitter) is found on single fiber EMG, and a decremental response in combined motor action potential (CMAP) amplitude to repeated stimulation over 5 Hz is highly suggestive of the disease *(34)*. For patients without limb involvement, proximal nerves should be used, and where available, small facial nerves/muscles. Phrenic nerve testing may also be useful in myasthenic crisis, and if stimulation here is anticipated, care must be taken to avoid disturbance of indwelling internal jugular catheters, which may be placed for plasmapheresis and will preclude testing in this area.

MANAGEMENT

Clinical Assessment

The initial management of the myasthenic patient with shortness of breath is directed toward assessing the adequacy of ventilation and possible need for immediate intubation. The patient's overall comfort level and the rapidity with which the dyspnea has developed are both important to assess. Rapid, shallow breathing, with inability to generate adequate tidal volumes, is an important danger sign of significant respiratory muscle fatigue. Diaphragmatic strength can be estimated by palpating for normal outward movement of the abdomen with inspiration; with severe weakness, inspiration is associated with spontaneous inward movement of the diaphragm (paradoxical respirations). The patient's ability to count from 1 to 25 in a single breath crudely and quickly assesses ventilatory reserve. The strength of the patient's cough should be observed. A wet, gurgled voice and pooled oropharyngeal secretions are the best clinical signs of significant dysphagia. When severe, weakness of the glottic and oropharyngeal muscles can lead to stridor, which is indicative of potentially life-threatening upper airway obstruction. The presence or absence of a gag reflex is a poor indicator of the patient's ability to swallow. Dysphagia is best screened for by asking the patient to sip three ounces of water; coughing is diagnostic of aspiration, and if present, the patient should be made nothing par oral (NPO) until swallowing can be formally assessed by videoflouroscopy or other means *(6,35)*. In the interim, patients should be fed with small-bore nasoduodenal tubes.

Pulmonary Function and Criteria for Intubation

The simplest and most direct way to evaluate respiratory function in patients with MG is frequent bedside measurement of vital capacity. Arterial blood gases are also important to monitor, but abnormalities (hypoxia and hypercarbia) usually develop late in the cycle of respiratory decompensation, and thus are not sensitive for detecting early ventilatory failure. As a general rule, intubation in myasthenic patients with impending respiratory failure should be performed before significant blood gas abnormalities develop. However, this is often difficult to accomplish in clinical practice.

Vital capacity (VC), the volume of exhaled air after maximal inspiration, is normally 60–70 mL/kg. Reduction of VC to 30 mL/kg is associated with a weak cough, accumulation of oropharyngeal secretions, atelectasis, and hypoxemia. A vital capacity of 15 mL/kg (approx 1 L) is generally considered the level at which intubation is required (Table 4). However, a number of other factors must also be considered, including the rate of respiratory deterioration, arterial blood gas values, and the

Table 4
Pulmonary Function Tests in Patients With Myasthenic Crisis

Test	Normal	Criteria for intubation	Criteria for weaning	Criteria for extubation
Vital capacity	>60 mL/kg	≥15 mL/kg	≥10 mL/kg	~25 mL/kg
Negative inspiratory force	>70 cm H_2O	<20 cm H_2O	≥20 cm H_2O	~40 cm H_2O
Positive expiratory force	>100 cm H_2O	<40 cm H_2O	≥40 cm H_2O	~50 cm H_2O

Adapted from refs. 2 and 6.

patient's overall comfort level and baseline vital capacity. In general, conservative early intubation is recommended because the early institution of positive pressure ventilation may prevent increasing degrees of atelectasis, and lead to earlier extubation (*see* Chapter 9). Noninvasive positive pressure ventilation (NPPV) may be considered by some clinicians as a temporizing measure to stabilize the patient and avoid intubation *(36)*. However this mode of ventilation does not protect against the risk of aspiration from upper airway and pharyngeal weakness and in practice discomfort from the mask precludes adequate rest for the patient. Nomori et al. have shown that MG patients fare better with pressure control ventilation via a mini-tracheostomy tube as compared to biphasic positive airway pressure (BIPAP) *(37)*.

We advocate admission to the Neurosciences Critical Care Unit (NSU) and serial measurements of VC (2–4 times daily) for all MG with dyspnea and reduced VC who do not require immediate intubation. Peak respiratory muscle pressures also provide valuable information and should be followed closely in these patients. Negative inspiratory force (NIF), normally <–70 cm H_2O (i.e., more negative than –70 cm H_2O), measures the strength of the diaphragm and other muscles of inspiration, and generally reflects the ability to maintain normal lung expansion and avoid atelectasis. Positive expiratory force (PEF), normally > 100 cm H_2O, measures the strength of the muscles of expiration, and correlates with strength of cough and the ability to clear secretions from the airway.

Criteria for intubation included VC less than 15 mL/kg, NIF < 20 cm H_2O, and PEF < 40 cm H_2O. These values, in the absence of hypoxia, fever, pneumonia, or other adverse medical conditions, may also be used to indicate readiness for weaning from mechanical ventilation *(5,6)*.

Ventilator and Airway Management

We prefer nasotracheal intubation to orotracheal intubation in MG patients because we believe it may be more comfortable and pose less risk of tube displacement. All cholinergic medications should be discontinued upon intubation, because they are unnecessary in an intubated patient and promote excessive secretions, mucous plugging, and atelectasis. The initial goals of mechanical ventilation are to promote lung expansion and provide rest. Early intubation and the use synchronized intermittent mandatory ventilation (SIMV) or assist-control (AC) modes with a high-pressure, high-volume ventilator strategy may reverse and limit progressive alveolar collapse and atelectasis. Larger tidal volumes (approx 15 mL/kg) are combined with lower rates (6–8 min) to maintain normal minute ventilation (6–10 L/min) and pCO_2 levels (approx 40 mmHg). Positive end-expiratory pressure (PEEP) is applied generously at levels of 5–15 cm H_2O, as long as peak airway pressures are maintained within acceptable limits (<40 cm H_2O). Because most patients in crisis do not have significant lung disease (e.g., acute respiratory distress syndrome) and have normal lung compliance, aggravation of pulmonary injury from barotrauma is not a major concern. However, as discussed in Chapter 9, lung tissue injury has been reported with this ventilatory strategy. In addition to these measures, aggressive pulmonary toilet, with fiberoptic bronchoscopy in some cases, is maintained to further prevent atelectasis and lung consolidation.

Because one of the immediate goals of ventilation in MG patients is to provide rest, intravenous sedation with short acting agents such as fentanyl, propofol, lorazepam, or dexmedetomidine should be administered liberally the first few days to avoid ventilator associated discomfort and anxiety. However, patients who are on intravenous sedatives should have such medications interrupted regularly to assess neurologic status *(38)*. This practice has been shown to reduce the duration of mechanical ventilation. While in a dedicated NSU this practice is standard of care, this may not be the case in other critical care units where a neurologist may be called for consultation.

Patients with longstanding myasthenic weakness and chronic CO_2 retention should be intentionally hypoventilated ($pCO_2 \geq 45$ mmHg). Overventilating to normal or reduced pCO_2 levels will result in alkalosis and renal serum bicarbonate wasting. This, in turn, will make it more difficult to successfully wean the patient, from the loss of the capacity to buffer and respiratory acidosis that will ensue when the patient is permitted to breath independently *(26)*.

Anticholinesterase Therapy

In our practice, anticholinesterase therapy is discontinued for as long as MG patients remain on mechanical ventilation to avoid excess secretions that may worsen atelectasis and lung consolidation. Others have used intravenous pyridostigmine in crisis patients. However, increased incidences of potentially lethal bradyarrhythmias may have resulted from this form of treatment *(7,39)*. When switching from oral to intravenous forms of medication, the physician should keep in mind dosing differences. Failure to adequately reduce corresponding intravenous to oral dose could result in a 30-fold medication overdose. Additionally, mechanical difficulties arise in attempting to administer the timed release form of pyridostigmine (Mestinon Timespan®) to patients receiving nasogastric/ duodenal tube feeds as this form of Mestinon cannot be crushed *(40)* (Table 5).

Weaning

Weaning the MG patient from mechanical ventilation should be initiated when: (1) strength is improving; (2) vital capacity exceeds 10 mL/kg; (3) NIF negatively exceeds –20 cm H_2O; (4) oxygenation is normal (FiO_2 40%); and (5) the patient is free of infection or other medical complications. We advocate weaning with daily trials (2–12 h) of continuous positive airway pressure (CPAP) and pressure support to levels of 5–15 cm H_2O *(6)*. These are not significantly different from parameters employed for other patients requiring mechanical ventilation where additional indices of readiness for spontaneous breathing trials include oxygenation (paO_2) greater than 60 mmHg on an inspired oxygen of less than or equal to 50% (*see* Chapter 9). Additionally, patients should be hemodynamically stable and not have elevated airway resistance (>20 cm H_2O/L/s) *(25)*. Pressure support is a preset level of pressure delivered with each inspiratory effort, which reduces the overall work of breathing; the level should be adjusted to attain spontaneous tidal volumes of 300–500 mL and a comfortable breathing pattern at a rate of 10–25 breaths per minute. Agitation or distress associated with an increased respiratory rate and decreasing tidal volume indicates tiring, at which point the weaning trial should be stopped and the patient returned to SIMV or AC for rest overnight. The number of hours that the patient tolerates CPAP, a reflection of endurance, should be considered the main outcome of the weaning trial. Arterial blood gases are most useful at the end of a weaning trial, when the patient becomes tired or uncomfortable, in order to determine whether hypoxia or hypercarbia is present. Once the patient is able to tolerate CPAP for prolonged periods (greater than 4 h), the level of pressure support can be gradually reduced by 1–3 cm H_2O each day, which allows the patient to gradually assume more of the work of breathing. In many instances, the weaning process is facilitated by giving low-doses of intravenous sedation (fentanyl, dexmedetomidine, or lorazepam) to patients who are anxious, agitated, uncomfortable, or "fighting" the ventilator *(6)*.

Table 5
Anticholinergic Drugs Used to Treat Myasthenia Gravis

Drug	Route	Dosage	Equivalent Onset	Maximal response	Dosage range
Pyridostigmine Bromide (Mestinon®)	PO[a]	60 mg	30–60 min	1–2 h	30–120 g q 3–8 h
	IM, IV[b]	2 mg	5–10 min	20–30 min	—
Pyridostigmine long-acting (Mestinon Timespan®)	PO	—	1–2 h	3–5 h	180 mg/d at night
Neostigmine bromide (Prostigmon®)	PO	15 mg	30 min	1 h	15–30 mg every 2–3 h
Neostigmine methylsulfate (Prostigmon® injectable)	IV[b]	0.5 mg	1–2 min	20 min	0.5–1 mg every 2 h
	IM	1.5 mg	30 min	1 h	1.5–3 mg every 2–3 h

[a]Can be given as a tablet or as a liquid.
[b]Equivalent IV dose of pyridostigmine or neostigmine is 1/30 of the oral dose.
From Marshall RS, Mayer SA *(40)*.

In individual patients, the ability of the patient to tolerate CPAP with minimal pressure support (5 cm H_2O) for extended periods (12–24 h) is probably the single best predictor of successful extubation. We restart anticholinesterase therapy at half the baseline dosage on the day of, or 1 d before, extubation. Fluctuating pulmonary function tests, excessive secretions, or concurrent medical problems (i.e., infection, cardiovascular instability) are relative contraindications to extubation. Extubation should always be performed early in the day, as some patients may require reintubation within the next 4–8 h.

Failed Weaning and Tracheostomy Placement

Previous analysis has identified risk factors present at baseline which are associated with prolonged intubation: (1) preintubation serum bicarbonate ≥ 30 mg/dL; (2) peak VC postintubation <25 m:/kg; and (3) age >50 yr *(2)*. With reference to VC, this is normally depressed the first 2 d after intubation and should only be used for prognostication thereafter. In our review of 73 patients with myasthenic crisis, the proportion of patients remaining intubated after 14 d with 0, 1, 2, or 3 of these risk factors was approx 0%, 20%, 50%, and 90%, respectively. Elevated serum bicarbonate concentration is probably a more reliable marker of chronic respiratory acidosis than preintubation pCO_2 levels, which may transiently normalize in some patients with increased respiratory effort. Although these three predictors of prolonged intubation need prospective validation, they may serve as clinically useful criteria for estimating the need for mechanical ventilation beyond 2 wk, the interval at which tracheostomy is usually performed (median 14 d in our series). The likelihood of successful extubation can also be judged using pulmonary function tests. Mean vital capacity at extubation was approx 25 mL/kg (1.75 L), NIF –40 cm H_2O, and PEF + 50 cm H_2O in our series *(41)*.

The median duration of crisis in most published clinical series is 2 wk. This is the point at which most clinicians perform tracheostomy in patients who require continued mechanical ventilation. Tracheostomy has several advantages over long-term intubation, including: (1) increased comfort; (2) reduced risk of permanent tracheolaryngeal injury; (3) increased ease of weaning from the ventilator (reduced dead space and less resistance to flow from the endotracheal tube); and (4) improved ability to manage and suction secretions.

Immunotherapy in the Intensive Care Unit

Plasmapheresis and Intravenous Immunoglobulin

The mainstay of immunotherapy for short-term improvement of myasthenic symptoms is plasmapheresis. The mechanism by which this achieves effect in myasthenia is both by removal of AchR Abs as well as other circulating complement components *(3,41)* and cytokines, which may give this treatment modality some theoretical advantage over IVIg. Although widely used and considered effective, plasmapheresis for crisis has not been compared with placebo in a controlled clinical trial. Others have compared plasmapheresis with intravenous immunoglobulin by means of a randomized, crossover trial *(42,43)* and retrospective analysis *(44)* and have shown improvement in clinical measures of MG as well as earlier time to extubation with early institution of plasmapheresis *(3,8,43,44)*. We institute plasmapheresis in almost all patients in crisis unless contraindicated by medical comorbidity. Our standard regimen is five exchanges of 2–3 L every 1–2 d. After about four or five sessions the decline in AchR Abs is not significantly further reduced *(13)*. A large bore central catheter is often necessary to facilitate the exchange of large volumes of plasma. Intravenous immunoglobulin, if administered, is dosed at 400 mg/kg/d for 5 d.

Steroids and Other Immunosuppressants

The use of steroids in acute crisis is controversial, as acutely they may worsen the degree of muscle weakness in the already decompensated patient. Furthermore, use of steroids may increase the rate of infection, precipitate hyperglycemia, and lead to secondary muscle wasting and steroid-induced myopathy. We initiate steroids (prednisone, 1 mg/kg) in patients who are in the midst of a prolonged crisis (over 2 wk) on the rationale that more aggressive immunosuppression will be necessary to control their disease and wean them from mechanical ventilation.

Steroid-sparing immunosuppressants such as azathioprine or cyclophosphamide may be begun at the discretion physician, but their effects are not complete for up to 6 mo, so it cannot be expected that these agents will reduce the duration of crisis.

COMPLICATIONS

Medical complications are undoubtedly the largest modifiable risk factor for prolonged intubation in myasthenic crisis. In our experience, all medical complications were associated with an excess number of days on mechanical ventilation *(2)*. Fever was the most common complication (70%), followed by pneumonia (50%), atelectasis (40%), anemia treated with transfusion, *C. difficile* diarrhea, and congestive heart failure. Complications of crisis were significantly more common in older patients *(9)*. Anemia treated with transfusion was associated with reduced hematocrit at the start of crisis, and in the majority of cases resulted from the combined effects of bedrest, hydration, and phlebotomy, rather than gastrointestinal bleeding. Based on these findings, we have developed management guidelines aimed at minimizing complications and decreasing the duration of crisis (Table 6). Given the high prevalence of atelectasis among patients in crisis, the importance of regular chest physical therapy and aggressive fiberoptic bronchoscopy for the treatment of severe atelectasis or lobar collapse deserves special emphasis.

Complications of plasmapheresis include pneumothorax and infection related to line placement, hypotension and congestive heart failure related to fluid shifts, and mild coagulopathy related to depletion of coagulation proteins. Hemolysis secondary to kinking in the tubing and rarely, air embolization may also occur *(4)*. Also, instances of phrenic nerve injury due to internal jugular cannulation attempts have been reported in the literature *(45–47)* that would be particularly devastating in a neuromuscular patient. We do not exchange patients with active fever or infection, or severe anemia.

Table 6
Ten Strategies to Minimize the Duration of Myasthenic Crisis

1. Perform *conservative early intubation* to prevent atelectasis, infiltrates, or worsening muscle weakness that might occur if intubation is delayed.
2. *Discontinue anticholinesterase medications* (i.e., pyridostigmine), which can aggravate secretions and mucous plugging, immediately upon intubation.
3. Initiate *plasmapheresis* as soon as possible. Insert a large bore central venous catheter to avoid delayed or incomplete treatments early in the course of crisis due to inadequate venous access.
4. Avoid or discontinue *medications* that can exacerbate myasthenic weakness.
5. Employ a *ventilator strategy* using large tidal volumes (~15 mL/kg) and generous levels of positive end expiratory pressure (5–15 cm H_2O), to expand collapsed alveoli and prevent   further atelectasis.
6. Perform *fiberoptic bronchoscopy* aggressively in patients with significant mucous plugging or lung collapse, to clear trapped secretions and promote lung reexpansion.
7. *Reserve full-course antibiotics* for culture-documented infections, to avoid *Clostridium difficile* infection.
8. *Discontinue intravenous sedation* daily and perform spontaneous breathing trials as soon h as possible.
9. Diagnose and treat *hypokalemia and hypophosphatemia*, which can exacerbate muscle weakness.
10. After 2 wk, perform *tracheostomy*, which facilitates weaning by reducing dead space and the extra work of breathing associated with an endotracheal tube.

Adapted from Mayer *(6)*.

PROGNOSIS

Although it can be life-threatening, with proper respiratory support, myasthenic crisis alone should never be fatal. The mortality of crisis has declined from over 40% in the early 1960s to approx 5% since the late 1970s *(2,20)*, primarily because of improvements in respiratory care and intensive care unit (ICU) management. In our experience, 4% of patients died during crisis, and another 5% died after extubation, for a total hospital mortality of 10% *(2)*. All deaths were the result of severe medical comorbidity (e.g., sepsis, myocardial infarction) rather than crisis *per se*. These data indicate that further reduction in the mortality rate of crisis is unlikely, and that future efforts should focus on reducing the duration of intubation and disability at hospital discharge *(6)*.

REFERENCES

1. Drachman D. Myasthenia gravis. *N. Engl. J. Med.* 1994;330:1797–1810.
2. Thomas CE, Mayer SA, Gungor Y, et al. Myasthenic crisis: clinical features, mortality, complications, and risk factors for prolonged intubation. *Neurology* 1997;48:1253–1260.
3. Pascuzzi R. Pearls and pitfalls in the diagnosis and management of neuromuscular junction disorders. *Semin. Neurol.* 2001;21:425–440.
4. Yavagal DR, Mayer SA. Respiratory complications of rapidly progressive neuromuscular syndromes: Guillain-Barre syndrome and myasthenia gravis. *Semin. Resp. Crit. Care Med.* 2002;23:221–228.
5. Fink ME. Treatment of the critically ill patient with myasthenia gravis. In: Ropper AH (ed). *Neurological and Neurosurgical Intensive Care*, 3rd ed. New York: Raven Press, 1993: 351–362.
6. Mayer SA. Intensive care of the myasthenic patient. *Neurology* 1997;48(Supp 5):S70–S75.
7. Saltis LM, Martin BR, Traeger SM, Bonfiglio MF. Continuous infusion of pyridogstigmine in the management of myasthenic crisis. *Crit. Care Med.* 1993;21:938–940.
8. Stricker RB, Kwiatkowska BJ, Habis JA, Kiprov DD. Myasthenic crisis: response to plasmapheresis following failure of intravenous gamma-globulin. *Arch. Neurol.* 1993;50:837–840.
9. Thomas CE, Mayer SA, Gungor Y, et al. Effect of age on the course and outcome of myasthenic crisis [abstract]. *Crit. Care Med.* 1996;24(suppl):A70.
10. Donaldson DH, Ansher M, Horan S, Rutherford RB, Ringel SP. The relationship of age to outcome in myasthenia gravis. *Neurology* 1990;40:786–790.
11. Lewis, JE, Wick MR, Scheithauer BW, Bernatz PE, Taylor WF. Thymoma. *Cancer* 1987;60:2727–2743.

12. Abramsky O, Aharanov A, Webb C, et al. Cellular immune response to acetylcholine receptor-rich fraction in patients with myasthenia gravis. *Clin. Exp. Immunol.* 1975;19;11–16.

13. Aharanov A, Tarrah-Hazdai E, Abramsky O, et al. Humoral antibodies to acetylcholine receptors in patients with myasthenia gravis. *Lancet* 1975;2:340–342.

14. Almon RR, Andrew CG, Appel SH. Serum globulin in myasthenia gravis: Inhibitor of bungarotoxin binding to acetylcholine receptors. *Science* 1974;186:55–57.

15. Bender AN, Ringel SP, Engel WH, et al. Myasthenia gravis: a serum fraction blocking acetylcholine receptors of human neuromuscular junction. *Lancet* 1975;1:607–609.

16. Lindstrom JM, Lennon VA, Seybold MR, et al. Experimental autoimmune myasthenia and myasthenia gravis. Biochemical and immunological aspects. *Ann. NY Acad. Sci.* 1976;274:254–174.

17. Richman DP, Antel JP, Patrick JW, Anrason BG. Cellular immunity to acetylcholine receptor in myasthenia gravis: Relationship to histocompatibility type and antigenic site. *Neurology* 1979;29:291–296.

18. Richman DP, Patrick J, Arnason BGW. Cellular immunity in myasthenia gravis: response to purified acetylcholine receptor and autologous thymocytes. *N. Engl. J. Med.* 1976;294:694–698.

19. Toyka KV, Drachman DB, Pestronk A, et al. Myasthenia gravis: Passive transfer from man to mouse. *Science* 1975;1990:397–399.

20. Cohen MS, Younger D. Aspects of the natural history of myasthenia gravis: Crisis and death. *Ann. NY Acad. Sci.* 1981;377:670–677.

21. Ferguson IT, Murphy RP, Lascelles RG. Ventilatory failure in myasthenia gravis. *J. Neurol. Neurosurg. Psychiatry* 1982;45:217–222.

22. Sellman MS, Mayer RF. Treatment of myasthenic crisis in late life. *South Med. J.* 1985;78:1208–1210.

23. Burke ME. Myasthenia gravis and pregnancy. *J. Perinat. Neonatal Nurs.* 1993;7:11–21.

24. Tanwani LK, Lohano V, Ewart R, Broadstone VL, Mokshagundam SP. Myasthenia gravis in conjunction with Graves' disease: A diagnostic challenge. *Endocr. Pract.* 2001;7:275–278.

25. Manthous, Hall JB. Liberation from mechanical ventilation, a decade in progress. *Chest* 1998;114:886–901.

26. Jenkins R, Witorsch P, Smyth NP. Aspects of treatment in myasthenia gravis. *South Med. J.* 1970;63:1127–1130.

27. Osserman KE, Genkins G. Studies in myasthenia gravis: Reduction in mortality rate after crisis. *JAMA* 1963;183:97–101.

28. Tether JE. Management of myasthenic and cholinergic crises. *Am. J. Med.* 1955;19:740–742.

29. Hoch W, McConville J, Helms S, Newsom-Davis J, Melms A, Vincent A. Auto-antibodies to the receptor tyrosine kinase MuSK in patients with myasthenia gravis without acetylcholine receptor antibodies. *Nat. Med.* 2001;7:365–368.

30. Lubke E, Freiburg A, Skeie GO, et al. Striational autoantibodies in myasthenia gravis patients recognize I-band titin epitopes. *J. Neuroimmunol.* 1998;81:98–108.

31. Howard FM Jr, Lennon VA, Finley J, Matsumoto J, Elveback LR. Clinical correlations of antibodies that bind, block, or modulate human acetylcholine receptors in myasthenia gravis. *Ann. NY Acad. Sci.* 1987;505:526–538.

32. Somnier FE, Engel PJ. The occurrence of anti-titin antibodies and thymomas: A population survey of MG 1970–1999. *Neurology* 2002;59:92–98.

33. Yamamoto AM, Gajdos P, Eymard B, et al. Anti-titin antibodies in myasthenia gravis; tight association with thymoma and heterogeneity of nonthymoma patients. *Arch. Neurol.* 2001;58:885–890.

34. Phillips LH 2nd, Melnick PA. Diagnosis of myasthenia gravis in the 1990s. *Semin. Neurol.* 1990;10:62–69.

35. DePippo KL, Holas MA, Reding MJ. Validation of the 3 oz water swallow test for aspiration after stroke. *Arch. Neurol.* 1992;49:1259–1261.

36. Gracey DR, Divertie MB, Howard FM. Mechanical ventilation for respiratory failure in myasthenia gravis: two-year experience with 22 patients. *Mayo Clin. Proc.* 1983;58:597–602.

37. Nomori H, Ishihara T. Pressure-controlled ventilation via a mini-tracheostomy tube for patients with neuromuscular diesase. *Neurology* 2000;55:698–702.

38. Kress JP, Pohlman AS, O'Connor MF, Hall JB. Daily interruption of sedative infusions in critically ill patients undertiong mecha nical ventilation. *N. Engl. J. Med.* 2000;342:1471–1477.

39. Berrouschot J, Baumann I, Kalichewski P. Therapy of myasthenic crisis. *Crit. Care Med.* 1997;25:1228–1235.

40. Marshall RS, Mayer SA. *On Call Neurology.* Philadelphia: WB Saunders; 1997:200.`

41. Thorlacius S, Mollnes TE, Garred P, et al. Plasma exchange in myasthenia gravis: changes in serum complement and immunoglobulins. *Acta. Neurol. Scand.* 1988;78:221–227.

42. Grob D, Arsura EL, Brunner NG, Namba T. The course of myasthenia gravis and therapies affecting outcome. *Ann. NY Acad. Sci.* 1987;505:472–499.

43. Ronager J, Ravngborg M, Vorstrup S. Clinical effects of high dose intravenous immunoglobulin compared to plasma exchange in patients with moderate to severe myasthenia gravis. American Academy of Neurology 51st Annual Meeting: Scientific Program, Scientific Sessions. 1999;52S:184–185.

44. Qureshi AI, Choundry MA, Akbar MS, et al. Plasma exchange versus intravenous immunoglobulin treatment in myasthenic crisis. *Neurology* 1999;52:629–632.

45. Depierraz B, Essinger A, Morin D, Goy JJ, Buchser E. Isolated phrenic nerve injury after apparently atraumatic puncture of the internal jugular vein. *Intensive Care Med.* 1989;15:132–134.
46. Hadeed HA, Braun TW. Paralysis of the hemidiaphragm as a complication of internal jugular vein cannulation: A report of a case. *J. Oral Maxillofac. Surg.* 1988;46:409–411.
47. Topaz O, Sharon M, Rechavia E, Mager A, Chetbuon I. Traumatic internal jugular vein cannulation. *Ann. Emerg. Med.* 1987;16:1394–1395.

27

Critical Care of Guillain-Barré Syndrome

Michel T. Torbey and J. Ricardo Carhuapoma

INTRODUCTION

Although the first description of what we now call Guillain-Barré syndrome (GBS) was portrayed by Osler in 1892 *(1)*, the fundamental features of the illness were not fully defined until after the advent of diagnostic lumbar puncture near the turn of the 20th century *(2)*. Because of its potential to cause respiratory failure and severe autonomic nervous system instability, it should be regarded as a potential neurological emergency that may rapidly require specialized intensive care *(3,4)*.

EPIDEMIOLOGY

Since the marked decline in the occurrence of poliomyelitis in the United States, GBS has become the major cause of acute flaccid paralysis in otherwise healthy individuals *(4,5)*. The worldwide incidence of GBS varies between 0.6 and 1.9 cases per 100,000/yr *(6–8)*. The disease attacks all ages with a minor peak frequency in young adults and a second larger one in the fifth through eighth decades of life *(6,9)*. The occurrence rate is slightly higher for men than for women, and higher for whites than for blacks *(6,7)*. Seasonal variability may reflect seasonal peaks of predisposing factors such as infections *(7,9,10)*. No familial or occupational triggers have been recognized.

PRECEDING ILLNESSES

After careful interrogation, often complaints of systemic nature can be elicited, such as "flu-like" symptoms or a diarrheal illness that occurs 1–3 wk before the onset of symptoms in two thirds of patients. Etiologic causality has been attributed to a variety of infectious agents including cytomegalovirus, Epstein-Barr and herpes simplex viruses, mycoplasma, influenza, and *Campylobacter jejuni* *(4,10–13)*. Other antecedent events include immunization, recent surgery, and renal transplantation *(4)*. GBS may also be associated with underlying well-defined systemic illnesses such as Hodgkin's disease, systemic lupus erythematosus, and infection with the human immunodeficiency virus *(4)*.

PATHOGENESIS

Several clinical and experimental observations support an immune-mediated mechanism for the clinical manifestations of the disease *(14,15)*. Evidence supporting the immune theory of peripheral nerve damage in GBS derives from neuropathologic observations such as perivascular infiltration of mononuclear cells in association with segmental demyelination and myelin splitting *(16,17)*. The strongest support for this immunopathogenesis in GBS was provided by the striking morphologic similarities that experimental allergic neuritis shares with GBS *(14)*.

From: *Current Clinical Neurology*
Critical Care Neurology and Neurosurgery
Edited by: J. I. Suarez © Humana Press Inc., Totowa, NJ

DIAGNOSTIC CRITERIA OF GUILLAIN-BARRÉ SYNDROME

Clinical Features

The main clinical features of GBS are weakness and areflexia (Table 1). Weakness evolves rapidly over days and usually ascends from lower to upper extremities in approx 50% of cases, whereas in 14% of them it descends from cranial nerves or upper extremities to the lower ones *(4)*. Dysesthesias of the feet and hands precede the weakness in most cases. Weakness does not usually progress for more than 1 mo, with 50% of patients reaching the nadir of their clinical course in 2 wk, 80% in 3 wk, and 90% in 1 mo *(18)*.

Physical Findings

Physical examination discloses symmetric limb weakness of both proximal and distal muscle groups, attenuation or loss of reflexes, and minimal objective sensory loss despite sometimes intense subjective paresthesias. Cranial nerves involvement may be present mainly in facial and oropharyngeal muscles *(4)*. Opthalmoparesis is unusual but is present in the Miller-Fisher variant of the disease *(19)*. Pupillary abnormalities are rare. When present, typically in the setting of ophthalmoparesis and ptosis *(4)*, they are the result of parasympathetic and sympathetic fibers involvement.

Laboratory Findings

Lumbar Puncture

Elevated spinal fluid protein without pleocytosis (albumino-cytologic dissociation) is characteristic of GBS. CSF protein is usually normal within the first 48 h after onset of symptoms but rises within 1 wk after the onset of the illness *(18)* and peaks in 3–4 wk, sometimes as high as 1800 mg/dL *(4)*. Cerebrospinal fluid (CSF) is usually acellular with ≤10 mononuclear cells; rarely 11–50 mononuclear leukocytes/mm^3 may be encountered *(18)*. CSF pleocytosis suggests that GBS may be a manifestation of an underlying systemic disease.

Routine Laboratory Work

Routine laboratory studies are usually normal with the exception of a mildly elevated erythrocyte sedimentation rate, occasionally hyponatremia and abnormal liver enzymes *(20,21)*.

Electrodiagnostic Studies

Delayed or absent F-waves may be the only electrophysiologic abnormality seen early in the course of the disease. Approximately 80% of patients will have evidence of nerve conduction slowing (<70% of the normal mean values) or conduction block at some point during their illness *(18)*. The yield of findings consistent with demyelinating neuropathy is usually increased by: (1) studying three or more motor nerves including late responses (F-waves and H-reflexes), (2) evaluating proximal nerve segments, and (3) performing precise measurements to determine whether partial conduction block and abnormal temporal dispersion exist *(18)*.

Early in the illness, needle EMG may only show reduced recruitment of muscle fibers. Denervation potentials may occur in the second week but are more common after the third week. In some patients, there is evidence of a primary axonal neuropathy as demonstrated by electrophysiological studies. These features of axonal loss include absent or severely reduced compound muscle action potentials amplitudes, relatively preserved conduction velocities, and late development of extensive muscle denervation. When present, these findings are usually considered to represent poor prognosis signs for motor function recovery *(22,23)*.

CLINICAL SPECTRUM

Over the past several years, our understanding of this syndrome has undergone significant evolution. Currently, GBS is considered a syndrome encompassing a group of interrelated forms of

Table 1
Diagnostic Criteria for Guillain-Barré Syndrome

I. Features required for the diagnosis
   Progressive motor weakness of more than one limb
   Areflexia
II. Features strongly supportive of the diagnosis
   Clinical features
       Symptoms and signs of motor weakness develop rapidly and cease to progress 4 wk
           into the illness.
       Symmetry is seldom absolute.
       Mild sensory symptoms or signs.
       Cranial nerve involvement (most common is facial nerve).
       Recovery usually begins 2–4 wk after progression stops.
       Presence of autonomic dysfunction.
       Absence of fever at the onset of symptoms.
   CSF features
       After the first week of symptoms, CSF protein is elevated or has been shown to rise
           on serial lumbar punctures.
       Counts of ≤ 10 leukocytes/mm^3 in CSF.
   Electrodiagnostic features
       Evidence of nerve conduction slowing or block at some point during the illness.
       Distal latencies may be increased to as much as three times normal.
       Conduction studies may not become abnormal until several weeks into the illness.
   Features casting doubt on the diagnosis
       Marked, persistent asymmetry of weakness.
       Persistent bladder or bowel dysfunction.
       Bladder or bowel dysfunction at onset.
       > 50 mononuclear leukocytes/mm^3 in CSF.
       Presence of polymorphonuclear leukocytes in CSF.
       Sharp sensory level.
   Features that rule out the diagnosis
       Diagnosis of botulism, myasthenia, poliomyelitis, or toxic neuropathy.
       Abnormal porphyrin metabolism.
       Recent diphteria infection.
       Occurrence of purely sensory syndrome.

From ref. *18*.

polyradiculoneuropathies that include an acute inflammatory demyelinating polyneuropathy (AIDP), an acute motor axonal neuropathy (AMAN), an acute motor sensory axonal neuropathy (AMSAN), and the Miller-Fisher syndrome (MFS). AIDP is the most prevalent form and accounts for 85–90% of cases *(24)*. In AMSAN, a more severe form of GBS, patients present with a fulminant onset of paralysis following a prodromal illness *(22)*. Pathologic findings indicate a severe primary insult to the axons of motor and sensory fibers *(23)*. AMAN, a less severe axonal form, has been described in children and young adults in northern China *(25)*. MFS is characterized by ophthalmoplegia, ataxia, and areflexia and has distinct immunologic and pathologic features *(19)*. It is usually triggered by certain *Campylobacter jejuni* strains that give rise to the characteristic pattern of antibodies to GQ1b ganglioside *(26)*.

SPECIFIC THERAPY

The decision to treat GBS is based on the severity and rate of progression of symptoms and length of time between symptom onset and the initial assessment. Patients who present with mild symptoms and little progression do not require specific therapy because their recovery is typically rapid and complete. Those patients who present several weeks after the onset of symptoms are the least likely to benefit from therapy *(5)*. However, the majority of patients present with early onset of moderate-to-severe progressive weakness and they are therefore candidates for therapy *(4)*.

Plasmapheresis

Three large multicenter controlled trials have demonstrated unequivocal benefit from PE in the treatment of GBS patients when it is used within the first 2 wk *(5,27,28)*. Within 1–2 wk after plasmapheresis (PE), secondary worsening may be seen in approx 10% of patients *(29)*. These relapses are thought to be due to persistent disease activity or to "antibody rebound"; additional treatments with PE may lead to renewed improvement *(30)*. A total of five PE sessions on alternate days is currently standard treatment. The actual amount of plasma removed varies from patient to patient but generally is 200–250 mL of plasma/kg body weight.

Side Effects

PE is reasonably safe when performed in institutions experienced in exchange procedures but it is not risk-free *(31)*. PE is contraindicated in patients in septic shock, myocardial infarction within the last 6 mo, marked dysautonomia, and active bleeding. Some of the reported side effects include vasovagal reactions, hypovolemia, allergic reactions, pneumothorax, hemolysis, and uncommonly, air embolization, and bleeding *(32)*. Anaphylactic reactions to fresh-frozen plasma have been reported. Currently the incidence of anaphylaxis is much lower with the increased use of albumin.

Intravenous Immunoglobulin

The risks associated with PE, its high cost, and the limited availability of PE facilities prompted the search for alternative treatments. Intravenous immunoglobulin (IVIgG) was introduced as an alternative in the treatment of GBS patients after evidence was collected by two trials that concluded that gamma globulin is as effective as PE *(20,33)*. A total of 400 mg/kg/d IVIgG for 5 d is a currently accepted therapeutic regimen. This treatment offers the additional advantage of simple administration and does not require specialized equipment or personnel. Because IVIgG infusion does not require central venous access and does not reduce the blood volume, it is generally preferred over PE in treatment of GBS in children and the elderly *(34,35)*.

Side Effects

In general IVIgG therapy is considered safe with only rare serious side effects *(36–38)*. A history of anaphylaxis to IVIgG is a contraindication for further therapy. However, if IVIgG treatment is necessary, pretreatment with hydrocortisone (1–2 mg/kg IV) will reduce the risk of another episode of anaphylaxis *(36)*. Patients with IgA deficiency frequently have anti-IgA antibodies and are at risk for anaphylactic shock after exposure to the small amount of IgA that frequently contaminates IVIgG *(39)*. IVIgG treatment in these individuals is generally contraindicated. Whether to test for IgA deficiency remains controversial because the syndrome is present only in 0.1% of the population *(40)*. Because IVIgG acts as an intravascular compartment expander because of its elevated oncotic pressure relative to plasma, its use is contraindicated in patients with severe congestive heart failure or renal insufficiency *(37)*. Patients with preexisting renal insufficiency are at increased risk for worsening renal function during IVIgG therapy *(41)*.

The most common side effects of IVIgG therapy are minor. Some patients experience headaches, fever, and mylagias. Severe headaches in the setting of IVIgG administration are frequently the result of aseptic meningitis *(42)*. "Flu-like" symptoms are self-limited and usually improve after reducing the infusion rate of IVIgG. Patients who experience these symptoms can be pretreated with antihistamines (diphendramine 50–75 mg) and acetaminophen (650 mg) administered because of future doses. Some patients receiving IVIgG for GBS treatment have transient increases in liver transami-

Table 2
Recommendations for Admission to the Neurologic
Critical Care Unit

Rapid progression of motor weakness including respiratory muscles
Presence of bulbar dysfunction and bilateral facial palsy
Autonomic dysfunction
Arrhythmia and bradycardia
Medical complications
    Deep vein thrombosis, pulmonary embolus
    Myocardial infarction
    Sepsis

nases. A reversible encephalopathy is occasionally observed and is believed to be due to vasospasm *(43)*. Thromboembolic events have been reported and may be due to increased plasma viscosity *(44)*. Therefore, patients should be maintained well hydrated.

Corticosteroids

Contrary to expectation, corticosteroids proved to be of no benefit in GBS in a large, double-blind, placebo-controlled, multicenter trial of methylprednisolone *(45)*. A continuing multicenter trial in the Netherlands is currently examining the efficacy of IVIgG alone vs IVIgG therapy combined with high-dose IV methylprednisolone. The study is based on pilot observations that suggested a beneficial interaction between IVIgG and steroids *(46)*.

NEUROLOGIC INTENSIVE CARE MANAGEMENT

Due to the complexity of care, GBS patients are likely to be best cared for in tertiary care centers with intensive care facilities and a multidisciplinary team of health care professionals who are familiar with the special needs of these patients. The progression and severity of the disease are variable. Admission to an intensive care unit and ventilatory support are needed in 33% of patients, who will often show hemodynamic instability and autonomic dysfunction *(5,9,27)*. Table 2 describes commonly used criteria currently for admission of patients to the neurosciences critical care unit (NSU).

Respiratory Failure

Adequate ventilation relies on effective expiratory force and inspiratory effort as well as on the ability of the patient to protect the airway. All of these factors may be compromised in GBS *(3,47–49)*. Clinical manifestations of respiratory failure include: (1) increased respiratory rate and use of accessory muscles, (2) weak shoulder shrug and head elevation, (3) absence of paradoxic inward movement of the abdominal wall muscles with inspiration, (4) complaints of air hunger, (5) inability to count to 20 on one breath *(50,51)*. Ventilatory failure may not correlate well with the general neuromuscular examination and may progress faster than the progression of weakness in these muscle groups. Table 3 summarizes the specific indications for intubation described by several authors *(52–54)*. Certainly no patient should have mechanical ventilation withheld because all these criteria are not met *(49,52)*. Current ICU practice is trending toward earlier intubation to minimize pulmonary complications and to avoid inherent risk of emergency intubation *(49,52)*.

Predictors of Mechanical Ventilation

Historically, blood gas analysis has not been particularly useful in deciding when a patient will require intubation and mechanical ventilation. Hypercarbia and hypoxemia are usually late occurrences. Hence, serial measurements of respiratory function (RF) are frequently advocated in patients with GBS. These measurements typically can reveal three patterns of RF decline: (1) gradual decline

Table 3
Recommendations for Intubation in GBS Patients

Clinical evidence of fatigue or severe oropharyngeal weakness
Respiratory function
    VC < 15–20 mL/kg or < 1 L
    Maximal inspiratory pressure < 30 cm H_2O
    Maximal expiratory pressure < 40 cm H_2O
    Reduction >30% of baseline VC
    PO_2 < 70 mmHg on room air

VC, vital capacity.

(<30% reduction in vital capacity [VC] over >24 h); (2) rapid decline (>30% reduction in VC in < 24 h); and (3) no decline *(54)*. The vast majority of patients without decline (86%) will not require ventilation. It is reasonable to recommend serial RF measurements during the period of disease progression to enable detection of significant decline *(53,54)*. If values are low, the tests should be repeated, ensuring full patient cooperation, before any significant changes in patient management. More frequent measurement may result in unnecessary fatigue *(55)*.

Several clinical and radiological abnormalities are more commonly reported in GBS patients who required MV. Clinical abnormalities included: (1) presence of bulbar dysfunction and bilateral facial palsy, (2) autonomic dysfunction, (3) shorter time to peak disability following the onset of symptoms. Radiographic abnormalities included: (1) pulmonary infiltrates, (2) atelectasis, and (3) pleural effusion *(53)*. These infiltrates are often multifocal in distribution despite the high frequency of significant bulbar weakness and risk of aspiration.

Modes of Ventilation

There is currently no evidence favoring any specific ventilatory mode in the treatment of patients with GBS requiring mechanical ventilatory support (*see* Chapter 9). Both synchronized intermittent mechanical ventilation (SIMV) and pressure support (PS) modes are used. Careful attention should be paid to provide adequate minute ventilation when using any mode of assisted ventilation. Both of these modes of ventilatory support have intrinsic potential disadvantages when used in this type of neuromuscular patients. Although arguably, the unassisted breaths in SIMV may induce fatigue and weakness of ventilatory muscles. During PS mode of ventilation, the potential inability to trigger the ventilator because of weakness and the intrinsic incapacity of this ventilatory mode to detect changes in lung compliance can lead to hypoventilation. In both situations, increasing ventilatory support is recommended *(56)*. Noninvasive methods of mechanical ventilation such as continuous positive airway pressure (CPAP) or bilevel positive airway pressure (BIPAP) have a limited role in patients with severe GBS and borderline pulmonary mechanics. In patients with bulbar weakness, the use of these modalities is particularly limited as upper airway collapse may increase airway resistance *(57)*. Additionally these modes of ventilation do not provide any airway protection against aspiration.

Indications for Weaning

Weaning from MV is considered when patient's general condition starts improving. Several clinical criteria should be met before extubation: (1) forced vital capacity (FVC) > 10 mL/kg, (2) negative inspiratory force (NIF) greater than 20 cm of H_2O, and (3) satisfactory oxygenatory and ventilatory functions. Extubation with direct laryngoscopic visualization or after a cuff test may be desirable in cases of prolonged intubation.

Tracheostomy

Approximately one third of patients no longer need intubation after 2 wk *(52)*. In some patients with absent motor responses and widespread fibrillation early in the course of the disease, intubation is anticipated for more than 2 wk *(56)*. In these patients early tracheostomy is desirable to avoid complications such as glottic and subglottic stenosis associated with prolonged intubation *(58)*. As opposed to head trauma patients, in whom early tracheostomy has been shown to be beneficial *(59)*, current practice involves waiting until the end of the second week of MV in patients with neuromuscular disease with rapidly resolving illness *(60)*.

Autonomic Dysfunction

Dysautonomia is an important cause of death in severe GBS *(61)* (*see also* Chapter 10). The risk of dysautonomia is high in patients with tetraplegia, respiratory failure, or bulbar involvement *(62)*. Frequent manifestations are sinus tachycardia *(61)* or bradycardia *(27)*, hypertension *(5)*, and labile blood pressure *(61,63)*. The latter is a sensitive indicator of dysautonomia and a risk factor for cardiac arrest *(61,63)*. Patients who had labile blood pressure in the ICU should remain under prolonged cardiovascular monitoring to reduce the fatality risk after an early transfer to the ward. Daily pulse changes by more than 30 bpm predicted significant arrhythmia independently of labile blood pressure *(61)*.

Fluctuations in blood pressure and sinus arrhythmias are often self-limited and well tolerated, especially by young patients, and may not require specific treatment. In severe cases of dysautonomia placement of a temporary pacemaker may be needed. Rarely, a patient may require a permanent pacemaker. Hypotension is best managed with fluid administration. If hypotension is refractory to volume repletion, treatment with an alpha agonist, such as phenylephrine, a short-acting vasopressor, may be indicated. Hypertension may follow a hypotensive episode or may occur independently. Generally, no treatment is necessary unless there is evidence of end-organ injury or unless the mean arterial pressure exceeds 120 mmHg, when pharmacotheray may be warranted.

Patients should not be left unattended in the upright sitting position without properly assessing for postural hypotension. During endotracheal suctioning and during routine tracheostomy care, nurses and respiratory therapists must be aware of the risk of inducing cardiac arrhythmias. Other common problems are urinary retention or incontinence, gastroparesis, ileus, diarrhea, or constipation. Although these conditions are not life-threatening if not recognized or managed inappropriately, they can cause significant patient discomfort and have the potential of contributing to hemodynamic instability. Bladder dysfunction is best treated with intermittent bladder catherization. This method decreases the incidence of bladder infection compared with indwelling bladder catherization; however intermittent catherization can be anxiety provoking and poorly tolerated by some patients. Stool softeners should be given to all patients with GBS. If gastroparesis or ileus develops, then continuous or intermittent nasogastric suctioning may be necessary.

Nutrition in Guillain-Barré Syndrome

Enteral feeding should be instituted as soon as possible in any GBS patient admitted to the ICU (*see also* Chapter 14). Failure to achieve optimal nutritional support could lead to increase risk of infectious complications and of failure to wean from mechanical ventilation, because these patients are highly hypercatabolic *(64)*. Roubenoff and coworkers have estimated initial replacement at 30–40 kcal/kg nonprotein calories and 2.0–2.5 g protein/kg *(64)*.

The respiratory quotient obtained by indirect calorimetry provides important information about substrate utilization and caloric expenditure. Weekly 24-h urine samples should be done to calculate nitrogen balance and estimate protein needs. Weekly estimation of serum transferrin concentration instead of albumin is indicated in light of the common administration of albumin in the course of plasmapheresis.

Enteral nutrition should always be considered first when designing the administration of nutritional support. Contraindications to enteral nutrition are vomiting, intestinal obstruction, ileus, and bowel ischemia. In those situations, parenteral nutrition can be initiated until these contraindications have improved or completely resolved. Central parenteral nutrition is the preferred method for delivery; however, if only required for a short time, then peripheral parenteral nutrition could be considered adequate.

Formulations of enteral supplements vary in their caloric density, osmolality, and fat content. Full-strength formulas are usually initiated unless there is delayed gastric emptying or the patient presents with severe protein-caloric malnutrition. Isotonic feeding should be used in these situations. Gastric emptying is usually facilitated when the enteral formulas used are isotonic and relatively low in fat. Minimizing administration of opiates or other sedatives as well as the concurrent administration of metoclopramide and may facilitate gastric emptying.

When short-lasting assisted feeding is entertained, a nasogastric tube (NGT) is usually well-tolerated. However, prolonged usage of NGT is associated with nasopharyngeal ulceration and with a higher incidence of aspiration pneumonia (65). Hence, if prolonged feeding is anticipated, percutaneous endoscopic gastrostomy (PEG) or jejunostomy (PEJ) are recommended to minimize patient discomfort and to reduce the risk of aspiration (66). Recently, it was demonstrated that with patients with possible gastroparesis or motor neuron disease a gastro-jejunostomy tube is associated with lower risk of aspiration pneumonia (67).

Pain Control

Pain management is an integral part of the overall care in the conscious GBS patients. Pain in GBS has dual origin and may require a combination of therapy. The most common type of pain in these patients originates deep in the lower back as well as in lower extremities and correlates with the distribution of motor loss (68). This type of neuropathic pain may be related to inflammation and nerve root entrapment and can initially be alleviated by frequent repositioning. If it persists nonsteroidal anti-inflammatory drugs are often effective. Ketorolac administered initially as an intramuscular injection of 30 mg and than 15–30 mg IM every 6 h often gives substantial analgesia. If a patient reports cramp-like pain in specific muscle groups, narcotics may be needed to provide appropriate patient comfort after other causes of pain have been excluded (e.g., deep venous thrombosis) (68).

Another type of pain has been described as paresthesia or causalgia associated with hyperesthesia and a constant burning sensation. This pain is also localized in the extremities (69). This peripheral neuralgia-like pain is related to alteration in spontaneous discharges in demyelinated sensory nerve. Nortriptyline may be an effective alternative but if symptoms of autonomic dysfunction are present it should be avoided. Mexiletine has been reported to be effective in the treatment of this pain syndrome; however, proarrhythmic effects may limit its use in some patients. Valproic acid and gabapentin have proven effective in treatment of neuropathic pain in other neurologic syndromes and may also be used in this setting. Carbamazepine, given as 100 mg every 8 h, was successful in improving pain symptoms and was narcotic dose-sparing in a randomized clinical trial (70). This clearly benefits the ventilator-weaning phase in certain GBS patients because it decreases the requirement for opiates keeping patients pain-free and less sedated.

Psychological Support

GBS patients may suffer from feelings of hopelessness and isolation (4). Such reactions may interfere with medical therapy. Awareness of this problem by the health care team first, followed by appropriate and formal psychological support will enhance the effects of any therapeutic intervention tailored for these patients. All conversations in the patients room should be directed at or include the patient. If the patient is intubated and unable to speak, a reader board or other communicating device should be provided to help alleviate the intense sense of isolation they later report. Ventilated patients fear accidental disconnection from the ventilator or, when being weaned, inability to efficiently breath without the complete support of the ventilator (71). Some patients struggle with wishes to "give up" or flee and react with excessive dependence or obsession (4). In the patient who experiences prolonged paralysis or difficulties copying with his or her illness, formal psychologic/psychiatric intervention is indicated.

General Intensive Care Unit Care

All GBS patients admitted to the ICU are at risk of developing other general ICU complications. Due to their immobility they are at risk of developing deep vein thrombosis (DVT). Subcutaneous heparin at 5000 U administered every 12 h and sequential air compression devices should be started to reduce the risk of this complication. In very obese patient an inferior vena cava filter may perhaps be of additional benefit. Turning patients frequently and applying pressure pads helps prevent pressure sores and nerve pressure palsies. Positioning the patient in the lateral decubitus position or the "frog-leg" position has been found to increase patient comfort during the acute phase of certain neuromuscular diseases *(56)*. Physical therapy should be started as early as is safe, because it reduces the risk of contractures, prevents venous stasis, and contributes to the patient's overall well-being.

LONG TERM OUTCOME

The majority of patients make a good recovery, usually over weeks to months, but some patients may take 1.5 to 2 yr to reach their "optimal functional state" *(4)*. Four factors correlate with poor outcome: 1) age greater than 60 yr; 2) rapid progression to severe weakness (7 d or less); 3) need for ventilatory support; and the most powerful of these predictors; 4) a mean distal motor amplitude of 20% of normal or less *(72,73)*.

Approximately 15% of patients recover without any residual deficits *(74)*. Another 50–65% are restored to nearly normal function and can return to work with minimal residual symptoms such as mild distal weakness and numbness. Severe residual deficits, such as motor weakness or proprioceptive loss that impairs ambulation occur in approximately 10% of GBS patients. The overall mortality rate varies between 2.4% and 6.4% *(5,9,27)*; but in patients requiring mechanical ventilation, the mortality rate might reach 15–30% *(4)*. Despite close monitoring in the ICU, acute mortality is 3–8%, most commonly from dysautonomia, sepsis, acute respiratory distress syndrome, or pulmonary emboli *(74)*. A total of 3% of patients are estimated to experience one or more acute relapses after complete or nearly complete recovery *(75)*.

CONCLUSION

GBS patients are well known to deteriorate clinically and very often require admission to the ICU. Reasons for admission to the ICU include need for close respiratory monitoring, respiratory failure, pulmonary embolus, and dysautonomia. An increased awareness of these complications is needed for all medical personnel who will be caring for GBS patients to improve outcome and their quality of life.

ACKNOWLEDGMENTS

Dr. Torbey is supported in part by a postdoctoral fellowship award from the Mid-Atlantic affiliate of the American Heart Association. Dr. Carhuapoma is partly supported by a Daland Fellowship for Clinical Research Award from the American Philosophical Society.

REFERENCES

1. Osler W. *The Principles and Practice of Medicine.* New York: Appleton, 1892:777–778.
2. Asbury AK. Guillain-Barre syndrome: Historical aspects. *Ann. Neurol.* 1990;27:S2–S6.
3. Hund EF, Borel CO, Cornblath DR, Hanley DF, McKhann GM. Intensive management and treatment of severe Guillain-Barre syndrome. *Crit. Care Med.* 1993;21:433–446.
4. Ropper A, Wijdicks E, Truaux B. *Guillain-Barre Syndrome.* Philadelphia: FA Davis; 1991.
5. Plasmapheresis and acute Guillain-Barre syndrome. The Guillain-Barre syndrome Study Group. *Neurology* 1985;35:1096–1104.

6. Schonberger LB, Hurwitz ES, Katona P, Holman RC, Bregman DJ. Guillain-Barre syndrome: Its epidemiology and associations with influenza vaccination. *Ann. Neurol.* 1981;9:S31–S38.

7. Larsen JP, Kvale G, Nyland H. Epidemiology of the Guillain-Barre syndrome in the county of Hordaland, Western Norway. *Acta. Neurol. Scand.* 1985;71:43–47.

8. Alter M. The epidemiology of Guillain-Barre syndrome. *Ann. Neurol.* 1990;27:S7–S12.

9. Dowling PC, Menonna JP, Cook SD. Guillain-Barre syndrome in Greater New York-New Jersey. *JAMA* 1977;238:317–318.

10. Baoxun Z, Yinchang Y, Huifen H, Xiuqin L. Acute polyradiculitis (Guillain-Barre syndrome): An epidemiological study of 156 cases observed in Beijing. *Ann. Neurol.* 1981;9:S146–S148.

11. Ropper AH. Campylobacter diarrhea and Guillain-Barre syndrome. *Arch. Neurol.* 1988;45:655–656.

12. Dowling PC, Cook SD. Role of infection in Guillain-Barre syndrome: Laboratory confirmation of herpesviruses in 41 cases. *Ann. Neurol.* 1981;9:S44–S55.

13. Dowling P, Menonna J, Cook S. Cytomegalovirus complement fixation antibody in Guillain-Barre syndrome. *Neurology* 1977;27:1153–1156.

14. Hartung HP, Heininger K, Schafer B, Fierz W, Toyka KV. Immune mechanisms in inflammatory polyneuropathy. *Ann. NY Acad. Sci.* 1988;540:122–161.

15. Cook S, Dowling P. The role of autoantibody and immune complexes in the pathogenesis of Guillain-Barre syndrome. *Ann. Neurol.* 1981;9:S163–S170.

16. Asbury AK, Arnason BG, Adams RD. The inflammatory lesion in idiopathic polyneuritis. Its role in pathogenesis. *Medicine (Baltimore)* 1969;48:173–215.

17. Prineas JW. Pathology of the Guillain-Barre syndrome. *Ann. Neurol.* 1981;9:S6–S19.

18. Asbury AK, Cornblath DR. Assessment of current diagnostic criteria for Guillain-Barre syndrome. *Ann. Neurol.* 1990;27:S21–S24.

19. Fisher C. Unusual variant of acute idiopathic polyneuritis (syndrome of ophthalmoplegia, ataxia and areflexia). *N. Engl. J. Med.* 1956;255:57.

20. Randomised trial of plasma exchange, intravenous immunoglobulin, and combined treatments in Guillain-Barre syndrome. Plasma Exchange/Sandoglobulin Guillain-Barre Syndrome Trial Group. *Lancet* 1997;349:225–230.

21. Posner JB, Ertel NH, Kossmann RJ, Scheinberg LC. Hyponatremia in acute polyneuropathy. Four cases with the syndrome of inappropriate secretion of antidiuretic hormone. *Arch. Neurol.* 1967;17:530–541.

22. Feasby TE, Gilbert JJ, Brown WF, Bolton CF, Hahn AF, Koopman WF, et al. An acute axonal form of Guillain-Barre polyneuropathy. *Brain* 1986;109(Pt 6):1115–1126.

23. Griffin JW, Li CY, Ho TW, Tian M, Gao CY, Xue P, et al. Pathology of the motor-sensory axonal Guillain-Barre syndrome. *Ann. Neurol.* 1996;39:17–28.

24. Rees JH, Soudain SE, Gregson NA, Hughes RA. Campylobacter jejuni infection and Guillain-Barre syndrome. *N. Engl. J. Med.* 1995;333:1374–1379.

25. McKhann GM, Cornblath DR, Griffin JW, Ho TW, Li CY, Jiang Z, et al. Acute motor axonal neuropathy: a frequent cause of acute flaccid paralysis in China. *Ann. Neurol.* 1993;33:333–342.

26. Willison HJ, Veitch J, Paterson G, Kennedy PG. Miller Fisher syndrome is associated with serum antibodies to GQ1b ganglioside. *J. Neurol. Neurosurg. Psychiatry* 1993;56:204–206.

27. Efficiency of plasma exchange in Guillain-Barre syndrome: Role of replacement fluids. French Cooperative Group on Plasma Exchange in Guillain-Barre syndrome. *Ann. Neurol.* 1987;22:753–761.

28. Plasma exchange in Guillain-Barre syndrome: one-year follow-up. French Cooperative Group on Plasma Exchange in Guillain-Barre Syndrome. *Ann. Neurol.* 1992;32:94–97.

29. Kleyweg RP, van der Meche FG. Treatment related fluctuations in Guillain-Barre syndrome after high-dose immunoglobulins or plasma-exchange. *J. Neurol. Neurosurg. Psychiatry* 1991;54:957–960.

30. Rudnicki S, Vriesendorp F, Koski CL, Mayer RF. Electrophysiologic studies in the Guillain-Barre syndrome: Effects of plasma exchange and antibody rebound. *Muscle Nerve* 1992;15:57–62.

31. Couriel D, Weinstein R. Complications of therapeutic plasma exchange: a recent assessment. *J. Clin. Apheresis* 1994;9:1–5.

32. Bouget J, Chevret S, Chastang C, Raphael JC. Plasma exchange morbidity in Guillain-Barre syndrome: results from the French prospective, randomized, multicenter study. The French Cooperative Group. *Crit. Care Med.* 1993;21:651–658.

33. van der Meche FG, Schmitz PI. A randomized trial comparing intravenous immune globulin and plasma exchange in Guillain-Barre syndrome. Dutch Guillain-Barre Study Group. *N. Engl. J. Med.* 1992;326:1123–1129.

34. Uldry PA, Bogousslavsky J, Regli F. Guillain-Barre syndrome in a 93-year-old woman: Rapid improvement of neurologic function following intravenous immunoglobulin. *Schweiz. Arch. Neurol. Psychiatry* 1991;142:301–305.

35. Zafeiriou DI, Kontopoulos EE, Katzos GS, Gombakis NP, Kanakoudi FG. Single dose immunoglobulin therapy for childhood Guillain-Barre syndrome. *Brain Dev.* 1997;19:323–325.

36. NIH consensus conference. Intravenous immunoglobulin. Prevention and treatment of disease. *JAMA* 1990;264:3189–3193.

37. Ratko TA, Burnett DA, Foulke GE, Matuszewski KA, Sacher RA. Recommendations for off-label use of intravenously administered immunoglobulin preparations. University Hospital Consortium Expert Panel for Off-Label Use of Polyvalent Intravenously Administered Immunoglobulin Preparations. *JAMA* 1995;273:1865–1870.

38. Misbah SA, Chapel HM. Adverse effects of intravenous immunoglobulin. *Drug Saf.* 1993;9:254–262.
39. Burks AW, Sampson HA, Buckley RH. Anaphylactic reactions after gamma globulin administration in patients with hypogammaglobulinemia. Detection of IgE antibodies to IgA. *N. Engl. J. Med.* 1986;314:560–564.
40. Cassidy JT, Nordby GL. Human serum immunoglobulin concentrations: prevalence of immunoglobulin deficiencies. *J. Allergy Clin. Immunol.* 1975;55:35–48.
41. Ellie E, Combe C, Ferrer X. High-dose intravenous immune globulin and acute renal failure. *N. Engl. J. Med.* 1992;327:1032–1033.
42. Sekul EA, Cupler EJ, Dalakas MC. Aseptic meningitis associated with high-dose intravenous immunoglobulin therapy: Frequency and risk factors. *Ann. Intern. Med.* 1994;121:259–262.
43. Voltz R, Rosen FV, Yousry T, Beck J, Hohlfeld R. Reversible encephalopathy with cerebral vasospasm in a Guillain-Barre syndrome patient treated with intravenous immunoglobulin. *Neurology* 1996;46:250–251.
44. Silbert PL, Knezevic WV, Bridge DT. Cerebral infarction complicating intravenous immunoglobulin therapy for polyneuritis cranialis. *Neurology* 1992;42:257–258.
45. Double-blind trial of intravenous methylprednisolone in Guillain-Barre syndrome. Guillain-Barre Syndrome Steroid Trial Group. *Lancet* 1993;341:586–590.
46. Treatment of Guillain-Barre syndrome with high-dose immune globulins combined with methylprednisolone: A pilot study. The Dutch Guillain- Barre Study Group. *Ann. Neurol.* 1994;35:749–752.
47. Hughes RA, Kadlubowski M, Hufschmidt A. Treatment of acute inflammatory polyneuropathy. *Ann. Neurol.* 1981;9:S125–S133.
48. Andersson T, Siden A. A clinical study of the Guillain-Barre Syndrome. *Acta. Neurol. Scand.* 1982;66:316–327.
49. Loh L. Neurological and neuromuscular disease. *Br. J. Anaesth.* 1986;58:190–200.
50. Tobin MJ, Perez W, Guenther SM, Semmes BJ, Mador MJ, Allen SJ, et al. The pattern of breathing during successful and unsuccessful trials of weaning from mechanical ventilation. *Am. Rev. Respir. Dis.* 1986;134:1111–1118.
51. Grinman S, Whitelaw WA. Pattern of breathing in a case of generalized respiratory muscle weakness. *Chest* 1983;84:770–772.
52. Ropper AH, Kehne SM. Guillain-Barre syndrome: Management of respiratory failure. *Neurology* 1985;35:1662–1665.
53. Lawn ND, Fletcher DD, Henderson RD, Wolter TD, Wijdicks EF. Anticipating mechanical ventilation in Guillain-Barre syndrome. *Arch. Neurol.* 2001;58:893–898.
54. Chevrolet JC, Deleamont P. Repeated vital capacity measurements as predictive parameters for mechanical ventilation need and weaning success in the Guillain-Barre syndrome. *Am. Rev. Respir. Dis.* 1991;144:814–818.
55. Borel CO, Guy J. Ventilatory management in critical neurologic illness. *Neurol. Clin.* 1995;13:627–644.
56. Fulgham JR, Wijdicks EF. Guillain-Barre syndrome. *Crit. Care Clin.* 1997;13:1–15.
57. Vincken W, Elleker G, Cosio MG. Detection of upper airway muscle involvement in neuromuscular disorders using the flow-volume loop. *Chest* 1986;90:52–57.
58. Lanza DC, Parnes SM, Koltai PJ, Fortune JB. Early complications of airway management in head-injured patients. *Laryngoscope* 1990;100:958–961.
59. Koh WY, Lew TW, Chin NM, Wong MF. Tracheostomy in a neuro-intensive care setting: Indications and timing. *Anaesth. Intensive Care* 1997;25:365–368.
60. Plummer AL, Gracey DR. Consensus conference on artificial airways in patients receiving mechanical ventilation. *Chest* 1989;96:178–180.
61. Winer JB, Hughes RA. Identification of patients at risk of arrhythmia in the Guillain-Barre syndrome. *Q. J. Med.* 1988;68:735–739.
62. Raphael JC, Masson C, Morice V, Brunel D, Gajdos P, Barois A, et al. [The Landry-Guillain-Barre syndrome. Study of prognostic factors in 223 cases]. *Rev. Neurol.* 1986;142:613–624.
63. Pfeiffer G, Schiller B, Kruse J, Netzer J. Indicators of dysautonomia in severe Guillain-Barre syndrome. *J. Neurol.* 1999;246:1015–1022.
64. Roubenoff RA, Borel CO, Hanley DF. Hypermetabolism and hypercatabolism in Guillain-Barre syndrome. *JPEN* 1992;16:464–472.
65. Ciocon JO, Silverstone FA, Graver LM, Foley CJ. Tube feedings in elderly patients. Indications, benefits, and complications. *Arch. Intern. Med.* 1988;148:429–433.
66. Cogen R, Weinryb J. Aspiration pneumonia in nursing home patients fed via gastrostomy tubes. *Am. J. Gastroenterol.* 1989;84:1509–1512.
67. Strong MJ, Rowe A, Rankin RN. Percutaneous gastrojejunostomy in amyotrophic lateral sclerosis. *J. Neurol. Sci.* 1999;169:128–132.
68. Ropper AH, Shahani BT. Pain in Guillain-Barre syndrome. *Arch. Neurol.* 1984;41:511–514.
69. Connelly M, Shagrin J, Warfield C. Epidural opioids for the management of pain in a patient with the Guillain-Barre syndrome. *Anesthesiology* 1990;72:381–383.
70. Tripathi M, Kaushik S. Carbamezapine for pain management in Guillain-Barre syndrome patients in the intensive care unit. *Crit. Care Med.* 2000;28:655–658.

71. Eisendrath SJ, Matthay MA, Dunkel JA, Zimmerman JK, Layzer RB. Guillain-Barre syndrome: psychosocial aspects of management. *Psychosomatics* 1983;24:465–475.
72. McKhann GM, Griffin JW, Cornblath DR, Mellits ED, Fisher RS, Quaskey SA. Plasmapheresis and Guillain-Barre syndrome: Analysis of prognostic factors and the effect of plasmapheresis. *Ann. Neurol.* 1988;23:347–353.
73. Cornblath DR, Mellits ED, Griffin JW, McKhann GM, Albers JW, Miller RG, et al. Motor conduction studies in Guillain-Barre syndrome: description and prognostic value. *Ann. Neurol.* 1988;23:354–359.
74. Ropper AH. The Guillain-Barre syndrome. *N. Engl. J. Med.* 1992;326:1130–1136.
75. Wijdicks EF, Ropper AH. Acute relapsing Guillain-Barre syndrome after long asymptomatic intervals. *Arch. Neurol.* 1990;47:82–84.

28

Less Common Causes of Quadriparesis and Respiratory Failure

Michel T. Torbey, Jose I. Suarez, and Romergryko Geocadin

INTRODUCTION

After the more common illnesses that lead to weakness and respiratory failure have been excluded, establishing the definitive diagnosis leading to weakness and respiratory failure becomes more challenging. In this chapter, we present the less common conditions that lead to quadriparesis and respiratory failure. These diseases have distinct clinical presentations and mostly affect the peripheral nerves, the neuromuscular junction and muscles. Early recognition may lead to successful management. We present an overview of these diseases, their clinical presentation and management with emphasis on critical care.

TETANUS

Epidemiology

Incidence is estimated to be between 500,000 to 1 million cases per year worldwide *(1)*. The majority of the cases occur in developing countries *(2)*. In the United States (US), there were 124 cases of tetanus reported between 1995 and 1997 *(2)*. Several tetanus risk factors have been identified. These include wounds and lacerations, intravenous drug use, diabetes, and lack of immunization *(2)*. Groups at risk in the United States include the elderly, Hispanics, African Americans, those with low income, and those without military service *(2)*. The mortality of tetanus in the United States is 11% *(2)*.

Pathophysiology

Clostridium tetani, a spore-forming Gram-positive bacillus, has been implicated in the pathophysiology of tetanus. The spores are highly resistant and can survive indefinitely in tissue *(3)*. When they germinate into mature bacilli, they form two types of toxins: tetanolysin and tetanospasmin.

The role of tetanolysin in clinical tetanus is uncertain. It may contribute to an anaerobic environment by damaging viable tissue *(3)*. As for tetanospasmin, it is primarily responsible for the clinical manifestations of tetanus. It enters peripheral nerves and travels to the central nervous system (CNS) via the axonal retrograde transport system. It then enters presynaptic neurons and disables neurotransmitter release, most importantly, the inhibitory neurotransmitters γ-aminobutyric acid (GABA) and glycine *(3)*. This results in a disinhibition of end-organ neurons, such as motor neurons and those of the autonomic nervous system *(3)*. This accounts for the muscle spasms and the autonomic instability seen with tetanus. Recovery involves synthesis of new presynaptic components and their transport to distal axon *(3)*.

From: *Current Clinical Neurology*
Critical Care Neurology and Neurosurgery
Edited by: J. I. Suarez © Humana Press Inc., Totowa, NJ

Clinical Features

Four clinical forms of tetanus have been reported: generalized, local, cephalic, and neonatal. In the US and other developed countries, generalized tetanus is the most common form, occurring in 80% of cases *(2)*. The most common initial symptom (50–75% of cases) is trismus or "lockjaw" secondary to masseter muscle spasm *(4)*. Facial muscle contraction can result in *Risus sardonicus*, the "ironical smile of tetanus." Nuchal rigidity and dysphagia is also seen in the initial phase of the disease. As the disease spreads, generalized muscle spasms occur, either spontaneously or to minor stimuli. Opisthotonus is classically seen with tetanus *(5)*. Unfortunately mental status is spare and spasms are experienced with severe pain. Cranial nerve palsies occur uniquely in cephalic tetanus. The seventh cranial nerve is most often involved, followed by cranial nerves VI, III, IV, and XII *(6)*.

Diagnosis

No laboratory tests can diagnose or rule out tetanus, therefore the diagnosis is made on clinical grounds. *C. tetani* cultures from wound may be positive in those without tetanus and cultures may be negative in those with tetanus. As an aid in clinical diagnosis, Apte and Karnad described a bedside "spatula test" for tetanus with 94% sensitivity and 100% specificity *(7)*. The test consists of a spatula that is carefully inserted into the pharynx. If the patient gags and tries to expel the spatula, the test is negative for tetanus; if the patient bites the spatula because of reflex masseter spasm, the test is positive for tetanus *(7)*. Emergency airway access must be assured while performing this test.

Therapy and Critical Care of Tetanus

The mainstay of tetanus therapy involves providing supportive care for respiration, autonomic instability, muscle spasms, and neutralizing tetanospasmin or removing the source of the toxin.

Respiratory Failure

In the acute phase, the most common cause of death is acute respiratory failure secondary to diaphragmatic paralysis or laryngeal spasms *(3)*. With intensive medical intervention, including the use of paralysis and mechanical ventilation, mortality rate of tetanus has improved. Early tracheotomy is preferred to avoid laryngeal spasms precipitated by the presence of an endotracheal tube and to facilitate long-term ventilatory support.

Autonomic Instability

Autonomic instability occurs several days after the onset of generalized spasms with a fatality rate of 11–28% *(8,9)*. It manifests as labile hypertension, tachycardia, and fever. Dysrhythmias and myocardial infarction are the most common fatal events *(8)*. Treatment of autonomic instability is challenging because no therapeutic regimen has proven to be universally effective.

Alpha- and beta-blockers can be used with caution. Unopposed alpha blockade can result in reflex worsening of tachycardia; unopposed beta blockade can result in worsening hypertension and an increased risk of sudden death *(9,10)*. Labetalol is recommended as a balanced agent, but case reviews have shown poor results with this agent, possibly because of its predominate beta effects *(3,9,11)*.

Other agents that modulate sympathetic output (clonidine) or which blunts catecholamine release (magnesium) have yielded variable success *(12,13)*. Morphine and fentanyl centrally decrease sympathetic outflow and generally produce good control of hypertension and tachycardia *(9,14)*. They have the additional benefit of providing sedation. Fentanyl may be superior to morphine because it does not depress the myocardium nor does it induce histamine release. Epidural anesthesia has also been successful in controlling autonomic instability *(15)*.

Muscle Spasm

With the sparing of the mental status, spasms are usually experienced with severe pain. Several agents have been used with varied success. Benzodiazepines are the drug of choice due to their

GABA-agonist and sedative properties. Doses up to 3400 mg of diazepam and 1440 mg of midazolam given over 24 h have been reported *(14)*. Dantrolene and intrathecal baclofen have been used *(16,17)*. For severe cases, paralytics may be needed. Vecuronium is an ideal agent for immediate and long-term control because of its minimal cardiovascular effects *(18)*. Succinylcholine should be avoided in the late phase of the disease because of the risk of hyperkalemia *(19)*. This side effect does not occur for 4 d and peaks at 14 d after the onset of disease *(20)*.

Neutralizing Agents

Human tetanus immunoglobulin (HTIG) is given to neutralize circulating tetanospasmin. It cannot inactivate toxin already within neurons. The preferred dose is 500 IU given once a day due to its prolonged half-life (25 d) *(3,21)*.

Metronidazole is the drug of choice to prevent on-going production of toxin *(3,21,22)*. It penetrates vascularly compromised wounds and abscesses better than does penicillin, the former drug of choice *(22)*. Furthermore, penicillin has GABA-antagonist activity, which may potentiate the effects of tetanospasmin. In addition to administering antibiotics, dirty wounds, abscesses, or devitalized tissue must be cleaned, drained, or excised to decrease the bacterial load.

Other Supportive Care

Because of the patients' sensitivity to environmental stimuli, they should be placed in a quiet, dark environment, minimizing patient manipulation. Owing to the recurrence of tetanus in nonimmunized survivors, it is recommended to vaccinate all survivors *(23)*.

GLYCOGEN STRORAGE DISEASE TYPE II (ACID MALTASE DEFICIENCY)

Epidemiology

Acid maltase deficiency (AMD) is an autosomal recessive glycogen storage disorder. It is considered a static myopathy associated with fixed weakness, rather than symptoms and signs associated with exercise intolerance *(24)*. There are three recognized clinical subtypes of AMD: (1) a severe infantile form (also known as Pompe's disease), (2) a juvenile-onset type, (3) and an adult-onset variant. Fifteen percent of patients with glycogen storage disease have AMD, however, the frequency of AMD is low, occurring in less than 1 in 100,000 newborns *(24)*.

Clinical Features

The adult-onset form of AMD usually begins in the third or fourth decade *(25–27)*. Symptoms are usually slowly progressive. Rare patients have scapuloperoneal distribution of weakness *(25)*. Weakness is asymmetric in approx 8% of cases *(27)*. Muscle atrophy is proportionate to the degree of muscle weakness and has been noted in approx 20% of patients *(27)*. Facial or tongue weakness occurs in 13%, whereas macroglossia is apparent in 8% *(27)*. Deep tendon reflexes have been reported as normal in 62%, diminished in 31%, and absent in 8% *(27)*.

Diagnosis

Laboratory Features

Deficiency of alpha-glucosidase (lysosomal acid maltase) activity can be demonstrated in muscle fibers, fibroblasts, leukocytes, lymphocytes, and in urine *(28)*. There is usually an inverse correlation between residual acid maltase activity and clinical severity *(29)*. Serum creatine kinase (CK) levels are elevated in all forms of the disease but to variable degrees *(24)*. The infantile form is associated with the highest CK levels, but these are still usually less than ten times the upper limit of normal. In adults with acid maltase deficiency, the CK levels can be normal *(24)*.

Electrophysiologic Features

Sensory and motor nerve conduction are typically normal in AMD *(25–27)*. In advanced disease, however, the compound muscle action potential (CMAP) amplitude may be reduced. Needle electromyography (EMG) reveals abnormalities such as fibrillation potentials and positive sharp waves especially in the paraspinal muscles. Fasciculation and profuse complex repetitive discharges potentials can be observed. Myotonic or pseudomyotonic potentials have been reported in nearly 30% of patients without any evidence of clinical myotonia *(27)*. Voluntary motor unit action potentials (MUAPs) demonstrate reduced MUAP durations and amplitudes, whereas the number of polyphasic potentials is increased. An early recruitment pattern can be documented in cooperative individuals especially in weaker muscles *(27)*.

Histopathological Features

The characteristic light microscopic feature of AMD is vacuole formation within type I and II fibers *(25–27)*. These vacuoles are secondary lysosomes; hence react strongly to periodic acid-Schiff (PAS) stain and to acid phosphatase. Glycogen also can be found free in the cytoplasm. Fiber size variation is common as is fiber splitting. In severe disease, muscle fiber atrophy and connective tissue proliferation in the endomysial regions may be present *(30)*. Glycogen accumulations can be observed in anterior horn cells, bulbar nuclei, and Schwann cells, accounting for the superimposed neurogenic findings in some patients *(30,31)*.

The gene encoding for acid maltase is located on chromosome 17q21–23 *(29,32)*. Missense, nonsense, and frame-shift mutations have been identified in the alpha-glucosidase gene in cases of infantile-, childhood-, and adult-onset AMD *(29,32)*. These mutations lead to a decrease in acid maltase activity *(29)*.

Therapy and Critical Care

Unfortunately, there is no specific treatment of AMD other than supportive therapy for associated cardiorespiratory complications.

Cardiac

Several cardiac abnormalities have been reported with AMD, such as: (1) arrhythmias and other electrocardiographic abnormalities, and (2) hypertrophic cardiomyopathy. Therefore an electrocardiogram (EKG) and echocardiogram should be part of the work-up for any patient with suspected AMD. An EKG can demonstrate left axis deviation, short PR interval, large QRS complexes, inverted T waves, ST depression, or persistent sinus tachycardia in the severe and mild forms of AMD *(27)*. Wolff-Parkinson-White syndrome has been reported in patients with infantile and adult forms of the disease *(33)*. Echocardiogram shows diffuse cardiac hypertrophy with normal mitral flow curve. Despite the presence of severe and diffuse hypertrophy, the pump function and the ventricular filling are not compromised *(34)*. Sudden death cases have been reported in the infant form of AMD resulting from massive lysosomal accumulation of glycogen in the heart *(35)*. Patients with any of these abnormalities need to be closely monitored.

Respiratory

Respiratory muscle involvement in AMD, although slowly progressive most of the time, is the most common cause of early death *(29)*. Diaphragmatic weakness is the most common etiology of respiratory failure *(36)*. Pulmonary function tests are consistent with a restrictive pattern with decreased forced vital capacity, reduced maximal inspiratory and expiratory pressures, and early fatigue of the diaphragm *(37)*. Not all patients require mechanical ventilation. Noninvasive positive pressure ventilation (NIPPV) is a more common method of ventilatory support *(36)*.

Diet

The role of low carbohydrate and ketogenic diets is still being debated. Studies evaluating the benefits of a high-protein diet have produced contradictory results. A recent study reported that four of 16 patients treated with a high-protein diet demonstrated improvement in muscle and respiratory function *(38)*.

Gene Therapy

There has been interest in correction of the defect with gene therapy. Using recombinant DNA techniques alpha-glucosidase activity was restored in vitro in fibroblasts, myoblasts, and myotubes *(39,40)*. The application of gene therapy has not been studied in the clinical arena.

PERIODIC PARALYSIS

Epidemiology

The periodic paralyses (PPs) are a rare group of disorders linked by their distinct clinical features. They are classically divided into two major categories based on serum potassium levels during a paralytic attack: hypokalemic periodic paralysis (HypoKPP) and hyperkalemic periodic paralysis (HyperKPP). Hypokalemic periodic paralysis is the most common form and estimated to have a prevalence of 1:100,000 *(41)*. They are inherited in an autosomal dominant manner with rare sporadic cases.

Clinical Features

Clinical presentation can be dramatic, with severe episodic focal or generalized weakness. The weakness is caused by an abnormality in sodium or chloride channels resulting in failure of action potential propagation along the muscle membrane. The two forms of PP can be differentiated by the duration of the attacks, provocative features, and serum potassium levels during attacks. In HypoKPP, the attacks are often precipitated by a high-carbohydrate meal and tend to be of long duration (many hours), whereas in HyperKPP, attacks can be precipitated by fasting or by rest after exercise and tend to be of short duration. Patients are usually asymptomatic between attacks.

Symptoms in HyperKPP begin in early childhood, although the HypoKPP form does not develop until puberty. In HyperKPP, attacks are initiated by fasting and may be terminated by carbohydrate intake. Conversely in HypoKPP, excessive carbohydrates may precipitate attacks. Most patients with HyperKPP develop myotonia. This is almost never present in HypoKPP. In most myotonic patients, this stiffness is worse in the cold.

Skeletal muscle only is involved, with respiratory muscles rarely involved to the point of respiratory failure *(42)*. There are no sensory changes or alterations in level of consciousness. Muscles are flaccid, and reflexes are decreased or absent. Muscles most commonly affected by the myopathy are in the lower body and limbs, proximal greater than distal.

Patients have a full recovery. In long-standing disease, however, mild-to-moderate weakness may become permanent. Frequency and severity of the attacks is highly variable, depending on the severity of the disease. Some patients may have resolution of symptoms by the fifth or sixth decade.

Diagnostic Evaluation

Careful clinical evaluation can lead to the diagnosis of PP. In HypoKPP, it is important to document a low serum K^+ concentration during the paralytic attacks. In cases where there is clinical uncertainty, provocative tests may be useful. In HyperKPP the serum K^+ concentration is usually elevated during an attack, although it can be normal in some patients. Secondary form of PP must be excluded. Thus, gastrointestinal, adrenal, and renal diseases should be excluded. Thyrotoxicosis, another secondary cause of HypoKPP, should also be ruled out.

Laboratory Features

Abnormal laboratory findings during an attack include a decrease or increase of serum potassium level from patient's baseline (although the level still may be in the normal range). EKG changes are related to the altered potassium levels. These include sinus bradycardia and T wave changes *(43)*. Serum CK concentration may be elevated between attacks and worsen after a major attack. Thyroid function tests also must be done to rule out thyrotoxic periodic paralysis. In patients with HypoKPP, if serum potassium is abnormally low, PP may be secondary rather than primary. In these cases, renal and gastrointestinal causes must be considered.

Provocative Tests

These tests should only be performed in a monitored setting. Patients should be admitted to a Neurosciences Critical Care Unit (NSU) and be monitored for at least 12 h following the tests. Provocative testing should not be done in patients with abnormal potassium levels, thyrotoxicosis, or renal and adrenal disease, even when the patient is asymptomatic because of the potential morbidity to the patient.

HypoKPP

Oral glucose, usually 5 g/kg, is given to a total of 100 g. If oral glucose does not provoke an attack intravenous glucose may be given for a total of 3 g/kg over 1 h. If necessary insulin may be given IV up to 0.1 U/kg at 30 and 60 min into the glucose infusion. The serum potassium should be measured every 15–30 minutes for 3 h. The test result is positive if the patient becomes weak. CMAP amplitudes may be decreased or absent during the weakness. Serum potassium levels should be 3.0 mmol/L or less. A negative test result does not, however, rule out HypoKPP because patients may be refractory at times *(41,44)*.

HyperKPP

In a monitored setting, 2–10 g KCl (40–120 mmol) in an unsweetened solution should be given, preferably in the morning, in a fasting state, and immediately after exercise. An attack should occur in 1–2 h. Alternatively, the patient can use a bicycle ergometer for 30 min (pulse 120–160 beats/min) followed by absolute bedrest. Ten to 20 min after the onset of rest, weakness should begin. CMAPs following exercise should show progressive decrease in amplitude. Corresponding serum K^+ concentration show an increase during exercise and a decrease to the pre-exercise level after exercise *(41)*.

Electrodiagnostic Features

Some distinguishing electrodiagnostic features may be found when the patient is asymptomatic. When performed during an attack, the EMG findings may reveal myotonia (more often in HyperKPP) or progressive reduction in motor unit recruitment. In addition CMAP shows a progressive reduction in amplitude. With disease progression, EMG findings may show myopathic changes even between attacks *(45)*.

Histopathological Features

In both HyperKPP and HypoKPP, weakness during an attack is triggered by depolarization and inexcitability of the skeletal muscle. Recently the genetic basis of periodic paralysis has been more clearly delineated. The abnormality in HyperKPP has been linked to an abnormality in the alpha subunit of the sodium channel of skeletal muscle linked to chromosome *17q (46–48)*. The failure of normal inactivation of this sodium channel initially causes membrane hyperexcitability (myotonia), followed by depolarization, causing muscle inexcitability and paralysis. The abnormality in HypoKPP has been linked to a mutation in the dihydropyridine receptor, an alpha1 subunit of the L-type calcium channel of the skeletal muscle, on chromosome *1q31-32 (49,50)*.

In the initial phase of the disease muscle biopsy results may be normal. After frequent attacks of periodic paralysis, microscopy may reveal vacuolated fibers with typical pathologic changes of tubular aggregates *(51)*. Occasional necrosis is also seen. This degenerative pathology most likely contributes to irreversible proximal limb weakness in some individuals.

TREATMENT

Treatment of periodic paralysis can be divided into abortive and prophylactic therapy. Treatment of the periodic attacks is guided by their frequency and their intensity. The rational for therapy is that reducing attack frequency reduces the chances of developing a fixed progressive myopathy. Figure 1 describes the diagnostic workup and the treatment of PP.

HypoKPP Treatment

ABORTIVE

Oral potassium supplementation is effective in blunting the severity and shortening the duration of an acute attack of weakness. Intravenous potassium should be avoided unless the oral route is precluded. Because of the transient worsening of the hypokalemia when KCl is given with glucose or normal saline, the preferred diluent for intravenous potassium is 5% mannitol *(52)*.

PROPHYLACTIC

Dietary manipulation aimed at maximizing potassium retention can be helpful in preventing attacks of weakness. Thus a low salt (2.3 g/d), low carbohydrate (60–80 g/d) diet is recommended, as is the avoidance of large carbohydrate meals. The mainstay of pharmacologic therapy is the carbonic anhydrase inhibitor. Traditionally these have included mainly acetazolamide (ACZ). If ACZ proves ineffective, patients should be switched to dichlorophenamide. Nephrolithiasis is associated with the use of ACZ. Hence, a renal ultrasound or Kidneys-ureter-bladder (KUB) radiologic examination should be performed at the start of the treatment. Patients intolerant of the carbonic anhydrase inhibitors should try potassium-sparing diuretics *(52)*.

HyperKPP Treatment

ABORTIVE

A quick and practical approach is the use of inhaled beta-agonists, such as metaproterenol nebulizers *(41)*. Alternatively, oral glucose and subcutaneous insulin can be used. In situation of life-threatening hyperkalemia, intravenous calcium gluconate is administered.

PROPHYLACTIC

Frequent carbohydrate rich intakes can help prevent hyperkalemia. As with HypoKPP, the carbonic anhydrase inhibitors are the first line of treatment to prevent attacks in HyperKPP. The second-line drugs are thiazide diuretics.

BOTULISM

Epidemiology

Botulism is a paralyzing disease caused by the neurotoxin of the bacterium *Clostridium botulinum* *(53)*. Since 1991, the numbers of cases of wound botulism have increased dramatically *(54)*. Nearly all of these new cases have occurred in IV drug users. The organism has been cultured from the abscesses of IV heroin users, and from sinus aspirate specimen from a patient in whom botulism developed following intranasal cocaine abuse *(55)*.

Clinical Features

The clinical spectrum of botulism continues to expand with the discovery of previously unknown forms. There are now five clinical categories of botulism: (1) classic or foodborne *(56)*; (2) wound

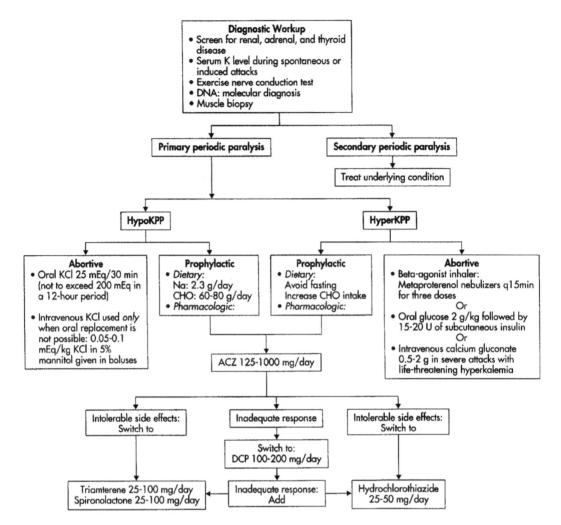

Fig. 1. Treatment or periodic paralysis. HypoKPP, Hypokalemic periodic paralysis; HyperKPP, Hyperkalemic periodic paralysis; ACZ, acetazolamide; CHO, carbohydrate; DCP, dichlorophenamide. From ref. *52* with permission.

botulism *(57,58)*; (3) infant botulism *(59)*; (4) the hidden form, the adult variation of infant botulism; and (5) inadvertent botulism, an unintended consequence of the treatment with botulinum toxin A.

The clinical presentations of severe botulism are stereotypical *(60)*. Within 2–36 h after ingestion of contaminated food, signs and symptoms related to oculobulbar muscle weakness develops. The signs and symptoms include blurring of vision, diplopia, ptosis, ophthalmoplegia, dysarthria, and dysphagia. These cranial nerve abnormalities are followed by a descending pattern of weakness affecting the upper limbs, then lower limbs, and in severe cases, respiratory muscle. Limb and ocular weakness are usually bilateral but can be asymmetric.

Sensory system and mentation are usually spared, although there have been occasional reports of sensory abnormalities *(61)*. Autonomic signs and symptoms such as constipation, dry mouth, postural hypotension, urinary retention, and pupillary abnormalities are commonly seen in botulism.

The time of convalescence in severe cases may take weeks or months *(62)*. The long recuperation (weeks or months) probably results from nerve terminal sprouting at motor end plates *(62)*. Recovery of autonomic function may take longer than that of neuromuscular transmission *(63)*.

Pathophysiology

Classic or foodborne botulism is an intoxication caused by ingestion of a preformed neurotoxin of the bacterium *Clostridium botulinum (56)*. Botulinum toxin inhibition of acetylcholine release affects the parasympathetic and the sympathetic systems as well as the neuromuscular junction (NMJ) *(64)*. The NMJ involvement is presynaptic; the toxin prevents the release of Ach at motor nerve terminals. The size of each quantum of Ach is normal in botulism, but the number of quanta released by nerve stimulation is below the threshold for activation.

Diagnosis

Laboratory Features

Diagnosis is established with the detection of toxin in patient's serum, stool, or wound. The suspected food, if still available, should also be tested. In many patients, laboratory tests are not confirmatory, especially when the collection of the specimens has been deferred for days after the onset of symptoms. If the delay in securing serum samples is more than 2 d after ingestion of the toxin, the chances of obtaining a positive test result is less than 30%. Only 36% of stool culture results are positive after 3 d *(65)*.

Electrodiagnostic Features

Several electrophysiological findings have been reported in botulism *(66)*: (1) sensory nerve amplitudes, velocities, and latencies are normal; (2) motor conduction velocities are normal. The amplitude of the motor action potential (MAP) after a single nerve stimulus is reduced in many affected muscles. (3) A decremental response of the MAP to slow rates of nerve stimulation (2–3 Hz) is seen infrequently; (4) post-tetanic facilitation (PTF) can be found in some affected muscles. The degree of PTF in botulism is usually between 30% and 100% *(67)*. PTF may be absent in severely affected muscles; (5) needle EMG studies reveal an increased number of brief polyphasic motor unit action potentials and spontaneous denervation potentials; (6) single-fiber EMG studies typically, but not consistently, reveal increased jitter and blocking, which become less marked following activation *(68,69)*. The most consistent abnormality is a small evoked MAP in response to a single supramaximal nerve stimulus in a clinically affected muscle.

Critical Care and Treatment

Treatment of severe botulism consists mainly of supportive medical and nursing care with special attention to respiratory status. With improvement in critical care management, fatality rates have dropped from 50% of documented cases during much of this century to 9% in recent years *(70)*.

Respiratory Care

Physicians should carefully observe patients for progression of limb and respiratory muscle weakness. Elective intubation should be considered for those at risk for respiratory failure. No specific intubation criteria have been established. Recovery from botulism is prolonged and usually complete. Most patients will not require a tracheostomy. NSU teams should be especially vigilant in their management, because recovery from botulism is common.

Autonomic Instability

Autonomic signs and symptoms are commonly seen in botulism (*see also* Chapter 10). Patients should be placed on stool softeners to avoid constipation. A foley insertion or intermittent catheterization should be attempted. Patients with severe postural hypotension may require vasopressor therapy. Recovery of autonomic function may take longer than that of neuromuscular transmission *(63)*.

Antitoxin Administration

This remains a controversial therapy for lack of efficacy in many cases and the associated 2% risk of allergic reactions *(71)*. To be of benefit, antitoxin must be given early, while the toxin is still in the blood and before it is internalized and bound at the nerve terminal.

Ach Release Promoters

Guanidine and 4-aminopyridine (4-AP) have been reported to improve ocular muscle and limb muscle strength in some patients without any benefit for respiratory paralysis *(72,73)*. These two drugs enhance the release of Ach from nerve terminals. The serious side effects of guanidine such as bone marrow suppression and nephritis are dose and time related. Although these side effects have not been reported when it has been administered for botulism, patients should be carefully monitored. 4-AP therapy can be complicated by the development of seizures. The experience with both drugs is limited and results are variable. Steroids, plasmapheresis, and intravenous immune globulin have not proven to be effective therapies in botulism.

ACUTE INTERMITTENT PORPHYRIA

Epidemiology

Acute intermittent porphyria (AIP) is an autosomal dominant disease of porphyrin metabolism manifested by recurrent attacks of abdominal pain and neurologic dysfunction. It results from a deficiency of porphobilinogen (PBG) deaminase. Symptoms rarely appear until puberty, and in most cases they begin in the second to fourth decade of life. Females outnumber males in symptomatic cases *(74)*.

Clinical Features

The clinical features are usually observed in the context of an acute exacerbation of the porphyria, with abdominal pain, vomiting, tachycardia and sometimes central nervous system (CNS) manifestations including anxiety, agitation, psychosis, cranial nerve palsies, psychosis, depression, confusion, coma, and seizures. Porphyric attacks may be precipitated by several drugs (Table 1) or by infections. Attacks may leave the patient with residual peripheral nerve or psychiatric dysfunction. The neuropathy usually starts in the arms, with symmetrical or asymmetrical weakness, followed by facial weakness and proximal weakness in the lower limbs. Autonomic features are frequent; sensory symptoms are absent or very mild compared with motor signs. Tendon reflexes are diminished or absent, sometimes with preservation of ankle jerks. Even with optimum management, a severe acute attack of AIP carries a significant mortality *(74)*.

Diagnosis

Laboratory Features

The diagnosis is usually elicited by the detection of porphyrin precursors delta amino-levulonic acid (ALA) and porphobilinogen in the urine. The fecal pigment coproporphyrin levels are elevated during attacks of neuropathy. The definitive test for this disease is to compare the activity of PBG deaminase in the patient's erythrocytes with that of relatives. Family members with this disease have enzyme levels that are about half those of unaffected family members *(75)*.

Electrophysiological Features

In electrophysiological studies, motor nerve conduction velocities (MNCV) are normal or slightly reduced, with a reduction of the amplitude of motor evoked responses *(76)*. EMG usually shows active denervation with profuse fibrillation potentials.

Therapy and Critical Care of Acute Intermittent Porphyria

The mainstay of management of this disease is the avoidance of factors known to precipitate acute attacks such as drugs, hormones, infections, and starvation. The most common precipitant of an acute attack of AIP is the administration of a drug that induces hepatic delta-ALA synthetase activity. Table 1 reports the different drugs that should be avoided. Respiratory failure and bulbar paralysis may require tracheal intubation, respiratory support, or gastric feeding.

Table 1
Medications in Acute Intermittent Porphyria

Drugs to be avoided				
Anticonvulsants	*Tranquilizers*	*Sedatives*	*Antibiotics*	*Other*
Barbiturates	Chlordiazepoxide	Barbiturates	Sulfonamides	Alcohol
Phenytoin	Meprobamate	Gluthetimide	Griseofulvin	Ergots
Methosuximide		Methylprylon	Dapsone	Estrogens
Primidone				Progestins
Trimethadione				
Drugs demonstrated safe				
Analgesics	*Antihypertensives*	*Sedatives*	*Antibiotics*	*Other*
Salicylate	Propranolol	Chloral hydrates	Penicillins	Digoxin
Opiates		Bromides	Tetracycline	Corticosteroids
Meperidine			Nitrofurantoin	
Acetminophen				

Suppression of Porphyrin Synthesis

This is achieved by the administration of high carbohydrate diet or hematin.

Diet

Patient is provided with 450–600 g of carbohydrate daily, either PO or parenterally, during the attack. Especially if parenteral glucose solutions are used, serum electrolytes should be followed closely because of the frequent association of SIADH with porphyria *(75)*.

Hematin

Hematin, like carbohydrate, lowers hepatic delta-ALA synthetase levels experimentally. I has shown promising results when administered IV at a dosage of 80–100 mg daily in adults. To avoid phlebitis, hematin should be administered through a central catheter or infused into a large peripheral vein slowly over 15–20 min *(75)*.

Abdominal Pain

Several agents have been used for relief of abdominal pain. Among those, chlorpromazine is highly effective for the abdominal pain. Doses must be titrated for each individual patient to avoid oversedation. A dose of 50 mg IM may be repeated every 3–4 h as needed. Opiates may be added as necessary. One must be careful not to depress respiration excessively in patients with severe neuropathies and respiratory compromise. Frequent disimpaction may be needed.

Psychosis

Chlorpromazine or other phenothiazines may be used safely to control psychiatric manifestations. Acute and chronic depression may occur, and patients should be evaluated for suicide risk.

Seizures

The treatment of seizures may be very difficult in these patients because many drugs cannot be used. If the seizures are associated with an acute attack, diazepam, 5 mg IV, or lorazepam 2–4 mg IV, may be sufficient, although repeated IV doses may be required until the attack is aborted. Clonazepam in low doses (0.5–1 mg po thrice daily) is probably safe for chronic administration.

Autonomic Instability

Labile hypertension or postural hypotension may accompany the autonomic nervous system disorders associated with AIP. Labile hypertension usually requires no treatment. Postural hypotension requires careful maintenance of intravascular volume.

ORGANOPHOSPHATE INTOXICATION

Epidemiology

Organophosphates are a class of compound that irreversibly inhibits cholinesterases, including acetylcholinesterases (AchE) *(77)*. Their potential use in chemical warfare continues to be a serious concern. Acute organophosphate intoxication is most commonly the result of suicide attempts *(78,79)*. Organophosphate poisoning as result of accidental insecticide exposure is much less frequent in the United States.

Pathophysiology

Organophosphates are irreversible inhibitors of AchE. The resultant phosphorylated enzyme is extremely stable. The return of AchE activity depends on the synthesis of new enzyme *(77)*. Organophosphates may inhibit other enzymes including neurotoxic esterase, responsible for the delayed polyneuropathy occasionally seen some weeks after exposure *(80)*. This polyneuropathy, often associated with a myelopathy, is much more likely to occur with subacute and chronic exposure than in response to a single large dose, as in suicide attempt *(81)*.

The irreversible inhibition of AchE results in a complex set of physiological and clinical changes related to excessive amounts of Ach at the NMJ as well as CNS cholinergic and peripheral and autonomic nervous system muscarinic synapses *(82)*. The prolonged exposure of the postsynaptic Ach receptors results in a prolonged endplate potential and desensitization of the postsynaptic membrane. The prolonged endplate potential contributes to the repetitive muscle action potentials in response to a single nerve stimulus *(83)*. The desensitization is in large part responsible for the decremental response occurring with organophosphate intoxication *(83)*.

Clinical Features

The number and severity of abnormalities reflect the degree of intoxication *(83)*. Symptoms may begin within 3 h of exposure and progress to death within 10 h if the intoxication was severe. The wide range of symptoms can be summarized into two types: muscarinic and nictonic.

The muscarinic symptoms reflect the AchE inhibition at autonomic synapses. These include miosis, conjunctival hyperemia, rhinorrhea and drooling, bronchospasms with wheezing and coughing, increased bronchial secretion with airway obstruction, respiratory distress, pulmonary edema, laryngeal spasms, sweating, bradycardia, hypotension, and loss of bowel and bladder control.

The nicotinic effects reflect AchE inhibition at the NMJ. The initial skeletal muscle symptoms of fasciculations and cramps reflect the early stimulatory phase and coincide with axonal backfiring. Fasciculations are first seen in the eyelids, spread to the face and calves, and then become generalized. This occurs during the first 24 h and is followed by weakness or paralysis, depending on the severity of the intoxication. Paralysis involves all skeletal muscles, including those of respiration, with labored, shallow, rapid breathing. Respiratory failure and cyanosis ensue; weakness of the tongue and pharyngeal muscles further enhances respiratory failure by virtue of airway obstruction.

Other symptoms have been reported secondary to the accumulation of Ach at central cholinergic synapses. These include anxiety, restlessness, emotional lability, insomnia and excessive dreaming. Severe intoxication ultimately results in confusion, ataxia, dysarthria, and absent reflexes and may progress to coma, tonic-clonic seizures.

With prompt initial diagnosis and therapeutic intervention, the maximum clinical features are attained within the first 3 or 4 d, at which time recovery begins. In most patients, complete recovery is expected within 1–3 wk, depending on the severity of intoxication and the effectiveness of the initial therapy *(79)*. Death is usually secondary to respiratory failure often associated with cardiovascular collapse. In the absence of any significant complication recovery occurs within 1 wk.

Diagnosis

Prompt diagnosis is essential to initiate appropriate therapy early in the course of the disease to shorten the duration and decrease the severity of the illness. The rarity of the syndrome in the United States makes it an exceptionally challenging diagnostic problem.

Laboratory Features

Serum levels of organophosphates and cholinesterase activity are the most important laboratory studies in the initial diagnosis. Serum cholinesterase is markedly decreased early in the course and remains so for a long time. Serum organophosphates levels, initially elevated, decrease rapidly over the first 48 h as they are cleared from the blood to other body tissues *(78)*.

Electrophysiological Features

They are the most sensitive indicators of intoxication severity and the recovery process. In addition, they represent the only mode of quantifying the organophosphate inhibitions of AchE at cholinergic synapses. These features include: (1) repetitive firing of the single evoked compound muscle action potential (CMAP); and (2) distinctive CMAP abnormalities in response to repetitive nerve stimulation referred to as the decrement-increment and decrement phenomena *(78)*. The CMAP with repetitive discharges is seen early and virtually always present. The decrement increment response occurs early or late in the course of the intoxication and may be associated with little or no clinical weakness. The decrement phenomenon occurs with more severe intoxications and may be profound at higher rates of repetitive stimulation. The degree of decrement with this latter phenomenon actually reflects the severity of the weakness and the subsequent improvement in the decrement heralds the onset of clinical recovery.

Therapy and Critical Care of Organophosphate Toxicity

Specific Critical Care Issues

Careful monitoring of blood pressure, vital capacity, and mental status in an NSU setting is recommended *(78)*. Depending on the severity of intoxication endotracheal intubation and mechanical ventilation may be required. Removing the patients from further exposure is very important. Gastric lavage with water is essential in order to remove as much as possible of the ingested poison. Along with activated charcoal, cathartics should be given repeatedly for several days. Contamination of skin and mucous membranes requires frequent washing. Although seizures are rare anticonvulsant therapy is advised.

Specific Pharmacologic Therapy

Atropine is primarily effective in treating the muscarinic side effects. It has no action on the NMJ dysfunction. It is recommended to use atropine in doses of 1–2 mg every hour to control excessive pulmonary or bronchial secretion over the first 4–5 d.

Cholinesterase reactivators may be used. Pralidoxime is the one usually used. Prompt utilization would be essential, since phosphorylated AchE becomes resistant to reactivation within a few hours. Failure of reactivation is common and is usually related to delayed initiation of therapy and failures of some organophosphates to be antagonized by oximes. If used in severe intoxication, 1 g of pralidoxime is given IV at a rate less than 500 mg/min. If weakness persists after 20 min, this dosage may be repeated. Pralidoxime has some side effects, including abdominal discomfort, headaches, dizziness, diplopia, nervousness, and malaise *(83)*.

Benzodiazepines, such as midazolam, are useful as sedation in the treatment of the induced CNS hyperirritability. They also assist in the process of mechanical ventilation, as do opiod analgesics such as fentanyl *(78)*.

SNAKE, SPIDER, AND SCORPION ENVENOMATION

Snake Envenomation

In North America, approx 2500 individual experience a poisonous snake bite each year. More than 95% of these are from pit vipers, including rattlesnakes, moccasins, cotton mouth, and copperheads *(84)*.

Clinical Features

The Ebers Papyrus (ca. 1550 BC) recorded the first symptoms reported by a patient bitten by a snake "I am as cold as water and then again as hot as fire. All my body sweats, and I tremble. My eyesight is not steady, and I cannot see for the sweats pours over my face." The clinical course of snakebite is variable and unpredictable because of factors that involve both the biting snake and the bitten human. The two most important factors are the intrinsic toxicity of the venom and the amount injected. The numerous toxins present in snake venoms virtually guarantee that any serious snake bite will show evidence of injury to several organ systems.

Nearly all physicians experienced in treating snakebites stress the various clinical classifications of bites as neurotoxic, hematotoxic, myotoxic. However, a common theme in the clinical picture is the development of cranial nerve palsy. These are characteristically manifested as ptosis and ophthalmoplegia with blurred vision and diplopia, difficulty in swallowing with an inability to handle oral secretions, slurred speech, weakness of facial muscles, and occasionally loss of the sense of taste or smell. The pupils usually are dilated and respond sluggishly to light. This syndrome is accompanied by drowsiness, sometimes with mental confusion and euphoria. Flaccid paralysis affects all muscle groups in no particular order and is accompanied by loss of reflexes. There is no pain on passive movement or pressure. Breathing becomes shallow and diaphragmatic; coma and convulsions may precede death. The onset of this syndrome may be as soon as 3 min after a bite or as late as 24 h *(85)*.

Treatment

ANTIVENINS

Antivenins in adequate doses usually neutralizes life-threatening systemic effects of snake venoms; they are less effective against local effects *(86)*. There are no firm indications for initiating antivenin therapy. Ptosis, occulomotor palsy, slurred speech, and dysphagia are common early signs of envenoming and are indications for antivenin therapy. It is usually administered intravenously diluted with crystalloid or glucose solution. Antivenin is most effective if begun within 4 h after a bite, however some venom effects such as coagulopathy may be reversed even after 24 h *(86)*. Total response of the patient rather than a single parameter should determine the quantity of antivenin given. Doses of 400–500 mL may be needed.

Acute anaphylaxis is a complication of antivenin therapy and appropriate precaution should be taken. About 70–80% of patients who receive antivenin develop serum sickness *(86)*. Venum antigen levels in plasma and in urine are most significant in determining severity of envenoming, whereas aspirate from the bite site or venom deposited on skin or clothing is better for identification of the snake species.

RESPIRATORY PARALYSIS

The respiratory paralysis caused by venom neurotoxins may be difficult to reverse with antivenin therapy. Edrophonium hydrochloride counteracts the NMJ blocking action of some venom more rapidly than antivenin, hence may be administered concomitantly with antivenin therapy *(87)*. Intermittent positive pressure ventilation with or without a tracheostomy is often needed. Artificial respiratory support may be needed for up to 48 h in some cases and for more than 10 d on others *(88)*.

OTHER LIFE-THREATENING COMPLICATIONS

Hypovolemic shock usually responds to antivenin in adequate dosage plus IV fluids. In severe cases vasopressors may be required. A coagulation profile should be obtained on all patients hospitalized for snakebite and repeated in 6–8 h in all but clearly trivial envenoming. It usually responds favorably to antivenin therapy. Supplemental fresh-frozen-plasma, cryoprecipitate, and platelets may be helpful. Renal failure requires correction of electrolyte imbalance and often dialysis. Bacterial infections are uncommon. Local tissue damage and rhabdomyosis may result from impairment of circulation or the direct effect of the venom on tissues or both. If intracompartment pressure reaches 30 mmHg, fasciotomy should be considered *(86)*. When intense swelling involves the hand, digit dermotomy often is beneficial in preventing impairment of function. Periodic measurement of circumference of a bitten limb is usually necessary to determine the presence and progression of swelling. Creatine kinase and lactic dehydrogenase levels should be followed. Examination of urine and plasma for myoglobin may also be helpful.

Spider Envenomation

Black widow spiders are the most common type of spider bites *(89)*. They are found throughout North America, except the extreme north *(89)*. Spiders usually bite when they are disturbed. They usually prefer warm, dark, dry places outdoors or in basement and garages. The venom lacks human cytotoxic agents, so there is no local tissue injury *(84)*. The neurotoxin acts on the presynaptic membrane of the NMJ, opening cation channels that result in the release and decreased reuptake of Ach *(84)*. This causes severe muscle cramping.

Clinical Features

Following spider bites, patients experience only a pricking sensation that fades almost immediately. This is usually followed, 30 min later, by an uncomfortable sensation in the bitten extremity. A "target" or "halo" lesion may appear at the bite site. This local manifestation is specific for black widow and it fades within 12 h of the bite *(89)*. Although significant symptoms usually develop within 1 h, it may be delayed as many as 6–12 h. Patient will experience proximal muscle cramping.

Patients often experience dysautonomia that include nausea, vomiting, malaise, sweating, hypertension, tachycardia, and a vague feeling of dysphoria. Sweating patterns may be unique, involving exclusively the upper lip or even one side of the upper lip or the tip of the nose. Untreated symptoms wax and wane over 36–72 h. Although the pain fades, some patients describe malaise or sensation of not feeling "right" for 2–4 wk *(89)*.

Management

With modern supportive care, death rarely results from a black widow spider bite. The cornerstone of treatment is analgesia. Symptomatic care also includes maintenance of adequate hydration and treatment of severe hypertension.

PAIN CONTROL

Analgesics should be administered in doses sufficient to relieve pain. Oral medications may be sufficient for patients experiencing minor discomfort. Intravenous opiods, such as morphine or meperidine, are reserved for severe pain. Benzodiazepines are used as adjunctive therapy to analgesics. Patients who have severe pain refractory to opiod analgesics should receive horse serum-derived antivenin, which offers rapid, complete relief of pain *(89)*.

HYPERTENSION

In most cases, adequate analgesia alleviates hypertension. Although severe hypertension is rare, but if present despite analgesia, nitroprusside or antivenin should be considered. Acute hypersensitivity reactions to antivenin have resulted in death. Therefore, only those experiencing severe pain that cannot be controlled by opioid analgesics or those who have life-threatening hypertension and tachycardia that are not controlled with supportive care should be considered candidates for antivenin *(89)*.

Scorpion Stings

The only scorpion species of medical importance in the United States is the Arizona bark scorpion *(84)*. Toxins in its venom interfere with activation of sodium channels and enhance firing of axons.

Clinical Features

Local pain is the most frequent symptom. Cytotoxic effects are absent; there is no erythema, swelling or blanching. Peripheral motor neuron and cranial nerve manifestations often appear. These include muscle fasciculation, tongue fasciculation, facial twitching, and rapid disconjugate eye movements. When victims experience a severe reaction, they frequently exhibit agitation, extreme tachycardia, salivation, and respiratory distress. The respiratory distress probably is owing to a combination of excess salivation, loss of pharyngeal muscle tone, and uncoordinated contraction of the diaphragm and intercostals muscles.

Management

Mechanical ventilation may be required in some patients. Patients may be managed with supportive care (analgesia, sedation, airway support, ventilation, and supplemental oxygen administration). Antivenin therapy may reduce the need for airway and ventilatory support mostly in children. Symptoms severity in adults rarely justifies the risk of antivenin administration and usually resolve over 12–48 h *(84)*.

TICK PARALYSIS

Epidemiology

Tick paralysis has been well known in domestic and wild animals in Australia and South Africa. It was first recognized in humans in the late 19th century *(90)*. Human cases are best known in Australia but have been reported from North America and South Africa. In North America, the west and the southeast regions of the United States and British Columbia in Canada have been sources of most of the cases. The offending tick differs from continent to continent. The North American tick is *Dermacentor andersoni (91)*.

Pathophysiology

Ticks are arachnids. When in immature forms, both males and females feed by sucking blood from hosts, but only adult females feed. Adult ticks may survive several years between feedings. Paralysis is caused only by the bite of a pregnant female tick. It was initially postulated that a substance produced by the tick and injected into the host induced the paralysis *(90)*. No infectious agent has been identified in tickborne paralysis. A toxin present in the salivary glands of pregnant female ticks is the paralytic agent *(92)*. Repeated exposure to tick bite may result in resistance to subsequent bites *(91)*.

Clinical Features

Children are much more commonly involved than adults. Dark haired persons are said to be more susceptible, but in fact dark hair may only allow the tick to remain obscure *(93)*. Two or more days after attachment of the tick, weakness begins. The pattern of weakness has been described as ascending. Rarely, only localized weakness such as unilateral facial paralysis has occurred *(94)*. The weakness progresses over 2 or more days. At maximum evolution, the weakness is symmetrical and flaccid, and there is diffuse areflexia. Pupils remain reactive, and sensorium remains clear in the absence of compounding factors, such as untreated respiratory insufficiency. The patient is afebrile unless a secondary infection is present. The sensory examination is normal, although some patients have reported a tingling sensation.

The tick is commonly found in the hair of the scalp. It is engorged from feeding on the host's blood, and more than one may be present. The tick should be removed. Following removal of the tick, weakness may progress for some hours but is generally beginning to improve somewhat by 24 h. Full recovery is frequently noted by 3–11 d after tick removal, but one case with leg weakness persisting 6 mo has been reported *(95)*. Blood and cerebrospinal fluid (CSF) studies are normal.

Electrophysiological Features

Motor nerve conduction studies show slow velocities and normal distal latencies *(95)*. CMAP are abnormally low or low normal in amplitude at the time of maximum clinical deficit. Sensory nerve action potential have been of normal amplitude at the time of the maximum motor deficit. There is no abnormal dispersion of the action potentials between distal and proximal stimulation sites. F waves have been normal. Repetitive motor nerve stimulation at frequencies up to 50 Hz has produced no decrement in the amplitude of CMAP. Following removal of the tick, CMAP amplitudes begin increasing and may double in 3–4 d. Sensory action potentials have been noted to increase in amplitude following tick removal despite having been "normal" initially *(96)*.

Treatment

Removal of the tick is the most successful therapy for tick bite. Many methods of removal have been devised, but the preferred method is by using forceps pressed to the sides of the mouth. A levering and lifting motion of the forceps will detach the tick *(97)*. The body of the tick should not be squeezed. Attention should also be placed on the respiratory signs of airway compromise and some patients may need to be placed on sustaining life support.

CRITICAL ILLNESS POLYNEUROPATHY AND MYOPATHY

Epidemiology

Critical illness polyneuropathy (CIP) and myopathy (CIM) are neuromuscular disorders that have been documented in patients admitted to general intensive care units (ICU) *(98–107)*. Their incidence has been found to range from 33% to 44% in critically ill patients and is responsible for failure-to-wean from mechanical ventilation in these patients *(99)*. The true incidence in the NSU is not known because most of the studies reported thus far have been carried out in ICU. However, owing to the severity of illness that many NSU patients experience it is expected that some of them will develop CIP and CIM. These disorders should be entertained in all patients deemed "difficult-to-wean." We describe the key clinical, diagnostic, and management features of these conditions.

Pathophysiology

The etiology of CIP and CIM has been linked to two possible factors: (1) Severe sepsis or systemic inflammatory response syndrome (SIRS); or (2) a combination of sepsis or SIRS and neuromuscular blocking agents (NMA) or steroids *(98,99,102,105,106)*. SIRS includes the presence of two or more of the following findings: body temperature >38°C or <36°C; hear rate >90 beats/min; tachypnea (respiratory rate >20 breaths/min) or hyperventilation as determined by $PaCO_2$ <32 mmHg; and alteration in the white blood cell count (count >12,000/mm^3, count <4000/ mm^3, or the presence of more than 10% of immature neutrophils) *(99)*. Other conditions that have been postulated as etiologic factors include nutritional status, severity of underlying illness, and interaction between medications used in the ICU. More evidence has emerged regarding neuromuscular dysfunction in CIP and CIM patients prior to the development of the disease *(98,102)*. There is a fall in CMAP within 2 wk of SIRS onset, which may be associated to decreased bioenergetic reserves. Also in patients with CIM the muscle may be unresponsive to direct stimulation, which may be related to diminished sodium currents. Another interesting finding is the inflammatory reaction found in muscle and nerve biopsy specimens in this patient population, which implies some sort of humoral or cellular immune response. The association between SIRS and CIP and CIM has been recently investigated in a longitudinal observational prospective study in mechanically ventilated patients in an ICU *(99)*. The authors found that after multivariate analysis, the presence of SIRS and the APACHE III score were significantly related to the risk of developing these conditions. There appears to be three different subgroups of patients: low-risk group (APACHE III score ≤ 70 and no SIRS) with a probability of 8% for developing CIP or CIM; high risk group (APACHE III score > 85 and SIRS) with a probability of 72%; and a medium-risk group (includes patients in between low and high risk) with a probability of 28% of developing these disorders. These findings provide useful information for NSU clinicians regarding identification of patients at risk, determination of long-term prognosis, and management.

Clinical Presentation

The clinical features basically include patients who are difficult to wean from mechanical ventilation, and who also have tetraparesis and muscle wasting on examination. These patients usually present with severe sepsis or multiorgan failure. Although the administration of NMA or steroids is not the cause of CIP or CIM, these agents may be harmful to muscles exacerbating the condition *(98,99)*. This has been shown in patients with status asthmaticus treated with steroids and NMA.

Diagnosis

The diagnosis is essentially established by EMG studies *(98,99,103)*. Measurement of serum CK concentrations and analysis of muscle biopsy specimens can also be helpful. Because the majority of patients are diagnosed within 2–3 wk after initiation of mechanical ventilation, an EMG should be performed 10–12 d after *(99)*. Based on the combination of these tests a classification has been proposed *(98)*: *Polyneuropathy*, which includes CIP and distal motor axonopathy. In CIP, EMG findings include axonal degeneration of motor and sensory fibers, serum CK is normal, and muscle biopsy reveals denervation atrophy. In distal axonal axonopathy, EMG shows "myopathic" motor unit potentials, serum CK is normal, and muscle biopsy demonstrates denervation atrophy. *Neuromuscular transmission defect*, which is given by transient NMJ blockade. In this situation EMG reveals abnormal repetitive nerve stimulation, whereas serum CK and muscle biopsy are normal. *CIM* has been related to the administration of steroids and NMA, and asthma. EMG findings consist of "myopathic" motor unit potentials. Serum CK is elevated and muscle biopsy reveals a myopathy with myosin loss. Another two conditions related to CIM include disuse or cachectic myopathy and the so-called necrotizing myopathy of intensive care. The former presents with normal EMG, serum CK, and normal or type 2 fiber atrophy in muscle biopsy, whereas the latter presents with abnormal spontaneous activity in muscle by EMG, markedly elevated serum CK, and panfascicular muscle fiber necrosis by muscle biopsy.

Management

There is no specific management for CIP and CIM. However, from the discussion above it seems logical to expect a decrease in the incidence of these conditions with better and more aggressive treatment of sepsis and multiorgan failure. Supportive general and respiratory care is essential because most of these patients will eventually recover despite persistent EMG abnormalities *(100)*. There has been one retrospective study that reported on the administration of intravenous immunoglobulins in this patient population *(107)*. Although there was some indication of clinical improvement, the nature of the study and the lack of validation preclude us from recommending this treatment.

REFERENCES

1. Centers for Disease Control. Progress toward the global elimination of neonatal tetanus, 1988–1993. *MMWR* 1994;43:885–894.
2. Centers for Disease Control. Tetanus Surveillance-United States, 1995–1997. *MMWR* 1998;47:1–13.
3. Bleck T, Brauner J. Tetanus. In: Scheld W, Whitely R, Durack D (eds). *Infections of the Central Nervous System*, 2nd ed. Philadelphia: Lippincott-Raven, 1997:629–653.
4. Stoll BJ. Tetanus. *Pediatr. Clin. North Am.* 1979;26:415–431.

5. Hsu SS, Groleau G. Tetanus in the emergency department: A current review. *J. Emerg. Med.* 2001;20:357–365.
6. Jagoda A, Riggio S, Burguieres T. Cephalic tetanus: A case report and review of the literature. *Am. J. Emerg. Med.* 1988;6:128–30.
7. Apte NM, Karnad DR. Short report: the spatula test: A simple bedside test to diagnose tetanus. *Am. J. Trop. Med. Hyg.* 1995;53:386–387.
8. Trujillo MH, Castillo A, Espana J, Manzo A, Zerpa R. Impact of intensive care management on the prognosis of tetanus. Analysis of 641 cases. *Chest* 1987;92:63–65.
9. Wright DK, Lalloo UG, Nayiager S, Govender P. Autonomic nervous system dysfunction in severe tetanus: current perspectives. *Crit. Care Med.* 1989;17:371–375.
10. King WW, Cave DR. Use of esmolol to control autonomic instability of tetanus. *Am. J. Med.* 1991;91:425–428.
11. Domenighetti GM, Savary G, Stricker H. Hyperadrenergic syndrome in severe tetanus: Extreme rise in catecholamines responsive to labetalol. *BMJ* 1984;288:1483–1484.
12. Sutton DN, Tremlett MR, Woodcock TE, Nielsen MS. Management of autonomic dysfunction in severe tetanus: the use of magnesium sulphate and clonidine. *Intensive Care Med.* 1990;16:75–80.
13. Brown JL, Sinding H, Mathias CJ. Autonomic disturbance in severe tetanus: failure of parenteral clonidine to control blood pressure. *J. Infect.* 1994;29:67–71.
14. Moughabghab AV, Prevost G, Socolovsky C. Fentanyl therapy controls autonomic hyperactivity in tetanus. *Br. J. Clin. Pract.* 1996;50:477–478.
15. Southorn PA, Blaise GA. Treatment of tetanus-induced autonomic nervous system dysfunction with continuous epidural blockade. *Crit. Care Med.* 1986;14:251–252.
16. Farquhar I, Hutchinson A, Curran J. Dantrolene in severe tetanus. *Intensive Care Med.* 1988;14:249–250.
17. Brock H, Moosbauer W, Gabriel C, Necek S, Bidal D. Treatment of severe tetanus by continuous intrathecal infusion of baclofen. *J. Neurol. Neurosurg. Psychiatry* 1995;59:193–194.
18. Fassoulaki A, Eforakopoulou M. Vecuronium in the management of tetanus. Is it the muscle relaxant of choice? *Acta. Anaesthesiol. Belg.* 1988;39:75–78.
19. Martyn JA, White DA, Gronert GA, Jaffe RS, Ward JM. Up-and-down regulation of skeletal muscle acetylcholine receptors. Effects on neuromuscular blockers. *Anesthesiology* 1992;76:822–843.
20. John DA, Tobey RE, Homer LD, Rice CL. Onset of succinylcholine-induced hyperkalemia following denervation. *Anesthesiology* 1976;45:294–299.
21. Sanford JP. Tetanus—forgotten but not gone. *N. Engl. J. Med.* 1995;332:812–813.
22. Ahmadsyah I, Salim A. Treatment of tetanus: an open study to compare the efficacy of procaine penicillin and metronidazole. *BMJ* 1985;291:648–650.
23. Spenney JG, Lamb RN, Cobbs CG. Recurrent tetanus. *South Med. J.* 1971;64:859 passim.
24. Amato AA. Acid maltase deficiency and related myopathies. *Neurol. Clin.* 2000;18:151–165.
25. Barohn RJ, McVey AL, DiMauro S. Adult acid maltase deficiency. *Muscle Nerve* 1993;16:672–676.
26. Engel AG, Gomez MR, Seybold ME, Lambert EH. The spectrum and diagnosis of acid maltase deficiency. *Neurology* 1973;23:95–106.
27. Felice KJ, Alessi AG, Grunnet ML. Clinical variability in adult-onset acid maltase deficiency: Report of affected sibs and review of the literature. *Medicine (Baltimore)* 1995;74:131–135.
28. Wokke JH, Ausems MG, van den Boogaard MJ, Ippel EF, van Diggelene O, Kroos MA, et al. Genotype-phenotype correlation in adult-onset acid maltase deficiency. *Ann. Neurol.* 1995;38:450–454.
29. Reuser AJ, Kroos MA, Hermans MM, Bijvoet AG, Verbeet MP, Van Diggelen OP, et al. Glycogenosis type II (acid maltase deficiency). *Muscle Nerve* 1995;3:S61–S69.
30. Engel A, Hirschorn R. Acid maltase deficiency. In: Engel A, Franzini-Armstrong C (eds). *Myology.* New York: McGraw Hill, 1994:1533–1553.
31. Gambetti P, DiMauro S, Baker L. Nervous system in Pompe's disease. Ultrastructure and biochemistry. *J. Neuropathol. Exp. Neurol.* 1971;30:412–430.
32. Raben N, Nichols RC, Boerkoel C, Plotz P. Genetic defects in patients with glycogenosis type II (acid maltase deficiency). *Muscle Nerve* 1995;3:S70–S74.
33. Bulkley BH, Hutchins GM. Pompe's disease presenting as hypertrophic myocardiopathy with Wolff- Parkinson-White syndrome. *Am. Heart J.* 1978;96:246–252.
34. De Dominicis E, Finocchi G, Vincenzi M, Calvelli M, Ronconi G, Angelini C, et al. Echocardiographic and pulsed Doppler features in glycogen storage disease type II of the heart (Pompe's disease). *Acta. Cardiol.* 1991;46:107–114.
35. Metzl JD, Elias ER, Berul CI. An interesting case of infant sudden death: severe hypertrophic cardiomyopathy in Pompe's disease. *Pacing Clin. Electrophysiol.* 1999;22:821–822.
36. Mellies U, Ragette R, Schwake C, Baethmann M, Voit T, Teschler H. Sleep-disordered breathing and respiratory failure in acid maltase deficiency. *Neurology* 2001;57:1290–1295.
37. Servidei S, DiMauro S. Disorders of glycogen metabolism of muscle. *Neurol. Clin.* 1989;7:159–178.
38. Bodamer OA, Leonard JV, Halliday D. Dietary treatment in late-onset acid maltase deficiency. *Eur. J. Pediatr.* 1997;156 Suppl 1:S39–S42.

39. Nicolino MP, Puech JP, Kremer EJ, Reuser AJ, Mbebi C, Verdiere-Sahuque M, et al. Adenovirus-mediated transfer of the acid alpha-glucosidase gene into fibroblasts, myoblasts and myotubes from patients with glycogen storage disease type II leads to high level expression of enzyme and corrects glycogen accumulation. *Hum. Mol. Genet.* 1998;7:1695–1702.

40. Pauly DF, Johns DC, Matelis LA, Lawrence JH, Byrne BJ, Kessler PD. Complete correction of acid alpha-glucosidase deficiency in Pompe disease fibroblasts in vitro, and lysosomally targeted expression in neonatal rat cardiac and skeletal muscle. *Gene Ther.* 1998;5:473–480.

41. Lehmann-Horn F, Rudel R. Channelopathies: the nondystrophic myotonias and periodic paralyses. *Semin. Pediatr. Neurol.* 1996;3:122–139.

42. Riggs JE. The periodic paralyses. *Neurol. Clin.* 1988;6:485–498.

43. Sansone V, Griggs RC, Meola G, Ptacek LJ, Barohn R, Iannaccone S, et al. Andersen's syndrome: a distinct periodic paralysis. *Ann. Neurol.* 1997;42:305–312.

44. Hayward L, Brown RH. Periodic paralysis and related mytonic diseases. In: Feldman E (ed). *Current Diagnosis in Neurology*. St. Louis: Mosby-Year Book, 1993:353–356.

45. Gutmann L. Periodic paralyses. *Neurol. Clin.* 2000;18:195–202.

46. Feero WG, Wang J, Barany F, Zhou J, Todorovic SM, Conwit R, et al. Hyperkalemic periodic paralysis: rapid molecular diagnosis and relationship of genotype to phenotype in 12 families. *Neurology* 1993;43:668–673.

47. Cannon SC. Sodium channel defects in myotonia and periodic paralysis. *Annu. Rev. Neurosci.* 1996;19:141–164.

48. Cummins TR, Sigworth FJ. Impaired slow inactivation in mutant sodium channels. *Biophys. J.* 1996;71:227–236.

49. Fontaine B, Vale-Santos J, Jurkat-Rott K, Reboul J, Plassart E, Rime CS, et al. Mapping of the hypokalaemic periodic paralysis (HypoPP) locus to chromosome 1q31-32 in three European families. *Nat. Genet.* 1994;6:267–272.

50. Greenberg DA. Calcium channels in neurological disease. *Ann. Neurol.* 1997;42:275–82.

51. Fardwau M, Tome F. Congenital myopathies. In: Engel A, Franzini-Armstrong C (eds). *Myology*. New York: McGraw-Hill, 1994:1516–1519.

52. Tawil R. Periodic paralysis. In: Johnson R, Griffin J, McArtur J (eds). *Current Therapy in Neurologic Disease*, 6th ed. St. Louis: Mosby Year Book, 2002:422–424.

53. Cherington M. Botulism: clinical and therapeutic observations. *Rocky Mt. Med. J.* 1972;69:55–58.

54. Wound botulism—California, 1995. *MMWR* 1995;44:889–892.

55. Kudrow DB, Henry DA, Haake DA, Marshall G, Mathisen GE. Botulism associated with Clostridium botulinum sinusitis after intranasal cocaine abuse. *Ann. Intern. Med.* 1988;109:984–985.

56. Schantz EJ, Johnson EA. Botulinum toxin: The story of its development for the treatment of human disease. *Perspect. Biol. Med.* 1997;40:317–327.

57. Burningham MD, Walter FG, Mechem C, Haber J, Ekins BR. Wound botulism. *Ann. Emerg. Med.* 1994;24:1184–1187.

58. Mandler RN, Maselli RA. Stimulated single-fiber electromyography in wound botulism. *Muscle Nerve* 1996;19:1171–1173.

59. Pickett J, Berg B, Chaplin E, Brunstetter-Shafer MA. Syndrome of botulism in infancy: Clinical and electrophysiologic study. *N. Engl. J. Med.* 1976;295:770–772.

60. Cherington M. Botulism. *Semin. Neurol.* 1990;10:27–31.

61. Goode GB, Shearn DL. Botulism: a case with associated sensory abnormalities. *Arch. Neurol.* 1982;39:55.

62. Duchen LW, Strich SJ. The effects of botulinum toxin on the pattern of innervation of skeletal muscle in the mouse. *Q. J. Exp. Physiol. Cogen. Med. Sci.* 1968;53:84–89.

63. Jenzer G, Mumenthaler M, Ludin HP, Robert F. Autonomic dysfunction in botulism B: A clinical report. *Neurology* 1975;25:150–153.

64. Girlanda P, Vita G, Nicolosi C, Milone S, Messina C. Botulinum toxin therapy: Distant effects on neuromuscular transmission and autonomic nervous system. *J. Neurol. Neurosurg. Psychiatry* 1992;55:844–845.

65. Woodruff BA, Griffin PM, McCroskey LM, Smart JF, Wainwright RB, Bryant RG, et al. Clinical and laboratory comparison of botulism from toxin types A, B, and E in the United States, 1975–1988. *J. Infect. Dis.* 1992;166:1281–1286.

66. Cherington M. Electrophysiologic methods as an aid in diagnosis of botulism: A review. *Muscle Nerve* 1982;5:S28–S29.

67. Gutmann L, Bodensteiner J, Gutierrez A. Electrodiagnosis of botulism. *J. Pediatr.* 1992;121(5 Pt 1):835.

68. Chaudhry V, Crawford TO. Stimulation single-fiber EMG in infant botulism. *Muscle Nerve* 1999;22:1698–703.

69. Girlanda P, Dattola R, Messina C. Single fibre EMG in 6 cases of botulism. *Acta. Neurol. Scand.* 1983;67:118–123.

70. Brown LW. Infant botulism. *Adv. Pediatr.* 1981;28:141–157.

71. Black RE, Gunn RA. Hypersensitivity reactions associated with botulinal antitoxin. *Am. J. Med.* 1980;69:567–570.

72. Davis LE, Johnson JK, Bicknell JM, Levy H, McEvoy KM. Human type A botulism and treatment with 3,4-diaminopyridine. *Electromyogr. Clin. Neurophysiol.* 1992;32:379–383.

73. Oh SJ, Halsey JH, Jr., Briggs DD, Jr. Guanidine in type B botulism. *Arch. Intern. Med.* 1975;135:726–728.

74. Kappas A. The porphyrias. In: Scriver C (ed). *The Metabolic Basis of Inherited Disease*. New York: McGraw-Hill, 1989:1305–1365.

75. Sagar S. Toxic and metabolic disorders. In: Samuels M (ed). *Manual of Neurologic Therapeutics*, 5th ed. Boston: Little, Brown, 1994:299–301.

76. Albers JW, Robertson WC Jr, Daube JR. Electrodiagnostic findings in acute porphyric neuropathy. *Muscle Nerve* 1978;1:292–296.

77. Taylor P. Anticholinesterase agents. In: Gilman A, Goodman L, Rall T, Murad F (eds). *The Pharmacological Basis of Therapeutics*, 7th ed. New York: Macmillan, 1985:110–129.
78. Besser R, Gutmann L, Dillmann U, Weilemann LS, Hopf HC. End-plate dysfunction in acute organophosphate intoxication. *Neurology* 1989;39:561–567.
79. Wadia RS, Sadagopan C, Amin RB, Sardesai HV. Neurological manifestations of organophosphorous insecticide poisoning. *J. Neurol. Neurosurg. Psychiatry* 1974;37:841–847.
80. Lotti M, Becker CE, Aminoff MJ. Organophosphate polyneuropathy: pathogenesis and prevention. *Neurology* 1984;34:658–662.
81. Cherniack MG. Organophosphorus esters and polyneuropathy. *Ann. Intern. Med.* 1986;104:264–266.
82. Namba T, Nolte CT, Jackrel J, Grob D. Poisoning due to organophosphate insecticides. Acute and chronic manifestations. *Am. J. Med.* 1971;50:475–492.
83. Gutmann L, Besser R. Organophosphate intoxication: Pharmacologic, neurophysiologic, clinical, and therapeutic considerations. *Semin. Neurol.* 1990;10:46–51.
84. Bond GR. Snake, spider, and scorpion envenomation in North America. *Pediatr. Rev.* 1999;20:147–150.
85. Watt G, Padre L, Tuazon L, Theakston RD, Laughlin L. Bites by the Philippine cobra (Naja naja philippinensis): Prominent neurotoxicity with minimal local signs. *Am. J. Trop. Med. Hyg.* 1988;39:306–311.
86. Minton SA. Neurotoxic snake envenoming. *Semin. Neurol.* 1990;10:52–61.
87. Watt G, Theakston RD, Hayes CG, Yambao ML, Sangalang R, Ranoa CP, et al. Positive response to edrophonium in patients with neurotoxic envenoming by cobras (Naja naja philippinensis). A placebo-controlled study. *N. Engl. J. Med.* 1986;315:1444–1448.
88. Patten BR, Pearn JH, DeBuse P, Burke J, Covacevich J. Prolonged intensive therapy after snake bite. A probable case of envenomation by the rough-scaled snake. *Med. J. Aust.* 1985;142:467–469.
89. Clark RF, Wethern-Kestner S, Vance MV, Gerkin R. Clinical presentation and treatment of black widow spider envenomation: a review of 163 cases. *Ann. Emerg. Med.* 1992;21:782–787.
90. Kincaid JC. Tick bite paralysis. *Semin. Neurol.* 1990;10:32–34.
91. Njau BC, Nyindo M, Mutani A. Immunological responses and the role of the paralyzing toxin in rabbits infested with Rhipicephalus evertsi evertsi. *Am. J. Trop. Med. Hyg.* 1986;35:1248–1255.
92. Stone BF, Neish AL, Wright IG. Immunization of rabbits to produce high serum titres of neutralizing antibodies and immunity to the paralyzing toxin of Ixodes holocyclus. *Aust. J. Exp. Biol. Med. Sci.* 1982;60 Pt 4:351–358.
93. Andersen RD. Colorado tick fever and tick paralysis in a young child. *Pediatr. Infect. Dis.* 1983;2:43–44.
94. Pearn J. Neuromuscular paralysis caused by tick envenomation. *J. Neurol. Sci.* 1977;34:37–42.
95. Donat JR, Donat JF. Tick paralysis with persistent weakness and electromyographic abnormalities. *Arch. Neurol.* 1981;38:59–61.
96. Swift TR, Ignacio OJ. Tick paralysis: Electrophysiologic studies. *Neurology* 1975;25:1130–1133.
97. Tibballs J, Cooper SJ. Paralysis with Ixodes cornuatus envenomation. *Med. J. Aust.* 1986;145:37–38.
98. Bolton CF. Critical illness polyneuropathy and myopahty. *Crit. Care Med.* 2001;29:2388–2390.
99. de Letter MAC, Schmitz PIM, Visser LH, et al. Risk factors for the development of polyneuropathy and myopathy in critically ill patients. *Crit. Care Med.* 2001;29:2281–2286.
100. Hund EF, Fogel W, Krieger D, DeGeorgia M, Hacke W. Critical illness polyneuropathy: Clinical findings and outcomes of a frequent cause of neuromuscular weaning failure. *Crit. Care Med.* 1996;24:1328–1333.
101. Latronico N, Fenzi F, Recupero D, et al. Critical illness myopathy and neuropathy. *Lancet* 1996;347:1579–1582.
102. Bolton CF. Sepsis and the systemic inflammatory response syndrome: neuromuscular manifestations. *Crit. Care Med.* 1996;24:1408–1416.
103. Schwarz J, Planck J, Briegel J, Straube A. Single-fiber electromyography, nerve conduction studies, and conventional electromyography in patients with critical-illness polyneuropathy: evidence for alesion of terminal motor axons. *Muscle Nerve* 1997;20:696–701.
104. Hund E. Myopathy in critically ill patients. *Crit. Care Med.* 1999;27:2544–2547.
105. Hund E. Critical illness polyneuropathy. *Curr. Opin. Neurol.* 2001;14:649–653.
106. Hund E. Neurological complications of sepsis: critical illness polyneuropathy and myopathy. *J. Neurol.* 2001;248:929–934.
107. Mohr M, Englisch L, Roth A, et al. Effects of early treatment with immunoglobulin on critical illness polyneuropathy following multiple organ failure and gram-negative sepsis. *Intensive Care Med.* 1997;23:1144–1149.

29

Infections of the Central Nervous System

Ronald G. Riechers, II, Abel D. Jarell, and Geoffrey S. F. Ling

INTRODUCTION

The central nervous system (CNS) is typically regarded as a privileged environment in the human body because of the innate protection afforded by the blood brain barrier. Nevertheless, various microbial pathogens are capable of infecting the nervous system, particularly in the immunocompromised host. Generally, CNS infections can be broadly categorized into infections of the meninges (meningitis), parenchyma (encephalitis), abscesses, granulomatous infections, and fungal infections. This chapter covers the epidemiology, diagnosis, pathophysiology, treatment, and outcome of these general categories of CNS infections.

MENINGITIS

Epidemiology

There are two main forms of meningitis: septic and aseptic. Septic meningitis is defined as a bacterial infection of the meninges, whereas aseptic meningitis is either an infectious or inflammatory process involving the meninges in which no bacterial pathogen is identified. Making a distinction in the type of meningitis is important because the incidence and severity of each vary markedly, and their treatment is different. Septic meningitis is typically more severe with a greater propensity for causing lasting neurological sequelae. In 1995, there were 5755 cases of septic meningitis reported. Aseptic meningitis typically has a more benign clinical course. Approximately 10,000 cases are reported each year with some studies estimating that up to 75,000 cases occur yearly (1).

Recent case studies demonstrate an increasing rate of nosocomial meningitis with reports that nosocomial meningitis accounts for up to 28–40% of total meningitis cases. The median age for all types of meningitis is 25 yr. In a recent retrospective case review of adult meningitis, excluding neurosurgical patients, the mean age was 50. Interestingly, the authors of this study also noted a slight male predominance. Meningitis in the pediatric age group tends to occur as a result of respiratory dissemination of bacteria among children in close quarters. Owing to this airborne method of spread, bacterial meningitis is often seen in outbreaks (1–3).

Signs/Symptoms

Meningitis is an acute febrile illness with a classic clinical triad of symptoms: fever, headache, and meningismus (stiff neck). The onset of symptoms usually occurs within hours to days of infection. Associated findings include general malaise, photophobia, nausea, vomiting, mental status changes, focal neurologic findings, and seizures. While the classic triad of findings is thought to be diagnostic for meningitis, in certain age groups parts or all of the triad may be absent. In the elderly, who have a diminished capability to develop a fever, the peak temperature may be low grade, and

From: *Current Clinical Neurology*
Critical Care Neurology and Neurosurgery
Edited by: J. I. Suarez © Humana Press Inc., Totowa, NJ

photophobia or signs of meningeal irritation such as stiff neck are some times not observed either. Often, mental status changes may be the only presenting complaint. A recent report found that fever was seen in 97% of cases, nuchal rigidity in 87%, headache in 66%, nausea in 55%, confusion in 56%, and decreased level of consciousness in 51%. Specific physical examination findings include Kernig's and Brudzinski's signs—indications of meningeal irritation. Brudzinski's sign is elicited by passively flexing the patient's neck with observation of reflexive leg flexion. Kernig's sign is seen when the patient's neck flexes as a result of passive leg extension and hip flexion. Focal neurologic findings may also be elicited on examination. Approximately 15% of all patients with meningitis have focal findings, and this proportion increases to 40% in elderly patients. Other findings that often present on initial evaluation include the more ominous signs of increased intracranial pressure (ICP) such as papilledema, unilateral dilated pupil, opthalmoparesis, and the Cushing response (hypertension and bradycardia). These findings are more likely observed in patients who present in an obtunded state *(1,3–6)*.

Pathophysiology

Four main pathophysiologic mechanisms explain the development of meningitis. The most common mechanism leading to infection of the meninges is colonization of the nasopharynx with subsequent translocation of bacteria into the bloodstream, resulting in bacteremia and meningeal seeding. This mechanism requires that bacteria survive the host's complement-mediated immunologic defenses within the bloodstream. Bacteria that are successful in accomplishing this feat usually do so because of the presence of a protective polysaccharide capsule. Next, the bacteria must cross the blood-brain barrier, and finally, they need to replicate within the cerebrospinal fluid (CSF). A second mechanism of infection is parameningeal spread of bacteria from head and neck infections. Common parameningeal infections include sinusitis, otitis media and externa, mastoiditis, and, less frequently, dental infections. Sinus and dental infections are of particular importance to the intensivist because they are commonly undetected reservoirs of bacteria. Other pathophysiologic mechanisms of meningitis particularly relevant to the critical care clinician are invasive neurosurgical procedures or other trauma leading to disruption of the meninges. Finally, rupture of a brain abscess into the subarachnoid space may result in meningitis *(7)*.

The severity of meningitis is due to several factors. First, the CNS is a well-protected organ system with a bony skeletal encasement that allows little room for expansion during a localized inflammatory process. The Monro-Kellie doctrine dictates that, given the rigidly enclosed intracranial space and its defined components consisting of brain matter, CSF, and blood, when there is expansion of any one component, there must be compensatory contraction of another. If compensation is incomplete, pressure (ICP) within this closed space will increase. Because the liquid components in the intracranial compartment are noncompressible, excessive ICP can result in neuronal damage and, ultimately, brain herniation. Second, because of the blood brain barrier, the CNS is poorly penetrated by antibiotics making treatment difficult. Finally, the immune system employed in the CNS does not possess the complete armamentarium of defensive components, thus limiting its ability to thoroughly protect against invading infectious pathogens. The bactericidal response of the immune system to infection eventually leads to bacterial killing, but before all of the virulent bacteria are eliminated, potentially detrimental effects may ensue *(1)*.

The inflammatory process occurs in response to bacterial cell wall components such as lipopolysaccharide, peptidoglycan and teichoic acid. Inflammatory mediators subsequently cause brain edema and localized tissue injury. The key circulating factors orchestrating the inflammatory process are most likely interleukin-1 (IL-1), IL-6, and tumor necrosis factor (TNF). The primary mechanisms leading to brain edema in meningitis are fourfold: (1) increased permeability of the blood-brain barrier mediated by CNS inflammation (vasogenic edema); (2) toxins released by both bacteria and neutrophils resulting in intracellular edema (cytotoxic edema); (3) syndrome of inappropriate antidiuretic hormone (SIADH) secondary to inflammation (cytotoxic edema); and (4) resistance to CSF outflow (interstitial edema). SIADH can complicate as many as 50% of cases of meningitis *(7,8)*.

Pathogens

Pathogens that cause meningitis are varied and depend on many factors including the type of meningitis (aseptic vs septic), patient age, and comorbid medical conditions. Aseptic meningitis is primarily an infectious process caused by viral pathogens, however, it can be caused by drugs and autoimmune disorders. Viral pathogens are many and include the Enteroviruses (echovirus, cocksackie A and B, poliovirus, and so on) and certain arboviruses. Enteroviruses account for 55–70% of aseptic meningitis cases. Specific pathogen identification is often unnecessary for many reasons. Viral meningitis is typically self-limited, and no viral-specific therapies exist. Also, these pathogens are of less importance to the intensivist given their generally benign nature *(1,6)*.

Septic meningitis is an infection of the meninges caused by bacteria. The most common bacterial pathogens in all age groups are as follows: *Streptococcus pneumoniae* (47%), *Neisseria meningitidis* (25%), Group B *Streptococcus* (GBS) (12%), *Listeria monocytogenes* (8%), and *Haemophilus influenzae* (7%). In adults, the distribution of pathogens is similar to that seen in the general population except that the incidence of both GBS and *H. influenzae* is lower, and Gram-negative rods such as *E. coli* occur more frequently. *S. pneumoniae* is spread via respiratory droplets, thus there is often a concomitant pneumonia. *N. meningitidis* tends to occur in adolescents in outbreaks, frequently in college dormitories and military barracks because of close contact and respiratory dissemination. Diabetics, elderly patients (age >60), immunocompromised patients, and alcoholics demonstrate a higher frequency of Listerial meningitis. *H. influenzae* used to be a frequent cause of meningitis with significant morbidity in the past. However, since the introduction of the Hib vaccine, its incidence has markedly decreased. GBS, a constituent of the normal vaginal flora, is a pathogen often seen in neonatal meningitis. Neonates acquire this microbe from passage through the birth canal; thus GBS is a rare cause of adult meningitis. Certain clinical conditions predispose patients to other less common pathogens. Staphylococcal meningitis (*S. aureus* and *S. epidermidis*) is seen in patients with indwelling catheters, intraventricular shunts, head trauma and those postoperative from neurosurgical procedures. Gram-negative rods such as *Proteus*, *Pseudomonas*, *Serratia*, and *Flavobacteria* are seen with increased frequency in mechanically ventilated patients. In general, Gram-negative bacteria make up a higher percentage of nosocomial meningitis, 39% of cases vs 3% of community-acquired cases. Also, Gram-negative meningitis mostly occurs as a result of meningeal seeding from bacteremia, thus these patients may be septic on presentation *(1,3,6–8)*.

Diagnosis

As mentioned previously, history and physical examination are typically very suggestive of the diagnosis of meningitis in most patients. Nevertheless, all suspected meningitis patients warrant a thorough workup to include, at a minimum, complete blood cell count, blood chemistries, blood cultures and lumbar puncture (LP) with an analysis of CSF cell count, glucose, protein, Gram stain, and culture. General laboratory findings in meningitis include elevated white blood cell (WBC) count with neutrophilia and a left shift as well as occasionally hyponatremia. Blood culture results may be positive in up to 50% of cases. Any patient with a suspected CNS infection requires a lumbar puncture as part of the general work up. This is especially true in the case of suspected meningitis as the LP is likely to be the most important tool in making the diagnosis *(1,6)*.

Prior to lumbar puncture, any patient with focal neurological signs or papilledema should have a CT scan of the head to rule out mass lesions. Findings on LP that are indicative of a diagnosis of bacterial meningitis include: elevated opening pressure (> 200 mm H_2O), elevated protein (100–500 mg/dL), decreased glucose (<40% of serum levels), elevated WBC count (100–10,000/μL) with more than 60% neutrophils. The findings typically seen in viral meningitis include elevated protein, normal glucose, and elevated WBC (but usually not as high as in bacterial meningitis) with mononuclear or lymphocytic predominance, unless early on in the course. CSF obtained from lumbar puncture should be sent for Gram stain evaluation and culture. The Gram stain is positive in 60% of cases, and cultures are positive in 75%. An extremely important consideration is that this yield is dramatically decreased if the LP is performed more than 1 hour after the administration of antibiotics. The following constellation of CSF findings on LP when occurring together have been found to have a 99% positive predictive value for bacterial meningitis: glucose less than 34 mg/dL, CSF:serum glucose ratio greater than 0.23, WBC count >2000 WBC/mm^3. Bacteria-specific testing is available for some pathogens using latex agglutination but is of unclear benefit. In patients with suspected fungal meningitis or immunocompromised patients, CSF India ink stains should be performed to look for the encapsulated *Cryptococcus*. Also, specific antigen assays are available for *Cryptococcus* and *Neisseria*. Typical neuroimaging findings in meningitis include meningeal enhancement on gadolinium-enhanced magnetic resonance imaging (MRI) scan; however, this finding is nonspecific and may be seen in many pathologic processes and even after LP *(1,4,5,9–11)*.

Treatment

General management of the patient with meningitis begins with a detailed neurological examination. Patients with meningitis requiring intensive care usually do so because of airway compromise secondary to altered mental status, elevated ICP, or recurrent seizures (*see also* Chapters 5, 9, and 25). In obtunded patients, suspicion should be high for elevated ICP, and if any clinical signs of increased ICP are present, the patient should have an ICP monitoring device placed. Normal ICP is in the range of 2–10 mmHg. Drowsiness occurs in the 15–40 mmHg range, and pupillary dilatation may occur at approx 30 mmHg. Treatment of elevated ICP should be initiated when ICP reaches and is sustained above 15 mmHg as described elsewhere in this book. Treating the lower end of increased ICPs has been shown to improve outcome. This is most likely due to preventing the occurrence of plateau waves, which are sustained ICP elevations that increase the likelihood of herniation and death. The initial treatment of increased ICP begins with certain bedside practices. First, the head of bed should be elevated to 30 degrees. Also, care should be taken to minimize patient agitation, especially while performing chest physiotherapy and tracheal suctioning as each of these procedures alone can exacerbate elevated ICP. If the patient has a tracheostomy, the clinician should be aware of the ties around the patient's neck securing the device in place are often the cause of elevated ICP owing to inadvertent over-tightening. Active treatments for elevated ICP include intubation with hyperventilation, IV mannitol, and barbiturate coma. Hyperventilation works by lowering cerebral blood flow in response to hypocarbia. The initial response occurs within 30 s of hyperventilation, but this method generally loses effectiveness in 24–48 h. Mannitol lowers ICP by osmotically drawing fluid out of the interstitium and promoting diuresis. Barbiturate coma is a last resort treatment for refractory elevated ICP and works by lowering cerebral metabolism and thus blood flow. Seizures, especially when prolonged or recurrent, result in neuronal damage from ischemia and therefore require aggressive treatment *(8,12)*.

Fortunately, most patients with meningitis are stable from a cardiovascular standpoint. Important exceptions include patients with *Neisseria* meinigitis who may develop meningococcemia and patients with Gram-negative meningitis. In both of these situations of bacteremia, septic shock may ensue from lipopolysaccharide-induced systemic inflammatory response. Other treatments include control of fever and correction of fluid and electrolyte abnormalities. Hyperthermia will increase cerebral metabolism and may exacerbate neurological damage *(7,13)*.

SIADH is a well-described complication of CNS infections. The neurointensivist must be vigilant of its occurrence in patients with meningitis. Clinically, body weight, serum and urine electrolytes, and urine output should be followed. If present, SIADH will lead to increased total body water and hyponatremia. Both of these conditions contribute to cerebral edema, elevated ICP, and lowering of the seizure threshold. When detected, SIADH should be managed by fluid restriction and judicious use of hypertonic saline with a target serum osmolarity of more than 285–290 mmol/kg. Fluid management is exceedingly difficult in this situation when patients may also be septic and hypotensive. One should consider use of central venous pressure or pulmonary artery pressure (e.g., Swan-Ganz catheter) monitoring to guide appropriate fluid resuscitation based on overall volume status *(8,12)*.

Another adjunctive treatment to be considered in patients with meningitis is dexamethasone. Based on experimental evidence, dexamethasone provides an important block to the inflammatory pathways that lead to the majority of parenchymal brain injury. In infants and children, dexamethasone therapy reduces the incidence of neurological sequelae from bacterial meningitis. However, clinical studies in adults have failed to demonstrate a clear benefit in all patients. If considered, it may be helpful for patients with a high infectious load or increased ICP *(1,12,14,15)*.

Specific antimicrobial therapy should be directed at identified pathogens. However, in those patients with suspected bacterial or fungal meningitis, empiric IV antibiotic coverage is indicated when positive lumbar puncture results (elevated WBC count, elevated protein, decreased glucose) are obtained. Empiric antibiotic coverage is initiated based on the patient's age and clinical factors related to the development of meningitis. In patients aged 18–50, therapy should be initiated with a third-generation cephalosporin such as ceftriaxone. Third-generation cephalosporins provide good coverage of the typical pathogens such as *S. pneumoniae* and *N. meningitidis*. In patients older than 50 yr of age, ampicillin should be added to provide coverage of *Listeria monocytogenes* in addition to the aforementioned pathogens. In those patients who develop meningitis following head trauma or invasive neurosurgical procedures, empiric antibiotic coverage should be initiated with vancomycin and ceftazidime to provide coverage of *Staphylococcus* species and Gram-negative bacteria in addition to the typical pathogens. Finally, in immunocompromised patients, appropriate empiric antibiotic coverage should include ampicillin and ceftazidime to cover Gram-negative bacteria and *L. monocytogenes*. Once specific pathogens have been identified, a focused antibiotic regimen and duration of therapy can be determined. Table 1 details the antibiotic regimen and duration of therapy for specific pathogens *(5,7,17)*.

Complications/Outcome

Septic meningitis is unequivocally a neurologic emergency not only because of its high mortality but also because of its high likelihood for severe complications. Complications occur as a result of the host immune response as well as the primary infection. The host immune response along with the intrinsic characteristics of the CNS discussed above can lead to increased ICP. Elevation of ICP can subsequently cause a watershed infarction from decreased cerebral perfusion or a herniation syndrome. Moreover, alteration of cerebrovascular autoregulation also contributes to the risk of cerebral infarction. The primary infection often causes arteritis or septic venous thrombosis, both of which can result in cerebral infarction. Cerebritis, also a result of the primary infection, causes directs neuronal damage. These complications comprise the brunt of post-meningitis morbidity and also account for a significant portion of the mortality *(8)*.

Mortality figures for meningitis vary depending on age, pathogen, and comorbid medical conditions. For all age groups, the overall case fatality rate is less than 10% with higher levels in the elderly. Risk factors for increased mortality rate include age >59 yr of age, obtundation on admission, and seizures within 24 h of onset. In adult-specific studies, the overall mortality was found to be 18% even with appropriate antibiotic therapy. In this study, the case fatality rate for common adult pathogens was 24% for *S. pneumoniae* and 40% for *L. monocytogenes*. *N. meningitidis* is associated with a lower case-fatality rate of approx 3%. This rate is substantially higher when patients have concomitant meningococcemia, especially with skin findings of coagulopathy such as purpura fulminans. In an evaluation of mortality rates for nosocomial versus community acquired meningitis, nosocomial meningitis was associated with a 35% mortality rate, whereas community acquired infection had a 25% mortality rate *(3,4,7)*.

Table 1
Common Antibiotic Regimen for Treatment of Meningitis

Pathogen	Primary antibiotic	Secondary antibiotic	Duration of therapy	Notes
S. pneumoniae (PCN sens.)	Pen. G 4 mill. U IV q 4 h	Vanco 15 mg/kg IV q 6–12 h + Rifampin 600 mg PO or IV qd (for severe PCN allergy)	10–14 d	Max. vanco dose of 2–3 g per day, high dosage secondary to low CSF penetration of vancomycin
S. pneumoniae (PCN reis.)	Ceftriaxone 2.0 g IV q 12 h + vancomycin	Meropenem (limited clinical experience)	10–14 d	Ceftriaxone + vanco synergistic even w/ inc. MIC to ceftriaxone
N. meningitidis	Pen. G 4 mill. UIV q 4 h		7–10 d	Consider prophylaxis for family members and close contacts
L. monocytogenes	Ampicillin 2.0 g IV q 4 h + gentamicin 2 mg/kg loading dose then 1.7 mg/kg IV q 8 h	TMP/SMX 15– 20 mg/kg divided q 6–8 h (for PCN allergic)	14–21 d	Follow gentamicin levels
Gram-negative bacilli	Ceftazidime 2.0 g IV q 4 h + gentamicin 2 mg/kg loading dose then 1.7 mg/kg IV q 8 h	Aztreonam, cipro, meropenem	21 d	Follow gentamicin levels; for post-surgical cases of coliform or Pseudomonas consider intrathecal gentamicin 4 mg into lateral ventricles q 12 h

Adapted from Quagliarello, et a., 1997 *(5)* and Sanford Guide to Antimicrobial Therapy *(17)*. PCN, penicillin; TMP/SMX, trimethoprim/sulfamethoxazole; cipro, ciprofloxacin; MIC, minimum inhibitory concentration.

ENCEPHALITIS

Epidemiology

Encephalitis is characterized by either direct viral infection of the brain parenchyma or postinfectious autoimmune parenchymal inflammation. It occurs less frequently than meningitis. Encephalitis tends to occur with seasonal peaks in the winter and summer when certain pathogens are more common. Arboviral encephalitis cases peak in late summer and early fall, and it affects all age groups. Herpes virus encephalitis is also seen in all age groups. Most arboviruses affect persons of all ages with notable exceptions being La Cross virus, which tends to afflict children; and St. Louis virus, which afflicts adults older than 50 yr of age. Furthermore, arboviral encephalitis cases tend to occur in epidemics. Its significance for critical care clinicians is its ability to cause coma and alteration of mental status. Risk factors include exposure to infected persons, cat or wild animal bites, arthropod bites in endemic regions, as well as travel to endemic regions *(6,18)*.

Signs/Symptoms

Early in the clinical course, the signs and symptoms of encephalitis are similar to those of meningitis. Initially, patients experience fatigue, malaise, fever, headache, and possibly gastroenteritis with some pathogens. Patients subsequently develop signs of parenchymal cerebral dysfunction including altered mental status, focal neurological deficits and possibly seizures. In some cases, a meningoencephalitis syndrome will be present with patients having meningeal signs in addition to the above. Post infectious encephalomyelitis presents with identical symptoms as infectious encephalitis. Historical clues include recent respiratory infection or immunization. Many clinical and historical features are idiosyncratic for certain pathogens and thus can be helpful in diagnosis. For example, herpes encephalitis may present with prominent behavioral changes, psychosis or amnesia. Rabies encephalitis is often characterized by high fevers with temperatures of 105°–107°F, hydrophobia, agitation, and hallucinations. Japanese B encephalitis may present with parkinsonian features and rapidly progress to acute respiratory failure. Patients with eastern equine encephalitis will often have excessive salivation, high fever, convulsions, and a rapidly progressive course. Tremor and other involuntary movements are frequently seen in patients with western equine encephalitis *(6,18)*.

Pathophysiology

Encephalitic patients are infected via multitudinous routes. The encephalitis-causing viruses can be contracted via respiratory droplets, fecal-oral transmission, body fluids, and animal or insect bites. The virus disseminates through the bloodstream and localizes in the CNS. Notable exceptions to this pathway are the herpes and rabies viruses, which spread within neurons. The viral inflammatory response in addition to the detrimental effects of viral intracellular inhabitation result in pathophysiologic changes, which include neuronal necrosis, edema, and even hemorrhage with certain pathogens. These changes are often irreversible and may result in permanent damage. Certain pathogens have a predilection for affecting specific areas of the brain. In *Herpes simplex* virus (HSV) encephalitis, lesions tend to localize to the inferior and medial temporal lobes, the orbital-frontal cortex and the limbic structures. The involvement of these structures has importance to its clinical presentation, often characterized by hallucinations and behavioral abnormalities. The arboviruses predominantly affect the cortical gray matter, thalamic nuclei, and brainstem. Japanese B virus infects brainstem nuclei and basal ganglia structures, which contributes to its clinical presentation, often characterized by movement disorders *(18)*.

Pathogens

The most common pathogens in encephalitis are viral. In the United States, Herpes simplex virus (HSV-1), arboviruses, enteroviruses, measles, and mumps account for almost all cases of viral encephalitis. HSV is the infectious etiology in 10% of the cases of encephalitis in the United States, and if left untreated has a mortality of 70%. One third of the reported cases are from primary infection, and the other two-thirds result from reactivation of latent virus. Arboviruses are the leading cause of encephalitis worldwide. They are spread via mosquito and tick bites, thus their incidence tends to peak during fall and late summer. The most prevalent arboviruses include St. Louis, eastern equine, western equine, California, Japanese, and of recent notoriety, the West Nile virus. St. Louis and La

Crosse virus are the most common arboviral causes of encephalitis in the United States. Japanese encephalitis occurs more frequently in the eastern hemisphere. Eastern equine encephalitis is perhaps the most severe encephalitis due to its rapidly progressive nature; fortunately, only about five cases per year occur in the United States. Enteroviruses cause encephalitis but more frequently cause aseptic meningitis. Cocksackie and echoviruses are the most common encephalitic enteroviruses. These viruses are contracted via the fecal-oral route, and their clinical syndrome may include gastroenteritis. Before the development of vaccination, poliovirus was a common cause of encephalitis and myelitis with significant morbidity and mortality. It is now a rare cause of disease in the United States. Rabies virus also used to be a common cause of fatal encephalitis prior to the institution of animal vaccination. It is contracted via bites from infected animals and causes a delayed onset of encephalitis. The rabies virus replicates in the muscle of the bitten area and then traverses the nerves supplying that muscle to and through the spinal cord until it finally reaches the brain. Other less common viral causes of encephalitis include adenovirus, paramyxoviruses (mumps, measles), lymphocytic choriomeningitis virus, and HIV. Immunosuppressed patients are at risk for development of encephalitis from pathogens such as Varicella zoster virus (VZV), Epstein-Barr virus (EBV), human herpes virus 6 (HHV-6), and cytomegalovirus (CMV) in addition to the traditional pathogens. Measles, once a common pathogen in encephalitis before routine immunizations, is rarely seen in clinical practice today. It occurs in three distinct forms—postinfectious encephalomyelitis, subacute sclerosing panencephalitis, and subacute measles encephalitis. Finally, a noninfectious cause in the differential diagnosis of encephalitis is acute disseminated encephalomyelitis. This is a demyelinating disease that occurs following infection or immunization *(18–20)*.

Diagnosis

As with most medical disorders, the diagnosis of encephalitis begins with a thorough history and physical examination. The historian should pay particular attention to clues such as recent travel to endemic areas and history of tick, mosquito, or animal bites. The examiner should look for evidence of bites. As part of the physical examination, a detailed neurologic examination is necessary to identify localizing findings. The presence of meningeal signs does not rule out encephalitis, because certain pathogens cause meningoencephalitis. Because patients with encephalitis by definition have signs of parenchymal cerebral infection, the next step in the evaluation should include neuroimaging to visualize the extent of CNS involvement. Neuroimaging studies are especially important to rule out mass lesions or infarction in patients who present with seizures or focal signs on neurologic examination. As a precaution for brain herniation, computed tomography (CT) scanning of the head should be performed prior to lumbar puncture in patients with suspected mass lesions. Head CT scanning primarily serves to rule out other processes but can be diagnostic in cases of HSV, demonstrating frontal and temporal hemorrhages. MRI will also demonstrate these lesions as hyperintensities in the temporal lobes. MRI is typically nonspecific in arboviral encephalitis, with the exceptions of eastern equine and Japanese B encephalitis where hyperintensities may be present in the basal ganglia and the thalamus. Notably, acute disseminated encephalomyelitis has an MRI appearance similar to multiple sclerosis *(6,9,18)*.

Upon completion of imaging studies, and if a head CT scanning rules out mass lesions, the workup should proceed with analysis of the CSF through lumbar puncture. Typical findings on LP include normal or slightly elevated opening pressure, mildly elevated protein, normal glucose, and mononuclear pleocytosis, defined as elevated WBC count with greater than 50% lymphocytes or monocytes. Important exceptions to this are CSF samples obtained early in the clinical course when there may be a neutrophilic predominance and in eastern equine encephalitis where the CSF leukocyte count is typically higher than in other encephalitides. In HSV encephalitis, RBCs may be present along with xanthochromia. Specific serologic tests are available for CSF including HSV polymerase chain reaction (PCR). The timing of CSF testing by HSV PCR is crucial because within the first 48 h of infection, it will be falsely negative. Within 2–10 d of infection, HSV PCR will be positive in nearly 100% of cases, but after 10 d, its positivity decreases precipitously. In cases where clinical features suggest HSV encephalitis but PCR is negative, brain biopsy may be necessary to establish the diagnosis. Identification of the pathogen is often for academic and epidemiologic purposes only, as few specific treatments exist for viral encephalitides other than HSV. Moreover, virus isolation from CSF is exceedingly difficult in cases of arboviral encephalitis. In addition to CSF serology, acute and convalescent blood titers and cultures may be valuable in pathogen identification. Blood cultures may identify a specific pathogen in arboviral infections, measles, or mumps. Stool virus isolation can identify enteroviral pathogens. EEG may be of value in the diagnosis of HSV encephalitis as periodic spike and slow wave complexes every 2–3 s may be seen over the temporal lobes either unilaterally or bilaterally. Indeed these discharges are seen in two-thirds of pathologically proven cases of HSV encephalitis. Rabies may be diagnosed via inoculation of saliva from the patient or the animal into the brain of a mouse. The Center for Disease Control (CDC) has established diagnostic criteria for confirmation of arboviral encephalitis as these illnesses are considered reportable diseases. The diagnosis requires a patient to present with a febrile illness and encephalitis during a period when arboviral transmission occurs along with at least one of the following: (1) fourfold or greater rise in viral antibody titers between acute and chronic sera; (2) viral isolation from blood, tissue or CSF; or (3) specific IgM in CSF *(6,16,18,21,22)*.

Treatment

In general, treatment options are limited in encephalitis. Herpes simplex virus is the only virus with available medical treatment. If encephalitis is suspected, IV acyclovir should be started immediately. Early initiation of this therapy is crucial because it not only may be life saving but also may prevent significant long-term neuropathologic sequelae. Acyclovir should be administered 10 mg/kg IV every 8 h for 10–14 d or until HSV PCR is negative. In patients with renal insufficiency, caution should be exerted as acyclovir is nephrotoxic. Some strains of HSV may be resistant to acyclovir, especially in immunocompromised patients. If acyclovir-resistant strains of HSV are identified, foscarnet should be used. Experimental use of interferon-gamma has been shown to be protective against neuronal cell death in HSV infection. In other viral encephalitides, treatment is only supportive. Acute disseminated encephalomyelitis often responds to high dose IV steroids but requires Neurosciences Critical Care Unit (NSU) care due to increased ICP and obtundation. NSU care is necessary in those patients with rapidly changing neurological status as airway management and ICP monitoring may be required *(18,22,23)*.

Prophylactic vaccination is the cornerstone of preventive therapy for viral encephalitis. As for both polio and rabies, the initiation of human and animal vaccinations, respectively, has significantly reduced the occurrence of these diseases. Currently, humans are only vaccinated for rabies if they work in high-risk professions, such as with wild animals or lab animals with endemic infection (e.g., bats) or following bites from suspected rabid animals. If bitten by a rabid animal, patients may also be given rabies immune globulin. A vaccine also exists for Japanese encephalitis *(18,24,25)*.

Complications/Outcome

Outcome from viral encephalitis is pathogen-dependent. HSV and eastern equine virus encephalitis have the worst outcomes with high mortality rates and neurological sequelae present in a significant percentage of survivors. HSV, if untreated, has a mortality rate of 70%, but with treatment, this figure drops to 20%. Nevertheless, even with treatment, only a third of patients recover with mild or no neurologic deficit. If rabies infection progresses to encephalitis, the mortality rate approaches 100%. St. Louis, La Crosse, and California encephalitis have a generally good prognosis. La Crosse virus encephalitis has less than 1% mortality, but a seizure disorder occurs in 6–13% of those afflicted. St. Louis encephalitis can be complicated during the acute phase by SIADH, and chronically

10% of survivors have long term sequelae of memory loss, headaches, chronic fatigue, and seizures. The mortality rate approaches 10–20% in patients with St. Louis encephalitis. Other arboviruses have higher mortality rates. Japanese encephalitis has a mortality rate of 20–40%, and fatalities typically occur within the first weeks of infection. Eastern equine encephalitis has a mortality rate of 50–75% with significant neurologic morbidity among survivors. Western equine encephalitis has a mortality rate of 5–10% with seizures and developmental delay commonly persisting in children who survive the disorder *(18,19,22,23)*.

BRAIN ABSCESS
Epidemiology

Brain abscess occurs less frequently than either meningitis or encephalitis; nonetheless, it remains an important clinical entity to the neurocritical care clinician. Patients with brain abscesses can be treated in the NSU both preoperatively and postoperatively. A brain abscess is defined as a focal intracerebral infection characterized by an encapsulated collection of pus within the brain parenchyma. Although rare, brain abscess is the most common suppurative intracranial process. The yearly incidence of brain abscess is 1.3 per 100,000 person years. This translates to 1500–2500 cases per year in the United States. Overall the incidence of brain abscess has decreased following the introduction of antibiotics. In one group, however, the incidence has increased—the immunocompromised. Brain abscesses affect males more frequently than females with ratios as high as 3:1. The risk factors for development of a brain abscess are multiple. First, head and neck infections can be complicated by development of CNS abscesses. Sinusitis, otitis (both media and externa), mastoiditis, and dental infections can all lead to the development of a CNS abscess when left untreated. A brain abscess may ensue following a penetrating head injury. Immunocompromised (especially solid organ transplant recipients) patients are at increased risk of intracranial abscess formation. Finally, endocarditis and other conditions that predispose to septic embolization can be the source of CNS abscesses *(20,26–28)*.

Signs/Symptoms

General complaints related to brain abscess include fever, headache, nausea, vomiting, and altered mental status. Other early symptoms can be related to the predisposing condition such as ear pain with otitis or sinus pain and congestion with sinusitis. Seizures also occur owing to parenchymal invasion. A classic triad of fever, headache and focal neurological deficit is described, however, this is found in fewer than half of patients with brain abscess. The presentation is typically nonspecific with only 50% of patients presenting with fever and up to 50% presenting with nausea alone. General physical exam may reveal findings of predisposing conditions. Papilledema may be seen on fundoscopic examination if the patient has elevated intracranial pressure. Neurological exam may reveal alterations in mental status and focal deficits based on location of the abscess. Indeed focal neurologic findings such as hemiparesis, hemisensory deficits, aphasia, or ataxia are seen in 33–50% of patients with brain abscess *(6,26–29)*.

Pathophysiology

Brain abscesses generally develop from invasion by local infection, hematogenous spread, or trauma; however, according to one study, as many as 63% of cases have no predisposing infection. Areas of pre-existing brain pathology such as previous stroke, intracerebral hematoma, or tumor may serve as a nidus for abscess formation. In the case of head and neck infections, the brain abscess develops as a result of localized infiltration of bacteria. The abscess develops as the local infection grows when left untreated. Consequently, location of the abscess is often related to location of the primary infection. For example, frontal sinusitis will generally lead to abscess development in the frontal lobes, whereas mastoiditis and otitis tend to spread to the temporal lobes. The valveless emissary veins that drain the head and neck allow retrograde flow of bacteria into the brain parenchyma. Head trauma, such as penetrating injuries, or neurosurgical procedures can predispose to development of brain abscess. When brain abscesses develop without primary head and neck infections or antecedent trauma, they may occur as the result of hematogenous spread. Endocarditis is the most commonly identified source for hematogenous spread, but congenital heart disease, pulmonary arteriovenous malformations (AVMs), lung or abdominal abscesses can also serve as sources. Brain abscesses resulting from hematogenous spread are often multiple and typically form at the gray-white junction *(26–28)*.

Regardless of the mechanism, brain abscesses develop in a series of radiographic and pathologic stages. The first stage is the "early cerebritis stage" occurring in the initial 1–3 d of infection and characterized by the direct inoculation of bacteria into the brain with surrounding focal area of inflammation and edema. The "late cerebritis stage" follows on days 4–9 and is characterized by the development of a central necrotic focus. The "early capsule stage" occurs on days 10–14 and is characterized by the appearance of a ring-enhancing capsule with peripheral fibrosis and gliosis. The final stage, the "late capsule phase," appears beyond day 14 and is characterized by a well-formed capsule established by host defense mechanisms *(26–28)*.

Pathogens

The pathogens causing brain abscesses are predominantly bacterial and as many as 60% are polymicrobial. The isolated organisms are typically related to predisposing conditions. Aerobic bacteria are slightly more frequently isolated than anaerobic bacteria. Overall, streptococcal species are the most commonly identified pathogens and are seen in approx 70% of cases. Microaerophyllic streptococci and anaerobic bacteria typically cause brain abscesses that arise from sinus and dental infections. Similar pathogens are identified in brain abscesses of otitic origin, however, additional consideration should be made for enterobacteriaceae and pseudomonas. *Staphylococcus aureus* is a common pathogen in abscesses occurring after head trauma or neurosurgical procedures. The microbiology of brain abscess is unique in immunocompromised patients in that specific pathogens are associated with the particular immune deficit. In general, patients with a neutrophil deficiency, whether in number or function, have a higher frequency of Gram-negative rod and fungal abscesses, whereas patients with T cell deficits acquire brain abscesses due to listeria, nocardia, cryptococcus and toxoplasma *(26–28)*.

Diagnosis

The diagnosis of brain abscess is based on a constellation of signs and symptoms in conjunction with radiographic imaging. Fever, signs of increased ICP, and focal findings on neurological examination are strong clues that a brain abscess is present. A history of recent sinusitis or ear infection is also an important clue. More so than in other infections of the CNS, radiographic imaging is crucial to confirming the diagnosis of brain abscess. The initial imaging modality used should be contrast-enhanced head CT scanning. This will demonstrate a hyper-dense ring-enhancing lesion with surrounding edema. The early cerebritis stage may appear as only an area of hypodensity due to edema. Magnetic resonance imaging is a helpful adjunct in the evaluation of brain abscess especially in the early cerebritis stage of infection. T2-weighted images will demonstrate an iso- or hyperintense center with surrounding edema. Following administration of gadolinium, the abscess will demonstrate ring-shaped enhancement of the abscess capsule. The appearance of these lesions may be very similar to necrotic metastatic lesions or other CNS tumors. In patients where the diagnosis is in question, nuclear medicine scans such as single photon emission computed tomography (SPECT) or positron emission tomography (PET) may be beneficial ancillary diagnostic tests. Neuroimaging may be diagnostic of abscess, but ultimately pathogen identification is necessary for initiation of appropriate antibiotic treatment. Stereotactic CT-guided needle aspiration provides the least invasive method of obtaining tissue and culture material. This procedure is relatively low risk with morbidity of 1% or less and mortality of 0.2%. Samples obtained during aspiration must be sent for Gram stain and aerobic and anaerobic cultures. In general, lumbar puncture is contraindicated in patients with brain abscess due to the risk of herniation in patients with elevated ICP and low yield of beneficial clinical information. Blood cultures should be performed in all patients with brain abscess, especially those with a suspected hematogenous source of infection *(11,27–29)*.

Treatment

Treatment of the abscess is twofold. First, intravenous antibiotic therapy should be empirically initiated based on the presumed source of the abscess and then tailored to the pathogen isolated during aspiration. A common empiric regimen used in the immunocompetent patient includes vancomycin, metronidazole, and cefotaxime. Table 2 provides more specific empiric antibiotic regimens based on location of presumed source of pathogen. Intravenous antibiotics are administered for a total of 6–8 wk. Some experts recommend oral antibiotic therapy following intravenous antibiotics; however, this is of unproven clinical benefit. Second, surgical drainage of all abscesses larger than 2.5 cm should be performed. Stereotactic abscess drainage is the procedure of choice for initial surgical management of brain abscess because it serves both diagnostic and therapeutic purposes. Stereotactic drainage revolutionized surgical management of brain abscess as it provides a minimally invasive method for removal of purulent material not only for culture but also for reduction of mass effect. Abscess excision with open craniotomy is now reserved for patients with abscesses that are multi-loculated, refractory to stereotactic drainage, or due to resistant pathogens such as fungi or *Nocardia*. Serial neuro-imaging should be performed at 2-wk intervals to follow response to treatment during the initial period of intravenous antibiotic treatment. The patient should then be followed with repeat neuro-imaging every 2–4 mo for 1 yr to evaluate for recurrence. Prophylactic anticonvulsants are also recommended because these patients are at high risk for seizure development. Other general treatment should be aimed at monitoring of ICP. Furthermore, airway management is critical in the NSU for patients with recurrent seizures or rapidly changing mental status. Steroids are generally contraindicated unless elevated ICP is present, because they may decrease antibiotic penetration into the abscess. In cases complicated by severely elevated ICP, the use of intravenous mannitol may be necessary *(26–30)*.

Complications/Outcome

Following introduction of antibiotics, the mortality of brain abscess has decreased precipitously. Currently, the mortality of brain abscess is less than 10%, even as low as 0% in some case studies. Predictors of poor outcome in brain abscess are rate of development of symptoms and level of consciousness at time of presentation. Immunocompromised patients are an important exception to the aforementioned mortality rates. These patients tend to have higher mortality rates even with appropriate antibiotic therapy, especially transplant patients where mortality approaches 90% *(20,27–29)*.

Morbidity in brain abscess is approx 50% with as many as 70% of survivors having a seizure disorder. In addition to seizures, brain abscess can be complicated by intraventricular rupture of the abscess leading to meningitis. This is a critical complication because it is associated with an 80% mortality rate. Another related condition that can either complicate brain abscess or form independently is the subdural empyema. A subdural empyema is a collection of pus that forms in the subdural space and is often a consequence of sinus or ear infection. It is diagnosed on neuroimaging, however, its size is often underestimated by current imaging techniques. It requires emergent surgical intervention, which usually involves drainage through a burr hole. Finally, although rare, brain abscesses may be complicated by epidural abscess formation or septic venous thrombophlebitis *(26–29)*.

Table 2
Recommended Antimicrobial Regimens for Brain Abscess

Source of abscess	Location	Typical pathogens	Antibiotic regimen
Sinus infection	Frontal lobe	*Streptococci* (microaerophilic and anaerobic), *Haemophilus* sp., *Bacteroides* sp., *Fusobacterium* sp.	PCN or third generation cephalosporin + metronidazole
Dental infection	Temporal lobe	*Streptococci, Bacteroides fragilis*	PCN + metronidazole
Otogenic infections (otitis media and mastoiditis)	Temporal lobe, cerebellum	*Bacteroides* sp., *Streptococci, Enterobacteriaceae, Pseudomonas aeruginosa*	PCN + ceftazidime + metronidazole
Metastatic spread	Multiple lesions typically at gray-white junction, often occurring in MCA distribution but can be in any vascular territory	Dependent on source	
Endocarditis		Viridans *Streptococci, S. aureus*	Nafcillin or vancomycin + metronidazole + third generation cephalosporin
Lung abscess		*Streptococci, Actinomyces* sp., *Fusobacterium* sp.	PCN + metronidazole + ceftazidime
Urinary sepsis		*Enterobacteriaceae, Pseudomonaceae*	PCN + metronidazole + ceftazidime +
Abdominal abscess		*Streptococci, Enterobacteriaceae,* anaerobes	PCN + metronidazole + ceftazidime
Penetrating head trauma	Dependent on location of injury	*Staphylococcus aureus, Clostridium* sp., *Enterobacteriaceae*	Nafcillin or vancomycin + third generation cephalosporin
Neurosurgical procedure	Dependent on site of procedure	*Staphylococci, Enterobacteriaceae Pseudomonaceae*	Vancomycin + cerftazidime

Adapted from Mathiesen GE, et al., 1997 *(26)* and Calfee WP, et al., 2000 *(27)*. PCN, penicillin; MCA, middle cerebral artery.

NOSOCOMIAL CENTRAL NERVOUS SYSTEM INFECTIONS

Nosocomial infections of the CNS are generally rare without predisposing risk factors such as invasive neurosurgical procedures. However, for the NSU clinician, invasive procedures are daily occurrences. Whether they are postoperative craniotomy patients or patients with cerebral edema and ICP monitors in place, all have a common denominator of iatrogenic violation of the normal barrier to infection. The two most common nosocomial CNS infections are meningitis and CSF shunt infections. Meningitis typically occurs as a sequela of neurosurgical wound infection. CSF shunt infections occur following either shunt placement or ICP monitor placement. The rates of nosocomial CNS infections have generally been low but highly variable, ranging from as low as 7/100,000 discharges to as high as 84/100,000 discharges. The most recent figures show an incidence of 1.41 surgical site infections per 100 craniotomies and 3.9 surgical site infections per 100 CSF shunt operations *(31)*.

Nosocomial meningitis is almost exclusively postsurgical and occurs after violation of the external barriers of the CNS. Indeed the two most important risk factors for development of nosocomial meningitis are recent neurosurgical procedure and presence of a neurosurgical device. Other notable risk factors for deep wound infections (meningitis and abscess) include emergency surgery, CSF leakage or drainage, Glasgow Coma Scale (GCS) score less than 10, total shaving of the wound, and early reoperation. Contiguous spread of infection is important in the pathogenesis of nosocomial meningitis with spread occurring from either wound infection or other proximal infection such as sinusitis. Nosocomial meningitis has a different clinical presentation from community-acquired meningitis. Symptoms are insidious in onset and include meningismus and altered level of consciousness. These symptoms are, however, common in the normal postoperative period as patients recover from anesthesia. Often the only clue to the diagnosis is a prolonged recovery period following surgery. The microbiology of nosocomial meningitis, like its clinical presentation, differs from community-acquired meningitis. The most common pathogens in nosocomial meningitis are *S. aureus*, Gram-negative 11bacilli including *Pseudomonas*, and coagulase-negative *Staphylococci*. The diagnosis of nosocomial meningitis is based on evaluation of CSF cell count, protein, glucose, Gram stain and culture. The treatment of nosocomial meningitis is IV antibiotics. Initially, empiric therapy is administered with subsequent tailoring of the regimen based on culture results and antibiotic sensitivity. Appropriate initial empiric therapy of nosocomial meningitis is a combination of vancomycin and cytazidime. Vancomycin provides adequate coverage of both methicillin-resistant and susceptible *Staphylococcus*, and ceftazidime covers Gram-negative pathogens including *Pseudomonas*. Prevention of nosocomial meningitis is crucial and multifaceted. Attention must be paid to aseptic surgical technique, clean operative environment, and finally, choice of antimicrobial prophylaxis. There is no clear consensus for surgical antibiotic prophylaxis, but options include third generation cephalosporins, vancomycin, cloxacillin, clindamycin, and aminoglycosides. The majority of neurosurgeons favor cefazolin 1 g IV before skin incision for most routine surgical procedures in immunocompetent patients. In patients with a penicillin allergy, vancomycin is the preferred prophylactic surgical antibiotic *(31,32)*.

CSF shunt infections occur more frequently than nosocomial meningitis and are a challenging clinical entity because therapy involves removal of a device that is often critical to the patient's health. The higher rate of infection is likely related to the key role that normal CSF flow plays in infection prevention by carrying pathogens away from brain to be eliminated. There are multiple pathogenetic factors causing CSF shunt infections. First, with an external draining device the ventricular catheter creates a pathway from the scalp to the ventricles. Second, the uneven surface of the shunt allows for bacterial adherence. Third, when a shunt malfunctions, normal CSF flow is interrupted. Finally, shunts have poor leukocyte adherence and subsequently impaired phagocytosis occurs within them. Moreover, certain pathogens have virulence factors that increase their ability to infect shunts. Coagulase-negative *Staphylococci* adhere to foreign bodies avidly and produce an extracellular slime that protects them from host defenses. The bacteria infecting shunts likely colonize the wound at the time of surgery and then spread proximally within the system *(31)*.

The clinical presentation of CSF shunt infections is dependent on the site of infection within the shunt system. There are three main presentations—systemic infection, focal infection, and shunt malfunction. The most sensitive sign of shunt infection is fever. Systemic symptoms include anorexia, pain, malaise, and lethargy. However, patients in shunt failure are known to present with a wide variety of nonspecific signs and symptoms that are often seemingly unrelated to the indwelling catheter. Focal signs of infection include erythema and purulent drainage at the implantation site. In general patients with shunt malfunction present with signs and symptoms of elevated ICP including headache, nausea, vomiting, and altered mental status. When the infection spreads to the ventricles, the patient develops ventriculitis. Patients with ventriculitis will present with the above signs of increased ICP, but they typically lack meningeal signs. The predominant pathogens causing CSF shunt infection are coagulase-negative *Staphylococci* and *S. aureus*. Other less common pathogens are Gram-negative bacilli, *Streptococci*, and normal skin flora. The diagnosis of CSF shunt infection is made by evaluation of CSF obtained from a shunt tap. Elevated WBC count in the CSF is the most critical laboratory finding. A WBC count more than 100 cells/mm^3 has a positive predictive value of 89%. Treatment of CSF shunt infections requires both IV antibiotics and removal of the shunt. Empiric antibiotic therapy should be initiated with vancomycin given the high proportion of infections owing to coagulase-negative staphylococci. Antibiotic therapy can then be further directed based on Gram stain and culture. Ideally, the infected shunt should be removed with subsequent replacement delayed owing to the high risk of reinfection. An external draining device is used in the interim while the infection is being treated with antibiotics. Ultimately, the decision to remove the infected shunt is based on the original problem necessitating shunt placement and the clinical condition of the patient *(31,33)*.

ICP monitoring devices also serve as portals for infection and, similar to CSF shunts, must be removed if infection develops. Previously, the duration of ICP monitoring was felt to directly correlate with development of infectious complications. However, recent studies have shown that duration of monitoring does not significantly affect risk of infection *(34)*.

Prevention of CSF shunt contamination is critical given the role initial colonization plays in subsequent infection. Meticulously sterile operative technique is the sine qua non of successful prevention of shunt infection. Recent data has emerged showing that preoperative shaving of the shunt site increases risk of infection. Perioperative antibiotics are controversial in prevention of CSF shunt infection, and no clinical consensus for their use exists *(31,35)*.

A rare but important clinical complication associated with CSF shunt infection is shunt nephritis. Shunt nephritis occurs owing to deposition of antigen-antibody complexes in the glomerular basement membrane in chronic shunt infection. Patients present with the nephrotic syndrome. Shunt nephritis is treated by treating the underlying infection *(31)*.

FUNGAL CENTRAL NERVOUS SYSTEM INFECTIONS

Fungal CNS infections are rare except in immunocompromised patients. With the increasing numbers of immunosuppressed persons due to AIDS, organ transplantation, and cancer chemotherapy, fungal pathogens are identified with increasing frequency *(20)*.

The clinical syndromes of fungal CNS infection are similar to bacterial disease and include meningitis, meningoencephalitis, and abscess formation. The pathogenesis of fungal infections depends on their form at the time of infection. In the yeast form (single cell), the organisms tend to reach the meninges via hematogenous seeding. In the hyphal form (filamentous, multicellular), the organisms tend to spread via local invasion from infection of contiguous sites. The clinical presentation of fungal CNS infections differs from that of bacterial infections in that most patients have a subacute course with symptoms developing over several weeks. The exception to chronic progression is when patients with fungal infections with filamentous fungi present with acute stroke due to invasion of blood vessel walls by fungal hyphae. A distinct geographic predilection for certain fungal pathogens exists. *Coccidiodes immitis* is found predominately in the southwestern United States. *Histoplasma capsulatum* is found in the Ohio and Mississippi valleys. *Blastomyces dermatitidis* is found in the Midwestern and Mideastern states. Other fungal pathogens including *Cryptococcus neoformans*, *Candida*, *Aspergillus*, and *Zygomycetes* are found throughout the world *(36)*.

Diagnosis of fungal CNS infections is based on clinical features and CSF analysis, except in the case of granuloma or abscess formation where biopsy and drainage of the lesion may be necessary. CSF findings are similar to those of bacterial meningitis with elevated WBC count, elevated protein, and low glucose levels. The difference is that in fungal infections there is usually a lymphocytic predominance. Fungi are difficult to isolate from CSF via culture, and often multiple large volume taps are necessary to provide enough CSF for culture. More valuable in establishing the diagnosis of CNS fungal infection is the use of antibody testing of the CSF. Specific antibodies chosen for analysis should be based on clinical suspicion taking into consideration patient characteristics and geographic location *(36)*.

Primary treatment of fungal CNS infection is amphotericin B. Amphotericin is the treatment of choice, because most fungal pathogens are sensitive to amphotericin, resistance is rare, and CNS penetration is good. Unfortunately, amphotericin B is associated with significant toxicity. Fever, chills, nausea, vomiting, anaphylaxis, thrombocytopenia, headache, seizures are some of the many reported untoward effects. Fever and chills occur in approx 50% of patients but may be minimized by pretreating with acetaminophen. Renal toxicity is one of the more common amphotericin B side effects with approx 80% of patients affected. In most patients, renal function returns to normal during therapy. In spite of this, patients generally are left with some degree of compromised glomerular filtration. The extent of which is based on total dose received. Occasionally, additional therapy with flucytosine may be recommended. Patients who develop fungal CNS infections will likely require lifelong prophylactic therapy with fluconazole *(36,37)*.

REFERENCES

1. Coyle PK. Overview of acute and chronic meningitis. *Neurol. Clin.* 1999;17:691–710.
2. Durand ML, Calderwood SB, Weber DJ, et al. Acute bacterial meningitis in adults: A review of 493 episodes. *N. Engl. J. Med.* 1993;328:21–28.
3. Hussein AS, Shafran SD. Acute bacterial meningitis in adults: A 12 year review. *Medicine (Baltimore)* 2000;79:360–368.
4. Schuchat A, Robinson K, Wenger JD, et al. Bacterial meningitis in the United States in 1995. *N. Engl. J. Med.* 1997;337:970–976.
5. Quagliarello VJ, Scheld WM. Treatment of bacterial meningitis. *N. Engl. J. Med.* 1997;336:708–716.
6. Rajnik M, Ottolini MG. Serious infections of the central nervous system: Encephalitis, meningitis, and brain abscess. *Adol. Med.* 2001;11:401–425.
7. Spach DH, Jackson LA. Bacterial meningitis. *Neurol. Clin.* 1999;17:711–735.
8. Roos KL, Scheld WM. The management of fulminant meningitis in the intensive care unit. *Infect. Dis. Clin. North Am.* 1989;3:137–152.
9. Hasbun R, Abrahams J, Jekel J, Quagliarello VJ. Computed tomography of the head before lumbar puncture in adults with suspected meningitis. *N. Engl. J. Med.* 2001;345:1727–1733.
10. Zunt JR, Marra CM. Cerebrospinal fluid testing for the diagnosis of central nervous system infection. *Neurol. Clin.* 1999;17:675–689.
11. Wong J, Quint DJ. Imaging of central nervous system infection. *Semin. Roentgenol.* 1999;34:123–143.
12. Rauf SJ, Roberts NJ. Supportive management in bacterial meningitis. *Inf. Dis. Clin. North Am.* 1999;13:647–659.
13. Kilpatrick MM, Lowry DW, Firlik AD, Yonas H, Marion DW. Hyperthermia in the neurosurgical intensive care unit. *Neurosurgery* 2000;47:850–855.
14. Tunkel AR, Wispelwey B, Scheld WM. Bacterial meningitis: Recent advances in pathophysiology and treatment. *Ann. Intern. Med.* 1990;112:610–623.
15. Thomas R, Le Tulzo Y, Bouget J, et al. Trial of dexamethasone treatment for severe bacterial meningitis in adults. *Intensive Care Med.* 1999;25:475–480.
16. Roos KL. Pearls and pitfalls in the diagnosis and management of central nervous system infectious diseases. *Semin. Neurol.* 1998;18:185–196.
17. Gilbert DN, Moellering RC, Sande MA. *The Sanford Guide to Antimicrobial Therapy*, 31st ed. Hyde Park, VT: Antimicrobial Therapy, 2001: 2–45.
18. Roos KL. Encephalitis. *Neurol. Clin.* 1999;17:813–833.
19. Arboviral infections of the central nervous system—United States, 1996–1997. *MMWR* 1998;47:517–542.
20. Singh N, Hasain S. Infections of the central nervous system in transplant recipients. *Transpl. Infect. Dis.* 2000;2:101–111.
21. Akhan SC, Coskunkan F, Mutlu B, Gundes S, Vahaboglu H, Willke A. A probable case of herpes simplex encephalitis despite negative PCR findings. *Infection* 2001;29:359–361.
22. Schmutzhard E. Viral infections of the CNS with special emphasis on herpes simplex infections. *J. Neurol.* 2001;248:469–477.
23. Villarreal EC. Current and potential therapies for the treatment of herpes virus infections. *Prog. Drug. Res. (Spec)* 2001;185–228.
24. Strady C, Hung Nguyen V, Jaussaud R, Lang J, Lienard M, Strady A. Pre-exposure rabies vaccination: strategies and cost-minimization study. *Vaccine* 2001;19:11–12.

25. Wilde H, Khawplod P, Hemachudha T, Sitprija V. Postexposure treatment of rabies infection: Can it be done without immunoglobulin? *Clin. Infect. Dis.* 2001;34:477–480.

26. Mathiesen GE, Johnson JP. Brain abscess. *Clin. Infect. Dis.* 1997;25:763–781.

27. Calfee DP, Wispelwey B. Brain abscess. *Semin. Neurol.* 2000;20:353–360.

28. Davis LE, Baldwin NG. Brain abscess. *Curr. Treat. Options Neurol.* 1999;1:157–166.

29. Calfee DP, Wispelwey B. Brain abscess, subdural empyema, and intracranial epidural abscess. *Curr. Infect. Dis. Rep.* 1999;1:166–177.

30. Sarma S, Sekhar LN. Brain-stem abscess successfully treated by microsurgical drainage: a case report. *Neurol. Res.* 2001;23:855–861.

31. Morris A, Low DE. Nosocomial bacterial meningitis, including central nervous system shunt infections. *Infect. Dis. Clin. North Am.* 1999;13:735–750.

32. Korinek AM. Risk factors for neurosurgical site infections after craniotomy: A prospective multicenter study of 2944 patients. The French Study Group of Neurosurgical Infections, the SEHP, and the C-CLIN Paris-Nord. Service. Epidemiologie Hygiene et Prevention. *Neurosurgery* 1997;41:1073–1079.

33. Bell WO. Management of infected cerebrospinal fluid shunts in children. *Contemp. Neurosurg.* 1992;14:6–16.

34. Winfield JA, Rosenthal P, Kanter RK, Casella G. Duration of intracranial pressure monitoring does not predict daily risk of infectious complications. *Neurosurgery* 1993;33:424–431.

35. Horgan MA, Piatt JH. Shaving the scalp may increase the rate of infection in CSF shunt surgery. *Pediatr. Neurosurg.* 1997;26:180–184.

36. Davis LE. Fungal infections of the central nervous system. *Neurol. Clin.* 1997;17:761–782.

37. Bennett JE. Antimicrobial agents: antifungal agents. In: Hardman JG, Limbird LE, Goodman AG (eds). *Goodman and Gilman's The Pharmacologic Basis of Therapeutics*, 10th ed. New York: McGraw-Hill, 2001:1295–1312.

30

Neuro-Ophthalmologic Evaluation of the ICU Patient

Eroboghene E. Ubogu and R. John Leigh

HOW THE NEURO-OPHTHALMOLOGIC EXAMINATION CAN CONTRIBUTE TO EVALUATION OF THE ICU PATIENT

Common questions posed by patients who have been admitted to a neurosciences critical care unit (NSU) include: (1) If the patient is unresponsive, what is the cause—a structural lesion above or below the tentorium, metabolic or toxic disorder? (2) Is the patient deteriorating—especially following a procedure? (3) Are therapeutic interventions indicated? (4) What is the prognosis? Careful and systematic examination of the patient's eyelids, optic fundi, pupils, and eye movements often provide important clues that help resolve these issues (1–3).

EXAMINATION OF THE EYELIDS

Recall the four main forces that determine the position of the eyelids. The main upward force is owing to the levator palpebrae superioris muscle; Müller's muscle makes a smaller contribution. Elastic forces due to the tendons and ligaments that surround the lids cause the lids to passively close; the orbicularis oculi muscle contracts during forceful lid closure. In the unconscious patient, the eyelids are usually closed and reclose slowly if the examiner pulls back the lids and then suddenly releases them. Forceful lid closure occurs in mild stupor and in patients pretending to be unconscious. Whenever unresponsive patients show intermittent eye opening with lid twitches, consider epileptic seizures. An underrecognized syndrome in patients with acute stroke, especially with right-sided parietal-lobe infarction, is *cerebral ptosis (4)*. Such patients may be alert and cooperative, yet unable to open their eyelids (unlike eye-opening apraxia, for example in progressive supranuclear palsy, when spontaneous eye opening occurs). Limitation of upward gaze and ipsilesional horizontal gaze deviation may also be present. "Eyes-open coma" (spastic eyelids) has been reported in unresponsive patients who show spontaneous vertical eye movements, no horizontal eye movements, and large brainstem infarction (5). In conscious patients, lid retraction may be a sign of posterior commissure lesions (1), or thyrotoxicosis. Test the corneal reflex. It is often preserved when other brainstem reflexes are in abeyance. In patients who have been left in a vegetative state following cardiac arrest, synkinetic jaw movements (corneomandibular response) are quite common.

THE OPTIC FUNDI

Always examine the optic fundi of NSU patients (2). In patients with small pupils, dilating drops can be given, but only after examining and documenting the pupillary responses. (Also make it clear to the patient's caregivers that the pupillary responses will be abnormal for a few hours.) Papilledema

From: *Current Clinical Neurology*
Critical Care Neurology and Neurosurgery
Edited by: J. I. Suarez © Humana Press Inc., Totowa, NJ

is an important finding, but may be absent in older individuals with increased intracranial pressure. Look for hyperemia of the disc and note that vessels approaching the disc edge may be obscured by swollen, opaque nerve fibers. Papilledema with a hypertensive fundus (e.g., presence of hard exudates) suggests hypertensive encephalopathy. Visible hemorrhages may occur at several locations. Intraretinal hemorrhages occur with papilledema. Pre-retinal (subhyaloid) hemorrhages, which may layer due to gravity, lie between the retina and vitreous; they classically occur with rapid increases of intracranial pressure, such as occurs with subarachnoid hemorrhage and head trauma. Subretinal hemorrhages, which are characteristically dark, lie between the retina and choroid, and occur following ocular trauma. Retinal infarcts (soft exudates) are encountered in vasculitis but also occur in intravenous drug abusers, due to septic emboli. Patients who have suffered massive trauma may show "cumulus cloud" infiltrates due to fat embolism. Ischemic fundi following head and neck trauma may reflect interruption of carotid circulation by dissection.

THE PUPILS

Recall pertinent anatomy of the innervation of the pupils (2,3). Note that a light stimulus applied to each eye will cause both pupils to constrict. This means that, in ambient light, anisocoria implies an efferent problem that most commonly is due to oculomotor nerve palsy, Horner's syndrome, or malfunction of the pupil itself from eye drops, previous trauma or surgery. Horner's syndrome's may be present in almost 50% of cases of carotid dissection (6), but diagnosis may be difficult because the ptosis is minor (and often masked by senile changes), and anhydrosis may be difficult to detect.

Consider pupillary abnormalities in terms of size, shape, and reaction to light. First note the resting size of the pupils in room light. If they are very small (pinpoint), consider administrating naloxone immediately to reverse narcotic intoxication. Also consider brain imaging to detect pontine or cerebellar hemorrhage (7). Symmetrically large pupils may be due to local, or systemic, atropine-like agents (such as might be given during cardiopulmonary resuscitation), and also tricylic antidepressants and other agents (8,9) Large unresponsive pupils also occur with midbrain lesions such as traumatic hemorrhage (10), or following transtentorial herniation. Persistently large pupils after noxious stimuli (ciliospinal reflex) may be observed in pentobarbital coma (11).

Pupils that are oval or irregular may reflect prior trauma or surgery, but in the setting of intracranial hemorrhage, suggest midbrain infarction and a poor prognosis (12).

Test the pupillary reaction to a bright penlight. If the pupils are equal in ambient light, it is possible to assess the relative function of each optic nerve, use the swinging flashlight test, in which the direct and consensual responses are compared. Reactions of small pupils are often difficult to detect, even with a magnifying glass. Many patients in metabolic coma will have small but sluggishly responsive pupils. In patients with unequal pupils (anisocoria), it becomes important to determine if the response of the larger pupil is impaired or absent. Pupils that are unequal in room light by more than about 1.5 mm may be due to eye drops, but the main concern is compression of the oculomotor nerve by herniating temporal lobe or other mass lesion, including posterior-communicating artery aneurysm. To differentiate between pharmacologic mydriasis and oculomotor nerve dysfunction, apply 1% pilocarpine drops. A pupil that does not constrict with pilocarpine has received atropinic eye drops.

EXAMINATION OF THE POSITION AND MOVEMENTS OF THE EYES

In examining the eye movements in unconscious patients, address the following questions: (1) Are the eyes "straight"? (2) If there is a deviation, is it exo, eso, or vertical? (3) Is there a conjugate gaze deviation? (4) Are there any spontaneous eye movements? (5) What reflex eye movements can be induced by head rotation or caloric stimulation?

Deviations of the Visual Axes

Most normal subjects have a horizontal deviation (phoria) during sleep. Thus, an exo or eso deviations may not be pertinent to the diagnosis of coma. However, a horizontal deviation in which there is limited motion of one eye often indicates a palsy. Thus, during reflex eye movements (*see* below), incomplete abduction suggests that an esotropia is the result of abducens palsy, whereas limited adduction suggests that an exotropia is due either to internuclear ophthalmoplegia or a third cranial nerve palsy. Vertical deviations should always be regarded as abnormal, and may be due to a skew deviation (interruption of prenuclear, otolithic inputs to motoneurons) or fourth nerve palsy. Restrictive ophthalmopathy, particularly blow-out fracture of the orbit, may be the mechanism in patients who have suffered head trauma.

Complete oculomotor nerve palsy causes pupillary dilatation, ptosis and deviation of the eye down and out. Pupillary involvement is an early sign of uncal herniation, and impairment of eye movements usually follows *(13)*. Vertical misalignment may be due to skew deviation or trochlear nerve palsy; the latter is common following head trauma. Bilateral abducens palsy occurs when increased intracranial pressure compromises the nerves as they pass through the petroclinoid ligament. Occasionally, skew deviation and internuclear ophthalmoplegia occur in metabolic encephalopathy *(14,15)*, or with drug intoxication *(16–19)*. The differential diagnosis of complete ophthalmoplegia includes botulism, brainstem stroke, drug intoxications, Wernicke's encephalopathy, pituitary apoplexy, myasthenia gravis, and Guillain-Barré and Miller Fisher syndromes.

Conjugate Deviations of Gaze

Horizontal gaze deviations in unconscious patients are common and may provide important clues as to the localization of the disease process (Table 1). Destructive lesions (e.g., infarction) affecting one cerebral hemisphere may cause an ipsilateral gaze deviation, especially with large, more posterior, right-sided locations. The eyes are directed away from the hemiparesis. Such patients may be stuporous, but are seldom unconscious unless there is substantial mass effect. Rarely, the gaze deviation with hemispheric disease is contralateral to the lesion ("wrong-way deviation"); classically, this occurs with thalamic processes *(20)*, and rarely with disease at other sites, such as subfrontal hemorrhage *(21,22)*. Usually, it is possible to drive the eyes across the midline with a vestibular stimulus when a gaze deviation is the cause of a hemispheric lesion.

When conjugate gaze deviation occurs with lesions below the pontomesencephalic junction (site of putative ocular motor decussation), then the eyes are usually directed away from the side of the lesion and toward the hemiparesis. The latter is typically seen with pontine lesions and, in such patients, the eyes usually cannot be induced to cross the midline with vestibular stimuli.

Intermittent deviation of the eyes and head turning are often because of seizure activity. At the beginning of each attack, gaze is usually deviated contralateral to the side of the seizure focus *(1)*; it may be followed by nystagmus with contralaterally directed quick phases. Toward the end of the attack, gaze drifts to an ipsilateral (paretic) position. Seizures are an important cause of unresponsiveness in an NSU setting, and it is important to dedicate a few minutes examination in any unconscious patient with a gaze deviation to determine whether it is sustained or intermittent.

Tonic *downward deviation* of the eyes, often accompanied by convergence, occurs in thalamic hemorrhage *(23)*, and with lesions affecting the dorsal midbrain. It also occurs as a late effect following unilateral caloric stimulation in patients with coma due to sedative drugs *(24)*. Forced downward deviation of the eyes has also been reported in patients feigning coma *(25)* or seizures.

Tonic *upward deviation* of the eyes occurs in unconscious patients following hypoxic-ischemic insult *(26)*. No pathologic lesions may be found in the midbrain, but those patients that survive may

Table 1
Acute Deviations of the Eyes

Sustained horizontal conjugate deviation
Ipsilateral ("looks away from the hemiparesis"): destructive
    lesions (e.g., infarcts), especially with large,
    posterior,and right-sided location
Contralateral ("wrong-way"—"looks toward the hemiparesis"):
    thalamic lesions; rarely with other supratentorial disease;
    pontine lesions
Intermittent horizontal conjugate deviation
Usually a manifestation of epileptic seizures
Sustained upward gaze deviation
Following hypoxic-ischemic insult
Drugs' effects and oculogyric crisis
Sustained downward deviation
Thalamic hemorrhage
Lesions compressing the dorsal midbrain,
    such as hemorrhage, tumor, and hydrocephalus

---

develop downbeat nystagmus. It has been suggested that upward drift in these patients is due to decreased inhibition of the upward vertical vestibulo-ocular reflex, due to loss of cerebellar Purkinje cells *(27)*. Upward deviation also occurs as a component of oculogyric crisis, and this may be encountered in the NSU as a side effect of certain drugs, especially neuroleptic agents *(28,29)*.

Spontaneous Eye Movements in Coma

Slow conjugate or disconjugate *roving eye movements* are similar to the eye movements of light sleep (but slower than the rapid movements of paradoxical or REM sleep). They imply that brain stem gaze mechanisms are intact.

Ocular bobbing consists of repetitive rapid downward movement of the eyes followed by a slower return to the primary position *(30,31)* (Table 2). Reflex horizontal eye movements are often absent. Classic ocular bobbing is a sign of intrinsic pontine lesions, usually hemorrhage, but it has also been reported with cerebellar lesions that secondarily compress the pons, as well as in metabolic or toxic encephalopathy. An *inverse* form of ocular bobbing is described in which the downward movement is slow and the return to midposition is rapid; this has also been called *ocular dipping (32)*. Reverse bobbing consists of an initial rapid deviation of the eyes upward and a slow return to the horizontal *(33)*. Finally, *reverse dipping* or *converse bobbing* has been used to describe a slow upward drift of the eyes followed by a rapid return to primary position *(31)*. These variants of ocular bobbing are less reliable for localization of the lesion. The report that some patients have shown several types of bobbing suggests a common underlying pathophysiology *(34--36)*. Because the pathways that mediate upward and downward eye movements differ anatomically, and probably pharmacologically, it seems possible that these movements represent a varying imbalance of mechanisms for vertical gaze. Rarely, large-amplitude pendular vertical oscillations occur in acute brain stem stroke *(37)*; this *acute vertical myoclonus* may be similar to acquired pendular nystagmus. Repetitive vertical eye movements, including variants of ocular bobbing, that contain convergent-divergent components ("pretectal pseudobobbing") usually indicate disease affecting the dorsal midbrain *(38,39)*.

Ping-pong gaze consists of slow, horizontal, conjugate deviations of the eyes that alternate every few seconds *(40)*. Ping-pong gaze usually occurs in association with bilateral infarction of the cerebral hemispheres, or of the cerebral peduncles *(41)*. Sometimes oscillations with a similar periodicity to ping-pong gaze can be induced as a transient phenomenon, by a single, rapid, horizontal head

Table 2
Spontaneous Eye Movements in Unconscious Patients

Term	Description	Significance
Ocular bobbing	Rapid, conjugate, downward movement; slow return to primary position	Pontine strokes; other structural, metabolic, or toxic disorders
Ocular dipping or inverse ocular bobbing	Slow downward movement; rapid return to primary position	Unreliable for localization; follows hypoxic-ischemic insult or metabolic disorder
Reverse ocular bobbing	Rapid upward movement; slow return to primary position	Unreliable for localization; may occur with metabolic disorders
Reverse ocular dipping or converse bobbing	Slow upward movement; rapid return to primary position	Unreliable for localization; pontine infarction and with AIDS
Ping-pong gaze	Horizontal conjugate deviation of the eyes, alternating every few seconds	Bilateral cerebral hemispheric dysfunction
Periodic alternating gaze deviation	Horizontal conjugate deviation of the eyes, alternating every 2 min	Hepatic encephalopathy; disorders causing periodic alternating nystagmus and unconsciousness or vegetative state
Vertical "myoclonus"	Vertical pendular oscillations (2–3 Hz)	Pontine strokes
Monocular movements	Small, intermittent, rapid monocular horizontal, vertical, or torsional movements	Pontine or midbrain destructive lesions, perhaps with coexistent seizures

Source: ref. *1.*

537

rotation, in patients with bilateral hemispheric disease *(42)*. *Periodic alternating gaze deviation*, in which conjugate gaze deviations change direction every 2 min, is reported in hepatic encephalopathy *(43)*. This phenomenon is related to periodic alternating nystagmus in conscious patients, in which quick phases are present *(1)*.

Rapid, small amplitude, vertical eye movements may be the only manifestation of epileptic seizures in patients who have coexistent brain stem injury *(44)*. Rapid, monocular eye movements with horizontal, vertical, or torsional components occurring in coma, may also indicate brain stem dysfunction.

Identification of patients who are conscious but quadriplegic (the *locked-in* or *de-efferented state*) depends upon identifying preserved voluntary vertical eye movements *(2,45)*. This syndrome is typically caused by pontine infarction with a variable loss of voluntary and reflex horizontal movements, so that eyelid or vertical eye movements may be the only means of communication in the acute illness. The locked-in syndrome is also reported with midbrain lesions, in which case ptosis and ophthalmoplegia may be associated *(46)*.

Reflex Eye Movements in Coma

Eye movements may be elicited in unconscious patients either by head rotation (the *doll's head* or *oculocephalic* maneuver) or by caloric stimulation *(1,2,47,48)*. Head rotation mainly stimulates the labyrinthine semicircular canals—the vestibulo-ocular reflex (VOR) *(42,47,48)*. Head rotations should not be performed in unconscious patients unless there is certainty that no neck injury or abnormality is present. Both horizontal and vertical rotations should be tested. If small-amplitude head rotations are performed, the adequacy of the VOR can be evaluated by observing the optic disc of one eye with an ophthalmoscope *(49)*; if the VOR is working normally, the disc should remain stationary during head movements.

Caloric irrigation of the external auditory meatus causes convection currents of the vestibular endolymph that displace the cupula of a semicircular canal; thus, this procedure also tests the VOR. The canal stimulated depends upon the orientation of the head; with the head elevated 30 degrees from supine position, the horizontal canals are principally stimulated. Prior to caloric stimulation, always check that the tympanic membrane is intact. Large quantities (100 mL or more) of ice water may be required. Caloric stimulation with ice water may sometimes be a more effective stimulus than head rotation, perhaps due to the sustained nature of the stimulus but also to the arousing effect of the cold water. Combined cold caloric stimulation and head rotation may be the only effective stimulus in the deeply unconscious patient, producing tonic deviation of the eyes toward the irrigated ear, if the brainstem is intact.

In testing reflex eye movements in unresponsive patients, it is important to note (1) the magnitude of the response and whether or not the ocular deviation is conjugate; (2) the dynamic response to position-step head rotations; and (3) the occurrence of any quick phases of nystagmus, particularly during caloric stimulation. Impaired abduction suggests sixth nerve palsy; impaired adduction implies either internuclear ophthalmoplegia or third nerve palsy. Sometimes, impaired adduction to vestibular stimulation may be observed in patients with metabolic coma *(14)*, or drug intoxication *(18,19)*. Vertical responses may be impaired with disease of the midbrain *(50)*, or bilateral lesions of the medial longitudinal fasciculus. Pontine lesions may abolish the reflex eye movements in the horizontal plane but spare the vertical responses. Loss of all conjugate horizontal eye movements except for abduction of one eye constitutes the "one-and-a-half" syndrome *(1)*. When reflex eye movements are present in an unresponsive patient, the brainstem is likely to be structurally intact. When reflex eye movements are abnormal or absent, the cause may be structural disease, profound metabolic coma, or drug intoxication *(51)*. Intoxication with a variety of medications may lead to partial or total loss of reflexive eye movements. Metabolic disturbances can cause restriction of reflex eye movements, but usually only with profound coma *(52)*. When used in combination with other clinical signs, especially pupillary light responses and motor responses, reflex eye movements have been helpful in evaluating the outcome of coma *(53,54)*.

Quick phases of nystagmus are usually absent in acutely unconscious patients and their presence, without a tonic deviation of the eyes, raises the possibility of *feigned coma*. In patients who are stuporous but uncooperative, caloric nystagmus may be helpful way of inducing eye movements that cannot be initiated voluntarily. For example, in a patient with a pineal tumor, retraction nystagmus was produced by caloric stimulation *(55)*. Patients who survive coma but who are left in a *persistent vegetative state*, with severe damage of the cerebral hemispheres but preservation of the brain stem, regain quick phases with caloric or rotational stimulation *(42)*. Caloric nystagmus has been reported in patients with neocortical death and an isoelectric electroencephalogram *(56)*. Eye movements have been studied in normal subjects during syncope *(57)*; both downbeat nystagmus and tonic upward deviation may occur, so that these findings—when transient—need not imply structural lesions.

REFERENCES

1. Leigh RJ, Zee DS. *The Neurology of Eye Movements*, 3rd ed. (Text/CD). New York: Oxford University Press, 1999.
2. Miller NR, Newman N, (eds). *Walsh and Hoyt's Clinical Neuro-ophthalmology*, 5th ed., vol 1. Baltimore: Lippincott, Williams and Wilkins, 1998.
3. Plum F, Posner JB. *The Diagnosis of Stupor and Coma*, 3rd ed. Philadelphia: FA Davis, 1981.
4. Averbuch-Heller L, Stahl JS, Remler BF, Leigh RJ. Bilateral ptosis and upgaze palsy with right hemispheric lesions. *Ann. Neurol.* 1996;40:465–468.
5. Keane JR. Spastic eyelids. Failure of levator inhibition in unconscious states. *Arch. Neurol.* 1975;32:695–698.
6. Biousse V, Touboul PJ, D'Anglejan-Chatillon J, Levy C, Schaison M, Bousser MG. Ophthalmologic manifestations of internal carotid artery dissection. *Am. J. Ophthalmol.* 1998;126:565–577.
7. St.Louis EK, Wijdicks EF, Li H. Predicting neurologic deterioration in patients with cerebellar hematomas. *Neurology* 1998;51:1364–1369.
8. Cordova S, Lee R. Fixed, dilated pupils in the ICU: another recoverable cause. *Anaesth. Intens. Care* 2000;28:91–93.
9. Rizzo MA, Fisher M, Lock JP. Hypermagnesemic pseudocoma. *Arch. Intern. Med.* 1993;153:1130–1132.
10. Ropper AH, Miller DC. Acute traumatic midbrain hemorrhage. *Ann. Neurol.* 1985;18:80–86.
11. Andrefsky JC, Frank JI, Chyatte D. The ciliospinal reflex in pentobarbital coma. *J. Neurosurg.* 1999;90:644–646.
12. Fisher CM. Oval pupils. *Arch. Neurol.* 1980;37:502–503.
13. Keane JR. Bilateral ocular motor signs after tentorial herniation in 25 patients. *Arch. Neurol.* 1986;43:806–807.
14. Caplan LR, Scheiner D. Dysconjugate gaze in hepatic coma. *Ann. Neurol.* 1980;8:328–329.
15. Fisher M. Ocular skew deviation in hepatic coma. *J. Neurol. Neurosurg. Psychiatry* 1981;44:458.
16. Cook FF, Davis RG, Russo LS, Jr. Internuclear ophthalmoplegia caused by phenothiazine intoxication. *Arch. Neurol.* 1981;38:465–466.
17. Donhowe SP. Bilateral internuclear ophthalmoplegia from doxepin overdose. *Neurology* 1984;34:259.
18. el-Mallakh RS. Internuclear ophthalmoplegia with narcotic overdosage. *Ann. Neurol.* 1986;20:107.
19. Rizzo M, Corbett J. Bilateral internuclear ophthalmoplegia reversed by naloxone. *Arch. Neurol.* 1983;40:242–243.
20. Fisher CM. Some neuro-ophthalmological observations. *J. Neurol. Neurosurg. Psychiatry* 1967;30:383–392.
21. Pessin MS, Adelman LS, Prager RJ, Lathi ES, Lange DJ. "Wrong-way eyes" in supratentorial hemorrhage. *Ann. Neurol.* 1981;9:79–81.
22. Sharpe JA, Bondar RL, Fletcher WA. Contralateral gaze deviation after frontal lobe haemorrhage. *J. Neurol. Neurosurg. Psychiatry* 1985;48:86–88.
23. Fisher A, Knezevic W. Ocular and ocular motor aspects of primary thalamic haemorrhage. *Clin. Exp. Neurol.* 1985;21:129–139.
24. Simon RP. Forced downward ocular deviation. Occurrence during oculovestibular testing in sedative drug-induced coma. *Arch. Neurol.* 1978;35:456–458.
25. Rosenberg ML. The eyes in hysterical states of unconsciousness. *J. Clin. Neuro-ophthalmol.* 1982;2:259–260.
26. Keane JR. Sustained upgaze in coma. *Ann. Neurol.* 1981;9:409–412.
27. Nakada T, Kwee IL, Lee H. Sustained upgaze in coma. *J. Clin. Neuro-ophthalmol.* 1984;4:35–37.
28. Leigh RJ, Foley JM, Remler BF, Civil RH. Oculogyric crisis: A syndrome of thought disorder and ocular deviation. *Ann. Neurol.* 1987;22:13–17.
29. Sachdev P. Tardive and chronically recurrent oculogyric crises. *Mov. Disord.* 1993;8:93–97.
30. Fisher CM. Ocular bobbing. *Arch. Neurol.* 1964;11:543–546.
31. Mehler MF. The clinical spectrum of ocular bobbing and ocular dipping. *J. Neurol. Neurosurg. Psychiatry* 1988;51:725–727.
32. Ropper AH. Ocular dipping in anoxic coma. *Arch. Neurol.* 1981;38:297–299.
33. Titer EM, Laureno R. Inverse/reverse ocular bobbing. *Ann. Neurol.* 1988;23:103–104.
34. Brusa A, Firpo MP, Massa S, Piccardo A, Bronzini E. Typical and reverse bobbing: A case with localizing value. *Eur. Neurol.* 1984;23:151–155.

35. Goldschmidt TJ, Wall M. Slow-upward ocular bobbing. *J. Clin. Neuro-ophthalmol.* 1987;7:241–243.
36. Rosenberg ML, Calvert PC. Ocular bobbing in association with other signs of midbrain dysfunction. *Arch. Neurol.* 1986;43:314–315.
37. Keane JR. Acute vertical ocular myoclonus. *Neurology* 1986;36:86–89.
38. Keane JR. Pretectal pseudobobbing. Five patients with 'V'-pattern convergence nystagmus. *Arch. Neurol.* 1985;42:592–594.
39. Noda S, Ide K, Umezaki H, Itoh H, Yamamoto K. Repetitive divergence. *Ann. Neurol.* 1987;21:109–110.
40. Ishikawa H, Ishikawa S, Mukuno K. Short-cycle periodic (ping-pong) gaze. *Neurology* 1993;43:1067–1070.
41. Larmande P, Dongmo L, Limodin J, Ruchoux M. Periodic alternating gaze: A case without any hemispheric lesion. *Neurosurgery* 1987;20:481–483.
42. Leigh RJ, Hanley DF, Munschauer FEI, Lasker AG. Eye movements induced by head rotations in unresponsive patients. *Ann. Neurol.* 1983;15:465–473.
43. Averbuch-Heller L, Meiner Z. Reversible periodic alternating gaze deviation in hepatic encephalopathy. *Neurology* 1995;45:191–192.
44. Simon RP, Aminoff MJ. Electrographic status epilepticus in fatal anoxic coma. *Ann. Neurol.* 1986;20:351–355.
45. Larmande P, Henin D, Jan M, Elie A, Gouaze A. Abnormal vertical eye movements in the locked-in syndrome. *Ann. Neurol.* 1982;11:100–102.
46. Meienberg O, Mumenthaler M, Karbowski K. Quadriparesis and nuclear oculomotor palsy with total bilateral ptosis mimicking coma. A mesencephalic "locked-in syndrome"? *Arch. Neurol.* 1979;36:708–710.
47. Buettner UW. Ocular motor dysfunction in stupor and coma. *Baillieres Clin. Neurol.* 1992;1:289–300.
48. Buettner UW, Zee DS. Vestibular testing in comatose patients. *Arch. Neurol.* 1989;46:561–563.
49. Zee DS. Ophthalmoscopy in examination of patients with vestibular disorders. *Ann. Neurol.* 1978;3:373–374.
50. Uematsu D, Suematsu M, Fukuuchi Y, Ebihara S, Gotoh F. Midbrain locked-in state with oculomotor subnucleus lesion. *J. Neurol. Neurosurg. Psychiatry* 1985;48:952–953.
51. Rosenberg M, Sharpe J, Hoyt WF. Absent vestibulo-ocular reflexes and supratentorial lesions. *J. Neurol. Neurosurg. Psychiatry* 1975;38:6–10.
52. Hanid MA, Silk DB, Williams R. Prognostic value of the oculovestibular reflex in fulminant hepatic coma. *BMJ* 1978;1:1029.
53. Levy DE, Plum F. Outcome prediction in comatose patients: Significance of reflex eye movement analysis. *J. Neurol. Neurosurg. Psychiatry* 1988;51:318.
54. Mueller-Jensen A, Neunzig HP, Emskotter T. Outcome prediction in comatose patients: Significance of reflex eye movement analysis. *J. Neurol. Neurosurg. Psychiatry* 1987;50:389–392.
55. Singh BM, Strobos RJ. Retraction nystagmus elicited by bilateral simultaneous cold caloric stimulation. *Ann. Neurol.* 1980;8:79.
56. Nayyar M, Strobos RJ, Singh BM, Brown-Wagner M, Pucillo A. Caloric-induced nystagmus with isoelectric electroencephalogram. *Ann. Neurol.* 1987;21:98–100.
57. Lempert T, von Brevern M. The eye movements of syncope. *Neurology* 1996;46:1086–1088.

31

Management of the Patient With Mitochondrial Disease in the Neurosciences Critical Care Unit

Julio A. Chalela

INTRODUCTION

The term *mitochondrial disorder* (MD) encompasses a group of diseases that result from the structural, biochemical, or genetic derangement of mitochondria. In simple terms, MDs are disorders of deficient cellular energy production *(1)*. The role of MD in aging and in a wide variety of systemic and neurologic disorders is increasingly recognized *(2)*. Mitochondrial disorders may present as independent syndromes, complicate other medical disorders, or occur as complication of therapies used to treat other disorders *(1)*. Most patients with MD are not diagnosed on initial presentation but present with recurrent episodic symptoms that elude diagnosis for months to years.

Mitochondrial disorders may originate in the neurosciences critical care unit (NSU) as a result of medications, or may be latent and triggered by unrelated systemic conditions (fever, acidosis, infection). In addition, what appear to be common variety diseases (status epilepticus, stroke) requiring admission to the NSU may actually represent unrecognized forms of MDs. This chapter focuses on specific MD syndromes that may require admission to the NSU. A detailed explanation of the pathogenesis of mitochondrial dysfunction is beyond the scope of this text, but a brief overview of the role of mitochondria in disease is provided to help the reader understand the approach to MDs in the NSU.

PATHOGENESIS OF MITOCHONDRIAL DISEASE

The pathogenesis of MD is complex and multifactorial. Similar disorders may originate from a wide variety of different cellular alterations and the correlation between the abnormal phenotype and the clinical syndrome is poor *(3)*. The field of mitochondrial molecular genetics expands vertiginously and our current understanding of MD is incomplete.

Several unique features of mitochondria make this structure vulnerable to malfunction *(3–5)*. Mitochondrial deoxyribonucleic acid (DNA) mutates more than ten times as frequently as nuclear DNA and has no introns, so a random mutation will usually affect a coding DNA sequence. DNA in the mitochondria lacks a repair mechanism. In addition, DNA in the mitochondria is exposed to reactive oxygen species generated from oxidative phosphorylation. Mitochondrial DNA is inherited primarily maternally, and does not recombine; mutations thus accumulate sequentially through maternal lineage. The proportion of mutant DNA required for the expression of a particular phenotype (the threshold effect) varies from person to person and within the same person over time.

Mitochondrial disorders are considered primary MDs when they affect mitochondrial DNA or nuclear genes that encode subunits of the respiratory chain complexes *(5)*. Secondary MDs include

From: *Current Clinical Neurology*
Critical Care Neurology and Neurosurgery
Edited by: J. I. Suarez © Humana Press Inc., Totowa, NJ

those that are caused by, or associated with mutations in nuclear genes that encode nonrespiratory chain mitochondrial proteins or dysfunction or deficiency in other proteins that may in turn affect respiratory chain activity. It was formerly believed that MDs were transmitted exclusively on a maternal fashion. However, such assumption was based on studies that lacked the sensitivity to detect small concentrations of paternal DNA. The ratio of mitochondrial DNA molecule number in sperm to that in ova is estimated at 1:70–1000. Thus, MDs may be transmitted via paternal lineage albeit very rare *(5,6)*.

Mitochondrial defects fall into four major categories: large scale rearrangements (large segments of the genome are deleted), transmitter RNA gene defects (point mutations or insertions or deletions of single base pairs), protein-coding gene point mutations, and ribosomal ribonucleic acid (RNA) gene point mutation *(6–8)*. Abnormalities of mitochondrial structure may occur in the absence of disease, and mutations that may cause disease in an individual may be innocuous in an individual of different race or age. Specific biochemical criteria must be met before ascribing pathogenic status to an identified change *(3)*. A strict correlation exists between the proportion of mutant DNA and the functional consequence.

Regardless of the defect that accounts for the MD, all MDs ultimately lead to deficient function of the respiratory chain, abnormal oxidation-phosphorylation, and increased production of reactive oxygen species. The consequences of mitochondrial dysfunction are more evident in organs with high metabolic rates such as the heart, brain, and muscle *(1,9)*. The clinical manifestations are heterogeneous and identical mutations may lead to a wide variety of syndromes in different individuals. For instance the A3243G mutation which may cause the syndrome of mitochondrial encephalomyopathy with lactic acidosis and stroke-like episodes (MELAS) may also be associated with chronic external progressive ophthalmoplegia *(8,10)*.

A common histopathologic feature of patients with defects of mitochondrial DNA is the presence of so-called ragged red fibers in skeletal muscle. The ragged red fibers represent areas of focal mitochondrial proliferation. It is hypothesized that such proliferation represents an effort to compensate for impaired respiratory chain function within a muscle segment. It is believed that neurotropin 4 is the mediator of mitochondrial proliferation *(3)*.

CLINICAL AND LABORATORY PRESENTATION OF MITOCHONDRIAL DISORDERS

Mitochondrial diseases can affect almost any system in the human body *(1,4,11)*. The clinical and laboratory abnormalities of MDs are listed in Tables 1 and 2. The presence of a multisystemic disorder of undetermined etiology is the most important clue to presence of MD *(1)*. Thus, the presence of strokes and migraines in a patient with lactic acidosis, cardiomyopathy, and diabetes should alert the clinician to the possibility of a MD. A maternal history of a similar disorder is useful but one must bear in mind that paternal transmission may occur, and that *de novo* mutations, or mutations related to drug exposure may occur. The presentation may be organ-specific or may be multisystemic, and fatal or nonfatal. The spectrum of severity varies, with some patients presenting with isolated fatal lactic acidosis at birth and others developing mild, benign, proximal myopathy later in life. In most cases the disease follows a progressive course over years before reaching a plateau or leading to death.

Laboratory Findings

Biochemical Evaluation

The diagnosis of a MD relies heavily on laboratory findings, as the clinical features are often indistinguishable from other disorders (*see* Table 2) The presence of lactic acidosis in a patient not in shock or in sepsis is the most common laboratory abnormality *(12)*. Lactate levels in MD are raised both at rest and after exercise *(12)*. Lactic acid and pyruvic acid may be normal in the serum but elevated in the cerebrospinal fluid *(13)*. Lactate-to-pyruvate ratios of more than 20 are abnormal. Levels may rise dramatically after alcohol consumption or after administration of propofol, meperi-

Table 1
Clinical Manifestations of Mitochondrial Disease

Neurologic
 Myopathy, neuropathy, ataxia, stroke, seizures, encephalopathy, myelopathy,
  sensorineural hearing loss, ophthalmoplegia, dystonia, dementia, migraines
Ophthalmic
 Retinitis pigmentosa, cataracts, ptosis, optic atrophy
Otorynolaryngologic
 Hearing loss, increased susceptibility to aminoglycoside-induced hearing loss
Cardiac
 Hypertrophic cardiomyopathy, dilated cardiomyopathy, heart block
Pulmonary
 Idiopathic fibrosis, pulmonary hypertension, restrictive lung disease
Gastrointestinal
 Episodic nausea and vomiting, dysphagia, pancreatitis, hepatic dysfunction
Metabolic endocrine
 Diabetes Mellitus, thyroid disorders, hypoparathyroidism, hypoadrenalism,
  hypogonadism
Renal
 Renal tubular acidosis, acute renal failure, glomerulopathy
Musculoskeletal
 Myalgias, poor exercise tolerance
Hematologic
 Sideroblastic anemia, pancytopenia

Table 2
Laboratory Abnormalities in Mitochondrial Disease

Lactic acidemia
Elevated lactate, pyruvate and alanine in the serum
Elevated lactate in the spinal fluid
Elevated aminoacids, glucose, lactate, pyruvate, and phosphate in the urine
Elevated creatine kinase
Sideroblastic anemia, pancytopenia
EKG evidence of conduction block
Myopathic potentials on electromyography
Axonal and demyelinating neuropathy on nerve conduction studies
Basal ganglia calcifications
Abnormal phosphorus-31 nuclear magnetic resonance spectroscopy
Defective oxidative phosphorylation on mitochondrial enzyme studies
Molecular genetic evidence of mitochondrial-DNA mutation

dine, clonazepam, and nucleoside analogues *(1)*. Pancreatic enzymes may be elevated in patients
with pancreatic involvement and diabetes mellitus can occur as a consequence of impaired insulin
secretion *(4)*. Urine measurements of pyruvate, lactate, glucose, phosphate, or amino acids may detect defects in the renal tubular cells.

Pulmonary Evaluation

 Pulmonary function tests may show reduced forced vital capacity, maximum minute ventilation,
and inspiratory and expiratory pressures. Spirometric maneuvers alone will rarely induce fatigue and
patients with isolated fatigue owing to MD usually have normal spirometry. Arterial blood gases may

be normal at rest but after exercise a mixed respiratory failure may become evident *(14,15)*. Bilateral, diffuse, reticular interstitial infiltrates on chest X-ray have been described *(14)*.

Cardiac Evaluation

Cardiac evaluation in the patient with MD is mandatory as the myocardium with its high basal metabolic rate is particularly susceptible to MDs *(5)*. The EKG may reveal conduction abnormalities (typical of Kearns-Sayre syndrome), Wolf-Parkinson-White syndrome, or signs of left ventricular hypertrophy. Echocardiography may reveal left ventricular hypertrophy or dilated cardiomyopathy.

Neuroimaging Evaluation

Computed tomography (CT) and magnetic resonance imaging (MRI) of the brain are an essential part of the workup of patients with MD. Computed tomography evidence of symmetric hypodense areas in the basal ganglia, particularly in the putamen or increased signal in the putamen on T2-weighted MRI are suggestive of Leigh disease. Baso-ganglionic hemorrhages, indistinguishable from hypertensive hemorrhages may occur *(16)*. Elevated lactate levels and decreased in the *N*-acetylaspartate /creatine ratio may be seen on proton magnetic resonance spectroscopy *(6)*. Subcortical strokes in the posterior circulation may be seen in patients with MELAS. Basal ganglia calcifications are suggestive of MELAS or Kearns-Sayre syndrome. Diffuse white matter changes are common in patients with Kearns-Sayre syndrome. Cerebral blood flow studies in patients with MELAS are usually normal and arteriography fails to reveal any vasculopathy *(17)*.

Magnetic Resonance Spectroscopy

Phosphorus-31 nuclear magnetic resonance spectroscopy is a noninvasive method used to assess muscle metabolism. Resting and postexercise levels of phosphocreatine, adenosine diphosphate, and inorganic phosphate are measured. The ability of the muscle to generate adenosine triphosphate (ATP) is extrapolated. In MDs, the resting phosphocreatine levels are reduced and rapidly decline after exercise. In addition, the postexercise recovery of phosphocreatine, adenosine diphosphate, and inorganic phosphate is prolonged *(1)*.

Muscle Biopsy and Mitochondrial Enzymology

When the clinical examination and the laboratory findings suggest MD a muscle biopsy is often performed to confirm the diagnosis. The characteristic finding on light microscopy is ragged, red fibers (RRF), which represent subsarcolemmal proliferation of mitochondria that can be detected with trichrome and succinate dehydrogenase staining *(9)*. The absence of RRF does not exclude a MD, as some mutations are not associated with RRF *(3)*. Mitochondrial enzymatic studies can be performed to determine the metabolic capabilities of oxidative phosphorylation. After isolating mitochondria from tissue, the function of each complex is assessed using a variety of complex inhibitors and substrates. The test may locate specific abnormalities within the mitochondria directing treatment. If the diagnosis of MD is still not clear, performing genetic analysis of mitochondrial DNA in muscle or leukocytes may aid. The genome is screened for the most common type of mutations using *in situ* hybridization or the whole genome is sequenced. Because the concentration of mutated DNA varies in different cell divisions, it is possible to miss a MD if a cell line with "diluted" DNA is studied.

CLINICAL SYNDROMES REQUIRING NEUROINTENSIVE CARE

The systemic or the neurologic presentation of MDs may lead to admission to the critical care unit. A striking feature of MDs is their clinical heterogeneity, ranging from single-organ involvement to severe multisystem disease. For the neurointensivist, four particular syndromes associated with MDs are of interest: neuromuscular respiratory failure, stroke (ischemic and hemorrhagic), status epilepticus, and the encephalomyelopathy of Leigh disease.

Neuromuscular Respiratory Failure

Mitochondrial myopathies usually present with slowly progressive muscle weakness, myalgias, exercise intolerance, external ophthalmoplegia, or a facioscapulohumeral syndrome *(18)*. Kearns-Sayre syndrome, MELAS, myoclonic epilepsy with ragged-red fibers (MERFF), and isolated deficiencies of complexes II, III, and IV may manifest with muscle weakness *(14,18)*. In some cases, gradual progression of weakness may culminate in ventilatory failure and in others abrupt bellows failure may lead to intubation. In patients with unrecognized mitochondrial myopathy low doses of sedatives may trigger respiratory failure *(1)*. Respiratory insufficiency in MDs is due to a combination of muscle weakness and reduced respiratory drive to hypoxia and hypercapnia. The underlying mechanism for the reduced ventilatory drive is unclear but cytochrome *c* oxidase deficiency may be involved *(15)*.

Clinical Presentation

The clinical presentation is similar to that of other neuromuscular disorders that can lead to respiratory failure. Patients present with progressive limb weakness that later involves the neck flexors and extensors, the bulbar muscles, the intercostal muscles, and the diaphragm. History of poor exercise tolerance and recurrent visits to the hospital with "bronchitis" or pneumonia are common *(18)*. Atrophy of the chest muscles, deformity of the chest, clubbing of the fingers and toes, and signs of pulmonary hypertension are common. Brow sweating, staccato speech, inability to complete sentences, use of accessory muscles, and paradoxical inspiration signal impending respiratory failure. The inability to count to 20 on one breath usually indicates a reduced vital capacity (<15 mL/kg) *(19)*.

Laboratory

Although hypercapnia is believed to be the hallmark of neuromuscular respiratory failure, hypoxemia often precedes CO_2 elevation *(19)*. Because atelectasis and air space occupation (because of edema or infection) are not uncommon in neuromuscular respiratory failure and in MDs, it is not unusual to see hypoxemic or mixed respiratory failure. Thus, the alveolo-arterial gradient may be normal or widened and the clinician must be cautious about it's interpretation. Acidosis signals underlying lactic acidosis, CO_2 retention, or renal tubular defects *(20)*. The chest radiograph may show chest cage deformities, reticular interstitial infiltrates, atelectasis, areas of consolidation, or signs of pulmonary hypertension *(18)*.

Treatment

Treatment of the patient with MD presenting with respiratory failure is similar to the treatment of respiratory failure in other diseases (*see* Chapter 9). Intubation and mechanical ventilation is indicated in patients with marked bulbar weakness precluding coughing and clearing of secretions, patients with vital capacity (VC) less than 15 mL/kg, patients with hypercapnic and/or hypoxemic respiratory failure, negative inspiratory force of less than –25 cm H_2O, positive inspiratory force of less than 40 cm H_2O, or a decrease in VC of more than 55% from sitting to supine *(19)*. Treatment of underlying metabolic acidosis, infection, and fever is of utmost importance because they can worsen MDs. Drugs that can worsen MDs should be avoided, a list is provided in Table 3 *(1)*. An increased sensitivity to neuromuscular blockers is well recognized and those agents should be used judiciously if at all. Prolonged need for mechanical ventilation is common, and tracheostomy should be considered in patients intubated for 3 or more wk. Intermittent positive pressure ventilation via tracheostomy or bilevel positive airway pressure by nasal mask are useful therapeutic options once the patient is weaned or a tracheostomy is performed *(21,22)*.

Specific therapy is aimed at increasing ATP production by providing components of oxidative phosphorylation and/or inhibiting lactate production. Treatment with riboflavin or coenzyme Q has

Table 3
Agents With Potential Mitochondrial Toxicity

Propofol
Valproate
Barbiturates
Benzodiazepines
Aminoglycosides
Neuromuscular blockers
Meperidine
Blue dye used in enteral feeding
Aspirin
Dinitrophenol
Nitroprusside
Cocaine
Alcohol

been shown to increase maximum oxygen uptake, exercise tolerance, and reduce lactate *(1)*. Coenzyme Q may improve respiratory muscles strength in MDs *(23)*. Dichloroacetate has been used to treat the lactic acidosis seen in MDs by inhibiting the inactivation of pyruvate dehydrogenase leading to a decrease in the accumulation of pyruvate and the production of lactate. The prognosis in most cases of MD presenting with respiratory failure is poor with patients dying from complications of critical illness or from subsequent bouts of respiratory failure. A significant proportion of patients require long-term ventilatory support *(14,15,18)*.

Ischemic Stroke from Mitochondrial Disease

Ischemic stroke (IS) and less commonly intracranial hemorrhage (ICH) may complicate MDs *(16)*. The cause of strokes in patients with MDs is multifactorial. The concept of "metabolic stroke" has been proposed to explain the stroke-like lesions seen in MELAS. It is hypothesized that intact perfusion and substrate delivery are faced with defects in electron transport causing deficient ATP production and cellular injury. A mitochondrial angiopathy characterized by abnormal accumulation of mitochondria in endothelial and vascular smooth muscle cells has also been described *(24)*. In patients with cardiac involvement owing to MD, the stroke may be caused by cardioembolism. In patients with diabetes mellitus due to MD, small vessel ischemic disease, carotid occlusive disease, and diabetic cardiomyopathy with resulting cardioembolism are the main culprits. In patients with restrictive pulmonary disease with resulting pulmonary hypertension right to left shunts may facilitate paradoxical embolism and stroke.

Clinical Presentation

Of the clinically defined subtypes of MD that can cause stroke, MELAS is the best recognized *(24)*. The hallmark of this syndrome is the occurrence of stroke-like episodes that result in hemiparesis, hemianopia, cognitive decline, or cortical blindness. Focal or generalized seizures, migraine-like headaches, sensorineural hearing loss, and muscle weakness are common. Systemic disorders such as diabetes mellitus, ileus, pancreatitis, persistent lactic acidosis, and congestive heart failure are common. A maternal history of a similar disorder may be present but affected relatives may not have overt symptoms *(5)*.

Neuroimaging

Neuroimaging studies show radiolucent areas on CT scans and areas of hyperintense signal on T2-weighted or diffusion-weighted imaging. The lesions predominate in the parieto-occipital region and cerebellum and have a non-vascular distribution. Basal ganglia lesions with or without cortical involvement may also occur. The deep white matter is usually spared. Lesions are often transient or migratory. Vasogenic edema may complicate strokes in patients with MELAS *(25)*. Vasoreactivity of the cerebral blood vessels as determined by transcranial Doppler is normal *(17)*.

Treatment

Management of acute ischemic stroke and intracranial hemorrhage are discussed in detail elsewhere in this text (*see* Chapters 18 and 19). Patients should be admitted to stroke unit or NSU. Cardiac telemetry is essential to detect any rhythm or conduction disturbances that may need cardiac pacing or other interventions. Patients with IS in the setting of MD should be considered for thrombolysis if they meet the established criteria *(26)*. The clinician should not assume that the stroke is a "metabolic stroke" as this would negate the patient from the potential benefits of thrombolysis. Stroke in patients with MDs may be due to diverse etiologies including cardioembolism and carotid occlusive disease.

Airway protection is of paramount importance and endotracheal intubation should be considered in patients with Glasgow Coma Scale (GCS) score less than 8, in patients with impaired bulbar function, in patients with depressed level of consciousness and protracted vomiting, and in patients with significant compartment shifts and impending herniation. Blood pressure should be left untreated unless there is evidence of end-organ damage or the patient has received thrombolysis. In nonthrombolysis cases crystalloids and/or vasopressors should be used to keep blood pressure above 160/90 mmHg and optimize cerebral perfusion. Hyperglycemia and lactic acidosis should be corrected; as they tend to worsen MDs *(1)*. Acidosis causes cerebral vasodilatation and may lead to increased intracranial pressure. Dichloroacetate may control the acidosis, but in extreme cases bicarbonate infusions may be necessary. Gastric decompression using nasogastric or orogastric tubes, prokinetic agents, and stool softeners should be used to prevent the gastrointestinal complications of MDs *(1)*. If aspirin therapy is associated with worsening of the MD or recurrent stroke, consideration should be given to using an aspirin-free antiplatelet agent *(6)*. Drugs aimed at restoring the energy producing capacity of the mitochondria should also be instituted. As mentioned previously, all drugs known to trigger or worsen MDs should be avoided. Compartment shifts associated with clinical deterioration should be treated with elevation of the head of the bed at 30 degrees, osmotherapy, and/or hyperventilation. Hemicraniectomy and therapeutic hypothermia may be beneficial in selected cases.

Intracranial Hemorrhage

Intracranial hemorrhage is a rare manifestation of MDs and only a handful of cases have been reported *(16)*. An association with the G13513A mutation in *ND5* has been proposed *(16)*. The ICH seen in association with MDs is indistinguishable clinically and radiologically from hypertensive hemorrhages. Cerebral blood flow studies have shown cerebral hyperemia and it is possible that ICH in MDs has a similar pathophysiology to the hemorrhage seen in hyperperfusion syndrome after carotid endarterectomy.

Treatment of Intracranial Hemorrhage

Management of the patient with MD and ICH is similar to the management of spontaneous nonaneurysmal ICH (*see* Chapter 19). The author suggests following the American Heart Association guidelines *(27)*. Patients should be admitted to the NSU for close monitoring. Airway protection takes precedence, and intubation should be considered in all patients with GCS score of less than 8, patients with impaired bulbar function, patients with frequent vomiting and decreased level of consciousness, patients with frequent seizures, and patients in whom therapeutic hyperventilation is being contemplated. Blood pressure should be left untreated unless there is clear evidence of end-organ damage or the mean arterial pressure exceeds 130 mmHg. Nitroprusside should be avoided as it is toxic to mitochondria *(1)*. Labetalol, esmolol, hydralazine, or nicardipine, are useful therapeutic alternatives to nitroprusside. Hypotension should be corrected because it may worsen cerebral perfusion in the peri-hematoma region *(27)*. Volume replacement is the first line of approach, and volume status can be monitored with central venous pressure or pulmonary artery wedge pressure. Coexistent congestive heart failure may complicate fluid administration in MDs. If intracranial pressure monitoring is available, cerebral perfusion pressure should be kept above 70 mmHg.

Intracranial pressure should be monitored in all patients with GCS score less than 9 or any patient in whom deterioration is believed to be secondary to increased intracranial pressure *(27)*. Ventriculostomies are the procedure of choice when hydrocephalus is complicating the ICH. Increased intracranial pressure should be treated with a combination of general and specific measures. The general measures include elevating the head of the bed to 30–45 degrees, keeping the head centered to optimize venous drainage, controlling pain, treating fever, treating seizures, and suppressing cough. Specific measures include, osmotherapy, hyperventilation, neuromuscular paralysis, barbiturates, hypothermia, and hemicraniectomy *(27)*. There is no benefit of using steroids in ICH and steroids may have serious side effects in patients with MDs *(1)*. There are reports of narcotics worsening or triggering MDs, the author suggests using fentanyl, benzodiazepines, and/or butyrophenones cautiously. Neuromuscular blockers are best avoided particularly in patients with concomitant myopathy and/or neuropathy as prolonged paralysis may occur.

Patients with hepatic involvement due to MD may have abnormal synthetic liver function and coagulopathy requiring fresh frozen plasma. Early nutrition is crucial as starvation negatively affects respiratory chain function in MDs *(3)*. Nutritional needs should be adjusted to the patient's needs using either indirect calorimetry or nitrogen balance. As previously described, patients with MDs are at risk of developing gastrointestinal motility disturbances and measures aimed at ensuring adequate gastric emptying and gut motility should be instituted.

Surgical management of ICH is controversial, the author suggests following the guidelines published by the American Heart Association *(27)*. An increased sensitivity to anesthetics and a slow emergence from general anesthesia has been described in MDs and should be kept in mind when ICH patients with MD undergo surgical procedures such as hematoma resection *(1,15)*.

Status Epilepticus in Mitochondrial Disease

Status epilepticus (SE) may be the presenting manifestation of epilepsy in MDs *(11)*. General seizures are the cardinal symptoms of MERFF, and focal seizures are more common in patients with MELAS *(28)*. Myoclonic status, focal motor status, and generalized motor status can occur. Motor ictal symptoms appear to be exceedingly common. Such presentation is likely related to the marked excitability of the motor cortex observed in MDs *(28)*. Photosensitive discharges are frequent, likely related to the preferential distribution of lesions in the posterior parts of the brain.

Treatment of Status Epilepticus in Mitochondrial Disorders

With the exception of some specific points, management of SE in patients with MD is similar to SE management in non-MD patients *(29)* *(see* Chapter 25*)*. The multiple systemic problems that accompany MDs make the management more complicated. The initial care should involve stabilization of the airway with either ambu-bag ventilation (may suffice in the postictal period), or endotracheal/nasotracheal intubation and mechanical ventilation *(29)*. If needed a short acting neuromuscular blocker can be used to facilitate intubation. Arterial blood gases in the patient with MD and SE need to be interpreted cautiously. Lactic acidosis may result from the underlying MD or from the vigorous muscle activity. Adequate respiratory compensation argues in favor of chronic lactic acidosis due to MD. Respiratory acidosis may be secondary to the seizures, the medications used for seizure control, or to decreased respiratory drive linked to MD *(1,11,29)*.

Fever is common in patients with SE and does not always indicate acute infection *(29)*. Because fever is deleterious to most forms of cerebral injury and to MDs in general, passive cooling should be attempted. Acetaminophen should be used with caution, as hepatic dysfunction is common in MDs. Intravenous fluids and dopamine should be used to maintain adequate blood pressure and ensure cerebral perfusion. Infections should be treated aggressively avoiding aminoglycosides due to the increased risk of ototoxicity.

Electroencephalographic monitoring should be considered in patients in whom neuromuscular blockers have been administered, in patients who remain unconscious after administration of first line agents for seizure control, or in patients with refractory SE *(29)*. Because subtle SE and difficult-to-recognize seizures are common in MDs, electroencephalographic monitoring is particularly important *(28)*.

As in all cases of SE the main goal is to achieve prompt cessation of seizure activity. The drug of first choice for SE in MD is lorazepam, but if unavailable, diazepam is a useful alternative. Since lorazepam has a more prolonged anti-seizure effect it is the preferred agent *(29)*. Due to the increased sensitivity of patients with MDs to benzodiazepines the author suggests starting at a very low dose (0.1 mg/kg IV) and titrating the dose upward as needed. The physician should be prepared to intubate the patient at lower doses of benzodiazepines owing to the impaired ventilatory drive seen in MDs. The coexistence of liver dysfunction (common in MDs) may also alter the elimination kinetics of anticonvulsants and lead to prolonged sedation.

Phenytoin and fosphenytoin are the drugs of choice for maintaining a prolonged anti-seizure effect after seizure control with benzodiazepines, when benzodiazepines fail, and occasionally as initial therapy *(29)*. Caution must be exerted in patients with MD as cardiac conduction abnormalities are frequent and use of phenytoin could result in complete heart block *(4)*. Continuous electrocardiographic monitoring should be performed and a transvenous or external pacemaker should be readily available. In patients with liver dysfunction conversion of fosphenytoin to phenytoin may be impaired resulting in a delayed time to onset of clinical effect. Theoretically since fosphenytoin does not contain propylene glycol it is a better choice than phenytoin in patients with MD *(29)*.

If seizures are not terminated with benzodiazepines and/or phenytoin most physicians recur to intravenous barbiturates. Phenobarbital is as effective as the combination of benzodiazepines and phenytoin in controlling seizures but has more sedative effect. In the patient with MD phenobarbital may have negative effects as it inhibits the oxidative phosphorylation system and may lead to impaired energy production *(6)*. Other therapeutic options in patients with MD and refractory SE include midazolam intravenous continuous infusion, lidocaine infusion, and paraldehyde. Unfortunately paraldehyde is not available in the United States and lidocaine is limited by its potential toxicity. Midazolam via continuous infusion appears to be as effective as other therapeutic alternatives in controlling SE *(30)*. Midazolam has the advantage over barbiturates of producing less hypotension and having rapid clearance. Although there may be an increased sensitivity to benzodiazepines in MDs, midazolam is not known to be directly toxic to the mitochondria. If midazolam fails, thiopental or pentobarbital are potential therapeutic options with possible cerebral-protective effects *(29)*.

Valproate and propofol are two useful therapeutic options in patients with SE. Unfortunately both agents have been reported to cause mitochondrial dysfunction and respiratory chain disorders. Prolonged use of propofol has been reported to increase lactate levels by inducing transient abnormalities in oxidative phosphorylation *(20)*. Valproate has been reported to inhibit fatty acid oxidation and thereby increase lactate production and has also been known to cause a creatine-responsive myopathy. Thus, propofol and valproate probably should be avoided in patients with MD and SE *(31)*.

In SE associated with MDs specific therapy aimed at restoring the normal function of the respiratory apparatus should be instituted as soon as possible. Although the therapeutic efficacy of most agents is limited, the safety profile of the drugs is excellent, justifying a therapeutic trial in most cases. The majority of the agents used are not available in parenteral form, which may be an issue in the patient in SE in whom the oral route is not an option, and in whom ileus is often present *(5,11)*. Riboflavin, coenzyme Q, thiamine, vitamin E, ascorbic acid, ubiquinone, and dichloracetate have all been used with variable results *(6)*.

Leigh Disease

Leigh disease (LD) is a syndrome with several different clinical presentations and more than one possible etiologic mechanism. The disease is a progressive neurodegenerative disorder that typically starts in infancy or young adulthood but rarely may present during adulthood *(8)*.

Clinical Presentation

Clinical features include ophthalmoplegia, nystagmus, respiratory abnormalities, ataxia, hypotonia, tremor, seizures, spasticity, dementia, and developmental delay or regression. A slowly progressive course characterizes LD, but acute presentations and episodic exacerbations are not uncommon *(32)*. Occasionally, the LD phenotype maybe associated with the phenotype of other MDs such as MELAS or the syndrome of neurogenic muscular weakness, ataxia, and retinitis pigmentosa (NARP) *(3)*.

Neuroimaging

Leigh disease bears some resemblances but also some differences with Wernicke's encephalopathy; both produce necrotic lesions in the periaqueductal gray matter *(33)*. Focal, bilateral, symmetric necrotic areas in the thalamus and brainstem are the cardinal findings of LD. The mamillary bodies, often involved in Wernicke's encephalopathy are spared in LD. Involvement of the spinal cord is common in LD but not in Wernicke's encephalopathy. Hemorrhagic lesions occur in Wernicke's encephalopathy but not in LD.

Pathophysiology

Leigh syndrome comprises a heterogeneous group of MDs that affect the respiratory chain and lead to impaired ATP production. Multiple genetic defects have been identified including defects in the pyruvate dehydrogenase complex I, complex II, cytochrome c oxidase, and the ATPase component of the respiratory chain *(32)*. The cerebral gray matter with its unique metabolic rate is particularly susceptible to injury. Ultimately the defects lead to deficient ATP production and loss of function of the affected organs including the brain, liver, kidneys, and muscle *(32)*.

Diagnosis

The diagnosis of LD has traditionally been performed at autopsy. Recently, MRI has allowed for the diagnosis of LD to be done accurately pre-mortem. Hyperintense lesions on T2-weighted images involving the medulla oblongata extending down to the C1–C3 levels, the dorsal pons, the cerebral peduncles, substantia nigra, medial thalami, the putamen, and the deep white matter in the frontal and parietal lobes are characteristic *(34)*. Because subclinical involvement of the cervical spinal cord is common, neuroimaging studies in suspected cases of LD should include the spinal cord. In addition, proton magnetic resonance spectroscopy can aid in the diagnosis of LD by showing an elevated lactate peak in the brain *(34)*. Mitochondrial enzymology confirms the diagnosis and indicates the specific enzyme defect. Brainstem auditory evoked responses, somatosensory evoked responses, and blink responses may show evidence of intrinsic brainstem disease and help monitor the progression of the disease *(35)*.

Treatment

For the neurointensivist the most germane presentation of LD are encephalopathy (ranging from confusion to coma) and respiratory dysfunction due to myelopathy and/or brainstem involvement *(33)*. Decreased level of consciousness occurs secondary to involvement of the reticular activation formation in the brainstem and its more rostral projections to the diencephalon and other hemispheric centers mediating arousal and attention. It is usually associated with signs of brainstem and cerebellar dysfunction such as ophthalmoplegia, pupillary abnormalities, abnormal respirations, bilateral pyramidal signs, ataxia, and nystagmus. The symptoms may be triggered by an intercurrent infection or by excessive carbohydrate ingestion. Hypothermia may occur particularly in patients with lipoamide dehydrogenase deficiency *(34)*.

Management of the comatose patient is discussed in detail elsewhere in this text (*see* Chapter 16). Airway protection should be the first priority. In the mildly obtunded patient supplemental oxygen via a nasal cannula or a face mask with or without an oral airway may suffice. In more obtunded patients or patients with clinical and/or radiological evidence of brainstem and or cervical cord dysfunction, endotracheal or nasotracheal intubation may be needed. The presence of hypotension and quadraplegia suggests cervical cord involvement and should be treated with crystalloids or colloids and vasopressors. Thermal regulation abnormalities indicate diencephalic compromise. Hyperthermia should be treated with cooling blankets, fans, cold mist via the endotracheal tube, and cold intravenous or enteral fluids. Hyperlactatemia should be corrected if there is associated acidemia particularly if there is evidence of impaired cardiac contractibility or cardiac arrhythmias *(36)*. Intercurrent infections should be treated. The patient with quadraplegia due to myelopathy is at risk for deep venous thrombosis and subcutaneous heparin and pneumatic compression devices should be used. Both starvation and excessive caloric intake are potentially harmful and nutrition, ideally with an isocaloric, normoproteic diet should be instituted as soon as it is feasible. Thiamine supplementation should be instituted empirically as temporary benefit following administration of thiamine has been described *(37)*.

Respiratory dysfunction in the patient with LD can take several forms. The most severe form is complete aventilation associated with high cervical cord lesions. It requires prolonged mechanical ventilation and is almost invariably fatal. Bilateral vocal cord paralysis triggered by respiratory infection and presenting with stridor, inspiratory gasp, and hypoventilation has been described *(34)*. Intubation using a flexible laryngoscope and prolonged tracheostomy may be necessary. Other less ominous respiratory disorders seen in LD include ataxic respiration, Cheyne-Stokes respiration, and apneustic breathing *(34,38)*. Ataxic breathing is characterized by an erratic rate and depth of breathing, alternating with interspersed apnea episodes. It is indicative of a medullary lesion and is due to dysfunction of the dorsal respiratory neurons that control the rhythmicity of respiration. Unless it is impairing oxygenation and/or ventilation, ataxic breathing should be left untreated. Cheyne-Stokes respiration is characterized by a progressive increase and then a decrease in the depth of breathing with a subsequent brief period of apnea. In patients with LD it likely represents bilateral deep brain or brainstem injury. The prognosis of Cheyne-Stokes is not as ominous as previously thought. Last, patients may present with apneustic breathing characterized by sustained deep inspiration lasting a few seconds followed by a quick exhalation and a sustained postexpiratory pause. Apneustic breathing localizes to the inferior medial pontine region and carries an ominous prognosis. In the intubated patient withdrawing mechanical ventilation temporarily may allow identification of the respiratory pattern *(38)*.

Prognosis

Because the prognosis of LD is variable and some patients exhibit temporary improvement, the author suggests instituting supportive measures and following the patient clinically and with electrophysiology studies to determine progression or regression of the disease. Enzyme replacement, correction of any possible triggering factors, and cardiorespiratory support should be continued and the patient reassessed frequently. Based on the clinical and paraclinical findings (MRI and evoked responses), the clinician can establish a prognosis and aid the family in determining the level of care to be provided. A particularly ominous finding is a progressive increase in the interpeak latency of the brainstem somatosensory or auditory-evoked responses *(35)*.

REFERENCES

1. Clay AS, Behnia M, Brown KK. Mitochondrial disease. *Chest* 2001;120:634–648.
2. Graeber MB, Muller U. Recent developements in the molecular genetics of mitochondrial disorders. *J. Neurol. Sci.* 1998;153:251–263.
3. Hanna MG, Nelson IP. Genetics and molecular pathogenesis of mitochondrial respiratory chain diseases. *CMLS* 1999;55:691–706.
4. Flier JS, Underhill L. Mitochondrial DNA and disease. *N. Engl. J. Med.* 1995;333:638–644.
5. Johns JR. Mitochondrial DNA and disease. *N. Engl. J. Med.* 1995;333:638–644.

6. Leonard JV, Schapira AHV. Mitochondrial respiratory chain disorders I: Mitochondrial DNA defects. *Lancet* 2000;355:389–394.
7. Leonard JV, Schapira AHV. Mitochondrial respiratory chain disorders II: Mitochondrial DNA defects. *Lancet* 2000;355:389–394.
8. Schapira AHV. Mitochondrial disorders. *Curr. Opin. Neurol.* 2000;13:526–532.
9. Chinnery PF, Turnbull DM. Epidemiology and treatment of mitochondrial disorders. *Am. J. Med. Genet.* 2001;106:94–101.
10. Griggs RC, Karpati G. Muscle pain, fatigue, and mitochondriopathies. *N. Engl. J. Med.* 1999;341:1076–1078.
11. Howard RS, Russsell S, Losseff N, et al. Management of mitochondrial disease in the critical care unit. *QJM* 1995;88:197–207.
12. Dandurand R, Matthews PM, Arnold DL, Eidelman DH. Mitochondrial disease-pulmonary function, excercise performance, and blood lactate levels. *Chest* 1995;108:182–189.
13. Kimura S, Ohtuki N, Nezu A, Tanaka M, Takeshita S. Clinical and radiological improvements in mitochondrial encephalomyelopathy following sodium dichloroacetate therapy. *Brain Dev.* 1997;19:535–540.
14. Bargiela-Lemos A, Mosquera J, Mate A, Sirvent J. Myopathy with mitochondrial changes presenting as respiratory failure in two brothers. *Pediatr. Pulmonol.* 1999;27:213–217.
15. Barohn RJ, Clanton T, Sahenk Z, Mendell JR. Recurrent respiratory insufficiency and depressed ventilatory drive complicating mitochondrial myopathies. *Neurology* 1990;40:103–106.
16. Penniso-Besnier I, Reynier P, Asfar P, et al. Recurrent brain hematomas in MELAS associated with an ND5 gene mitochondrial mutation. *Neurology* 2000;55:317–318.
17. Molnar MJ, Valikovics A, Molnar S, et al. Cerebral blood flow and glucose metabolism in mitochondrial disorders. *Neurology* 2000;55:544–548.
18. Cros D, Palliyath S, DiMauro S, Ramirez C, Shamsia M, Wizer B. Respiratory failure revealing mitochondrial myopathy in adults. *Chest* 1992;101:824–828.
19. Borel CO, Guy J. Ventilatory management in critical neurologic illness. In: KG J (ed). *Neurologic Clinics.* Philadelphia: Saunders Company, 1995:627–644.
20. Cray SH, Robinson BH, Cox PN. Lactic acidemia and bradyarrhythmia in a child sedated with propofol. *Crit. Care Med.* 1998;26:2087–2092.
21. Guilleminault C, Phillip P, Robinson A. Sleep and neuromuscular disease: bilevel positive airway pressure by nasal mask as a treatment for sleep disordered breathing in patients with neuromuscular disease. *J. Neurol. Neurosurg. Psychiatry* 1998;65:225–232.
22. Pfeiffer G, Winkler G, Neunzig P, Wolf W, Thayssen G, Kunze K. Long-term management of acute respiratory failure in metabolic myopathy. *Intensive Care Med.* 1996;22:1406–1409.
23. Desnuelle C, Pellissier J, Serratrice G. Chronic progressive external ophtalmoplegia (CPEO) associated with diaphragmatic paralysis: succesful treatment with coenzyme Q (CoQ). *Neurology* 1988;38:102.
24. Tanahashi C, Nakayama A, Yoshida M, Ito M, Hashizume Y. MELAS with the mitochondrial DNA 3243 point mutation: a neuropathological study. *Acta. Neuropathol.* 2000;99:31–38.
25. Yoneda M, Maeda M, Kimura H, Fujii A, Katayama K, Kuriyama M. Vasogenic edema on MELAS: A serial study with diffusion-weighted MR imaging. *Neurology* 2001;53:2182–2184.
26. Adams HP, Brott TG, Furlan AJ, et al. Guidelines for thrombolytic therapy for acute stroke: A supplement to the guidelines for the management of patients with acute ischemic stroke. *Circulation* 1996;94:1167–1174.
27. Broderick JP, Adams HP, Barsan W, et al. Guidelines for the management of spontaneous intracerebral hemorrhage-A statement for healthcare professionals from a special Wwriting group of the stroke council, American Heart Association. *Stroke* 1999;30:905–915.
28. Canafoglia L, Franceschetti S, Antozzi C, et al. Epileptic phenotypes associated with mitochondrial disorders. *Neurology* 2001;56:1340–1346.
29. Lowenstein DH, Alldredge B. Status epilepticus. *N. Engl. J. Med.* 1998;338:970–976.
30. Prasad A, Worrall BB, Bertram EH, Bleck TP. Propofol and midazolam in the treatment of refractory status epilepticus. *Epilepsia* 2000;42:380–386.
31. Matsumoto J, Ogawa H, Maeyama R, et al. Successful treatment by direct hemoperfusion of coma possibly resulting from mitochondrial dysfunction in acute valproate intoxication. *Epilepsia* 1997;38:950–953.
32. Absalon MJ, Harding CO, Fain DR, Mack KJ. Leigh syndrome in an infant resulting from mitochondrial DNA depletion. *Pediatr. Neurol.* 2001;24:60–63.
33. Young GB, DeRubies DA. Metabolic encephalopathies. In: Young GB, Ropper AH, Bolton CF (eds). *Coma and Impaired Consciousness.* New York: McGraw-Hill, 1998:307–392.
34. Lin Y-C, Lee W-T, Wang P-J, Shen Y-Z. Vocal cord paralysis and hypoventilation in a patient with suspected Leigh disease. *Pediatr. Neurol.* 1999;20:223–225.
35. Araki S, Hayashi M, Yasaka A, Maruki K. Electrophysiologic brainstem dysfunction in a child with Leigh disease. *Pediatr. Neurol.* 1997;16:329–333.
36. Marino PL. The organic acidosis. In: Marino PL (ed). *The ICU Book,* 2nd ed. Baltimore: Williams & Wilkins, 1998:592–607.
37. Pincus JH, Itokawa Y, Cooper JR. Enzyme inhibiting factor in subacute necrotizing encephalomyelopathy. *Neurology* 1969;19:841–844.
38. North JB, Jennett S. Abnormal breathing patterns associated with acute brain damage. *Arch. Neurol.* 1974;31:338–342.

32

Neurocritical Care During Pregnancy and Puerperium

Panayiotis N. Varelas and Lotfi Hacein-Bey

INTRODUCTION

The obstetric practice occasionally mandates for admission of unstable patients to an critical care unit. The reasons that such a patient becomes critical can be linked either directly to the physiologic changes that occur during pregnancy and the puerperium or can be independent and coincident. Because of its complexity and importance for the functional outcome of the mother, the nervous system, if affected, requires specialized management that in the past had been offered by the consulting neurology or neurosurgery service. In many cases, a team that includes neuro-intensivists and obstetricians in the neurosciences critical care unit (NSU) may better deliver the specialized care. This new concept, although an attractive idea, is not supported yet by outcome data. This chapter encompasses all these clinical situations for which, as we suggest, NSU admission may be a reasonable alternative to the obstetrical or general critical care units.

PRE-ECLAMPSIA AND ECLAMPSIA

Pre-eclampsia (PREC)–eclampsia (EC) complex is one of the most common causes of maternal and fetal morbidity and mortality and a common ground of concern and debate for both obstetricians and neurologists.

PREC is defined as the constellation of newly diagnosed hypertension (relative increase of $\geq$ 15 mm Hg diastolic or $\geq$ 30 mmHg systolic or absolute $\geq$ 140/90 mmHg) after 20 wk gestation and either proteinuria (> 300 mg/24 h or $\geq$ 1+ in dipstick testing) or generalized edema (particularly in nondependant areas like hands and face) or both. Severe PREC is characterized by blood pressure > 160/110 mmHg, proteinuria 2 or 3 +, serum creatinine > 1.2 mg/dL, oliguria < 500 mL/24 h, headache with or without visual symptoms, epigastric pain, pulmonary edema, thrombocytopenia < 100,000/μL or increased aspartate or alanine transaminases. EC is defined as seizures occurring before, during, or after delivery. Although EC is usually preceded by PREC, in up to 38% of cases it can occur without symptoms or signs of the latter *(1)*.

Epidemiology and Pathophysiology

In the developed world the incidence for PREC is 6–8% of pregnancies and for EC 1:2000 deliveries, although in the developing countries the numbers are much higher. EC confers a 1.8% maternal mortality and a 35% complication rate and in the United States ranks only second to embolic events as cause of maternal mortality *(2)*. PREC and its sequelae account for 20–50% of obstetrical admissions in the NSU *(3)*. Risk factors include poor nutrition, nulliparity, diabetes, multiple gestation, extremes of maternal age (< 18 or > 35 yr), pre-existing hypertension, history of EC, family history, hydatidiform mole and hydrops fetalis *(4)*.

From: *Current Clinical Neurology*
Critical Care Neurology and Neurosurgery
Edited by: J. I. Suarez © Humana Press Inc., Totowa, NJ

The cause of PREC-EC is unknown. Pathophysiologic changes in the placental circulation, such as alteration of the ratio of prostacyclin/thromboxane, platelet activation/aggregation and endothelial damage with fibrin deposition, lead to placental ischemia, diffuse maternal vasospasm and microangiopathy with increased capillary permeability and tissue edema. The cerebral pathology includes capillary damage with disruption of the tight junctions and extravasation of fluids into the perivascular spaces, with resultant white matter edema and cortical micro or macro-hemorrhages. Owing to fibrin deposition and vasospasm, areas of infarction are not uncommon, usually seen in the parieto-occipital watershed zones *(4,5)*.

Clinical Presentation

Seizures are the hallmark of EC. They usually occur before childbirth or during labor, but in some women they occur as late as 10–23 d postpartum *(2,6)*. After the first 48 h postpartum, however, one should look for another cause because only 3% of women experience late seizures from EC *(7)*. Seizures are usually generalized tonic-clonic, but occasionally may have a focal onset, frequently over the face and in 10–49% of patients are multiple. Their onset does not correlate with the severity of PREC and in up to 20% of cases seizures occur without one component of the PREC triad *(8)*.

Headache, visual hallucinations, confusion, or coma are other symptoms associated with EC. Coma carries a poor prognosis and is thought to be due to intracerebral hemorrhage or severe generalized cerebral edema. Retinal artery vasospasm or retinal detachment occurs less frequently than transient cortical blindness (in 2.3% of eclamptic women). This can persist for up to 8 d and usually resolves completely *(4,9)*.

Radiographic Features

In most of EC cases the computerized tomography (CT) of the head is normal *(10)*, but in some it may reveal focal lesions, such as cerebral edema, subarachnoid or intraparenchymal hemorrhage or, in patients with cortical blindness, occipital symmetric hypodensities. The magnetic resonance imaging (MRI) may show reversible hypodensities in the basal ganglia, cerebral edema, border zone ischemia or the more characteristically multifocal curvilinear changes in the gray-white matter junctions of the parieto-occipital areas *(5)*. The underlying pathophysiology, explaining the similarity of these reversible lesions with those seen in hypertensive encephalopathy and posterior leukoencephalopathy syndrome, is unknown *(10,11)*.

Management

Evaluation of disease severity and of maternal and fetal complications is the initial steps in making the decision about admitting in the NSU and managing the patient with PREC. Patients should be admitted early, because the course of the disease is quite unpredictable and can progress rapidly. The management of patients with EC includes treatment of seizures and prevention of their recurrence, control of hypertension, timely delivery of the infant and avoidance of further complications. There is still debate about the first-line drug for treatment of seizures. Magnesium sulfate (Mg^{2+}) is the oldest medication used, but one can argue that since seizures are associated with hypertensive encephalopathy and decreased cerebral perfusion, antiepileptics and antihypertensives should also been used *(5)*.

Mg^{2+} has a short-lived antihypertensive effect, but increases cerebral blood flow through vasodilatory action from elevated prostacyclin production *(12)*. It also blocks the Ca^{2+} influx through the NMDA glutamate receptors, both pre- and postsynaptically, thus reducing neuronal excitability *(5,13)*. Two large studies showed superior Mg^{2+} effectiveness in preventing and treating seizures in pregnant women. In the Eclampsia Trial Collaborative Group, an international multicenter randomized study, Mg^{2+} was compared in one arm to diazepam and in the other to phenytoin in 1687 women with eclampsia. Mg^{2+} was shown to covey a 52% lower risk for recurrent seizures compared to diazepam and a 67% lower risk compared to phenytoin. Maternal and infant mortality did not differ.

Mg^{2+} was also superior to phenytoin in the need for ventilation, ICU admission and developing pneumonia *(14)*. Another randomized study compared Mg^{2+} to phenytoin for seizure prevention in 2138 patients with pregnancy-induced hypertension. Ten of 1089 patients assigned to phenytoin developed seizures versus 0/1049 assigned to Mg^{2+}, a significant difference. Only 19% of patients, however, met PREC criteria and all patients in the phenytoin arm that seized had low therapeutic levels of the drug *(15)*.

Although several Mg^{2+} treatment protocols exist, the one most used in eclampsia is 4–6 g IV bolus over 5 min, followed by 1–2 g/h IV infusion for at least 48 h postpartum. If the treatment is used prophylactically in PREC, it can be stopped after 24 h *(16)*. Half this dose should be used in patients with serum creatinine more than 1.3 mg/dL *(4)*. Careful monitoring of potential Mg^{2+} toxicity should be done preferentially in an NSU setting. Loss of patellar reflexes, increasing drowsiness and dysarthria, muscle weakness and respiratory depression, all should prompt for Mg^{2+} concentration measurement and discontinuation of the infusion. Calcium gluconate (1 g IV in 10% solution) should be given as an antidote in case of impending respiratory arrest. If seizures recur after Mg^{2+} is given, either an extra 1–2 g IV *(15)* or a loading dose of phenytoin (18 mg/kg IV at a maximum rate 50 mg/min) can be tried. A dark room with low noise, padded bed rails and continuous fetal monitoring are other important measures required.

Blood Pressure Control

The aim of blood pressure (BP) control is to bring it at a level < 170/110 and > 130/90. One should take into account the physiologic changes during pregnancy. Cardiac output normally increases by 30–50% by 25–32 wk gestation. Systolic blood pressure falls less than the diastolic (10–20% drop by 28 wk), resulting in widening of pulse pressure. During the third trimester, the blood pressure slowly increases without reaching prepregnancy values. Systemic vascular resistance and pulmonary vascular resistance are decreased by 20–30%, but the CVP and PAWP remain unchanged *(17)*. In EC patients, invasive BP monitoring is indicated, because of potentially large fluctuations with treatment. Hydralazine has been successfully used in patients with EC as a 5–10 mg IV dose, that can be repeated every 20–30 min. If there is a response, the dose can be repeated every 6 h, because the onset of action is within 10 min and the duration for 6–8 h. Labetalol is gaining popularity, because of more rapid onset of action and less reflex tachycardia than hydralazine. It can be given as a 10 mg IV dose that can be repeated or doubled in 10–15 min. Nifedipine is an acceptable oral agent that can be administered as a 10-mg sublingual dose. It can be repeated in 30 min and then given orally every 4–6 h *(18)*. Sublingual nifedipine and concomitant use of Mg^{2+} should be avoided due to the possibility of profound hypotension. The dose of the antihypertensive medications is lowered after delivery and in most cases the drugs can be stopped within the first 6 wk postpartum. If there is a need for longer treatment, a complete evaluation of other causes of hypertension should be done *(16)*. Ketanserin, a selective serotonin-2 receptor blocker lowers blood pressure and inhibits platelet aggregation in hypertensive patients. A randomized, controlled trial showed benefit in the prevention of PREC, when high risk women were taking the drug *(19)*. In another multicenter study, ketanserin showed similar efficacy to dihydralazine in reducing the blood pressure in PREC patients. Ketanserin may have fewer side effects than hydralazine, cause a more gradual reduction in blood pressure and avoid any significant change in cardiac output *(20)*.

Intravascular Volume

Volume status of the EC patient should be carefully assessed. These patients are at higher risk for development of pulmonary edema. This complication occurs in up to 70% of PREC patients in the early postpartum period after excessive fluid administration *(21)*. Use of invasive monitoring should be individualized. Central venous pressure (CVP) should be kept < 5 mmHg *(16)*. CVP can be misleading, if used as the sole monitoring parameter. In a study of 18 patients with severe pregnancy-induced hypertension, CVP was unable to predict pulmonary artery wedge pressure (PAWP) *(22)*. In one study of 49 women with pulmonary artery catheterization, it was shown that severe PREC is a high cardiac output state associated with an inappropriately high peripheral resistance *(23)*. Eight of ten patients with severe PREC developed pulmonary edema in the postpartum period in another study. Five patients had elevated PAWP in addition to decreased plasma colloid osmotic pressure (COP), three patients had pulmonary capillary leak syndrome and two evidence of left ventricular failure *(24)*. Correlation of COP with PAWP gradient has been reported in critically ill patients and patients with PREC who developed pulmonary edema *(22,25)*. Albumin infusion in an effort to correct low COP in PREC patients, however, did not improve outcome *(26)*. Clark suggested that pulmonary artery catheterization is indicated in patients unresponsive to vasodilator therapy and those who frequently have high cardiac output and may need β-blockers or venodilators. Other indications are pulmonary edema with persistent hypoxemia unresponsive to diuresis and oliguria (< 100 mL over 4 h) not responding to fluid challenge *(27)*.

Intracranial Dynamics

Cerebral edema and elevated intracranial pressure management are not different from non-pregnant women (*see also* Chapter 5). Adequate oxygenation, hyperventilation, mannitol infusion, loop diuretics and correction of hyponatremia are general measures that can be taken, although their role in EC has not been tested in controlled studies *(10,17)*. The same is true for pyridoxal phosphate that promotes GABAergic synaptic activity, given as a 100 mg IV injection. In one study, pyridoxal normalized the electroencephalographic (EEG) abnormalities seen in EC *(28)*. Mannitol use during pregnancy should be judicious. It crosses the placenta and in animal studies has been shown to increase the risk for fetal dehydration, contraction of the blood volume, cyanosis, loss of amniotic fluid and bradycardia. Use of the drug in pregnant women has also been reported without ill effects, although it remains a FDA category C medication. The same is true for loop diuretics, like furosemide. In serious or life-threatening situations during pregnancy, both drugs can be used *(29)*. We suggest that mannitol be used in 0.25–0.5 g/kg of prepregnancy maternal weight every 4–6 h IV in such cases.

Termination of Pregnancy

Obstetricians decide the time of delivery. The patient should be hemodynamically stable and seizure free. The risk of prematurity should weight against the risks for intrauterine growth restriction for the fetus and continuation of the eclamptic process for the mother. If the blood pressure is controlled, pregnancy can be extended by an average of 2 wk *(30)*. Maternal and fetal guidelines for expedited delivery or conservative management of severe PREC remote from term have been previously published *(18)*. If the delivery is done before 32 wk, steroids are given to promote fetal lung maturity and in most centers elective caesarian section is advised. After 34 wk, vaginal delivery is the preferred method *(16)*.

HELLP SYNDROME

The HELLP syndrome is a laboratory-defined severe form of PREC, although up to 15% of patients may not have hypertension or proteinuria. The acronym stands for hemolysis (anemia, increased bilirubin, and schistocytes in blood smear), elevated liver enzymes and low platelets (< 100,000/ mm^3). It is associated with poor maternal (0–24%) and perinatal (8–60%) mortality due to multisystem involvement *(31)*. The incidence has been reported in 4–12% of severe PREC patients, with higher risk in white, older patients. In a retrospective analysis of 481 patients with HELLP syndrome the risk of recurrence in a subsequent pregnancy was 19–27% *(32)*.

Pathophysiology and Clinical Features

Fibrin capillary deposition, organ hypoperfusion, microangiopathic hemolysis and consumptive thrombocytopenia are the pathophysiologic mechanisms. The role of disseminated intravascular coagulopathy is controversial, although some patients have more widespread coagulation abnormality than simply thrombocytopenia. Clinically, it presents as severe PREC with nausea, vomiting and right upper quadrant pain. Hepatic hypoperfusion may lead to periportal and focal parenchymal necrosis that if complicated by subcapsular hemorrhage can progress to hepatic rupture. Patients with such clinical presentation should be evaluated by ultrasound of upper abdomen. Other complications include acute renal failure, adult respiratory distress syndrome, hypoglycemia, hyponatremia, diabetes insipidus and organ hemorrhage. The differential includes other microangiopathies with multisystem organ involvement. Fever is more common in thrombotic thrombocytopenic purpura (TTP) and low antithrombin III activity in PREC *(33,34)*.

Management

The treatment is similar to PREC, with prophylactic Mg^{2+} sulfate infusion and early delivery, as well as platelet and FFP transfusion. Plasma exchange with FFP has been successfully used if thrombocytopenia, hemolysis and organ dysfunction persist for more than 72 h postpartum *(35,36)*, although it is uncertain if the response to this treatment refers to HELLP or overlapping conditions such as TTP or hemolytic-uremic syndrome.

In a prospective, randomized study of 25 pregnant women with HELLP at 24–37 wk gestation, IV dexamethasone was administered as 10 mg every 12 h until delivery. In the treatment arm, the maternal platelets and urinary output increased significantly, the lactic dehydrogenase and alanine aminotransferase decreased over time and the entry-to-delivery interval was longer *(37)*. In another prospective randomized study of 40 patients with HELLP, IV dexamethazone was administered in 4 doses every 12 h (10 mg, 10 mg, 5 mg, and 5 mg). The treatment group had significantly lower mean arterial pressure at 22 h, increased urine output by 16 h, increased platelets by 24 h and decreased lactic dehydrogenase and aspartate aminotransferase by 36 h *(38)*. Although the number of patients enrolled in these studies is small, steroids seem to stabilize and improve the laboratory values and clinical status of the mother antepartum, reduce the need for transfusions, prolong the gestational age for delivery, with potential beneficial effect in fetal morbidity and mortality and hasten postpartum maternal recovery. Hepatic rupture needs immediate recognition, hemodynamic and blood product support, urgent delivery and surgical or interventional control of the bleeding point through hepatic artery branch ligation or embolization.

MYASTHENIA GRAVIS

Myasthenia gravis (MG) is a autoimmune disorder of the neuromuscular junction. Antibodies against the acetylcholine receptor (AchR) in the postsynaptic membrane of skeletal muscles are detected in up to 85% of MG patients (*see also* Chapter 26). They block the binding of the synaptically released acetylcholine and decrease the number of available receptors, reducing the safety factor for neuromuscular transmission. MG commonly affects women in the third decade of life who are in childbearing age *(39)*.

Clinical Course

Both MG and pregnancy interfere with each other. The course of MG during pregnancy is at best unpredictable. Although older series pertained that 41% of MG patients worsen during pregnancy, with only 29% improving and 32% remaining stable *(40)*, more recent studies give more promising outcomes, with only 19% of patients experiencing clinical worsening and the majority remaining stable or improving (59% and 22%, respectively) *(41)*. No correlation has been reported between the severity of MG before pregnancy and the risk for exacerbation during gestation. The first trimester and the puerperium are periods of MG exacerbation. The course in one pregnancy, however, does not predict the course in subsequent pregnancies *(41)*.

Conversely, MG may affect the course of pregnancy and the outcome of the fetus. Maternal antibodies crossing the placenta, block the function of the fetal nicotinic AchR isoform, leading to arthogryposis multiplex congenital *(42)* or more commonly to transient neonatal MG (NMG). Increased prevalence of premature labor in MG patients or the presence of congenital anomalies in their newborns, has not been confirmed *(41)*.

Management

The overall management of MG patients should not change during pregnancy (*see also* Chapter 26). An adjustment in medication dosage or schedule is occasionally necessary, because of increased glomerular filtration rate and excretion and a 40% increase in volume of distribution, especially in the last trimester. Acetylcholinesterase inhibitors, such as neostigmine 15–30 mg orally every 4–6 h and pyridostigmine 30–60 mg orally four to five times/d remain the mainstay of treatment. Breastfeeding should be avoided, because these drugs are excreted in milk *(43)*. Corticosteroids should be continued, if they were started before conception *(43)*. There is only a slight increased risk for cleft lip and palate, if taken during the first trimester *(44)* and at high dose an increased risk of premature rupture of membranes and infectious complications *(41)*. Prednisone, 40–80 mg orally daily, is usually recommended. The safety of other immunosuppressive drugs during pregnancy is unclear. Azathioprine crosses the placenta and there is evidence of teratogenicity in animals. In humans, at therapeutic doses (1–2.5 mg/kg/d orally), the drug has never been shown to contribute to higher abortion, prematurity, or malformation rate *(41)*. Cyclosporin A, carries a higher risk for spontaneous abortion, prematurity and small-for-dates *(45)*. It should be given only in intractable cases *(41)*. Methotrexate, on the other hand, should be avoided during pregnancy due to high risk for fetal abnormalities *(46)*. Thymectomy during pregnancy has beneficial results *(47)*, but the remission may take years to be evident *(48,49)*. Plasmapheresis (PLA) and intravenous immunoglobulins (IVIG) are effective treatments in MG crisis *(50,51)* and can be used in pregnancy, either alone or sequentially *(41)*. PLA may carry a risk for premature labor due to large hormonal shifts. It has been also successfully used in conjunction with steroids in a myasthenic patient who had two previous neonatal deaths due to multiple malformations. As the AchR antibodies fell, there were apparent fetal breathing movements. The infant had transient neonatal myasthenia, but no malformations *(52)*. There are no large series of IVIG use in pregnant myasthenics and for neonatal MG the results are conflicting. Mycophenolate mofetil has been used as a steroid sparing agent in non-pregnant myasthenic patients *(53)*. Although there is no experience with the agent in pregnant myasthenic patients, it has been used in a pregnant patient with kidney transplantation, in addition to steroids and tacrolimus. The child born had hypoplastic nails and short fifth fingers, but otherwise developed normally *(54)*. Myasthenic crisis is usually due to severe dysphagia and aspiration and in the NSU to neuromuscular junction blocking medications. The initial clinical manifestations of respiratory failure are subtle and can be missed if arterial gases and pulmonary function tests are not done. A compensated respiratory alkalosis ($PaCO_2$ 28–32 mmHg, HCO_3 18–21 mEq/L) and mild hypoxemia during supine position are normally seen during pregnancy. Increased tidal volume and minute ventilation (20–40% above baseline at term) and decreased functional residual capacity (10–25% at term) may decompensate the respiratory status of the myasthenic patient *(17)*. $PaO_2 < 60$ and $PaCO_2$ 45–50 mmHg, vital capacity less than 15 mL/kg and negative inspiratory force (NIF) < -25 cm H_2O are indications for elective intubation and positive pressure ventilation. Positive end-expiratory pressure of 5–10 mmHg is used in an effort to inflate the atelectatic regions and improve the shunting of blood. Due to decreased pulmonary compliance, plateau airway pressures more than 35 cm H_2O can be accepted without alveolar overdistension. Tracheostomy is performed if the patient requires naso- or orotracheal intubation for more than 2 wk, but by that time over 50% of myasthenics will be extubated *(55)*.

Fetal assessment tests, such as non-stress tests, fetal breathing or maternal perception of fetal movement can be unreliable in MG patients, because fetal movements may be affected. Five cases of MG and pre-eclampsia have been reported and pose therapeutic dilemmas. High dose steroids contribute to fluid retention and pulmonary congestion in PREC and Mg^{2+} is contraindicated in myasthenics, because of increasing neuromuscular blockade *(56)*. MG does not affect the smooth uterine muscles, but the striated muscles of the pelvic floor are involved and may fatigue during the expulsive efforts of the second stage of labor. Outlet forceps or vacuum extraction should be used in that case. Fatigue and relaxation of the muscles have been reported to contribute to pain-free, shortened labor, but also to increase postpartum hemorrhage. Careful monitoring of the respiratory function during labor for signs of fatigue and hypoventilation, as well as parenteral administration of medications, due to errant intestinal absorption, is also recommended *(39)*.

GUILLAIN-BARRÉ SYNDROME

Guillain-Barrésyndrome (GBS) is an uncommon autoimmune neurologic entity and the most common cause of acute neuromuscular generalized paralysis. The diagnosis is made when there is progressive areflexive weakness (usually starting in the lower extremities and preceded in 50% of patients by back pain or leg paresthesias), that extends proximally and reaches its nadir within 4 wk. Elevated protein without cells in the cerebrospinal fluid (after the first week), prolonged distal latencies and F-waves, and anti-ganglioside antibodies strengthen the diagnosis *(57,58)* (*see also* Chapter 27).

Epidemiology

Lower risk for GBS during pregnancy has been reported in a Swedish population (relative risk 0.86, 95% CI 0.4–1.84), but increased risk was found during 30 and 90 d postpartum (RR [95%CI], 2.21 [0.55–8.94] and 1.47 [0.54–3.99], respectively), suggestive of a putative hormonal role *(59)*. The increase of anti-inflammatory Th2 cytokines, that promote humoral immunity during pregnancy and the elevation of pro-inflammatory Th1 cytokines in the puerperium, may explain the different risk during these periods *(60)*. Fetal survival is close to 96%, but premature delivery is not uncommon in severe GBS cases. Unlike MG, there is no GBS involvement of the fetus or neonate, except for one reported case *(61)*. When the onset is on the third trimester, there is higher risk for respiratory failure that can contribute to higher maternal mortality. Ventilatory support has been reported in 35% of patients and mortality in up to 13% *(58,62)*. All these patients died after delivery and represented cases before 1971. Unlike PREC, premature delivery does not alter the course of the disease.

Management

The management of GBS in pregnancy should be done in a NSU and is similar to that in nonpregnant patients as discussed elsewhere in this book (*see also* Chapter 27). It is mainly supportive care until the patient regains her strength with the addition of treatments that may change the natural course of the disease. These include PLA or IVIG, but, interestingly, pregnancy was an exclusion criterion for enrollment in the largest randomized studies *(63,64)*. In case reports, GBS in pregnancy has been successfully treated with either IVIG alone within 2 wk from the onset of symptoms (0.4 g/kg/d for 5 d) *(65)* or with PLA alone (200–250 mL/kg over four to six sessions, up to 402 mL/kg over 4 wk) *(66)* or with a combination of IVIG-PLA *(61,67,68)*. If both are used, PLA should precede IVIG *(65)*. IVIG has also been used to treat the only reported newborn with congenital GBS born to a mother with GBS *(61)*.

Close monitoring of the respiratory function with assessment of FVC and the ability to cough and protect the airway is highly recommended in GBS patients. Even a small change in O_2 partial pressure may result in a large change in fetal oxygen saturation (because of a marked left shift on the fetal oxygen dissociation curve and the fact that the fetus is operating on the steep portion of the curve) and should be avoided *(17)*. The signs of respiratory failure are more insidious than in MG, because patients with autonomic dysfunction of the vagus nerve may lack the psychological feeling of breathlessness. If FVC is < 1.5 L, patient should be admitted in the NSU and if less than 15 mL/kg intubated and mechanically ventilated. Due to upper airway mucosal hyperemia during pregnancy, extra care should be taken when nasogastric or nasotracheal tubes are inserted due to higher risk for epistaxis and a smaller endotracheal tube should be available. Another reason for NSU admission is dysautonomia. The incidence in pregnancy is unknown. A temporary cardiac pacer is indicated in case of bradyarrythmias (usually after vagal stimulation following tracheal suction). Aortocaval compression from the growing uterus and hyperventilation that may compromise the placental perfusion should be avoided by using the left lateral decubitus position. During the third trimester up to 30% of pregnant women exhibit a significant systolic blood pressure drop just by laying supine. Patients with GBS dysautonomia may experience even more dramatic pressure fluctuations. The growing uterus also exacerbates gastrointestinal stasis and ileus, thus stool softeners are highly recommended. Fetal monitoring should be carried out as indicated and normal fetal activity is seen even during the periods of maximal maternal paralysis. GBS does not have an impact on uterine contraction or cervical dilatation and vaginal delivery with vacuum extraction is preferred, if the patient has inability to bear down.

Deep venous thrombosis (DVT) occurs in 0.11–0.36% of pregnancies and is up to 20 times higher during the first month postpartum compared to nonpregnant women, when the risk for pulmonary embolus (PE) is also the greatest *(69–71)*. The risk of DVT and PE in GBS patients was estimated between 2 and 13% *(72,73)*. There is no reported estimate when GBS and pregnancy coexist, but one may infer that it will be even higher. Thus, pregnant patients with GBS should be treated for potential thromboembolic disease, although the optimal treatment and duration are unclear. The treatment of DVT or PE during pregnancy is done initially with IV heparin for few days (PTT goal 1.5–2 times that of control) and then, either with warfarin with an INR goal 2–3 or SC unfractionated heparin or low-molecular-weight heparins (LMWH). The treatment continues until 36 wk (or ends when the patient becomes ambulatory), then IV heparin is used until 24 h before labor and restarted 12 h postdelivery. The risk for heparin-induced thrombocytopenia may be smaller in pregnancy *(74)*. Increased levels of factor VIII in pregnancy may lead to "heparin resistance" when the effect is monitored with PTT. For this reason the use of heparin assay (anti-Xa) with goal 0.3–0.4 U/mL has been recommended when the amount of heparin needed to reach a PTT 1.5 times control is > 18 U/kg/h *(75)*. LMWH, like heparin, do not cross the placenta and have gained popularity, but their safety and efficacy have not yet been adequately assessed in pregnancy *(76)*.

STROKE

The incidence of stroke in young women is higher than in men and this may be due to pregnancy. It carries significant morbidity and was the fifth cause of maternal death during 1980–1985 *(77)*. Specific pregnancy-related causes of stroke include eclampsia, choriocarcinoma, amniotic fluid embolism and postpartum angiopathy (Table 1). The diagnostic work-up of stroke in pregnancy is similar to that in nonpregnant women with the exception of radiological procedures. Abdominal shielding during CT and digital angiography in the embryogenetic period (first trimester; especially the first month) limits the amount of radiation given to an acceptable 2 mRads *(78)*.

Ischemic Stroke

Most of the strokes in pregnancy are attributed to arterial occlusion *(77)*. The incidence of ischemic stroke is estimated at 3.5/100,000/yr *(79)* or 4.3–26/100,000 deliveries *(77,80)*. Although pregnancy may increase the likelihood of cerebral infarction 13 times *(79)*, the relative risk is 0.7 during pregnancy and 8.7 during the puerperium, suggesting an increased risk only during the first 6 wk after delivery *(81)*.

Although the frequency of the various causes of ischemic stroke is not known *(see* Table 1), it is widely believed that the most common is eclampsia, accounting for 47% of cases *(80)*. In most cases, the focal neurologic deficits in eclampsia reverse within a few days, a fact arguing against a true cerebral ischemic necrosis and favoring cerebral edema from loss of autoregulation and low perfusion from severe vasospasm. Choriocarcinoma, a trophoblastic tumor associated with molar pregnancy, metastasizes in 20% of cases to the brain. The malignant cells invade the cerebral vessels,

Table 1
Causes of Stroke During Pregnancy

1. Ischemic
Watershed
    Severe hypotension, Sheehan's syndrome
Eclampsia
Choriocarcinoma
Angiopathies
    Infectious: syphilis, borreliosis, tuberculosis, malaria, chlamydia pneumoniae, herpes zoster, mycoses
    Inflammatory: collagen disorders, granulomatous angiitis of nervous system, sarcoidosis, Takayasu's
    Noninflammatory: dissection, postpartum cerebral angiopathy, Moya-Moya, fibromuscular dysplasia,
        atherosclerosis, subarachnoid hemorrhage, vascular malformation
Hematologic diseases
    Protein C, S, antithrombin III deficiency, factor V Leiden, homocystinuria, paraneoplastic
        coagulopathy, disseminated intravascular coagulation, thrombotic thrombocytopenic purpura, sickle
        cell disease, antiphospholipid antibodies, Sneddon's syndrome
Cardiac or pulmonary disorders
    Infective or marantic endocarditis, atrial myxoma, fibroelastoma, rheumatic heart disease, mitral
        valve prolapse, prosthetic valve, patent foramen ovale, amniotic fluid/ fat/air embolism, atrial septal
        aneurysm, atrial fibrillation, acute myocardial infarct, dilated cardiomyopathy, peripartum cardi
        omyopathy, hereditary hemorrhagic telengiectasia
Metabolic or channel dysfunction
    CADASIL, migraine
Air, fat, amniotic fluid embolism
2. Intracerebral hemorrhage
    Eclampsia, hypertension, cerebral venous and sinus thrombosis (*see* below), angiopathies (*see* above),
        choriocarcinoma, AVM, aneurysm, bacterial endocarditis, pituitary apoplexy, anticoagulation,
        cocaine abuse
3. Subarachnoid hemorrhage
    Aneurysm, AVM, eclampsia, angiopathies (*see* above), choriocarcinoma, cerebral venous and sinus
        thrombosis (*see* below), bacterial endocarditis, pituitary apoplexy, anticoagulation, cocaine abuse
4. Cerebral venous and sinus thrombosis
    Hematologic diseases (*see* above), volume depletion, brain, sinus or mastoid infection, eclampsia

Adapted from refs. *29, 78, 130, 131.*

resulting either in local thrombosis and/or distal embolization or pseudoaneurysm formation and intracranial bleeding. Amniotic fluid embolism is a rare complication of labor in multiparous women, presenting with respiratory failure or cardiogenic shock and leading to DIC. The neurological symptoms consist mainly of encephalopathy or seizures in 10–20% of cases. Paradoxical cerebral embolism can also occur, the incidence of which is unknown. It can be diagnosed on cytological examination of pulmonary artery catheter samples *(78,80)*. Postpartum cerebral angiopathy presents with severe headache, nausea, focal deficits and seizures in patients with or without hypertension few hours to a month after delivery. Multiple areas of segmental vessel narrowing thought to represent vasospasm than true inflammation are seen angiographically and improve within few days or weeks. Vasospastic drug administration, (especially ergot alkaloids), labile hypertension and pre-existing benign angiitis of the CNS are discovered but in many cases, no cause is found. The course is usually benign and nonrelapsing, although some cases lead to intracranial hemorrhage. Uncontrolled studies have reported good outcomes with a short course of high dose steroids *(82)*. Other causes of cardioembolic stroke include rheumatic heart disease recurrence associated with pregnancy (antibiotic prophylaxis is given before delivery) and peripartum cardiomyopathy, a rare dilating cardiomyopathy within the last month of pregnancy or 5-mo postpartum, leading to stroke in 5% of cases. Anticoagulation is recommended. Another reason for anticoagulation is cervical artery dissection, reported in 6–7% of cases of pregnancy-related stroke. Straining during delivery and hormonally mediated changes in the arterial wall are the implicated pathophysiologic mechanisms *(80,81)* (Fig. 1). Antiphospholipid antibodies syndrome can lead to spontaneous abortions, but transient ischemic attacks or true infarcts also occur during pregnancy or the puerperium, the incidence of which is not known. In a prospective, controlled study of women with antiphospholipid antibodies, no ischemic stroke was reported during pregnancy, but the presence of antibodies was a risk factor for adverse pregnancy outcome *(83)*. Low-dose heparin combined with aspirin in women with at least two fetal losses is recommended during pregnancy *(78)*.

The management of ischemic stroke during pregnancy rarely requires admission in the NSU. This is reserved for large strokes, with potentially increased ICP and need for respiratory or hemodynamic support. Although fibrinolysis has been considered a relative contraindication during pregnancy, it has been successfully used in cases of PE or cardiac valve thrombus *(84,85)*. Use of aspirin during the first trimester is controversial. There is a risk for fetal and maternal hemorrhage, premature closure of the ductus arteriosus, delay of the onset and prolongation of labor with its use in the third trimester. Low-dose aspirin (60–150 mg/d) during the second to third trimester; however, has been safely used in the CLASP trial *(78,86)*.

Reported maternal mortality after ischemic stroke is 0–25% and one third of patients have modified Rankin disability score less than 3. The risk for recurrence in subsequent pregnancies is estimated 2.3% within 5 yr and is higher during the postpartum period *(87)*. The decision to become again pregnant after a pregnancy-related stroke depends on the etiology and residual deficits that the patient has *(78,80)*.

Hemorrhagic Stroke

The incidence of SAH during pregnancy is estimated at 20/100,000 deliveries and that of ICH at 4.6/100,000 deliveries. This puts pregnant patients at higher risk for both *(80,81)*. The puerperium is the period when the risk for ICH is highest (RR 2.5 during pregnancy and 28.3 during the puerperium *(81)*.

The most common nontraumatic causes of SAH in pregnancy are aneurysms and arteriovenous malformations (AVM), in roughly equal proportions *(see* Table 1). In a retrospective study with 118 patients, 90% of aneurysmal bleeding occurred during pregnancy, 2% during labor, and 8% during postpartum, putting into question the older notion of frequent rupture during the strains of labor *(88)*. Advancing gestational age, hemodynamic and endocrine changes of pregnancy increase the risk of bleeding *(88–90)*. Causes of ICH during pregnancy included EC (44%), AVM, aneurysm and cavernous angioma (12.5% each) or were undetermined (19%) in a large retrospective study *(80)* *(see* Table 1). It is not clear whether pregnancy increases the risk of bleeding from an AVM. In a retrospective study of 451 women with AVMs, there was no increased rate of bleeding during pregnancy, with even distribution during gestation and the puerperium *(91)*. Another study, however, found 6% of AVM-related ICH occurring during labor and 94% during pregnancy *(88)*.

The treatment of SAH or ICH is not different during pregnancy *(see also* Chapters 19 and 20). Before and after securing the aneurysm the patients should stay in the NSU. Clipping of the aneurysm can be achieved in any stage of pregnancy and is associated with lower maternal and fetal mortality *(78,88)*. Successful endovascular treatment with GDCs has been recently reported in three patients during the third trimester *(92)*. Vasospasm can be treated with hypervolemia using crystalloids or colloids *(93)*. There are no data, however, supporting tripple H therapy in the pregnant population. Physiologic hemodilution normally occurs during pregnancy and pressors should be used with caution, since they diminish uteroplacental blood flow. Nimodipine has been safely used during pregnancy, but probably should be avoided due to teratogenic potential in animals *(93,94)*. There are no reported cases of balloon angioplasty for severe vasospasm. Delivery is preferred after the aneurysm is secured or before, if there are obstetrical indications. Cesarian section does not seem to add any

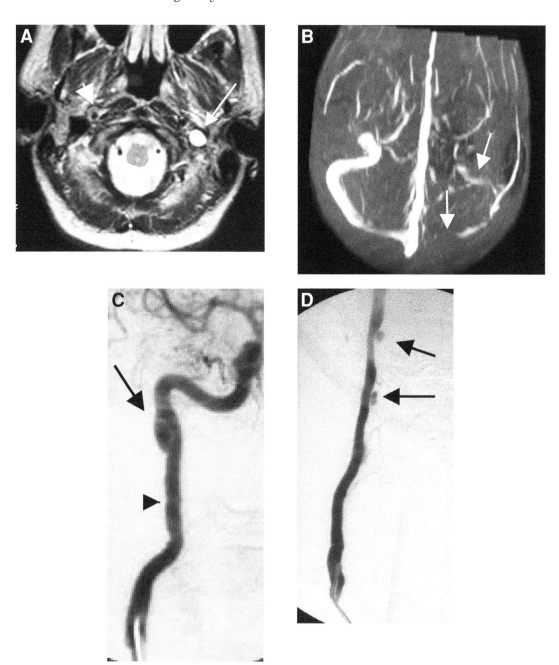

Fig. 1. A 38-yr-old female, 5 d postpartum, presented with severe right-sided neck pain and headache. **A:** MRI of the brain shows subacute thrombus in the left internal jugular vein (*arrow*). There is abnormal signal in the wall of the right petrous internal carotid artery (*arrowhead*). **B:** MRV of the brain shows absent or poor signal in the left transverse and sigmoid sinuses (*arrows*). **C:** Selective angiography of the right internal carotid artery (4A) showing a pseudo-aneurysm (*arrow*) at the junction between the cervical and petrous segments, and a "string-of-beads" pattern at the cervical level (*arrowhead*) consistent with fibromuscular dysplasia. **D:** Selective angiography of the right vertebral artery shows multiple pseudo-aneurysms (*arrows*).

benefit over vaginal delivery in unsecured aneurysms and is indicated in acute bleeding and for fetal salvage when the mother is moribund *(78,88)*. With vaginal delivery, epidural anesthesia, shortening of the second stage and low forceps should be used. The treatment of AVMs does not differ from that in non-pregnant women, except that stereotactic radiation is avoided. Cesarian section is reserved for obstetrical indications *(78)*.

SAH may result in 27–40% maternal mortality and may constitute the third most common cause of non-obstetric death in pregnancy *(78)*. Three of the six patients with ICH in a review of 50,700 records died *(77)*. The risk of another ICH in a subsequent pregnancy is not known *(78)*.

Cerebral Sinus Thrombosis

A high incidence of cerebral sinus thrombosis (CST) associated with pregnancy has been previously reported, usually without neuroimaging confirmation. In Mexico City, over 20 yr, 65% of CST were pregnancy-related *(95)* and in Toronto, 38% of infarctions during pregnancy were attributed to CST *(77)*. In India, the estimated incidence of CST is 200–500/100,000 deliveries *(96)*, which is 40–50 times higher than that in developed countries *(97)*.

Hormonal changes, blood stasis during the second stage of labor, volume depletion and hypercoagulability are various contributing factors *(see* Table 1). If EC complicates pregnancy, CST is usually attributed to DIC. In the rare case that CST occurs during pregnancy, protein S and antithrombin III deficiency must be accepted with scepticism and their serum concentration repeated several weeks after delivery, because they may be normally decreased during gestation *(94)*. CST occurs 1–4 wk after childbirth and follows an otherwise normal delivery. In developing countries it may occur soon after delivery at home or when there was insufficient prenatal care *(95,98)*. The diagnosis is made by MRI, angiography, MRV, or helical CT venography *(99)* *(see* Fig. 1).

Intravenous heparin to halt the thrombus propagation into cortical veins, fluid administration, antibiotics for infection and measures to reduce the elevated ICP are all used in CST. Oral anticoagulation is usually given for 6 mo in those patients with idiopathic venous thrombosis and indefinitely in those with a persistent or familial thrombophylic state. The risk for hemorrhagic conversion has been used as the major argument against anticoagulation and the only data from randomized studies are in non-pregnant populations *(100,101)*. In an uncontrolled study, 24% of patients with CST complicating pregnancy who received heparin died compared with 45% of untreated ones. One fatal hemorrhage occurred in the group with heparin *(102)*. More recently combined intra-thrombus rtPA and IV heparin in 12 patients showed encouraging results. Two had postpartum CST. The onset of symptoms was 23 and 21 d before treatment initiation. In one patient, there was partial flow restoration and all symptoms resolved. In the other patient, the infusion reduced the length of thrombus without flow restoration, but the seizures were controlled and she was discharged functionally independent *(103)*.

Mortality from CST is 10–50%, with lower percentages and better outcomes in more recent series *(99)*. Prophylactic anticoagulation during subsequent pregnancies is not indicated and recurrences are rare *(95,99)*.

PITUITARY APOPLEXY

Pregnancy increases the size of both the normal pituitary gland and any pituitary adenoma. Hemorrhage within the pituitary gland is called apoplexy (PA) and ischemic infarction of the gland leads to Sheehan's syndrome. Symptomatic PA occurs in only 2% and asymptomatic in 10–30% of patients harboring pituitary tumors *(93,104)*. Pregnancy may be a risk factor for PA in 25% of cases *(104)*. Only four cases during pregnancy had been reported, however, until 1990, three in prolactin and one in growth hormone–secreting adenomas *(104–108)*.

The role that other factors play in the development of PA is unclear, but anticoagulation, atheromatous emboli, angiography, diabetes, trauma or just the mere size of an hypervascular tumor have been usually implicated. Sheehan's syndrome occurs postpartum due to substantial postpartum hemorrhage and hypotension, but its incidence has decreased in the developed world.

The clinical presentation depends on the size and the direction of expansion of the hemorrhagic mass. The most frequent symptom is acute onset headache (76%) *(109)*. With supraclinoid extension the optic chiasm may be compressed leading to visual field deficits, the most characteristic of which is bitemporal heteronymous hemianopia (62%). Hypothalamic compression may also lead to autonomic dysfunction, deficient thermoregulation and various hormonal deficiencies. With lateral extension towards the cavernous sinus, cranial nerves III, IV, VI, and V1 or V2 divisions of the trigeminal nerve can be involved, leading to various degrees of ophthalmoparesis (40%) and pain. With extension into the subarachnoid space, SAH or "chemical" meningitis mimic can occur (16.8%) *(93)*. Alterations of mental status, even coma, are seen in 19.3% of patients. Sheehan's syndrome presents with panhypopituitarism (hypotension, hypoglycemia, and lactation failure). Thus, one should differentiate between these potentially lethal situations and although head CT scanning will reveal the enlarged hemorrhagic pituitary in most of the cases, MRI of the head with MRA will guide to the final diagnosis.

Management of PA is a medical emergency. Corticosteroids should be given in three to four times the normal dose (20 mg cortisol AM and 10 mg PM) during periods of stress to prevent Addisonian crisis. L-Thyroxine should also be given (0.1 mg orally daily), but mineralocorticoids are not required. Electrolyte and glucose derangements should be also corrected. Diabetes insipidus from compression of the pituitary stalk, hypothalamus or posterior pituitary gland may lead to profound water deficit and vasopressin or DDAVP should be supplemented *(109,110)*. Surgical resection of the compressing mass is indicated with involvement of the visual pathways or progression of the neurologic signs. Transphenoidal approach has been successfully used in pregnant women *(106)*. Bromocriptine is reserved for neurologically stable patients after the first trimester. For laboratory evaluation of endocrine emergencies, *see* Appendix.

STATUS EPILEPTICUS

The majority of epileptic women have an uneventful pregnancy or delivery and unchanged seizure frequency. Exacerbation of seizures can occur, however, in 37% of pregnant epileptics *(111,112)*. Status epilepticus during pregnancy is rare. In an extensive study of 153 pregnancies complicated by seizures, Knight and Rhind found two cases of SE out of 53,000 deliveries that took place over 20 yr *(112)*. In a recent review of the English language literature, 19 case reports were identified. SE was previously experienced in only 3/19 women, occurred in the third trimester in 74% of cases and episodes were equally split between multigravidas and primigravidas. Pregnancy did not appear to be a risk factor for SE in pregnant women without a history of epilepsy *(113)*. If a nonepileptic pregnant woman develops new onset seizures, EC should be excluded in the third trimester and similar causes of seizures (tumor, stroke, CNS infection, trauma, and hypoglycemia), as in nonpregnant women, should be sought *(114)*. There are many factors playing a role in the development of SE during pregnancy. Drug noncompliance, due to fear for teratogenicity and changes in drug level are among the most common. Increased plasma clearance of antiepileptic drugs with advancing gestation, has to be balanced against an increased ratio of unbound free to total drug level *(97,115–118)*. Thus, monthly free and not total drug levels have to be checked and appropriate changes in the dosage should be made *(119)*.

Although the fetus appears to be resilient to acidosis and hypoxia from a single maternal convulsion, repeated or continuous seizures, as in SE, are threatening for both mother and fetus *(120)*. With SE there is an estimated doubling of maternal mortality and 50% increased risk for spontaneous abortion *(97)*. In a 1982 review, 9/29 mothers with SE died and 14/29 fetuses died either *in utero* or shortly after birth *(121)*.

The SE treatment algorithm does not differ from that in non-pregnant women *(122,123)* and its goal is to stop the electrical and clinical seizure activity as soon as possible and support the mother and fetus *(93,120)* *(see also* Chapter 25). Additional measures are checks for urine protein, weight measurement and fetal monitoring. Administration of IV antiepileptic drugs should not be delayed because of concerns of teratogenic effects to the fetus even during the embryogenesis period. Medications, that are highly protein bound, should be initially administered in lower dose to avoid toxic free drug levels *(124)*. Reduced loading doses of phenytoin and valproic are used (10–15 mg/kg), but eventually full dosage can be given if seizures continue *(122,123)*. It is not known whether IV valproic load is safe in pregnancy, especially since high peak serum concentrations and combination with other antiepileptics have been implicated in teratogenicity. Data about midazolam use in SE are also lacking in pregnancy *(93)*. Delivery should be started only for obstetrical reasons. The neonate should be supported in the neonatal ICU, if benzodiazepines or barbiturates are given.

BRAIN DEATH

The clinical criteria for diagnosing brain death during pregnancy do not differ from those for nonpregnant women (*see also* Chapter 16). There are, however, several controversial ethical issues for supporting the mother until or beyond the fetus is viable (24 wk). Her wishes and, if never expressed, those of the biologic father of the fetus should be respected, as well as other important factors that play a role in decision making. The probability not only to reach a viable fetal status, but indeed deliver a healthy baby, that will be raised safely within the mother's family (with adoption as an alternative), should be taken into consideration *(125)*. The family should be informed in advance about the potentially significant cost for an endeavor with an often unpredictable outcome.

There are very few cases of successful delivery after maternal brain death. Dillon et al. reported a 23-wk pregnant patient who became brain dead due to status epilepticus and anoxia. She was supported until the 26th week when due to hypotensive episodes she delivered by Cesarean section a 930-g infant that survived *(126)*. Field et al. reported a brain dead patient at 22 wk, who, despite hemodynamic instability, ARDS, and infections delivered 63 d later a healthy 1440-g infant *(127)*. Bernstein et al. reported the longest duration of post-brain death support. Maternal death occurred at 15 wk gestation and she was supported for 107 d, when due to fetal distress she delivered a 1550 g infant *(128)*. Catanzarite et al. reported a patient who became brain dead due to posterior fossa AVM rupture at 25 wk. She was supported for 25 d and treated for ARDS and *Torulopsis glabrata* septicemia. Because of amnionitis, she delivered by Cesarean section a 1315-g infant, that despite fungal pneumonia and septicemia, survived *(129)*. Spike, in his excellent report, discussed the ethical issues regarding a 16.5 wk pregnant woman who died from an aneurysmal brainstem hemorrhage. At 31 wk, a healthy baby was delivered by Cesarean section *(125)*.

All these reports raise questions about the complex issues of maintaining the maternal body alive as far into gestation as possible. Continuous hemodynamic support and monitoring, use of pressors and IV fluids, monitoring of volume status with Swan-Ganz catheterization, continuous ventilatory support, enteral or parenteral nutrition with accurate estimation of resting energy expenditure, tocolytic treatment preferentially with Mg^{2+}, physiologic vasopressin infusion rates for diabetes insipidus, hydrocortisone and thyroxine replacement for the panhypopituitarism, glucose monitoring and insulin-need adjustments and treatment of infections, are few of the myriad maternal problems that should be addressed. In addition, continuous fetal monitoring, steroids for pulmonary maturation, amniocentesis when mother becomes septic and readiness for delivery and prolonged neonatal support are important issues for successful fetal outcome *(125–129)*. Finally, psychological support of the family and the medical and nursing staff involved in the care of a dead patient "used as a fetal container" *(125)* is often needed during the prolonged NSU course.

REFERENCES

1. Mushambi MC, Halligan AW, Williamson K. Recent developments in the pathophysiology and management of preeclampsia. *Br. J. Anaesth.* 1996;76:133–148.
2. Douglas KA, Redman CW. Eclampsia in the United Kingdom. *BMJ* 1994;309:1395–1400.
3. Mabie WC, Sibai BM. Treatment in an obstetric intensive care unit. *Am. J. Obstet. Gynecol.* 1990;162:1–4.
4. Ramin KD. The prevention and management of eclampsia. *Obstet. Gynecol. Clin. North Am.* 1999;26:489–503, ix.

5. Kaplan PW. Neurologic issues in eclampsia. *Rev. Neurol. (Paris)* 1999;155:335–341.

6. Brown CE, Cunningham FG, Pritchard JA. Convulsions in hypertensive, proteinuric primiparas more than 24 hours after delivery. Eclampsia or some other cause? *J. Reprod. Med.* 1987;32:499–503.

7. Miles JF Jr, Martin JN Jr, Blake PG, Perry KG Jr, Martin RW, Meeks GR. Postpartum eclampsia: A recurring perinatal dilemma. *Obstet. Gynecol.* 1990;76:328–331.

8. Porapakkham S. An epidemiologic study of eclampsia. *Obstet. Gynecol.* 1979;54:26–30.

9. Sibai BM. Eclampsia. VI. Maternal-perinatal outcome in 254 consecutive cases. *Am. J. Obstet. Gynecol.* 1990;163:1049–1054; discussion 1054–1055.

10. Thomas SV. Neurological aspects of eclampsia. *J. Neurol. Sci.* 1998;155:37–43.

11. Hinchey J, Chaves C, Appignani B, et al. A reversible posterior leukoencephalopathy syndrome. *N. Engl. J. Med.* 1996;334:494–500.

12. Belfort MA, Moise KJ Jr. Effect of magnesium sulfate on maternal brain blood flow in preeclampsia: A randomized, placebo-controlled study. *Am. J. Obstet. Gynecol.* 1992;167:661–666.

13. Borges LF, Gucer G. Effect of magnesium on epileptic foci. *Epilepsia* 1978;19:81–91.

14. Which anticonvulsant for women with eclampsia? Evidence from the Collaborative Eclampsia Trial. *Lancet* 1995;345:1455–1463.

15. Lucas MJ, Leveno KJ, Cunningham FG. A comparison of magnesium sulfate with phenytoin for the prevention of eclampsia. *N. Engl. J. Med.* 1995;333:201–205.

16. Walker JJ. Pre-eclampsia. *Lancet* 2000;356:1260–1265.

17. Lapinsky SE, Kruczynski K, Slutsky AS. Critical care in the pregnant patient. *Am. J. Respir. Crit. Care Med.* 1995;152:427–55.

18. Repke JT, Robinson JN. The prevention and management of pre-eclampsia and eclampsia. *Int. J. Gynaecol. Obstet.* 1998;62:1–9.

19. Steyn DW, Odendaal HJ. Randomised controlled trial of ketanserin and aspirin in prevention of pre-eclampsia. *Lancet* 1997;350:1267–1271.

20. Bolte AC, van Eyck J, Kanhai HH, Bruinse HW, van Geijn HP, Dekker GA. Ketanserin versus dihydralazine in the management of severe early-onset preeclampsia: Maternal outcome. *Am. J. Obstet. Gynecol.* 1999;180:371–377.

21. Sibai BM, Mabie BC, Harvey CJ, Gonzalez AR. Pulmonary edema in severe preeclampsia-eclampsia: Analysis of thirty-seven consecutive cases. *Am. J. Obstet. Gynecol.* 1987;156:1174–1179.

22. Cotton DB, Gonik B, Dorman K, Harrist R. Cardiovascular alterations in severe pregnancy-induced hypertension: Relationship of central venous pressure to pulmonary capillary wedge pressure. *Am. J. Obstet. Gynecol.* 1985;151:762–764.

23. Mabie WC, Ratts TE, Sibai BM. The central hemodynamics of severe preeclampsia. *Am. J. Obstet. Gynecol.* 1989;161:1443–1448.

24. Benedetti TJ, Kates R, Williams V. Hemodynamic observations in severe preeclampsia complicated by pulmonary edema. *Am. J. Obstet. Gynecol.* 1985;152:330–334.

25. Rackow EC, Fein IA, Leppo J. Colloid osmotic pressure as a prognostic indicator of pulmonary edema and mortality in the critically ill. *Chest* 1977;72:709–713.

26. Kirshon B, Moise KJ Jr, Cotton DB, et al. Role of volume expansion in severe pre-eclampsia. *Surg. Gynecol. Obstet.* 1988;167:367–371.

27. Clark SL, Cotton DB. Clinical indications for pulmonary artery catheterization in the patient with severe preeclampsia. *Am. J. Obstet. Gynecol.* 1988;158:453–458.

28. Brophy E, Brophy MH. Pyridoxal phosphate normalization of the EEG in eclampsia. *Electroencephalogr. Clin. Neurophysiol.* 1991;79:36.

29. Donaldson JO. Neurologic emergencies in pregnancy. *Obstet. Gynecol. Clin. North Am.* 1991;18:199–212.

30. Magee LA, Ornstein MP, von Dadelszen P. Fortnightly review: Management of hypertension in pregnancy. *BMJ* 1999;318:1332–1336.

31. Egerman RS, Sibai BM. HELLP syndrome. *Clin. Obstet. Gynecol.* 1999;42:381–89.

32. Sullivan CA, Magann EF, Perry KG Jr, Roberts WE, Blake PG, Martin JN Jr. The recurrence risk of the syndrome of hemolysis, elevated liver enzymes, and low platelets (HELLP) in subsequent gestations. *Am. J. Obstet. Gynecol.* 1994;171:940–943.

33. Helou J, Nakhle S, Shoenfeld S, Nasseir T, Shalev E. Postpartum thrombotic thrombocytopenic purpura: Report of a case and review of the literature. *Obstet. Gynecol. Surv.* 1994;49:785–789.

34. Weiner CP. Thrombotic microangiopathy in pregnancy and the postpartum period. *Semin. Hematol.* 1987;24:119–129.

35. Martin JN, Jr., Files JC, Blake PG, et al. Plasma exchange for preeclampsia. I. Postpartum use for persistently severe preeclampsia-eclampsia with HELLP syndrome. *Am. J. Obstet. Gynecol.* 1990;162:126–137.

36. Martin JN Jr, Perry KG Jr, Roberts WE, et al. Plasma exchange for preeclampsia: III. Immediate peripartal utilization for selected patients with HELLP syndrome. *J. Clin. Apheresis* 1994;9:162–165.

37. Magann EF, Bass D, Chauhan SP, Sullivan DL, Martin RW, Martin JN Jr. Antepartum corticosteroids: disease stabilization in patients with the syndrome of hemolysis, elevated liver enzymes, and low platelets (HELLP). *Am. J. Obstet. Gynecol.* 1994;171:1148–1153.

38. Magann EF, Perry KG Jr, Meydrech EF, Harris RL, Chauhan SP, Martin JN Jr. Postpartum corticosteroids: Accelerated recovery from the syndrome of hemolysis, elevated liver enzymes, and low platelets (HELLP). *Am. J. Obstet. Gynecol.* 1994;171:1154–1158.

39. Plauche WC. Myasthenia gravis in mothers and their newborns. *Clin. Obstet. Gynecol.* 1991;34:82–99.

40. Plauche WC. Myasthenia gravis. *Clin. Obstet. Gynecol.* 1983;26:592–604.

41. Batocchi AP, Majolini L, Evoli A, Lino MM, Minisci C, Tonali P. Course and treatment of myasthenia gravis during pregnancy. *Neurology* 1999;52:447–452.

42. Riemersma S, Vincent A, Beeson D, et al. Association of arthrogryposis multiplex congenita with maternal antibodies inhibiting fetal acetylcholine receptor function. *J. Clin. Invest.* 1996;98:2358–2363.

43. Daskalakis GJ, Papageorgiou IS, Petrogiannis ND, Antsaklis AJ, Michalas SK. Myasthenia gravis and pregnancy. *Eur. J. Obstet. Gynecol. Reprod. Biol.* 2000;89:201–204.

44. Fraser FC, Sajoo A. Teratogenic potential of corticosteroids in humans. *Teratology* 1995;51:45–46.

45. Pickrell MD, Sawers R, Michael J. Pregnancy after renal transplantation: severe intrauterine growth retardation during treatment with cyclosporin A. *BMJ* 1988;296:825.

46. Buckley LM, Bullaboy CA, Leichtman L, Marquez M. Multiple congenital anomalies associated with weekly low-dose methotrexate treatment of the mother. *Arthritis Rheum.* 1997;40:971–973.

47. Ip MS, So SY, Lam WK, Tang LC, Mok CK. Thymectomy in myasthenia gravis during pregnancy. *Postgrad. Med. J.* 1986;62:473–474.

48. Bril V, Kojic J, Ilse WK, Cooper JD. Long-term clinical outcome after transcervical thymectomy for myasthenia gravis. *Ann. Thorac. Surg.* 1998;65:1520–1522.

49. Eden RD, Gall SA. Myasthenia gravis and pregnancy: a reappraisal of thymectomy. *Obstet. Gynecol.* 1983;62:328–333.

50. Qureshi AI, Choudhry MA, Akbar MS, et al. Plasma exchange versus intravenous immunoglobulin treatment in myasthenic crisis. *Neurology* 1999;52:629–632.

51. Achiron A, Barak Y, Miron S, Sarova-Pinhas I. Immunoglobulin treatment in refractory myasthenia gravis. *Muscle Nerve* 2000;23:551–555.

52. Carr SR, Gilchrist JM, Abuelo DN, Clark D. Treatment of antenatal myasthenia gravis. *Obstet. Gynecol.* 1991;78:485–489.

53. Chaudhry V, Cornblath DR, Griffin JW, O'Brien R, Drachman DB. Mycophenolate mofetil: A safe and promising immunosuppressant in neuromuscular diseases. *Neurology* 2001;56:94–96.

54. Pergola PE, Kancharla A, Riley DJ. Kidney transplantation during the first trimester of pregnancy: Immunosuppression with mycophenolate mofetil, tacrolimus, and prednisone. *Transplantation* 2001;71:994–997.

55. Thomas CE, Mayer SA, Gungor Y, et al. Myasthenic crisis: Clinical features, mortality, complications, and risk factors for prolonged intubation. *Neurology* 1997;48:1253–1260.

56. Benshushan A, Rojansky N, Weinstein D. Myasthenia gravis and preeclampsia. *Isr. J. Med. Sci.* 1994;30:229–233.

57. Ho T, Griffin J. Guillain-Barre syndrome. *Curr. Opin. Neurol.* 1999;12:389–394.

58. Ropper AH. The Guillain-Barre syndrome. *N. Engl. J. Med.* 1992;326:1130–1136.

59. Jiang GX, de Pedro-Cuesta J, Strigard K, Olsson T, Link H. Pregnancy and Guillain-Barre syndrome: A nationwide register cohort study. *Neuroepidemiology* 1996;15:192–200.

60. Mack T, Weiner L, Gilmore W. Guillain-Barre syndrome, pregnancy, and the puerperium. *Epidemiology* 1998;9:588–590.

61. Luijckx GJ, Vles J, de Baets M, Buchwald B, Troost J. Guillain-Barre syndrome in mother and newborn child. *Lancet* 1997;349:27.

62. Nelson LH, McLean WT Jr. Management of Landry-Guillain-Barre syndrome in pregnancy. *Obstet. Gynecol.* 1985;65:25S–29S.

63. van der Meche FG, Schmitz PI. A randomized trial comparing intravenous immune globulin and plasma exchange in Guillain-Barre syndrome. Dutch Guillain-Barre Study Group. *N. Engl. J. Med.* 1992;326:1123–1129.

64. Randomised trial of plasma exchange, intravenous immunoglobulin, and combined treatments in Guillain-Barre syndrome. Plasma Exchange/Sandoglobulin Guillain-Barre Syndrome Trial Group. *Lancet* 1997;349:225–230.

65. Yamada H, Noro N, Kato EH, Ebina Y, Cho K, Fujimoto S. Massive intravenous immunoglobulin treatment in pregnancy complicated by Guillain-Barre syndrome. *Eur. J. Obstet. Gynecol. Reprod. Biol.* 2001;97:101–104.

66. Gautier PE, Hantson P, Vekemans MC, et al. Intensive care management of Guillain-Barre syndrome during pregnancy. *Intens. Care Med.* 1990;16:460–462.

67. Yaginuma Y, Kawamura M, Ishikawa M. Landry-Guillain-Barre-Strohl syndrome in pregnancy. *J. Obstet. Gynaecol. Res.* 1996;22:47–49.

68. Brooks H, Christian AS, May AE. Pregnancy, anaesthesia and Guillain Barre syndrome. *Anaesthesia* 2000;55:894–898.

69. Barbour LA. Current concepts of anticoagulant therapy in pregnancy. *Obstet. Gynecol. Clin. North Am.* 1997;24:499–521.

70. Weiner CP. Diagnosis and management of thromboembolic disease during pregnancy. *Clin. Obstet. Gynecol.* 1985;28:107–118.

71. Demers C, Ginsberg JS. Deep venous thrombosis and pulmonary embolism in pregnancy. *Clin. Chest. Med.* 1992;13:645–656.

72. Ferner R, Barnett M, Hughes RA. Management of Guillain-Barre syndrome. *Br. J. Hosp. Med.* 1987;38:525–528, 530.

73. Ropper AH. Critical care of Guillain-Barre syndrome. In: Ropper AH (ed). *Neurological and Neurosurgical Intensive Care*. 3d ed. New York: Raven Press, 1993:363–382.

74. Fausett MB, Vogtlander M, Lee RM, et al. Heparin-induced thrombocytopenia is rare in pregnancy. *Am. J. Obstet. Gynecol.* 2001;185:148–152.

75. Mc Phedran P. Venous thromboembolism during pregnancy. In: Burrow GN, Duffy TP (eds). *Medical Complications During Pregnancy*. Philadelphia: WB Saunders, 1999:97–109.

76. Bazzan M, Donvito V. Low-molecular-weight heparin during pregnancy. *Thromb. Res.* 2001;101:V175–V186.

77. Jaigobin C, Silver FL. Stroke and pregnancy. *Stroke* 2000;31:2948–2951.

78. Mas JL, Lamy C. Stroke in pregnancy and the puerperium. *J. Neurol.* 1998;245:305–313.

79. Wiebers DO, Whisnant JP. The incidence of stroke among pregnant women in Rochester, Minn, 1955 through 1979. *JAMA* 1985;254:3055–3057.

80. Sharshar T, Lamy C, Mas JL. Incidence and causes of strokes associated with pregnancy and puerperium. A study in public hospitals of Ile de France. Stroke in Pregnancy Study Group. *Stroke* 1995;26:930–936.

81. Kittner SJ, Stern BJ, Feeser BR, et al. Pregnancy and the risk of stroke. *N. Engl. J. Med.* 1996;335:768–774.

82. Ursell MR, Marras CL, Farb R, Rowed DW, Black SE, Perry JR. Recurrent intracranial hemorrhage due to postpartum cerebral angiopathy: Implications for management. *Stroke* 1998;29:1995–1998.

83. Out HJ, Bruinse HW, Christiaens GC, et al. A prospective, controlled multicenter study on the obstetric risks of pregnant women with antiphospholipid antibodies. *Am. J. Obstet. Gynecol.* 1992;167:26–32.

84. Turrentine MA, Braems G, Ramirez MM. Use of thrombolytics for the treatment of thromboembolic disease during pregnancy. *Obstet. Gynecol. Surv.* 1995;50:534–541.

85. Tissue plasminogen activator for acute ischemic stroke. The National Institute of Neurological Disorders and Stroke rt-PA Stroke Study Group. *N. Engl. J. Med.* 1995;333:1581–1587.

86. CLASP: A randomised trial of low-dose aspirin for the prevention and treatment of pre-eclampsia among 9364 pregnant women. CLASP (Collaborative Low-dose Aspirin Study in Pregnancy) Collaborative Group. *Lancet* 1994;343:619–629.

87. Lamy C, Hamon JB, Coste J, Mas JL. Ischemic stroke in young women: risk of recurrence during subsequent pregnancies. French Study Group on Stroke in Pregnancy. *Neurology* 2000;55:269–274.

88. Dias MS, Sekhar LN. Intracranial hemorrhage from aneurysms and arteriovenous malformations during pregnancy and the puerperium. *Neurosurgery* 1990;27:855–865; discussion 865–866.

89. Hunt HB, Schifrin BS, Suzuki K. Ruptured berry aneurysms and pregnancy. *Obstet. Gynecol.* 1974;43:827–837.

90. Robinson JL, Hall CS, Sedzimir CB. Arteriovenous malformations, aneurysms, and pregnancy. *J. Neurosurg.* 1974;41:63–70.

91. Horton JC, Chambers WA, Lyons SL, Adams RD, Kjellberg RN. Pregnancy and the risk of hemorrhage from cerebral arteriovenous malformations. *Neurosurgery* 1990;27:867–871; discussion 871–872.

92. Meyers PM, Halbach VV, Malek AM, et al. Endovascular treatment of cerebral artery aneurysms during pregnancy: Report of three cases. *AJNR* 2000;21:1306–1311.

93. Raps EC, Galetta SL, Flamm ES. Neuro-intensive care of the pregnant woman. *Neurol. Clin.* 1994;12:601–611.

94. Lamy C, Sharshar T, Mas J. Pathologie vasculaire cerebrale au cours de la grossesse et du post-partum. *Rev. Neurol. (Paris)* 1996;152:422–440.

95. Cantu C, Barinagarrementeria F. Cerebral venous thrombosis associated with pregnancy and puerperium. Review of 67 cases. *Stroke* 1993;24:1880–1884.

96. Srinivasan K. Cerebral venous and arterial thrombosis in pregnancy and puerperium. A study of 135 patients. *Angiology* 1983;34:731–746.

97. Donaldson J. Neurologic complications. In: Burrow G, Duffy T (eds). *Medical Complications During Pregnancy*. 5th ed. Philadelphia: WB Saunders, 1999:401–414.

98. Donaldson JO, Lee NS. Arterial and venous stroke associated with pregnancy. *Neurol. Clin.* 1994;12:583–599.

99. Bousser MG. Cerebral venous thrombosis: Nothing, heparin, or local thrombolysis? *Stroke* 1999;30:481–483.

100. Einhaupl KM, Villringer A, Meister W, et al. Heparin treatment in sinus venous thrombosis. *Lancet* 1991;338:597–600.

101. de Bruijn SF, Stam J. Randomized, placebo-controlled trial of anticoagulant treatment with low-molecular-weight heparin for cerebral sinus thrombosis. *Stroke* 1999;30:484–488.

102. Srinivasan K. Puerperal cerebral venous and arterial thrombosis. *Semin. Neurol.* 1988;8:222–225.

103. Frey JL, Muro GJ, McDougall CG, Dean BL, Jahnke HK. Cerebral venous thrombosis: Combined intrathrombus rtPA and intravenous heparin. *Stroke* 1999;30:489–494.

104. Onesti ST, Wisniewski T, Post KD. Clinical versus subclinical pituitary apoplexy: Presentation, surgical management, and outcome in 21 patients. *Neurosurgery* 1990;26:980–986.

105. Nagulesparan M, Roper J. Haemorrhage into the anterior pituitary during pregnancy after induction of ovulation with clomiphene. *Br. J. Obstet. Gynaecol.* 1978;85:153–155.

106. Lunardi P, Rocchi G, Rizzo A, Missori P. Neurinoma of the oculomotor nerve. *Clin. Neurol. Neurosurg.* 1990;92:333–335.

107. Hervet E, Barrat J, Pigne A, Darbois Y, Faguer C. [Prolactin adenoma. Hypophysectomy during pregnancy]. *Nouv. Presse Med.* 1975;4:2393–2395.

108. O'Donovan PA, O'Donovan PJ, Ritchie EH, Feely M, Jenkins DM. Apoplexy into a prolactin secreting macroadenoma during early pregnancy with successful outcome. Case report. *Br. J. Obstet. Gynaecol.* 1986;93:389–391.
109. Rolih C, Ober K. Pituitary apoplexy. *Endocrinol. Metabol. Clin. North Am.* 1993;22:291–302.
110. Oyesiku N. Pituitary tumors and Sheehan's syndrome in pregnant women. In: Loftus C (ed). *Neurosurgical Aspects of Pregnancy*: AANS, Rolling Meadows, IL, 1996:77–84.
111. Schmidt D, Canger R, Avanzini G, et al. Change of seizure frequency in pregnant epileptic women. *J. Neurol. Neurosurg. Psychiatry* 1983;46:751–755.
112. Knight AH, Rhind EG. Epilepsy and pregnancy: A study of 153 pregnancies in 59 patients. *Epilepsia* 1975;16:99–110.
113. Licht EA, Sankar R. Status epilepticus during pregnancy. A case report. *J. Reprod. Med.* 1999;44:370–372.
114. Michalsen A, Henze T, Wagner D, Schillinger H, Engels K. [Status epilepticus late in pregnancy—eclampsia or sub-arachnoid hemorrhage?]. *Anasthesiol. Intensivmed. Notfallmed. Schmerzther.* 1997;32:380–384.
115. Morrell MJ. The new antiepileptic drugs and women: Efficacy, reproductive health, pregnancy, and fetal outcome. *Epilepsia* 1996;37:S34–S44.
116. Lander CM, Eadie MJ. Plasma antiepileptic drug concentrations during pregnancy. *Epilepsia* 1991;32:257–266.
117. Nau H, Helge H, Luck W. Valproic acid in the perinatal period: decreased maternal serum protein binding results in fetal accumulation and neonatal displacement of the drug and some metabolites. *J. Pediatr.* 1984;104:627–634.
118. Yerby MS, Friel PN, McCormick K. Antiepileptic drug disposition during pregnancy. *Neurology* 1992;42:12–16.
119. Yerby MS, Friel PN, McCormick K, et al. Pharmacokinetics of anticonvulsants in pregnancy: alterations in plasma protein binding. *Epilepsy Res.* 1990;5:223–228.
120. Goetting MG, Davidson BN. Status epilepticus during labor. A case report. *J. Reprod. Med.* 1987;32:313–314.
121. Teramo K, Hiilesmaa V. Pregnancy and fetal complications in epileptic pregnancies: Review of the literature. In: Janz D (ed). *Epilepsy, Pregnancy and the Child.* New York: Raven Press, 1982:53–59.
122. Varelas PN, Mirski MA. Seizures in the adult intensive care unit. *J. Neurosurg. Anesthesiol.* 2001;13:163–175.
123. Dalessio DJ. Current concepts. Seizure disorders and pregnancy. *N. Engl. J. Med.* 1985;312:559–563.
124. Ryan G, Lange IR, Naugler MA. Clinical experience with phenytoin prophylaxis in severe preeclampsia. *Am. J. Obstet. Gynecol.* 1989;161:1297–1304.
125. Spike J. Brain death, pregnancy, and posthumous motherhood. *J. Clin. Ethics* 1999;10:57–65.
126. Dillon WP, Lee RV, Tronolone MJ, Buckwald S, Foote RJ. Life support and maternal death during pregnancy. *JAMA* 1982;248:1089–1091.
127. Field DR, Gates EA, Creasy RK, Jonsen AR, Laros RK, Jr. Maternal brain death during pregnancy. Medical and ethical issues. *JAMA* 1988;260:816–822.
128. Bernstein IM, Watson M, Simmons GM, Catalano PM, Davis G, Collins R. Maternal brain death and prolonged fetal survival. *Obstet. Gynecol.* 1989;74:434–437.
129. Catanzarite VA, Willms DC, Holdy KE, Gardner SE, Ludwig DM, Cousins LM. Brain death during pregnancy: Tocolytic therapy and aggressive maternal support on behalf of the fetus. *Am. J. Perinatol.* 1997;14:431–434.
130. Varelas P, Fayad P. Migraine and stroke. In: Cohen S (ed). *Management of Ischemic Stroke.* New York: Mc Graw-Hill, 2000:391–404.
131. Bodis L, Szupera Z, Pierantozzi M, et al. Neurological complications of pregnancy. *J. Neurol. Sci.* 1998;153:279–293.

33

Nursing Care in the Neurosciences Critical Care Unit

Janice L. Hickman

INTRODUCTION

The 1990s was designated the "Decade of the Brain" and was characterized by a virtual explosion in the knowledge base of the brain and neurological conditions as well as the treatment of these conditions. The 1990s provided the advancement of education for health care personnel who care for neurologically compromised patients, which allowed for the specialization in the care of these patients. However, it became evident that one of the ways to provide comprehensive care to the critically ill neurological patient is through collaborative practice and care. True collaborative practice dictates that nurse and physician work together as professional colleagues to jointly manage patients. Studies have shown that a close collegial working relationship between nurses and physicians is fundamental to excellent patient care delivery (1). Neurological conditions have serious consequences, not only for the patient but also for the family members. It is important that the family be involved in management of the patient. The family's ability to accept the patient's condition and adapt to it directly influences the emotional stability of the entire family, including the patient (2). Research shows that patients with strong family involvement appear to progress more rapidly and realistic outcomes are more readily accepted than in cases with little family involvement in the patient plan of care (3). The critical care environment enhances the use of the collaborative care model. In this chapter we will present the key elements of good nursing care to patients admitted to the neurosciences critical care unit (NSU) with various neurologic and systemic abnormalities.

NURSING CHALLENGES

The evolution of high technology in intensive care for patients who develop neurological conditions has dictated a new level of training for the staff who cares for these patients. Neurologic/neurosurgical critical care has become a specialized area that mandates a team that understands the pathophysiology and treatment of intracranial conditions (1). The neuroscience nurse must have strong assessment skills and a strong background in neuroanatomy and physiology to deliver quality care to the neurological critically ill patient population.

NEUROLOGIC ASSESSMENT

Nursing care of the neurologically compromised patient is based on highly developed nursing assessment skills. In order for the nurses to accurately ascertain where the patients' baseline neurological stability is they must know what to assess, the proper technology for assessment, and what it is they assess. These features combine to allow for appropriate intervention to take place if needed. The ability to detect changes, both obvious and subtle, is imperative in the care of a neurologically

From: *Current Clinical Neurology*
Critical Care Neurology and Neurosurgery
Edited by: J. I. Suarez © Humana Press Inc., Totowa, NJ

compromised patient. The baseline assessment is the marker that allows the nurse to detect any deviations that may warrant further corrective measures. This results from the fact that changes in neurological status may be rapid and dramatic, or very subtle, developing over minutes to days.

A neurological assessment should include level of consciousness (Fig. 1), orientation and cognition, pupillary signs, motor function, and vital signs. The frequency of neurological assessments in the NSU is every hour. The neurologic assessment is performed and documented on the neurologic flow sheet every hour (*see* Appendix) or more often if needed. Such documentation can also be carried out by entering information electronically using customized computer software programs. The Glasgow Coma Scale (GCS) is a commonly used tool to detect alterations of consciousness and can be obtained at the bedside very easily (Table 1). Besides these general principles of nursing care, there are other variables that need to be taken into account depending upon patients' underlying pathologies. We will now discuss some of the most common conditions that will present specific challenges to nurses.

Increased Intracranial Pressure

Patients who experience traumatic or nontraumatic cerebral injury are at risk for developing increased intracranial pressure (ICP). It is imperative for nurses caring for these patients to be aware of conditions increasing the risk. Because nurses provide continuous care to patients, they can be pivotal in preventing increased ICP. Neurologic assessment alerts the nurse to changes such increases in ICP. Accurate assessments consist of the patient's level of consciousness, orientation, pupillary reaction, and motor deficits. Rapid intervention can facilitate functions of compensatory mechanisms to decrease ICP preventing catastrophic effects (Fig. 2, Table 2).

Intracranial Pressure Monitoring Devices

ICP monitoring has been described in the literature since the 1960s. As technology increased, monitoring devices have been developed to obtain information about intracranial hemodynamics (*see also* Chapter 5).

The measurement of ICP has been commonplace in the management of the neurological patient. External ventriculostomy, which requires the insertion of a special catheter through a bur hole into the nondominant lateral ventricle of the brain, is a type of ICP monitoring (4). This is performed to control increases in ICP when the brain's ability to maintain normal intracranial compliance and elastance has been changed secondary to pathological processes. Once the ventriculostomy catheter is inserted into the lateral ventricle, it is connected to an external ventricular drainage system (EVD) of choice.

External ventriculostomy allows the practitioner to (1) drain cerebrospinal fluid (CSF) to reduce ICP; (2) continuously monitor ICP to assess the dynamic changes that can occur within the cranium; and (3) insert antibiotics directly into the CSF compartment.

When caring for a patient with a ventriculostomy the nurse has a number of responsibilities as will be delineated below. Following the insertion of the ventriculostomy catheter, the head of the bed is placed at a 20- to 30-degree elevation. Physicians caring for the patient should determine the specific pressure level at which the system will allow CSF drainage. The nurse measures the anatomical reference point that is usually taken from mid-ear, which corresponds with the intraventricular foramen and aligns the reference point to the 0-cm scale on the drainage system. The drip chamber of the collection system can then be positioned at the specified pressure level.

Neurological assessment and vital signs following this procedure should be performed every hour. When caring for a patient and EVD the following interventions should be performed: (a) the nurse should assess and document the incision site status; (b) the amount and color of the CSF in the drainage receptacle should be assessed and recorded hourly on the nursing flowsheet; (c) with each assessment the nurse should check that the ordered pressure level corresponds with the ventriculostomy flow chamber zero level at the patients reference point (5).

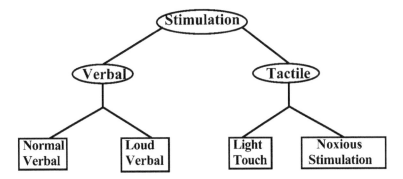

Fig. 1. Assessment of level of consciousness.

Anytime a patient is turned, the measuring point should be checked to assure it is at the proper level. When a patient is moved or taken out of bed for a procedure, the drainage system should be turned off until it can be returned to the position ordered *(6)*. Connecting a transducer to the system for periodic ICP readings may allow for its continuous or intermittent monitoring.

The ventricular system is a closed sterile system, so it should be handled with strict aseptic technique *(7)*. The insertion site should be clean, dry, and occlusive. The dressing should be changed as per institutional protocol, or when it is wet or soiled. If the dressing is noted to be dampened with CSF, the physician should be notified. The CSF system itself should be checked frequently for patency *(8)*.

The collection bag should be changed when the bag is three quarters full. If a CSF specimen needs to be obtained, it should be drawn from the CSF collection chamber using strict sterile technique. The sample port needs to be cleaned thoroughly with povidone-iodine before drawing the specimen.

There are risks in the use of external ventriculostomy for ICP monitoring. One of the most frequently cited is infection *(4)*. Infection may cause meningitis or ventriculitis. It is important that the closed system is preserved with as few interruptions as possible. Prophylactic antibiotics may be prescribed as preventive measure while the catheter is in place *(5)*.

Subarachnoid Hemorrhage

Intracranial Aneurysm

An aneurysm is considered to be a congenital developmental defect in the muscle layer of arteries, normally occurring at points of bifurcation *(9)*. The congenital weakness of the arterial wall results in a gradual outpouching of that segment of the artery over a period of years. When there is an increase in vascular pressure, to a certain point, the weakened ballooning section of the artery ruptures causing a subarachnoid hemorrhage (SAH).

Clinical Presentation

Aneurysms are commonly asymptomatic until a bleed occurs. Severe headache presents ("worst headache of my life") when the aneurysm starts to leak. Once the aneurysm ruptures, onset of symptoms is rapid and abrupt. Transient or sustained unconsciousness may be due to sudden increases in ICP, ischemia or necrosis of brain tissue. Patients may present with transient neurological deficits including numbness, aphasia, paresis, and nuchal rigidity (*see also* Chapter 20).

Nursing Considerations

The basics of treatment for a patient with SAH before surgery hinge on the prevention of rebleeding. Complete bed rest with a quiet environment promotes cardiovascular and neurologic

Table 1
Glasgow Coma Scale

The Glasgow Coma Scale is a practical mean of monitoring changes in the level of consciousness based upon eye opening and verbal and motor responses. The responsiveness of the patient can be expressed by the summation of the figures, the lowest score being three, the highest fifteen:

Eyes open	Spontaneously (eyes open, does not imply awareness)	4
	To speech (any speech, not necessarily a command)	3
	To pain (supraorbital pressure not used for stimulus)	2
	Never	1
Best verbal response	Oriented (to people, place, time)	5
	Confused speech (disoriented)	4
	Inappropriate (swearing, yelling)	3
	Incomprehensible sounds (moaning, groaning)	2
	None	1
Best motor response	Obeys commands	6
	Localizes pain (deliberate or purposeful movement)	5
	Withdrawal (moves away from stimulus)	4
	Abnormal flexion (decortication)	3
	Extension (decerebration)	2
	None (flaccidity)	1
	Total Score	___

stabilization. The head of the bed is elevated to 30 degrees to enhance cerebral venous return. If patients are alert, they should be instructed to avoid the Valsalva maneuver, and any other act that produces straining. Accurate neurological assessment is imperative for the nurse to precisely evaluate the patient's neurological status and detect any change that would mandate rapid interventions. It is also important for the nurse to closely monitor the patient's hemodynamic status. The minimum amount of monitoring for these patients should include ECG monitoring, with frequent measurements of the heart rate, respiratory rate and patterns, body temperature, blood pressure, and pulse oximetry. The patient's fluid status must also be documented closely. The goal is to maintain cerebral blood flow and prevent additional neurological injury from cerebral ischemia *(10)*. Effective volume resuscitation is imperative to control intracranial pressure and prevent further brain damage.

Cerebral vasospasm is a narrowing of the cerebral vasculature producing decreased blood flow within the brain and subsequent ischemia *(11)*. It is a significant cause of secondary brain injury, morbidity, and mortality after subarachnoid hemorrhage. Volume loading (hypervolemic-hemodilution therapy) to maintain cerebral perfusion beyond the area of vasospasm is used to bring the central venous pressures to greater than 8 mmHg or a pulmonary capillary wedge pressure of 12 mmHg or more. Hypertensive therapy with dopamine, or phenylephrine can be used to increase the systemic arterial pressure *(12)*. The use of this so-called triple H therapy (hypertension, hypervolemia, and hemodilution) has resulted in positive outcomes in patients with symptomatic vasospasm *(13)*. Nimodipine, which is a calcium channel blocker that has an affinity for cerebrovascular circulation and crosses the blood-brain barrier, is used to prevent vasospasm. Nursing staff should become familiar with this medication and recognize its most common adverse effect, hypotension that may lead to decreased cerebral perfusion pressure with subsequent ischemia.

Caring for patients with vasospasm can be very challenging. Knowledge of cerebral hemodynamic responses and advanced assessment skills are pivotal in assuring favorable clinical outcomes.

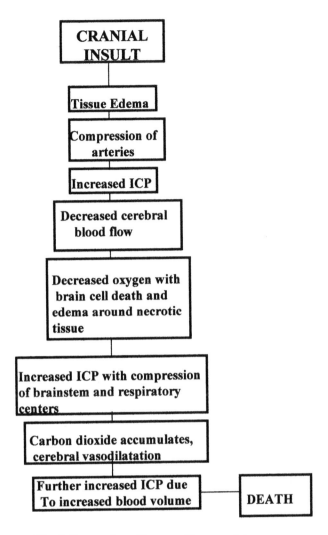

Fig. 2. Progression of increased intracranial pressure.

Traumatic Brain Injury

Traumatic brain injury (TBI) can occur from a variety of mechanisms including motor vehicle accidents, falls, assault, or sports injury. TBI may be classified based on severity, location, mechanism, GCS score, or the results of neuroimaging studies *(14)*. The management of the patient with traumatic brain injury requires intensive care management involving an intensivist and a nursing staff with expertise to provide appropriate care *(15) (see also* Chapter 22*)*.

Assessment

Patients that are in the NSU require frequent neurological evaluations. The nursing assessment should include level of consciousness, orientation, motor strength, pupillary reaction, and equality. If

Table 2
Nursing Interventions of Increased Intracranial Pressure

Maintain proper positioning
    Elevate head of bed 15–30 degrees
    Maintain neutral position of head and neck
    Avoid extreme hip flexion
Limit noxious stimuli
    Avoid "clustering" of nursing activity
    Limit painful procedures
    Avoid tension on any tubes
Control auditory stimuli
    Limit environmental noise
    Talk to patient quietly
    Limit visitors—explain to family why they must speak
      softly and avoid stimulating conversations
Prevent valsalva maneuver
    Give stool softeners to avoid constipation
    Avoid use of footboards
    Instruct patient to exhale whenever moving or turning in bed

the patient is undergoing ICP monitoring, those trends should also be assessed and charted. Other nursing responsibilities include evaluation of other systems. Patients must be followed very frequently for early detection of possible complications.

Respiratory management of traumatic brain injury patients includes airway management, hypoxia prevention, and determination of signs of pulmonary neurogenic edema, and pulmonary embolism *(16)*. The cardiovascular system should be monitored for complications including arrythmias and hypotension, and continuous electrocardiographic monitoring should be done and abnormalities treated accordingly *(17)*.

Deep venous thrombosis (DVT) is another serious complication in patients with TBI. The nurse should be aware of the patient's developing DVT. Use of antiembolism stockings, sequential compression wraps, lose dose heparin therapy have been shown to be the most effective combination for prevention of DVT. It is important that the nurses interrogate patients regarding calf or thigh pain or tenderness and perform vascular checks of the patients' extremities noting pulses, color, and temperature frequently, because DVT can lead to pulmonary embolisms. If pulmonary embolism occurs, chronic anticoagulation and/or a vena cava filter insertion is usually performed *(12)*.

Patients with TBI can also develop serious gastric complications. Stress ulcers that may lead to gastrointestinal hemorrhage are common occurrence. Use of H-2-blockers and sucralfate are used as preventative *(12)*. Nursing staff should review, medical orders to ensure that both DVT and gastric prophylactic measures are included in patients' care summary.

Acute Ischemic Stroke

Stroke is the third leading cause of death and the leading cause of disability among adult Americans *(18)*. The increased understanding of the pathophysiology of stroke has made healthcare workers aware that stroke is a "medical emergency." Until recently, there was no proven therapy for acute stroke victims. In the mid-1990s, the FDA approved the use of recombinant tissue plasminogin activator (rt-PA) intravenously for the treatment of acute ischemic stroke (AIS) patients *(19)* (*see also* Chapter 18).

There is a strict protocol for the screening of patients to decide whether they are candidates for thrombolysis. Treating physicians perform a baseline assessment, which includes time of onset of symptoms, pertinent medical history, and a neurological assessment for deficit. Coagulation studies are drawn and a head CT scan is performed. The onset of symptoms must be within a 3-h time limit.

If it is discovered that symptom onset is longer than 3 h, no rt-PA is administered. If the patient meets the clinical criteria and the symptoms are still present then thrombolytics are administered.

Nursing Interventions

Once patients receive the thrombolytic they are admitted to the NSU for close monitoring of intracranial bleeding or worsening of condition. Such monitoring should include hourly neurological assessment, vital signs, bleeding assessment and precautions, continuous electrocardiographic monitoring, and pulse oximetry to monitor oxygenation.

Detection of neurological changes is indicative of complications. Even though patients are carefully screened and selected to receive thrombolytics, they may still experience complications. Immediate recognition of these changes by the nurse is required for the appropriate intervention to occur.

NEUROLOGIC ASSESSMENT

Baseline neurologic assessment is used as a marker to detect any changes in level of consciousness, orientation, appropriate and clear speech, ability to follow commands, and motor strength.

The assessment schedule must be adhered to in the initial postthrombolytic therapy so that any changes that may indicate serious complications such as intracranial hemorrhage may be detected.

BLEEDING ASSESSMENT

Studies have shown that the most frequent adverse reaction related to the use of thrombolytics for AIS treatment is bleeding *(20)*. Intracranial hemorrhage (ICH) is usually associated with acute changes in neurologic status. The most common symptoms are a decreased level of consciousness, changes in motor examination, new onset of headache, and blood pressure changes.

If suspected of having ICH patients are taken to head CT scanning immediately and coagulation studies are done to rule out ICH. If this study confirms the presence of ICH, the neurosurgery team is consulted to evaluate patients' need for surgery to evacuate the ICH. Nursing staff should remain attentive to further changes in neurologic and systemic signs before, during, and following transportation of these patients from NSU to radiology suite and back to NSU.

VITAL SIGNS

The most important vital sign in patients with AIS is blood pressure. Inadequate pressure can compromise the amount of nutrients and oxygen required for adequate cerebral blood flow. Blood pressure should be monitored closely to avoid this. Specific guidelines and threshold determination for blood pressure treatment should be discussed with treating physicians as soon as patients are admitted to the NSU.

CARDIAC MONITORING

Patients should have continuous cardiac monitoring because there is a high incidence of cardiac arrhythmias after AIS. Arrhythmias are of concern because they may decrease cardiac stroke volume and compromise cerebral blood flow *(21)*.

RESPIRATORY MONITORING

The nurse should monitor the patients' oxygenation level by using pulse oximetry. If arterial desaturation occurs, treatment with supplemental oxygen should be instituted and its cause determined.

HYDRATION

In AIS patients, hydration should be watched closely. The nurse should monitor patients' intake and output closely, and carefully assess for symptoms of hypovolemia and electrolyte imbalance.

BLOOD GLUCOSE

Studies have shown that blood glucose in patients with AIS should be monitored closely and treated using a regular insulin sliding scale. These studies indicate that patients with elevated blood glucose develop larger infarctions than those with normal values *(22)*.

NUTRITION

It is important to assess AIS patient's nutritional status. Poor nutritional condition can impact their recovery process. Malnourished patients tend to recover more slowly and have an increased susceptibility to infection *(23)*. A swallowing evaluation for dysphagia should be done before the patient is given oral supplements or oral medication, preferably in the first 12 h following the event.

CEREBRAL EDEMA

All stroke patients are at risk for cerebral edema and increased intracranial pressure. Accordingly they should be monitored closely for signs and symptoms of increased ICP *(24)*. Nurses must be vigilant in the determination of patients' neurological status so that rapid intervention can be initiated if changes occur. Only intensive monitoring of these variables will help to detect changes that allow the healthcare team to initiate the appropriate interventions to enhance the recovery of AIS patients (Fig. 2).

Status Epilepticus

Recent epidemiologic studies suggest status epilepticus (SE) occurs in 100,000 to 150,000 people in the United States each year and is associated with substantial morbidity and mortality *(25)*. SE is the term used when there is continuing series of seizures without a recovery period in between the attacks. There are several types of SE including tonic, clonic, simple partial, absence, and complex partial seizures *(26)*. Studies have shown that the most common causes of SE are abrupt discontinuation of anticonvulsant drugs and acute brain insults. Hyponatremia, alcohol withdrawal, and fever are other known causes.

The most life-threatening form of this disorder is tonic clonic SE (also called generalized motor). It is a medical emergency because permanent brain damage and death are possible outcomes *(27)* (*see also* Chapter 25).

Nursing Considerations

AIRWAY MANAGEMENT

Patients who are in SE require aggressive airway management. Most patients who are in SE require the administration of sedatives and barbiturates that compromise their respiratory status. Often times these patients require intubation and mechanical ventilation. They should be suctioned frequently to prevent pneumonia and possible aspiration. Nursing staff should also refrain from starting oral feedings until adequate swallowing and level of consciousness are defined.

VITAL FUNCTIONS

The nurse caring for a patient in SE must frequently monitor vital signs and neurological status since the patient is administered high doses of anti-seizure drugs. High doses of sedatives and anticonvulsants are necessary to control the seizures. Loading doses of long-acting anticonvulsant medications, such as phenytoin must be administered by the intravenous route. Because of the potential for cardiac arrhythmias, patients should be monitored closely for cardiorespiratory depression. Intravenous benzodiazepines may be given as an adjunctive medication to control tonic-clonic seizures while a therapeutic serum concentration of long-acting anticonvulsants is being achieved. Therefore, respiratory monitoring is a must *(28)*.

PSYCHOSOCIAL CONSIDERATIONS

One of the greatest challenges that nursing staff in the NSU faces is the delivery of state of the art care within a humanistic environment *(29)*. To achieve this goal, it is required that we attend not only to the patients' needs but also to the needs of the families. Neurological illness has serious consequences. Because a majority of neurologic conditions bring about many psychological and emotional reactions in both patients and families, it is important for the entire team to work together to provide support and understanding to them. The role of the healthcare team should include conversing with the family frequently to determine how much they perceive is happening to the patient. The team should also recognize that often families need to be spoken to at regular intervals and will need information repeated at each meeting. It is equally important to become familiar with family dynamics and support systems. Many times understanding these issues will suffice to solve difficult interactions between families and NSU personnel. Relatives as well as patients (if able), should be encouraged to ask questions. Studies have shown that families who are given information frequently and consistently and are encouraged to visit cope better with the effects of a long-term neurologic illness *(30)*. Use of informational booklets and open visiting hours enhances family satisfaction and help meet their needs in this time of crisis. It is important that the team support families in their decision making process about patient care and management.

CONCLUSION

The care of the critically ill neuroscience patient continues to be enhanced due to advances in the field. The commitment to excellence has transpired through a collaborative effort by the neuroscience physician-nurse teams who continue to explore and research interventions that will result in positive outcomes for patients with neurologic conditions.

REFERENCES

1. Marshall SB, Marshall LF, Chesket RM. *Neuroscience Critical Care Pathophysiology and Patient Management*. Philadelphia: WB Saunders, 1990.
2. Michelson EL. The challenge of nurse-physician collaborative practices: improved patient care provisions and outcomes. *Heart Lung* 1988;17:390–391.
3. Aquilera DC, Messich JM. *Crisis Intervention: Theory and Methodology*, 6th ed. St Louis: CV Mosby, 1990.
4. Bader MK, Littlejohns L, Palmer S. Ventriculostomy and intracranial pressure monitoring: in search of a 0% infection rate. *Heart Lung* 1995;24:166–172.
5. Gibson I. Making sense of external ventricular drainage. *Nurs. Times* 1995;91:34–35.
6. Cummings R. Understanding external ventricular drainage. *J. Neurosci. Nurs.* 1992;24:84–87.
7. Pope W. External ventriculostomy: Practical application for the acute care nurse. *J. Neurosci. Nurs.* 1998;30:185–190.
8. Wisinger D, Mest-Beck L. Ventriculostomy: a guide to nursing management. *J. Neurosci. Nurs.* 1990;22:365–369.
9. Adams RD, Victor M. *Principles of Neurology*, 4th ed. New York: McGraw-Hill, 1989:667–675.
10. Arbour R. Aggressive management of intracranial dynamics. *Crit. Care Nurs.* 1998;18:30–40.
11. Hickey JV. *The Clinical Practice of Neurological and Neurosurgical Nursing*, 3rd ed. Philadelphia: JB Lippincott, 1992.
12. King WA, Martin NA. Critical Care of patients with subarachnoid hemorrhage. *Neurosurg. Clin. North Am.* 1994;5:767–787.
13. Ullman JS, Bederson JB. Hypertensive, hypervolemic, hemodilutional therapy for aneurysmal subarachnoid hemorrhage: Is it efficacious? YES. *Crit. Care Clin.* 1996;12:697–707.
14. Peterson PL, O'Heil BJ, Alcantara AL, et al. Initial evaluation and management of neuroemergencies. In: Cruz J (ed). *Neurological and Neurosurgical Emergencies*. Philadelphia: WB Saunders, 1998:1–20.
15. McNair ND. Traumatic brain injury. *Nurs. Clin. North Am.* 1999;34:637–659.
16. Cruz J, Miner ME, Allen SJ, et al. Continuous monitoring of cerebral oxygenation of acute brain injury. *Neurosurgery* 1991;29:743–749.
17. Cruz J, Mattiole C, et al. Severe acute brain injury. In Cruz J (ed). *Neurological and Neurosurgical Emergencies*. Philadelphia: WB Saunders, 1998:405–436.
18. Del Zoppo GJ, Yu JQ, Copeland BR, Thomas WS, Schneiderman J, Morrissey JH. Recombinant tissue plasminogen activator in acute ischemic stroke. *Ann. Neurol.* 1992;32:78–86.
19. Hund E, Grau A, Hacke W. Neurocritical care for acute ischemic stroke. *Neurol. Clin.* 1995;13:511–527.
20. The National Institutes of Neurological Disorders and Stroke rt-PA Stroke Study Group. Tissue plasminogen activator for acute ischemic stroke. *N. Engl. J. Med.* 1995;333:1581–1587.
21. Brott T, Lu M, Kothari R, et al. Hypertension and its treatment in the NINDS rt-PA Stroke Trial. *Stroke* 1998;29:1504–1509.
22. Matchar DB, Divine GW, Heyman A, Fenssner JR. The influence of hyperglycemia on outcome of cerebral infarction. *Ann. Inter. Med.* 1992;117:449–456.
23. Davalos A, Ricart W, Gonzalez-Huix F, et al. Effects of malnutrition after stroke on clinical outcome. *Stroke* 1996;27:1028–1032.
24. Davenport RJ, Dennis MS, Wellwood L, Warlow CP. Complications of acute ischemic stroke. *Stroke* 1996;27:415–420.
25. Fountain NB. Status epilepticus: risk factors and complications. *Epilepsia* 2000;41:S23–S30.

26. Engel J. Seizures, epilepsy, and the epilepsy pattern. In: *Contemporary Neurology Series*, vol. 3. Philadelphia: FA Davis, 1993.

27. Kernich KA. Seizures. In: Chernecky C, Berger B (eds). *Advanced and Critical Care Oncology Nursing.* Philadelphia: WB Saunders, 1998.

28. Marson AG, Kadir ZA, Chadwick, BW. New antiepileptic drugs: A systematic review of their efficacy and tolerability. *BMJ* 1996;313:1169–1174.

29. Henneman EA, McKenzie JB, Dewa CS. An evaluation of interventions for meeting the information needs of families of critically ill patients. *Am. J. Crit. Care* 1992;3:85–93.

30. Marsden C. Ethical issues in critical care. Real pressence. *Heart Lung* 1990;19:540–541.

34

Outcomes of Neurosciences Critical Care

Gene Sung

INTRODUCTION

Medical outcome research has gained significant prominence as healthcare providers work to determine the utility and efficacy of daily practice. Consequently, the outcome of neurosciences critical care is a topic of developing interest in the clinical neuroscience community. In fact, both outcomes research and neurosciences critical care are relatively new fields that are being defined and developed. We will attempt to discuss some of the key points pertaining these largely untapped areas.

NEUROSCIENCES CRITICAL CARE

Broadly defined, neurosciences critical care would include the rudimentary attempts at resuscitation and care throughout history. This definition would also refer to the care of patients after crude neurosurgical interventions such as trephination in ancient times. However, for the past hundred years it would steer us toward the care of patients during the polio epidemics and the care in the intensive care units (ICU) after modern neurosurgical operations.

Neurosciences critical care is a special area of clinical neuroscience that focuses on the neurologic and neurosurgical disorders that affect critically ill patients. These can be primary neurologic disorders or secondary to other systemic diseases and can affect either the central nervous system, the peripheral nervous system, or both. It includes understanding the effects of critical illness on the nervous system and the special vulnerabilities of the nervous system of patients in ICU and other emergency settings. It requires knowledge of the disorders that frequently occur in these settings, and the methods of diagnosis, assessment, treatment, management and prevention of further injury. Critical care and emergency neurology and neurosurgery also involve bridges into many medical and allied health specialties, including critical care medicine, emergency medicine, surgery, nursing and social work. Development of the specialty of critical care and emergency neurology and neurosurgery recognizes the special health needs of the population of critically ill patients with neurologic dysfunction, the characteristics of the nervous system in critically ill patients, and the need for interdisciplinary collaboration in this field.

The first neurosciences critical care programs in the United States were developed in the 1970s and the American Academy of Neurology section of Critical Care and Emergency Neurology was formed in 1989. The scope of care was varied and still is to this day. Efforts are now being made to better define the scope of practice and training for neurointensivists and to study the efficacy of neurosciences critical care.

The practice of neurosciences critical care is divided under the models of open vs closed neurosciences critical care units (NSU). The open model is that of a neurosciences critical care team that

From: *Current Clinical Neurology*
Critical Care Neurology and Neurosurgery
Edited by: J. I. Suarez © Humana Press Inc., Totowa, NJ

Table 1
Barthel Index: Highest Score 100

Variable	Scores	
	With help	Independent
1. Feeding	5	10
2. Moving from wheelchair to bed	5–10	15
3. Personal toilet	0	5
4. Getting on and off toilet	5	10
5. Bathing self	0	5
6. Walking on level surface	10	15
7. Ascend and descend stairs	5	10
8. Dressing	5	10
9. Controlling bladder	5	10
10. Controlling bowels	5	10

Modified from ref. *1*.

are consultants to the primary attending physician or team, usually a neurologist or neurosurgeon. The closed model has the neurosciences critical care team taking the primary responsibilities for each patient in the NSU and all other physicians playing more of a consultative role. Composition of these neurosciences critical care teams can vary from institution to institution and include neurologists, neurosurgeons, anesthesiologists and general intensivists. Often ancillary services are intimately involved in the team care as well and often round with the teams and participate in the decision-making process. For more details regarding the organization of NSU, refer to Chapter 2.

OUTCOMES

The ultimate outcome for life is death, and death is a frequent critical care outcome. Clinical studies in the ICU always must incorporate death and determining premature death or unusually frequent death compared to the norm. However, the first measure of outcome among those surviving critical illnesses is measured as function. One of the first measures of function is the Barthel Index *(1)* (Table 1), which measures the ability to perform the activities of daily living and was developed in 1965 to assess neuromuscular or musculoskeletal disorders. Functional scales are limited to gross assessments of the ability to perform tasks, but without an understanding of why the subject cannot perform the task.

As the field of physical medicine and rehabilitation has developed, new scales have been developed by physiatrists to monitor patient progress from a rehabilitation perspective. Since rehabilitation often starts in the ICU, these scales are sometimes used early in patient care. Probably the most widely used of these scales is the Functional Independence Measure (FIM) (Table 2), which consists of 18 items and is used by more than 100 rehabilitation institutions *(2)*.

In general critical care, severity of illness scales have been developed and used to help allocate resources, which are especially scarce in this area. The most popular scale used is the Acute Physiology, Age, Chronic Health Evaluation (APACHE) developed in 1981 and has had two major revisions since then *(3)*. The APACHE uses various physiological data to measure illness and has been used to help prognosticate mortality (Table 3). There have been several other scales developed. Unfortunately, the neurologic information incorporated in these scales is usually limited to the Glasgow Coma Scale (GCS).

The state of the art in outcome research expands upon physical function and now tries to measure health status as well as quality of life. Many researchers now use these terms interchangeably. Although not specifically designed for neurological diseases, these scales are important in the incorporation of nonphysical factors such as emotional and social dimensions of health. A commonly used

Table 2
Functional Independence Measure

Self-care
  Eating
  Grooming
  Bathing
  Dressing, upper body
  Dressing, lower body
  Perineal Care
Sphincter control
  Bladder management
  Bowel management
Mobility
  Transfer, bed, chair, wheelchair
  Transfer, toilet
  Transfer, tub or shower
Locomotion
  Walking
  Wheelchair
  Stairs
Communication
  Comprehension
  Expression
Social and cognitive skills
  Cooperation
  Problem solving

Modified from ref. *2*.

instrument is the Short-Form 36 Health Survey that came out of the Medical Outcomes Study *(4)*. This survey includes aspects of both physical health and mental health (Table 4).

Finally, one outcome that is increasingly important, and yet equally difficult to measure, is cost. The surrogate for actual cost of care is charges, but often this number has little relation to the actual cost of care. In patient outcomes research, in addition to the direct costs of care, it is also important to include the indirect costs that the patients bear, such as loss of employment or time spent by other caregivers.

OUTCOMES OF NEUROSCIENCES CRITICAL CARE

The latest trend in outcomes research is using a combination of scales, including a general functional scale, a global health status scale, and a disease-specific scale.Scales used to measure neurological diseases have been crude and not well developed, in part due to the few therapeutic interventions available for neurologic disease. As new therapies have been developed for neurologic disease, often, new outcomes scales have been developed to measure the efficacy of these therapies.

Head Injury

Besides mortality, for traumatic brain injury (TBI) patients, GCS *(5)* and the Glasgow Outcome Scale (GOS) *(6)* were the only measures available (Tables 5 and 6). To maintain reliability, the scales are very gross measures of disease. Both of these were designed for TBI evaluation and although not necessarily applicable to other disease processes, have often been used to measure coma of any etiology. In this patient population there have been attempts at improving the measurement of disease, but

Table 3
**Acute Physiology, Age, and Chronic Health
(APACHE)**

Temperature
Mean arterial pressure
Heart rate
Respiratory rate
Oxygenation
Arterial pH
Serum sodium
Serum potassium
Serum creatinine
Blood urea nitrogen
Urine output
Hematocrit
White blood cell count
Bilirubin
Albumin
Glasgow Coma Scale

Modified from ref. *3.*

Table 4
SF-36

Physical health
   Physical functioning
   Physical role
   Body pain
   General health
Mental health
   Vitality
   Social functioning
   Emotional role
   Mental health

Modified from ref. *4.*

are basically variations on the GCS, such as the Glasgow-Liege' scale *(7)*, the Innsbruck Coma Scale *(8)*, and Reaction Level Scale *(9)*, among others. None have surpassed the GCS in popularity, however. These primarily measure level of consciousness, one of the most common and glaring impairments in TBI patients. However, in a careful attempt to measure other deficits sustained by these individuals, the neurobehavioral rating scale was developed *(10)*. This scale divides 27 items into four factors or domains of "Cognition/Energy," "Metacognition," "Somatic/Anxiety," and "Language." "Later, a revision of the scale created a total of 29 items divided into the five factors of Intentional Behavior," "Lowered Emotional State," "Heightened Emotional State," "Arousal State," and "Language" *(11)*.

Acute Stroke

With the advent of thrombolytic and neuroprotective treatments in the field of stroke research, many new scales have been developed to evaluate deficit severity. This has led to the appearance of

Table 5
Glasgow Coma Scale: Score 3–15

Eye opening 1–4
Best verbal response 1–5
Best motor response 1–6

Modified from ref. *5.*

Table 6
Glasgow Outcome Scale

5   Good recovery
4   Moderate disability
3   Severe disability
2   Persistent vegetative state
1   Death

Modified from ref. *6.*

the Scandinavian Stroke Scale (SSS) *(12)*, National Institute of Health Stroke Scale (NIHSS) *(13)*, Canadian Neurological Scale *(14)*, European Stroke Scale *(15)*, and numerous others.These scales all take different components of the standard neurological exam and attempt to weight these in some fashion to obtain the most accuracy possible (the NIHSS is shown in Table 7 as an example). Not surprisingly, the scales are most frequently used in the countries in which they originated.

A commonly used functional scale in stroke studies is the Rankin scale, which is a test of physical ability *(16)*. And more recently, there have been efforts at developing disease-specific health status scales, such as the Stroke Impact Scale (SIS) in stroke *(17)*. The SIS includes the domains of physical, emotion, communication, and social participation to try to attain a measure of the broader consequences of stroke. In a specific type of stroke, subarachnoid hemorrhage, there was an evaluation of a group of patients who had been classified by their neurosurgeons as having had a good outcome *(18)*. The investigators found that all of the patients studied had significant negative outcomes when asked about psychosocial or neurobehavioral changes.

FUTURE DIRECTIONS OF NEUROSCIENCES CRITICAL CARE OUTCOMES RESEARCH

Unfortunately, because of the newness of neurosciences critical care and the many different outcome scales, there has been very little actual research in outcomes of this field.The studies done in the neurosciences critical care patients focus on the efficacy of new therapies and not the efficacy of the NSU care that the patients encounter. However, there has been some research in other areas that may be relevant to neurosciences critical care, which can then be used as evidence of outcomes or models for future research.

The first examples would be research in procedure-oriented care. There are numerous examples of the association of improved outcome with high patient volume; that is in difficult procedures, 'the more you do, the better you are.' This may be applicable to the critical care component of these patients, but these studies never delineate the contributions of the critical care versus that of the surgeon's skill. An example of this is a study on subarachnoid hemorrhage in New York state *(19)*, which revealed the improved mortality rates with higher surgical volumes. The postoperative care in the NSU likely contributed to the decrease in mortality, especially because many of the hospitals did not have dedicated neurointensive care units, but this could not be adequately assessed in this study.

Table 7
National Institute of Health Stroke Scale
(NIHSS): Score 0–42

Level of consciousness
Level of consciousness questions/orientation
Level of consciousness commands
Extraocular movements
Visual Fields
Facial palsy
Motor arm
Motor leg
Limb ataxia
Sensory test
Neglect
Dysarthria
Language

Modified from ref. *13*.

These issues have also been studied in TBI units. One of the best studies for our purposes attempted to determine the efficacy of trauma centers compared to general hospitals *(20)*. Examining only patients with severe injuries, the trauma centers consistently had improved mortality over general community hospitals. Because of studies like this, there has been the development of triage protocols that mandate paramedics to deliver severely injured patients to designated trauma centers.

In the field of stroke, there was a very remarkable study of the efficacy of stroke units and improved patient outcome *(21)*. The latest publication from this study documents the long-term benefits of patients who had been randomly assigned to care in a stroke unit, as opposed to the medicine wards. There was no difference in the medical therapies that were available and the initial care had only differed by the system of care that was in place in the specialty stroke unit.

CONCLUSION

The field of neurosciences critical care is in its infancy and outcomes research is only slightly older.As each of these field develops, there will need to be a better merger of these areas to study the work that is being done in neurosciences critical care unit and make changes based on these evaluations.These instruments will need to be able to measure function, physical and mental wellness, economic and process changes, and quality of life.

REFERENCES

1. Mahoney FI, Barthel DW. Functional evaluation: The Barthel Index. *Md. State Med. J.* 1965;14:61–65.
2. Granger CV, Hamilton BB. The uniform data system for medical rehabilitation report of first admissions for 1990. *Am. J. Phys. Med. Rehabil.* 1992;71:108–113.
3. Knaus WA, Zimmerman JE, Wagner DP, Draper EA, Lawrence DE. APACHE- acute physiologic and chronic health evaluation: A physiologically-based classification system. *Crit. Care Med.* 1981;9:591–597.
4. Ware JE, Sherbourne CD. The MOS 36-item short-form health survey (SF-36). Conceptual framework and item selection. *Med. Care* 1992;30:473–483.
5. Teasdale G, Jennett B. Assessment of coma and impaired consciousness. A practical scale. *Lancet* 1974;2(7872):81–84.
6. Jennett B, Bond M.Assessment of outcome after severe brain damage. *Lancet* 1975;1(7905):480–484.
7. Born JD.The Glasgow-Liege Scale. Prognostic value and evolution of motor response and brain stem reflexes after severe head injury. *Acta. Neurochir. (Wien)* 1988;91:1–11.
8. Benzer A, Mitterschiffthaler G, Marosi M, et. al. Prediction of non-survival after trauma: Insbruck Coma Scale. *Lancet* 1991;338(8773):977–978.

9. Starmark J-E, Stalhammar D, Holmgren E. The reaction level scale (RLS85). Manual and guidelines. *Acta. Neurochir.* 1988;91:12–20.
10. Levin HS, High WM, Goethe KE, et al.The neurobehavioural rating scale: assessment of the behavioural sequelae of head injury by the clinician. *J. Neurol. Neurosurg. Psychiatry* 1987;50:183–193.
11. McCauley SR, Levin HS, Vanier M, et al.The neurobehvioural rating scale-revised: sensitivity and validity in closed head injury assessment. *J. Neurol. Neurosurg. Psychiatry* 2001;71:643–651.
12. Scandinavian Stroke Study Group. Multicenter trial of hemodilution in ischemic stroke-background and study protocol. *Stroke* 1985;16:885–890.
13. Brott t, Adams HP, Olinger CP, et al.Measurements of acute cerebral infarction: a clinical examination scale. *Stroke* 1989;20:864–870.
14. Cote R, Battista RN, Wolfson C, Boucher J, Adam J, Hachinski V. The Canadian neurological scale: Validation and reliability assessment. *Neurology* 1989;39:638–643.
15. Hantson L, De Weerdt W, De Keyser J, et al.The european stroke scale. *Stroke* 1994;25:2215–2219.
16. Rankin J. Cerebral vascular accidents in patients over the age of 60. *Scott. Med. J.* 1957;2:200–215.
17. Duncan PW, Wallace D, Lai SM, Johnson D, Embretson S, Laster LJ. The stroke impact scale version 2.0. Evaluation of reliability, validity and sensitivity to change. *Stroke* 1999;30:2131–2140.
18. Buchanan KM, Elias LJ, Goplen GB. Differing perspective on outcome after subarachnoid hemorrhage: The patient, the relative, the neurosurgeon. *Stroke* 2000;46:831–838.
19. Solomon RA, Mayer SA, Tarmey JJ. Relationship between the volume of craniotomies for cerebral aneurysms performed at New York state hospitals and in-hospital mortality. *Stroke* 1996;27:13–17.
20. Clemmer TP, Orme JF Jr, Thomas FO, Brooks KA. Outcome of critically injured patients treated at Level I trauma centers versus full-service community hospitals. *Crit. Care Med.* 1985;13:861–863.
21. Indredavik B, Slordahl SA, Bakke F, Rokseth R, Haheim LL. Stroke unit treatment. Long-term effects. *Stroke* 1997;28:1861–1866.

Appendices A–N

Appendix A: Nursing Flowsheet in the Neurosciences Critical Care Unit at the University Hospitals of Cleveland follows p. 592.

Appendix B-1
Useful Hemodynamic Parameters

Parameter	Derivation	Normal range
RA, CVP	Measured	2–10 mmHg
RV	Measured	15–30/0–5 mmHg
PAS/PAD	Measured	15–30/8–15 mmHg
MAP, Mean arterial pressure	$diast + \dfrac{sys - diast}{3}$	80–95 mmHg
SVR, Systemic vascular resistance	$\dfrac{(MAP - CVP) \times 79.9}{CO}$	770–1500 dynes-s-cm^{-5}
PVR, Pulmonary vascular resistance	$\dfrac{(MPAP - PAOP) \times 79.9}{CO}$	20–120 dynes-s-cm^{-5}
SV, Stroke volume	$\dfrac{CO}{HR}$	55–100 mL
SV, Stroke volume index	$\dfrac{CI}{HR}$ or $\dfrac{SV}{BSA}$	35–60 mL/beat/m^2
LVSWI	$SVI \times (MAP - CVP) \times 0.0136$	42–62 g/m^2/beat
RVSWI	$SVI \times (MPAP - PAOP) \times 0.0136$	6–12 g/m^2/beat
CaO$_2$	$(Hgb \times 1.34) \, SaO_2 + (PaO_2 \times 0.0031)$	16–22 mL O$_2$/dL blood
CvO$_2$, Mixed venous O$_2$ content	$(Hgb \times 1.34) \, SvO_2 + (PvO_2 \times 0.0031)$	12–17 mL O$_2$/dL blood
C(a–v)O$_2$, AV O$_2$ difference	$CaO_2 - CvO_2$ $= (Hb \times 1.34)\,(SaO_2 - SaO_2)$	3.5–5.5 mL O$_2$/dL blood
CO, Cardiac output	$SV \times HR \quad \dfrac{VO_2}{C(a-v)\,O_2 \times 10}$	4–8 L/min CI, 2.7–4 L/min/m^2
DO$_2$, O$_2$ delivery	$CaO_2 \times CO \times 10$	700–1400 mL/min
VO$_2$, Oxygen consumption content	$C(a-v)\,O_2 \times CO \times 10$	180–280 mL/min

(continued on following page)

Appendix B-2 (*Continued*)
Useful Hemodynamic Parameters

Parameter	Derivation	Normal range
P_AO_2, Alveolar O_2 pressure	$\left(P_B - P_{H2O}\right) FIO_2 - \dfrac{PaCO_2}{0.8}$	
PaO_2, Arterial O_2 pressure	Measured	Room air: 80–100 mmHg
A-a gradient	$P_AO_2 - PaO_2$	Room air: 2–22 mmHg
	$\left[(713)\,FIO_2 - PaCO_2\,(1.25)\right] - PaO_2$	
CcO_2, Pulmonary end capillary O_2 content	$(Hbg \times 1.37 \times 1) + 0.0031\left[0.5\left(P_{ATM} - 47\right) - PaO_2\right]$ (Assumes 100% saturation of alveolar vessel blood)	
$\dfrac{Q_s}{Q_t}$ Shunt fraction	$\dfrac{\left(CcO_2 - CaO_2\right)}{\left(CcO_2 - CvO_2\right)}$	0.05
RQ, Respiratory quotient	$\dfrac{VCO_2}{VO_2}$	Normal: 0.8–0.85

Appendix C
Respiratory Parameters

Respiratory physiology

Alveolar ventilation: $VA = \dfrac{VCO_2}{PaCO_2}$ Normal: 4–6 L/min

Dead space: $\dfrac{VD}{VT} = \dfrac{P_aCO_2 - PECO_2}{PaCO_2}$ Normal: 0.2–0.4

Airway resistance: $Raw = \dfrac{Palv - Pmouth}{V}$ Normal: 1.5–2 cm H_2O/L/sec

Compliance $= \dfrac{\Delta\ Volume}{\Delta\ Pressure}$

a) Static compliance (Csta) $= \dfrac{VT}{Plateau\ pressure - PEEP}$ Normal: 50–85 mL/cm H_2O

b) Dynamic compliance (Cdyn) $= \dfrac{VT}{Peak\ Insp.\ Pressure - PEEP}$ Normal: 75–125 mL/cm H_2O

Predictors of successful mechanical ventilation weaning

Negative inspiratory force (NIF)	> –30 cm H_2O
Vital capacity (VC)	> 10 mL/kg
Minute volume	< 10 L/min
Inspiratory effort against occluded airway ($P_{0.1}$)	< –2 cm H_2O
Rapid shallow breathing index (RSBI)	< 105
RSBI = respiratory rate (*f*)/tidal volume (Vt)	
Compliance-rate-oxygen-pressure (CROP) index	> 13
CROP = Cdyn × NIF × (PaO$_2$/PA O$_2$/*f*	

Appendix D
Interpretation of Biochemical Results of Plasma and Urine with Renal Insufficiency

Parameter	Normal	Prerenal	Renal	Obstructive
Plasma				
Urea (mg/dL)	< 60	Slight↑	↑↑	↑↑
Potassium (mEq/Lt)	3.4.–5.0	Normal	↑↑	↑ or ↑↑
Creatinine (mg/dL)	0.5–1.2	Normal	↑↑	↑ or ↑↑
Osmolality (mosmol/kg)	285–300	Slight↑	↑↑	↑ or ↑↑
Urine				
Osmolality	400–1400	>400	285–295	260–330
Urine/plasma osmolality	>1.5:1	>2:1	1.1:1	1.1:1
Urine/plasma urea	>20:1	>10:1	<4:1	<4:1
Urine specific gravity	1000–1040	>1020	1010	1010
Creatinine clearance	90–120	Normal/slight↓	Low	Low

Appendix E
Renal Equations

Current body water (CBW) = 0.6 × current body weight (in Kg) [use 0.4–0.5 for female and cachectic patients]
Desirable body water (DBW) = [current Na^+/140] × CBW
Body water deficit (BWD) = DBW - CBW

$$\text{Calculated osmolarity} = 2 \times Na^+ \left(\text{mmol/L}\right) + \frac{\text{BUN (mmol/dL)}}{2.8} + \frac{\text{Glucose (mg/dL)}}{18}$$

Measured serum osmolality (mOsm/kg): normal values: 275–290 mOsm/kg
Osmolal gap = Serum osmolality measured–Serum osmolality calculated
Normal values: 0–5 mOsm/kg
Serum Anion Gap = $[Na^+]$–$[Cl^-]$–$[HCO_3^-]$
Expected anion gap in hypoalbuminemia = 3 × (albumin [g/dL])
Urinary anion gap= $[Na^+]$ + $[K^+]$–$[Cl^-]$–$[HCO_3^-]$ (may ignore HCO_3^- if pH < 6.5)
Urinary osmolar gap = measured urine osmolality – [2 × (urine sodium + urine potassium) + urinary glucose/18 – urinary urea nitrogen/2.8]

$$\text{Creatinine Clearance} = \frac{Ucr \times V}{P} = \frac{\left[\text{Urine creatinine (mg/dL)}\right] \times \left[\text{Urine volume (mL/d)}\right]}{\left[\text{Plasma creatinine (mg/dL)}\right] \times 1440 \text{ min/d}}$$

$$\text{Creatinine clearance} = \frac{140 - \text{Age (yr)}}{\text{Serum creatinine (mg/dL)} \times 72} \times \text{weight (kg)} \left(\times 0.85 \text{ if woman}\right)$$

$$\text{Fractional excretion of sodium (FeNa}^+\text{)} = \frac{\left(\text{Urine Na}\right) \times \left(\text{Plasma Cr}\right)}{\left(\text{Urine Cr}\right) \times \left(\text{Plasma Na}\right)}$$

< 1% in normal urine and prerenal azotemia

Appendix F
Calcium and Magnesium Preparations

	Dosage/form	Contents
Calcium preparations		
Parenteral		
Ca^{2+} gluconate (10%)	10 mL	93 mg Ca^{2+} (4.6 mEq)
Ca^{2+} gluceptate	5 Ml	90 mg Ca^{2+} (4.5 mEq)
Ca^{2+} chloride (10%)	10mL	272 mg Ca^{2+} (13.6 mEq)
Oral		
Ca^{2+} carbonate	Tablets	500 mg Ca^{2+}
Ca^{2+} gluconate	Tablets	500 mg Ca^{2+}
Ca^{2+} lactate	Tablets	650 mg Ca^{2+}
Ca^{2+} glubionate	Syrup	115 mg Ca^{2+}/5 mL
Magnesium preparations		
Parenteral		
Mg^{2+} chloride	1 g = 118 mg Mg^{2+} = 9 mEq	Loading: 1-2 g I.V. over 5–10 min
Mg^{2+} sulfate	1 g = 98 mg Mg^{2+} = 8 mEq	Maintenance: 0.5–2 g/h by infusion
Enteral		
Mg^{2+} oxide tablets	Tablets = 241 mg Mg^{2+} = 20 mEq	20–80 mEq/d in divided doses
Mg^{2+} gluconate tablets	500 mg tablet = 27 mg Mg^{2+} = 2.3 mEq	20–80 mEq/d in divided doses

Appendix G
Acid-Base Rules of Thumb

Metabolic acidosis $PaCO_2$	↓ 1.25 mmHg per mEq/L	Δ HCO_3 (± 5 mmHg)
Metabolic alkalosis $PaCO_2$	↑ 1.25 mmHg per mEq/L	Δ HCO_3 (± 5 mmHg)
Acute Resp acidosis HCO_3	↑ 1 mEq/L per 10mmHg	Δ $PaCO_2$ (± 3 mEq/L)
Chronic Resp acidosis HCO_3	↑ 4 mEq/L per 10 mmHg	Δ $PaCO_2$ (± 4 mEq/L)
Acute Resp alkalosis HCO_3	↓ 2 mEq/L per 10 mmHg	Δ $PaCO_2$ (± 3 mEq/L)
Chronic Resp acidosis HCO_3	↓ 4 mEq/L per 10 mmHg	Δ $PaCO_2$ (± 3 mEq/L)

Appendix H
Differential Diagnosis of Metabolic Acidosis

1. Increased serum anion gap
   Diabetic ketoacidosis
   Alcohol ketoacidosis (may have osmolal gap)
   Lactic acidosis
   Renal failure
   Intoxication with methanol and ethylene glycol
     (osmolal gap present)
   Paraldehyde (without osmolal gap)
   Salicylate
2. Normal serum anion gap
   Renal loss of HCO_3^- or proximal renal tubular acidosis (RTA 2): diagnosis made by
     documenting bicarbonaturia after IV administration of Na HCO_3
   Enhanced NH_4^+ excretion: negative urine anion gap or high urine osmolar gap or both.
   Look for gastrointestinal loss of HCO_3^- or acid gain
   Impaired NH_4^+ excretion or distal RTA:
     positive urine anion gap or urine osmolar gap < 100 mOsm/kg.
3. Treatment with $NaHCO_3$
   Correct severe metabolic acidosis (serum pH < 7.2)
   Normal serum anion gap metabolic acidosis
   Bicarbonate deficit (mEq/L) = [0.5 × body weight (Kg)] × [24–HCO_3^-]
   Monitor patients for pulmonary edema, hypokalemia, hypocalcemia.

Appendix I
Composition of Common Intravenous Solutions in the NSU

Solution	Na^+	Cl^-	K^+	Ca^+	Lactate	Kcal/L	mOsm/L
D5 water	0	0	0	0	0	170	252
D10 water	0	0	0	0	0	240	505
D50 water	0	0	0	0	0	1700	2530
0.45 NaCl	77	77	0	0	0	0	154
0.9% Nacl	154	154	0	0	0	0	308
3%NaCl	513	513	0	0	0	0	1026
Ringer' lactate	130	109	4	3	28	0	308
20% mannitol	0	0	0	0	0	0	1098

Appendix J
Serum Concentrations of Frequently Used Drugs in the NSU

Amikacin (peak/trough)	15–25/<10 µg/mL
Tobramycin (peak/trough)	5–8/<2 µg/mL
Gentamicin (peak/trough)	5–8/<2 µg/mL
Vancomycin (peak/trough)	30–40/5–10 µg/mL
Theophyline	10–20 µg/mL
Digoxin	0.5–2 ng/mL
Phenytoin	10–20 µg/mL
Phenobarbital	15–40 µg/mL
Carbamazepine	4–12 µg/mL
Valproic acid	50–100 µg/mL

Appendix K
Dosages in Renal Failure in the Neurosciences Critical Care Unit

Drug	Half–life in uremia (h)	Protein plasma binding	Vd	Dose for normal renal function	Method	GFR 10–50 mL/min	GFR <10 mL/min	Renal replacement therapy Hemo	Renal replacement therapy CRRT
Antiarrhythmics									
Amiodarone	14–120 d	96	70–140	200–400 mg q d	D	100%	100%	None	nd
Lidocaine	1.3–3	60–66	1.3–2.2	50 mg over 2 min repeat q 5 min x 3 then 1–4 mg/min	D	100%	100%	None	nd
Procainamide	5.5	15	2.2	350–400 mg q 3–4 h	I	q 6–12	q 8–24 h	200mg	Replace by blood level
Propafenone	Unknown	>95	3	150–300 mg q 8 h	D	100%	100%	None	nd
Antibacterial antibiotics									
Aminoglycosides									
Amikacin	17–150	<5	0.22–0.29	5 mg/kg q 8 h	D/I	30–70% q 12–18 h	20–30% q 24–48 h	Two thirds normal dose after dialysis	Dose for GRF 10–50 mL/min measure levels
Gentamicin	20–60	<5	0.23–0.26	1 mg/kg q 8 h	D/I	30–70% q 12 h	10–20% q 24–48 h	Two thirds normal dose after dialysis	Dose for GRF 10–50 mL/min measure levels
Tobramycin	27–60	<5	0.22–0.33	1 mg/kg q 8 h	D/I	30–70% q 12 h	10–20% q 24–48 h	Two thirds normal dose after dialysis	Dose for GRF 10–50 mL/min

(continued on next page)

Appendix K (Continued)
Dosages in Renal Failure in the Neurosciences Critical Care Unit

Drug	Half–life in uremia (h)	Protein plasma binding	Vd	Dose for normal renal function	Method	GFR 10–50 mL/min	GFR <10 mL/min	Renal replacement therapy Hemo	Renal replacement therapy CRRT
Cephalosporins									
Cefazolin	40–70	80	0.13–0.22	0.5–1 g q 6 h	I	q 12 h	q 24–48 h	0.5–1 g after dialysis	Dose for GRF 10–50 mL/min
Cefotaxime	15	37	0.15–0.55	1 g q 6 h	I	q 8–12 h	q 24 h	1 g after dialysis	1 g q 8–12 h
Ceftazidime	13–25	17	0.28–0.4	1–2 g q 8 h	I	q 24–48 h	q 48 h	1 g after dialysis	1 g q 12 h
Ceftizoxime	35	28–50	0.26–0.42	1–2 g q 8–12 h	I	q 12–24 h	q 24 h	1 g ater dialysis	Dose for GFR 10–50 mL/min
Ceftriaxone	12–24	90	0.12–0.18	0.2–1 g q 8–12 h	D	100%	100%	Dose after dialysis	Dose for GFR 10–50 mL/min
Cefuroxime	17	33	0.13–18	0.75–1.5 g q 8 h	I	q 8–12 h	q 24 h	Dose after dialysis	1 g q 12 h
Cephalothin	3–18	65	0.26	0.5–2 g q 6 h	I	q 6 h	q 12 h	Dose after dialysis	Dose for GFR 10–50 mL/min
Miscellaneous									
Aztreonam	6–8	55	0.1–2	1–2 g q 8–12 h	D	50–75%	25%	1 g after dialysis	Dose for GFR 10–50 mL/min
Clavulanic acid	6.5	30	0.3	100 mg q 4–6 h	D	100%	50–75%	Dose after dialysis	Dose for GFR 10–50 mL/min
Imipenem	4	13–21	0.17–0.3	0.25–1 g q 6 h	D	50%	25%	Dose after dialysis	500 mg q 8 h
Meropenem	7	Low	0.35	500–1000 mg q 6 h	D/I	250–500 mg q 12 h	250–500 mg q 24 h	Dose after dialysis	Dose for GFR 10–50 mL/min
Metronidazole	7–21	20	0.25–0.85	7.5 mg/kg q 6 h	D/I	100%	50%	Dose after dialysis	Dose for GFR 10–50 mL/min

(continued on next page)

Appendix K (*Continued*)
Dosages in Renal Failure in the Neurosciences Critical Care Unit

Drug	Half-life in uremia (h)	Protein plasma binding	Vd	Dose for normal renal function	Method	GFR 10–50 mL/min	GFR <10 mL/min	Renal replacement therapy Hemo	Renal replacement therapy CRRT
Pentamidine	118	69	55–462	4 mg/kg per day	I	q 24–36 h	q 48 h	None	None
Rifampin	9.2	30	0.9	600 mg q 6 h	D	50–100%	50%	None	Dose for GFR <10 mL/min
Sulbactam	10–21	30	0.25–0.5	0.75–1.5 g q 6–8 h	I	q 12–24 h	q 24–48 h	Dose after dialysis	750 mg q 12h
Vancomycin	200–250	10–50	0.47–1.1	500 mg q 6 h or 1g q 12 h	D/ I	500 mg q 24–48 h	500 mg q 48–96 h	Dose for GFR <10 mL/min	Dose for GFR of 10–50 mL/min
Penicillins									
Ampicillin	7–20	20	0.17–0.31	250 mg–2 g q 6 h	I	q 6–12 h	q 12–24 h	Dose	Dose for GFR
Penicillin G	6–20	50	0.3–0.42	0.5–4 million U q 6 h	D	75%	20–50%	Dose after dialysis	Dose for GFR of 10–5 mL/min
Piperacillin	3.3–5.1	30	0.18–0.30	3–4 g q 4 h	I	q 6–8 h	q 8 h	Dose after dialysis	Dose for GFR of 10–50 mL/min
Ticarcillin	11–16	45–60	0.14–0.21	3 g q 4 h	D/I	1–2 g q 8 h	1–2 g q 12 h	3 g after dialysis	Dose for GFR 10–50 mL/min
Quinolones									
Ciprofloxacin	609	20–40	2.5	500–750 mg q 12 h	D	50–75%	50%	250 mg q 12 h	200 mg q 12 h
Norfloxacin	8	14	<0	400 mg q 12 h	I	q 12–24 h	Avoid	na	na
Ofloxacin	28–37	25	1.5–2.5	400 mg q d	D	50%	25–50%	100 mg b.i.d.	300 mg q d

(continued on next page)

Appendix K (*Continued*)
Dosages in Renal Failure in the Neurosciences Critical Care Unit

Drug	Half–life in uremia (h)	Protein plasma binding	Vd	Dose for normal renal function	Method	GFR 10–50 mL/min	GFR <10 mL/min	Renal replacement therapy Hemo	Renal replacement therapy CRRT
Barbiturates									
Phenobarbital	117–160	40–60	0.7–1	50–100 mg b.i.d.–t.i.d.	I	q 8–12 h	q 12–16 h	Dose after dialysis	None
Benzodiazepines									
Diazepam	20–90	94–98	0.7–3.4	5–40 mg d	D	100%	100%	None	Unknown
Lorazepam	32–70	87	0.9–1.3	1–2 b.i.d–t.i.d.	D	100%	100%	None	Unknown
Ca channel blockers									
Nifedipine	6	97	1.4	10–20 mg q 6–8 h	D	100%	100 %	None	nd
Verapamil	2.4– 4	83–93	3–6	80 mg q 8 h	D	100%	100%	None	nd
Cardiac glycosides									
Digitoxin	210	94	0.6	0.1–0.2 mg q d	D	100%	100%	None	nd
Digoxin	80–120	20–30	5–8	1–1.5 mg load 0.25–0.5 mg q d	D/I	25–75% q 36 h	10–25% q 48 h	None	0.5 mg q 12 h
Miscellaneous cardiac drugs									
Amrinone	Unknown	20–40	1.3–1.6	5–10 µg/kg/min	D	100%	50–75%	nd	nd
Dobutamine	Unknown	Unknown	0.25	2.5–15 µg/kg/min	D	100%	100%	nd	nd
Milrinone	1.5–3	Unknown	0.25–0.35	15–75 ng/kg iv as load	D	100%	50–75%	nd	nd

From Bellomo R, Ronco C. *Acute Renal Failure in the Critically ill: Update in Intensive Care and Emergency Medicine Series*, vol. 20. New York: Springer Verlag, 1995 (reproduced with permission).

Appendix L
Various Tube Feedings

Pharmaceutical companies have designed standard tube feeding products as well as formulas for patients with various disease states. The formulas include those for patients with diabetes, pulmonary, hepatic, renal, elevated energy and protein needs, fluid restrictions, metabolically stressed and malabsorption conditions. For various formulas, refer to the following chart.

To compare various types of tube feeding products, *see* the following:

Types of formulas	Names of formulas
Nutritional complete supplement (1 Kcal/mL)	Boost, Ensure, NuBasic, Nutren 1.0, Resource Standard
Fiber containing supplement or tube feeding (1 Kcal/1 mL)	Boost with fiber, Ensure with fiber, NuBasic with fiber, Nutren 1.0 with fiber,
High-Protein oral supplement (1 cal/1 mL)	Boost High Protein, Ensure High Protein, NuBasics VHP, Promote, Replete
High-calorie supplement; nutritionally complete (1.5 cal/mL)	Boost Plus, Ensure Plus, Ensure Plus HN, NuBasics Plus, Nutren 1.5, Resource Plus
Oral supplement in pudding form	Boost Pudding, Ensure pudding
Powdered protein supplement (calcium caseinate)	Casec, Pro Mod
Glucose intolerance or diabetes formula, nutritionally complete oral and tube feeding	Choice dm liquid, Diabeti-Source, Ensure, Glucerna OS, Glucerna, Glytrol, Resource Diabetic
Ready to use blenderized tube feeding formulated from foods including meat, vegetables and fruit	Compleat Modified
High-calorie formula for tube feedings; nutritionally complete (1.5 cal/mL)	Comply, Ensure Plus, Nutren 1.5, Osmolite HN Plus, Resource Plus, IsoSource 1.5 Cal
Elemental liquid tube feeding formula (low fat); ready to use-form; unflavored (1 cal/mL)	Alitraq, Criticare HN, Peptamen, SandoSource Peptide, Tolerex, Vital HN, Vivonex Plus, Vivonex TEN, Optimental
High-calorie oral and tube feeding; nutritionally complete (2 cal/mL)	Deliver 2.0, NovaSource 2.0, NuBasics 2.0, Nutren 2.0, two Cal HN
Isotonic low-residue tube feeding; nutritionally complete with ultratrace minerals (1 cal/mL)	Isocal, IsoSource Standard, Osmolite, Nutren 1.0
High-nitrogen, isotonic low-residue tube feeding with ultratrace minerals; nutritionally complete (1 caL/mL)	Entrition HN, Isocal HN, IsoSource HN, Osmolite HN, Nutren 1.0
Higher calorie; nutritionally complete (1.2 cal/mL)	Isocal HN Plus, IsoSource HN, Osmolite HN Plus
Fiber containing tube and oral feeding. Nutritionally complete (children 1–10 yr)	Kindercal, Nutren Jr., Nutren Jr. with fiber, PediaSure, PediaSure with fiber, resource just for kids
High-calorie, high-nitrogen tube feeding with arginine (1.5 cal/mL)	Intensical

(continued on next page)

Appendix L (*Continued*)
Various Tube Feedings

Types of formulas	Names of formulas
MCT formulation for patients with fat malabsorption, nutritionally complete	Advera, Lipisorb
High-calorie formula for oral and tube feeding designed for people on renal dialysis, nutritionally complete (2 cal/mL)	Magnacal Renal, Nepro, NovaSource Renal
Modular source of medium chain triglycerides for patients unable to digest or absorb conventional fats	MCT oil
50% fat emulsion for special dietary use in oral or tube feeding formulas	Microlipid
Powdered carbohydrate supplement (maltodextrin)	Moducal, Polycose liquid, Polycose powder
Powdered supplement for tube feeding with major fat source as medium chain triglycerides (MCT); used for pediatric patients with fat malabsorption/maldigestion; nutritionally complete	Portagen
High-protein tube feeding formula with fiber; nutritionally complete; appropriate for wound healing patients (1 cal/mL)	Jevity Plus, IsoSource VHN, Promote with Fiber, Replete with Fiber, Protain XL
High-calorie, high-nitrogen, Low-carbohydrate supplement or tube feeding for patients with respiratory distress COPD; nutritionally complete (1.5 cal/mL)	NovaSource, Nutrivent, Oxepa, Pulmocare, Pulmonary, Respalor
Peptide-based liquid elemental diet; Nutritionally complete (1 cal/mL)	Altroq, Peptamen, Peptamen VHP, SandoSource Peptide, Subdue, Vital HN, Vivonex Plus, Vivonex TEN
Peptide-based liquid elemental diet; conc. calorie; nutritionally complete (1.5 cal/mL)	Peptamen 1.5, Subdue Plus
High-calorie, high-nitrogen supplement or tube feeding designed for trauma and burn patients; nutritionally complete (1.5 cal/mL)	Impact 1.5, Perative, Traumacal
Tube feeding with a blend of oat and soy fiber (3.4 g fiber/ 8 oz); nutritionally complete	FiberSource, FiberSource HN, Jevity, Jevity Plus, Nutren fl 1.0 with Fiber, ProBalance, Ultracal
Concentrated tube feeding with a blend of oat and soy fiber; Nutritionally complete; (1.2 cal/mL)	FiberSource, Jevity Plus, Ultracal HN Plus

Adapted from information provided by Mead Johnson Nutritionals.

Appendix M
Energy Requirements in Adult Patients

University Hospitals of Cleveland
Department of Nutrition Services
Standards of Clinical Nutritional Care
Nutritional Assessment Guidelines For Adults (18 yr or older)

Energy Needs for Adults

1. Harris Benedict Equation

BEE (Basal Energy Expediture)
In men:
BEE (kcal/d) = 66.5 + (13.8 × W) + (5.0 × H)–(6.8 × A)
In women:
BEE (kcal/d) = 655.1 + (9.6 × W) + (1.8 × H)–(4.7 × A)
Where: W = weight in kilograms
        H = height in centimeters
        A = age in years
The BEE value is multiplied by an activity factor and an injury factor to predict the total daily energy need.

a.	Activity Factor	Confined to Bed =1.2
		Out of Bed = 1.3
b.	Injury Factory	Surgery
		Minor = 1.0–1. 1
		Major = 1. 1–1.2
	Infection	Mild = 1.0–1.2
		Moderate = 1.2–1.4
		Severe = 1.4–1.8
	Trauma	Skeletal = 1.2–1.35
		Blunt = 1. 15–1.35
		Head trauma treated with steroids = 1.6
	Burns	Up to 20% body surface area (BSA) = 1.0–1.5
		20–40% BSA = 1.5–1.85
		Over 40% BSA = 1.85–1.95

References: The American Dietetic Association. Manual of Clinical Dietetics, 4th ed. Library of Congress. Chicago, IL, 1992; Grant A, DeHoog S. Nutritional Assessment and Support, 4th ed. Northgate Station. Seattle, WA, 1991.

2. Energy Needs Based on Weight and Activity Level (Healthy Persons)

	Sedentary	Moderate	Active
Overweight	20–25 kcal/kg	30 kcal/kg	35 kcal/kg
Normal	30 kcal/kg	35 kcal/kg	40 kcal/kg
Underweight	30 kcal/kg	40 kcal/kg	45–50 kcal/kg

Reference: The American Dietetic Association. Handbook of Clinical Dietetics, 2nd ed. Yale University Press. New Haven, CT, 1992.

3. Energy Needs Based on kcal/g (Healthy and Ill Persons)

Status	kcal/kg (IBW)
Basal energy needs	25–30
Ambulatory with wt. maintenance	30–35
Malnutrition with mild stress	40
Severe injuries and, sepsis	50–60
Extensive burns	80

Reference: Grant A, and DeHoog S. Nutritional Assessment and Support, 4th ed. Northgate Station. Seattle, WA, 1991.

Appendix N
Useful Neurologic Physiologic Parameters and Scales Commonly Used in the NSU
N1. Equations for Calculating Cerebral Metabolic Indices

Parameter (units)	Formula	Normal values (n = 72)		
CBF (mL/100 g/min)			54 + 12	52 + 12
CaO$_2$ (mL/dL)	$1.34 \times Hgb \times SaO_2 + 0.0031 \times paO_2$		9.6 ± 1.2	16.9+1.5
CjvO$_2$ (mL/dL)	$1.34 \times Hgb \times SjvO_2 + 0.0031 \times pjvO_2$		12.9 ± 1.3	
AVDO$_2$ (mL/dL)	$CaO_2\,(mL/dL) - CjvO_2\,(mL/dL)$	6.7 ± 0.8	6.3 ± 1.2	6.5 ± 1.8
CMRO$_2$ (mL/100 g/min)	$\dfrac{AVDO_2\,(mL/dL) \times CBF\,(mL/100\ g/min)}{100}$	3.3 ± 0.4		3.3 ± 0.6
O$_2$ER (%)	$\dfrac{AVDO_2\,(mL/dL) \times 100\%}{CaO_2\,(mL/dL)}$	34 ± 4		
AVDG (mL/dL)	$ArtGluc\,(mL/dL) - JVGluc\,(mL/dL)$	9.6 ± 1.7		11.0 ± 2.3
CMRG (mL/100 g/min)	$\dfrac{AVDG\,(mL/dL) \times CBF\,(mL/100\ g/min)}{100}$			5.5 ± 1.1
AVDL (mL/dL)	$ArtLact\,(mL/dL) - JVLact\,(mL/dL)$	−1.7 ± 0.9		−0.5 ± 0.9
CMRL (mL/100 g/min)	$\dfrac{AVDL\,(mL/dL) \times CBF\,(mL/100\ g/min)}{100}$			−0.23 ± 0.37
AI	$AI(\%) = \dfrac{AVDO_2\,(\mu mol/mL) \times 100\%}{6 \times AVDG\,(\mu mol/mL)}$			
AAI	$ANI(\%) = \dfrac{AVDL\,(\mu mol/mL) \times 100\%}{2 \times AVDG\,(\mu mol/mL)}$			

See Chapter 4 for definitions.

Appendix N2
Glasgow Coma Scale, Pupilary Gauge, Intracranial Pressure
and Cerebral Perfusion Pressure Derivation And Normal Values

Normal ICP 0-15	Document both at least every hour.
Normal CPP >70	

Calculate MAP	Calculate CPP
Systolic + (2x Diastolic)= MAP $\qquad\qquad$ 3	MAP-ICP=CPP

Glasgow Coma Scale

Eyes Open	Spontaneously		4
	To verbal stimulus		3
	To pain		2
	None		1
Best Motor Response	To Verbal	Follow Commands	6
	To Pain	Localizes	5
		Withdrawal	4
		Decorticates	3
		Decerebrates	2
		None	1
Best Verbal Response		Oriented	5
		Disoriented	4
		Inappropriate Words	3
		Incomprehensible Sounds	2
		None	1

Pupil Gauge

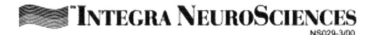

INTEGRA NEUROSCIENCES
NS029-3/00

© Integra Lifesciences Corporation 2002. Reprinted with permission.

Appendix N3
National Institutes of Health Stroke Scale (NIHSS)

1.a. Level of Consciousness:		6. Motor Function–Leg (right and left):	
0	Alert	0	No drift
1	Drowsy	1	Drift
2	Stuporous	2	Some effort against gravity
3	Comatose	3	No effort against gravity
		4	No movement
		X	Untestable

1.b. Ask patient the month and their age:		
0	Answers both correctly	7. Limb Ataxia:
1	Answers one correctly	
2	Both incorrect	

		0	Absent
		1	Present in 1 limb
		2	Present in 2 limbs
		X	Untestable

1.c. Ask patient to open and close eyes:		
0	Obeys both correctly	
1	Obeys one correctly	8. Sensory:
2	Both incorrect	0 Normal

		1	Partial loss
2. Best Gaze (only horizontal eye movement):		2	Dense loss
0	Normal		
1	Partial gaze palsy	9. Best Language:	
2	Forced deviation		

		0	No aphasia
		1	Mild to moderate aphasia
3. Visual Fields Testing:		2	Severe aphasia
		3	Mute

0	No visual field loss	
1	Partial hemianopia	
2	Complete hemianopia	10. Dysarthria:
3	Bilateral hemianopia	

		0	Normal articulation
		1	Mild to moderate slurring
4. Facial Strength:		2	Unintelligible
		X	Untestable

0	Normal	
1	Minor paralysis	
2	Partial paralysis	11. Neglect:
3	Complete paralysis	

		0	No neglect
		1	Partial neglect
5. Motor Function–Arm (right and left):		2	Complete neglect
0	No drift		
1	Drift		
2	Some effort against gravity		
3	No effort against gravity		
4	No movement		
X	Untestable	TOTAL NIHSS SCORE: _____(0–42)	

Appendix N4
Hunt-Hess Scale for Subarachnoid Hemorrhage (SAH)

Grade	Description
1	Asymptomatic or minimal headache and slight nuchal rigidity
2	Moderate-to-severe headache, nuchal rigidity, no neurological deficit other than cranial nerve palsy
3	Drowsiness, confusion, or mild focal deficit
4	Stupor, moderate to severe hemiparesis, possible early decerebrate rigidity and vegetative disturbances
5	Deep coma, decerebrate rigidity, moribund appearance

Note: Patients are moved into the next worst category if they have vasospasm on angiography or serious systemic disease, such as hypertension, diabetes, atherosclerosis, or chronic lung disease.
From Hunt WE, Hess RM. Surgical risk as related to time of intervention in the repair of intracranial aneurysms. Neurosurgery 1968;28: 14–20.

Appendix N5
World Federation of Neurological Surgeons (WFNS) Grading Scale for Patients with SAH

Grade	Description
1	Glasgow coma score 15, no motor deficit
2	Glasgow coma score 13 to 14, no motor deficit
3	Glasgow coma score 13 to 14, with motor deficit
4	Glasgow coma score 7 to 12, with or without motor deficit
5	Glasgow coma score 3 to 6, with or without motor deficit

From Drake CG. Report of World Federation of Neurological Surgeons committee on a universal subarachnoid hemorrhage grading scale. *J. Neurosurg.* 1988;68:985–986.

Appendix N6
Fisher Grading for Head CT Scanning in SAH

Fisher group	Blood on CT	No. of patients	Slight angiographic vasospasm	Severe angiographic vasospasm	Clinical vasospasm
1	No subarachnoid blood detected	11	2	2*	0
2	Diffuse or vertical layers+ <1 mm thick	7	3	0	0
3	Localized clot and/or vertical layer ≥ 1 mm	24	1	23	23
4	Intracerebral or intraventricular clot with diffuse or no SAH	5	2	0	0

Note: Measurements made in the greatest longitudinal and transverse dimension on a printed CT scan performed within 5 d of SAH.
*May actually be 0 since 1 patient was scanned late and 1 developed spasm only peripherally.
+Vertical layer refers to blood within the "vertical" subarachnoid spaces including the insular cistern, ambient cistern, and interhemispheric fissure.
From Fisher CM, Kistler JP, Davis JM. Relation of cerebral vasospasm to subarachnoid hemorrhage visualized by CT scanning. *Neurosurgery* 1980;6:1–9.

Appendix N7
Glasgow Outcome Scale

1	Death
2	Vegetative
3	Severe disability: dependent on others for all or part of care
4	Moderate disability: disabled but independent in activities of daily living
5	Good recovery: resumption of normal life despite minor neurological deficits

Appendix N8
The Barthel Index

Function	Score	Description
Feeding	10	Independent, able to apply any necessary device, eats in reasonable time.
	5	Needs help (e.g., cutting)
Wheelchair or bed transfers	15	Independent, including placing locks of wheelchair and lifting footrests
	10	Minimal assistance or supervision
	5	Able to sit but needs maximal assistance to transfer
Personal toilet (grooming)	5	Washes face, combs hair, brushes teeth, shaves (manages plug if using electric razor)
Toilet transfers	10	Independent with toilet or bedpan, handles clothes, wipes, flushes, or cleans pan
	5	Needs help for balance, handling clothes or toilet paper
Bathing self	5	Able to use bathtub or shower or take complete sponge bath without assistance
Walking	15	Independent for 50 yd, may use assistive devices, except for rolling walker
	10	Walks with help for 50 yd
	5	Independent with wheelchair for 50 yd, only if unable to walk
Stairs, ascending and descending	10	Independent, may use assistive devices
	5	Needs help or supervision
Dressing and undressing	10	Independent, ties shoes, fastens fasteners, applies braces
	5	Needs help, but does at least half of task within reasonable time
Bowel control	10	No accidents, able to care for collecting device if used
	5	Occasional accidents or needs help with enema or suppository
Bladder control	10	No accidents, able to care for collecting device if used
	5	Occasional accidents or needs help with device

Barthel Index (BI): total possible score is 100.

Appendix N9
Modified Rankin Score (RI)

0 = No symptoms at all
1 = No significant disability despite symptoms, patient is able to carry out all usual duties and activities
2 = Slight disability—patient is unable to carry out all previous activities, but able to look after own affairs without assistance
3 = Moderate disability—patient requiring some help, but able to walk without assistance
4 = Moderately severe disability—patient unable to walk without assistance and unable to attend to own bodily needs without assistance
5 = Severe disability—patient bedridden, incontinent requiring constant nursing care and attention
6 = Dead

Appendix N10
Intraventricular ICP Monitoring Setup

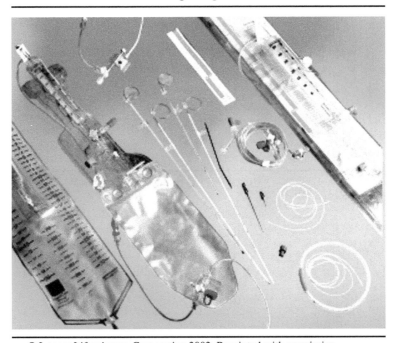

© Integra Lifesciences Corporation 2002. Reprinted with permission.

Appendix N11
Commercially Available Multi-Parameter Monitor

This machine displays intracranial pressure, cerebral perfusion pressure, and intra-cranial temperature simultaneously.

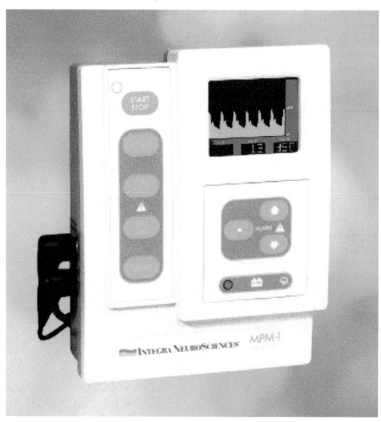

© Integra Lifesciences Corporation 2002. Reprinted with permission

Appendix N12
Commercially Available Brain Tissue Oxygen and Temperature Monitoring System

Brain tissue oxygenation (Pb_tO_2) probe and monitor with smart card calibration.

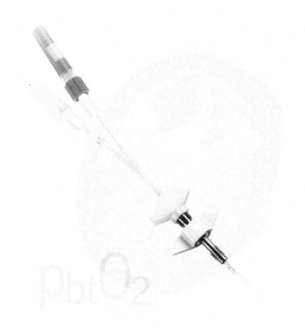

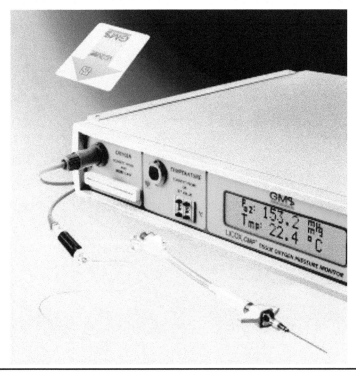

© Integra Lifesciences Corporation 2002. Reprinted with permission.

Index

Lightning Source UK Ltd.
Milton Keynes UK
UKHW051847211222
414258UK00003B/11

9 781617 3